Recipient Vessels in Reconstructive Microsurgery

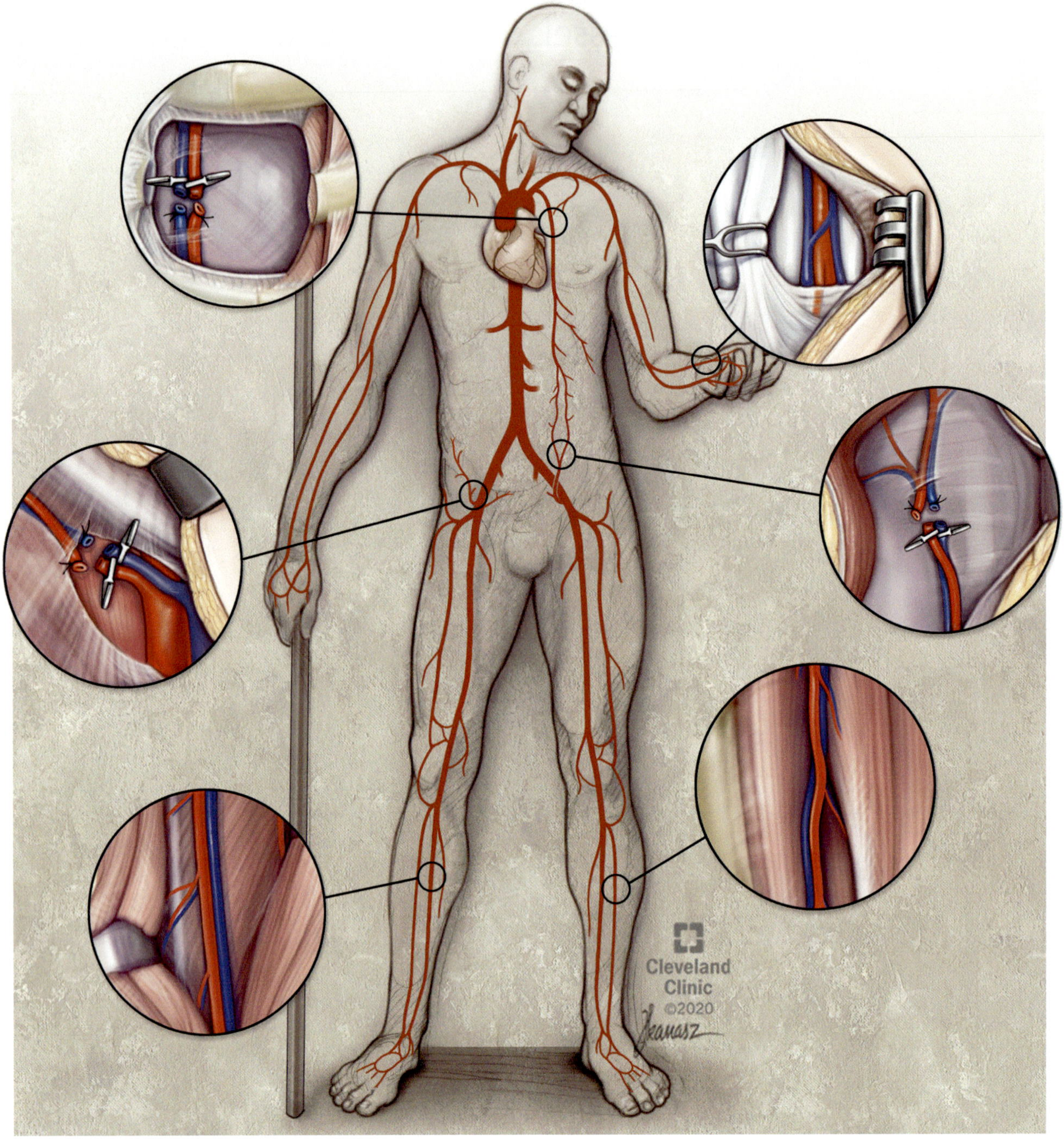
Cleveland Clinic
©2020

Raffi Gurunian • Risal Djohan
Editors

Recipient Vessels in Reconstructive Microsurgery

Anatomy and Technical Considerations

Springer

Editors
Raffi Gurunian
Department of Plastic Surgery
Cleveland Clinic
Cleveland, OH
USA

Cleveland Clinic Lerner College Of Medicine
Case Western Reserve University
Cleveland, OH
USA

Risal Djohan
Department of Plastic Surgery
Cleveland Clinic
Cleveland, OH
USA

Cleveland Clinic Lerner College Of Medicine
Case Western Reserve University
Cleveland, OH
USA

ISBN 978-3-030-75388-7 ISBN 978-3-030-75389-4 (eBook)
https://doi.org/10.1007/978-3-030-75389-4

This Springer imprint is published by the registered company Springer Nature Switzerland AG
The registered company address is: Gewerbestrasse 11, 6330 Cham, Switzerland

Preface

Recipient Vessels in Reconstructive Microsurgery: Anatomy and Technical Considerations is the product of my expertise and passion in anatomy and reconstructive microsurgery. I have been pursuing microsurgery for head to toe reconstruction for the past 30 years in Asia, Europe, and the USA. When performing microsurgical flaps, the overall tendency, especially among trainees, is to focus on the flap anatomy and dissection. An area of reconstructive microsurgery that has not been emphasized enough is the selection of recipient vessels and their surgical exposure for microvascular anastomosis. The approach I took was to cover more commonly used recipient sites and shed light on less frequently used ones combining anatomy and reconstructive microsurgery. The goal of this book is to highlight these aspects of reconstructive microsurgery with an emphasis on the recipient vasculature and to supplement the existing literature in this regard.

Chapters of this book have been contributed by eminent surgeons, both nationally and internationally. I am sincerely thankful to these authors and my co-editor Risal Djohan, MD, for their significant contributions to the creation of this book. The majority of chapters in this book were complemented with illustrations and videos to demonstrate applied anatomy and dissection technique for recipient site exposure. I would like to extend my special thanks to artist Joe Kanasz whose excellent medical illustrations depicted in this book enriched the content of several chapters.

I will be forever indebted to Dr. Richard Drake, head of the Anatomy Department, Cleveland Clinic, and his staff for their collaboration and cooperation. I am grateful to Susan Lopez who relentlessly worked on editing and labeling multiple images in this book. Also, I would like to thank my residents and microsurgery fellows who worked with me throughout the book's completion.

I hope this book, composed of forty-four chapters along with illustrations, figures, and videos, will be considered a significant resource in the armamentarium of reconstructive microsurgery for all plastic surgeons and microsurgeons in training and practice.

To my wife Aslin and my two beautiful daughters, Lia and Lena, this book is dedicated to you.

"...If you would like to be remembered,
leave something good behind..."

Cleveland, OH, USA — Raffi Gurunian

Contents

Part V Lower Extremity Reconstruction

Part VI Miscellaneous Special

Contributors

Dicle Aksoyler, MD Department of Plastic Surgery, International Medical Center of China Medical University Hospital, China Medical University, Taichung, Taiwan

Rachel E. Aliotta, MD Department of Plastic Surgery, Cleveland, OH, USA

Brendan Alleyne, MD Department of Plastic and Reconstructive Surgery, University of Pennsylvania, Cleveland, OH, USA

Oded Ben Amotz, MD Department of Orthopaedic Surgery, University of Pennsylvania, Philadelphia, PA, USA

Andrew R. Bauder, MD Division of Plastic Surgery, Department of Surgery, University of Pennsylvania, Philadelphia, PA, USA

Jonathan M. Bekisz, MD NYU Grossman School of Medicine, New York, NY, USA

Steven L. Bernard, MD Department of Plastic Surgery, Cleveland Clinic, Cleveland, OH, USA

Cleveland Clinic Lerner College of Medicine, Case Western Reserve University, Cleveland, OH, USA

Sarah N. Bishop, MD Department of Plastic Surgery, Cleveland Clinic, Cleveland, OH, USA

Cleveland Clinic Lerner College of Medicine, Case Western Reserve University, Cleveland, OH, USA

Alberto Bolletta, MD Department of Plastic Surgery, International Medical Service Center of China Medical University Hospital, China Medical University, Taichung, Taiwan

Stefanos Boukovalas, MD Department of Plastic Surgery, The University of Texas MD Anderson Cancer Center, Houston, TX, USA

Carter J. Boyd, MD NYU Grossman School of Medicine, New York, NY, USA

Philip S. Brazio, MD Plastic and Reconstructive Surgery, Stanford University, Palo Alto, CA, USA

Charles E. Butler, MD Department of Plastic Surgery, Charles B. Barker Endowed Chair in Surgery, The University of Texas MD Anderson Cancer Center, Houston, TX, USA

Edward I. Chang, MD Department of Plastic Surgery, The University of Texas MD Anderson Cancer Center, Houston, TX, USA

Hung-Chi Chen, MD, PhD, FACS Department of Plastic Surgery, International Medical Service Center of China Medical University Hospital, China Medical University, Taichung, Taiwan

Victor Chien, MD Chang Gung Memorial Hospital, Taoyuan, Taiwan

David Cholok, MD Division of Plastic & Reconstructive Surgery, Stanford University School of Medicine, Palo Alto, CA, USA

Marion Dietl, MD, MBA Department of Plastic Surgery, Academic Hospital of Feldkirch, Feldkirch, Austria

Michelle Djohan, MD Case Western Reserve University/MetroHealth Hospitals, Cleveland, OH, USA

Risal Djohan, MD, MBA Department of Plastic Surgery, Cleveland Clinic, Cleveland, OH, USA

Cleveland Clinic Lerner College of Medicine, Case Western Reserve University, Cleveland, OH, USA

Richard L. Drake, PhD Department of Anatomy, Cleveland Clinic Lerner College of Medicine, Cleveland, OH, USA

Gregory R. D. Evans, MD Department of Plastic Surgery, University of California, Irvine, Orange, CA, USA

Vahe Fahradyan, MD Department of Plastic Surgery, Cleveland Clinic, Cleveland, OH, USA

Jennifer E. Fligor, MD Department of Plastic Surgery, University of California, Irvine, Irvine, CA, USA

Michael Fritz, MD Head & Neck Institute, Cleveland Clinic, Cleveland, OH, USA

Bahar Bassiri Gharb, MD, PhD Department of Plastic Surgery, Cleveland Clinic, Cleveland, OH, USA

Cleveland Clinic Lerner College of Medicine, Case Western Reserve University, Cleveland, OH, USA

Lena Gurunian, BA Loyola Marymount University, Los Angelos, CA, USA

Lia Gurunian, BA Saddleback College, Mission Viejo, CA, USA

Raffi Gurunian, MD Department of Plastic Surgery, Cleveland Clinic, Cleveland, OH, USA

Cleveland Clinic Lerner College of Medicine, Case Western Reserve University, Cleveland, OH, USA

Nicholas T. Haddock, MD Department of Plastic Surgery, UT Southwestern Medical Center, Dallas, TX, USA

Geoffrey G. Hallock, MD Division of Plastic Surgery, St. Luke's Hospital, Sacred Heart Campus, Allentown, PA, USA

Matthew M. Hanasono, MD Department of Plastic Surgery, The University of Texas MD Anderson Cancer Center, Houston, TX, USA

Andrea Hanick, MD Head & Neck Institute, Cleveland Clinic, Cleveland, OH, USA

Austin Hembd, MD Department of Plastic Surgery, UT Southwestern Medical Center, Dallas, TX, USA

DeAsia D. Jacob, MD Department of Plastic Surgery, Cleveland, OH, USA

Alireza Hamidian Jahromi, MD Plastic and Reconstructive Surgery Department, Rush University Medical Center, Chicago, IL, USA

Matthew Joy, MD Division of Plastic Surgery, Department of Surgery, University of Pennsylvania, Philadelphia, PA, USA

David Kashan, MD Department of Plastic Surgery, Cleveland Clinic, Cleveland, OH, USA

Karlina Kegecik, BS Cleveland State University, Cleveland, OH, USA

Yoshihiro Kimata, MD, PhD Department of Plastic and Reconstructive Surgery, Okayama University, Graduate School of Medicine, Dentistry, and Pharmaceutical Sciences, Okayama-city, Okayama, Japan

Rebecca Knackstedt, MD, PhD Department of Plastic Surgery, Cleveland Clinic, Cleveland, OH, USA

Peter Kompatscher, MD Department of Plastic Surgery (emeritus status), Academic Hospital of Feldkirch, Feldkirch, Austria

Stephen J. Kovacs, MD Division of Plastic Surgery, Department of Surgery, University of Pennsylvania, Philadelphia, PA, USA

Katariina Laurila, MD Department of Plastic Surgery, Helsinki University Hospital, Helsinki, Finland

Christina Dami Lee, DO Department of Plastic Surgery, Cleveland Clinic, Cleveland, OH, USA

Gordon K. Lee, MD, FACS Plastic and Reconstructive Surgery, Stanford University, Palo Alto, CA, USA

L. Scott Levin, MD Division of Plastic Surgery, Department of Surgery, University of Pennsylvania, Philadelphia, PA, USA

Department of Orthopaedic Surgery, University of Pennsylvania, Philadelphia, PA, USA

Chih-Hung Lin, MD Chang Gung Memorial Hospital, Taoyuan, Taiwan

Ines C. Lin, MD, MSEd Division of Plastic Surgery, Department of Surgery, University of Pennsylvania, Philadelphia, PA, USA

Department of Orthopaedic Surgery, University of Pennsylvania, Philadelphia, PA, USA

Yee Cheng Low, MD Division of Plastic and Reconstructive Surgery, Department of Surgery, Lehigh Valley Health Network, Allentown, PA, USA

Samir Mardini, MD Division of Plastic Surgery, Department of Surgery, Mayo Clinic, Rochester, MN, USA

Hiroshi Matsumoto, MD, PhD Department of Plastic and Reconstructive Surgery, Okayama University, Graduate School of Medicine, Dentistry, and Pharmaceutical Sciences, Okayama-city, Okayama, Japan

Alexander F. Mericli, MD, FACS Department of Plastic Surgery, The University of Texas M.D. Anderson Cancer Center, Houston, TX, USA

Nathan F. Miller, MD University of Maryland/R Adams Cowley Shock Trauma Center, Baltimore, MD, USA

Arash Momeni, MD, FACS Division of Plastic & Reconstructive Surgery, Ryan-Upson Scholar in Plastic and Reconstructive Surgery, Director - Clinical Outcomes Research, Stanford University School of Medicine, Palo Alto, CA, USA

Lynn M. Orfahli, BM Department of Plastic Surgery, Cleveland Clinic, Cleveland, OH, USA

Cemile Nurdan Ozturk, MD Department of Head, Neck & Plastic Surgery, Roswell Park Comprehensive Cancer Center, Buffalo, NY, USA

Meenakshi Rajan, MD Department of Plastic Surgery, Cleveland Clinic, Cleveland, OH, USA

Antonio Rampazzo, MD, PhD Department of Plastic Surgery, Cleveland Clinic, Cleveland, OH, USA

Cleveland Clinic Lerner College of Medicine, Case Western Reserve University, Cleveland, OH, USA

Margaret S. Roubaud, MD Department of Plastic Surgery, The University of Texas MD Anderson Cancer Center, Houston, TX, USA

Pierre B. Saadeh, MD Hansjörg Wyss Department of Plastic Surgery at NYU Grossman School of Medicine, Plastic Surgery Service – Bellevue Hospital Center, New York, NY, USA

Joseph Scharpf, MD Head & Neck Institute, Cleveland Clinic, Cleveland, OH, USA

Loren S. Schechter, MD Plastic and Reconstructive Surgery Department, Rush University Medical Center, Chicago, IL, USA

The Center for Gender Confirmation Surgery, Weiss Memorial Hospital, The University of Illinois at Chicago, Chicago, IL, USA

Graham Schwarz, MD Department of Plastic Surgery, Cleveland Clinic, Cleveland, OH, USA

Isis Scomacao, MD Department of Plastic Surgery, Cleveland Clinic, Cleveland, OH, USA

Gokhan Sert, MD Department of Plastic Surgery, International Medical Center of China Medical University Hospital, China Medical University, Taichung City, Taiwan

Janki Shah, MD Head & Neck Institute, Cleveland Clinic, Cleveland, OH, USA

Deana Shenaq, MD Plastic and Reconstructive Surgery Department, Rush University Medical Center, Chicago, IL, USA

Andrea Sisti, MD Department of Plastic Surgery, Cleveland Clinic, Cleveland, OH, USA

Brandon C. Specht, DO Department of Plastic Surgery, Cleveland Clinic, Cleveland, OH, USA

Zvi Steinberger, MD Department of Orthopaedic Surgery, University of Pennsylvania, Philadelphia, PA, USA

Department of Hand and Microsurgery, Sheba Medical Center, Tel Hashomer, Israel

Jenna Rose Stoehr, BA Feinberg School of Medicine, Northwestern University, Chicago, IL, USA

Patrick Tassone, MD Department of Otolaryngology – Head & Neck Surgery, University of Missouri School of Medicine, Columbia, MO, USA

Erkki Tukiainen, MD Department of Plastic Surgery, Helsinki University Hospital, Helsinki, Finland

Fatma Betul Tuncer, MD Department of Plastic Surgery, Cleveland Clinic, Cleveland, OH, USA

Division of Plastic Surgery, University of Utah, Salt Lake City, UT, USA

Kavita T. Vakharia, MD Department of Plastic Surgery, Cleveland Clinic, Cleveland, OH, USA

Part I

Introduction

Recipient Vessels for Microsurgery

1

Raffi Gurunian

Introduction

Microsurgery is a powerful technique that provides the opportunity to utilize the best, and sometimes the only, available option to accomplish a particular reconstructive goal. Reconstructive microsurgical procedures consist of preparation of the recipient site, elevation of the microsurgical flap, transfer of the flap from the donor site to the recipient site, and revascularization through microvascular anastomoses [1–19].

Microvascular surgery is much more than performing microvascular anastomoses under the microscope. Considerable amount of critical thinking and careful planning is required in each and every microsurgical flap case. Patient comorbidities and potential donor site morbidities should be factored into selection of a proper microsurgical flap which is then tailored to the type, location, and size of the defect. During this planning stage, the length and caliber of the pedicle should be assessed taking into consideration the anatomic characteristics of the recipient site vessels. In some instances, the recipient vessel characteristics will alter the microsurgical flap choice.

"Which recipient vessels are we going to use for anastomosis?" and "how are we going to expose them?" are the two frequently asked questions in any microsurgical case. Selection of a proper recipient vessel that is workable is critical to the success of a microsurgical flap. This book is written with the goal of assisting readers in decision-making when selecting recipient vessels with an emphasis on surgical site exposure in various microsurgical flap reconstructions.

R. Gurunian (✉)
Department of Plastic Surgery, Cleveland Clinic, Cleveland, OH, USA

Cleveland Clinic Lerner College of Medicine, Case Western Reserve University, Cleveland, OH, USA
e-mail: gurunir@ccf.org

Preoperative Assessment

Clinical examination is the mainstay for assessment of most standard recipient site vessels from head to foot. A handheld Doppler is a useful adjunct tool. When suspicion arises, imaging studies, like color Doppler ultrasound, computed tomography angiography, or magnetic resonance angiography, may be warranted for confirming the existence and condition of recipient vessels, particularly in the presence of previous radiation and trauma. Essentially, any vessel may be used as a recipient as long as the flap pedicle can be matched to it (Fig. 1.1). A good example is the use of a perforating vessel, such as lumbar perforators or a posterior intercostal artery, for posterior trunk-free flap reconstruction [20, 21]. Imaging is recommended for identifying the location of these vessels when they are planned for microvascular anastomoses. In addition, imaging studies may be helpful to confirm the condition of recipient vessels in microsurgical reconstruction of upper and lower extremities. It is extremely important to ensure adequate perfusion in the foot or hand when a major contributing vessel, such as anterior or posterior tibial and radial or ulnar vessels, is going to be used as a recipient vessel. The reconstructive surgeon should be comfortable with performing end-to-side anastomosis and/or use of interpositional vein grafts if a need arises.

Every case should be evaluated individually based on the defect's characteristics and its anatomic location. It is important to note that in most cases the decision that any selected vessel be used as the recipient vessel is one that can be made intraoperatively. Therefore, unless the reconstructive surgeon ensures a viable recipient vessel, flap harvest should be delayed. For instance, if the superficial temporal vessels are going to be used for scalp reconstruction in a patient who has preexisting preauricular and temporal incision scars due to a previous neurosurgical procedure, it would be wise to first dissect those vessels to make sure a healthy workable artery and vein are available for microvascular anastomoses. Otherwise, one would need to expose the neck vessels as an

R. Gurunian, R. Djohan (eds.), *Recipient Vessels in Reconstructive Microsurgery*,
https://doi.org/10.1007/978-3-030-75389-4_1

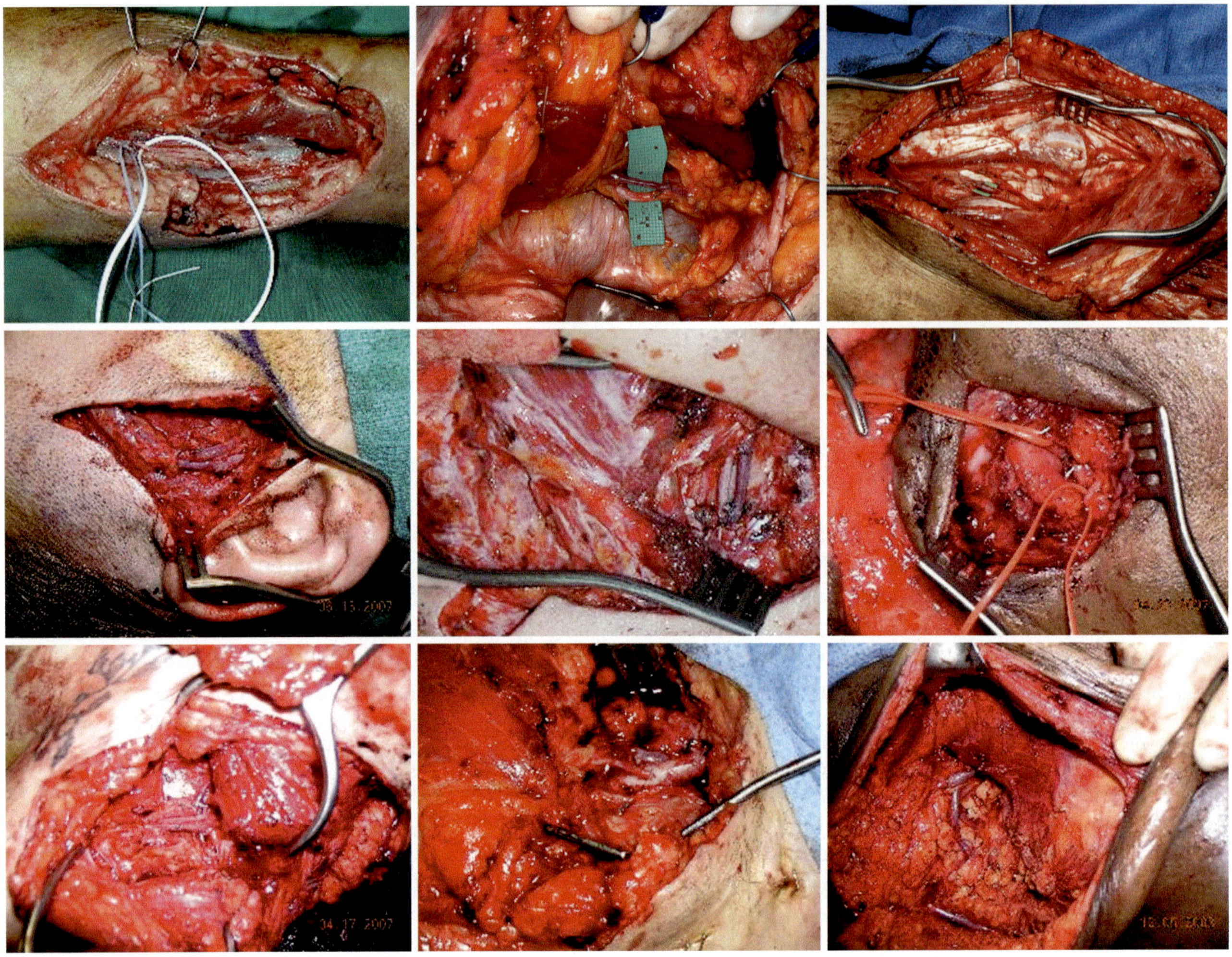

Fig. 1.1 Any vessel can be used as recipient as long as the flap pedicle can be matched to it. Some examples of recipient vessels: posterior tibial, deep inferior epigastric vessels, descending branch of the lateral circumflex femoral, (upper row from left to right), superficial temporal, internal thoracic, facial (middle row from left to right), ascending branch lateral circumflex femoral, femoral, thoracodorsal vessels (lower row from left to right)

alternative. Dimensions of the flap, as well as the pedicle length, should be modified to allow reach to the recipient neck vessels or use of interpositional vein grafts may be considered.

Typically, at any given location, preparation of recipient vessels in a standard microsurgical case should not take more than 30–45 minutes in experienced hands. That being said, in some instances, exposure and dissection will be relatively easier as recipient vessels are already exposed and readily available in the vicinity. In the event of previous trauma and radiation therapy when a recipient vessel is not readily available, plans should be made for arteriovenous loop grafts or vein grafts [13, 16]. All patients undergoing microsurgical flap reconstruction should be informed about the possibility of needing these techniques as part of the primary procedure or as a secondary means to salvage a flap.

Surgical Site Exposure

Reconstructive microsurgeons of today need to be anatomists who should know "head to toe" anatomy as it relates to flap dissection, as well as the recipient site vasculature. The surgical exposure techniques vary from location to location, but wide exposure in relation to the reconstruction site is required in most cases. Proper instrumentation should be available depending on the specifics of each case. Throughout my 30-year microsurgical experience, I have found self-

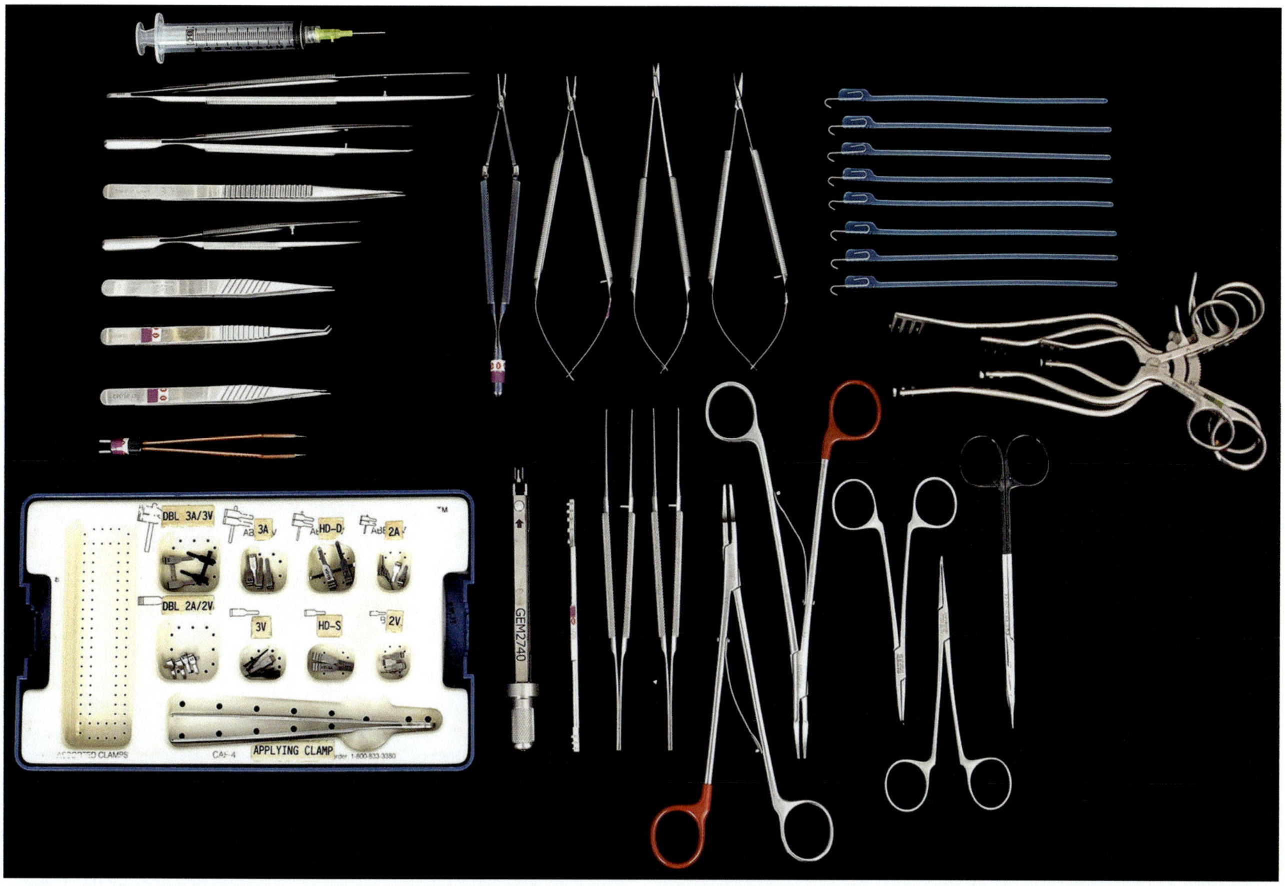

Fig. 1.2 Microsurgery instruments and accessory instruments that include self-retaining retractors in various sizes and forms, self-retracting hooks, nerve dissector, tenotomy scissors, bipolar cautery forceps, coupler, and microvascular clips

retaining retractors in various sizes and forms, self-retracting hooks, nerve dissectors, and tenotomy scissors as invaluable aids during recipient site exposure, as well as flap dissection (Figs. 1.2 and 1.3).

The principles of microsurgery should be applied in preparing the recipient vessels in each and every microsurgical case. Dissections should be performed patiently, tediously, and meticulously with minimal trauma in a relatively bloodless field. The final phase of vessel preparation should be done under the microscope prior to flap harvest. Arterial and venous adventitiectomies should be performed with great care and precision. Patency of arterial inflow and venous outflow should be confirmed prior to flap harvest. Finding out that the selected vessel does not have flow after the microsurgical flap is brought to the reconstruction site would increase the ischemia time that may jeopardize the microsurgical flap. Challenging intraoperative decisions have to be made to overcome these difficulties and identify back-up vessels. Vein or arterial grafts may be required to restore the perfusion in the microsurgical flap. Therefore, reconstructive microsurgeons should be comfortable harvesting saphenous veins and cephalic veins for arteriovenous loop graft reconstruction or to provide venous drainage.

Microvascular Anastomoses

One should enjoy performing microvascular anastomoses between the donor and recipient vessels. In order for this to happen, positioning of the surgical team, the microscope, and the vessel exposure should be optimal (Figs. 1.4 and 1.5). Vessel size match should be foreseen to minimize mismatch. Frequent cross-checking of the recipient vessel size with the flap pedicle or vice versa is helpful to reduce mismatch. Additional dissection may be required to select the vein, the artery, or its branches that are most suitable at the donor site, as well as the recipient site. Extra time spent outside the microscope may minimize the struggle under the microscope to match the vessel size discrepancy. End-to-side vessel anastomosis is always a viable option in case of significant vessel mismatch. Less significant mismatch can be overcome using techniques such as oblique transection of the vessel or creating a slit to increase lumen size of the smaller vessel. Telescoping the smaller recipient artery into the larger flap artery is a viable option in some cases. Venous mismatch can be easily circumvented using a coupler device. After perfusion into the flap is restored, one needs to make sure that there is no tension, kinking, torsion, or compression of the vessels. Considerable amount of experience is needed in each and every case to avoid these potential issues.

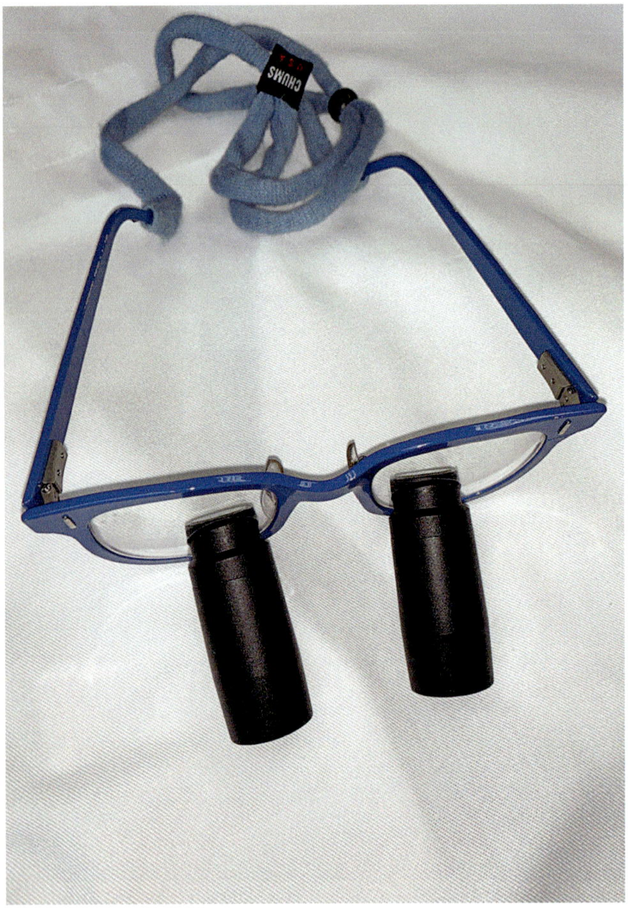

Fig. 1.3 Magnifying loupe × 4.5 that the editor prefers for pedicle dissection, recipient vessel preparation prior to using the microscope

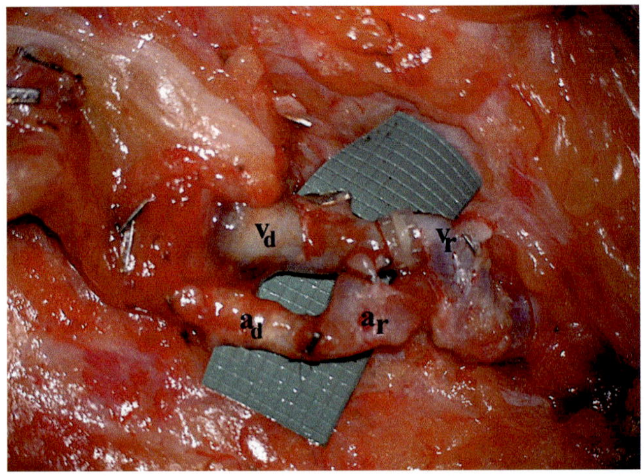

Fig. 1.5 Microvascular anastomoses completed between the superficial temporal vessels and the descending branch of the ALT flap for scalp reconstruction (vr, recipient vein; ar, recipient artery; vd, donor vein; ad, donor artery)

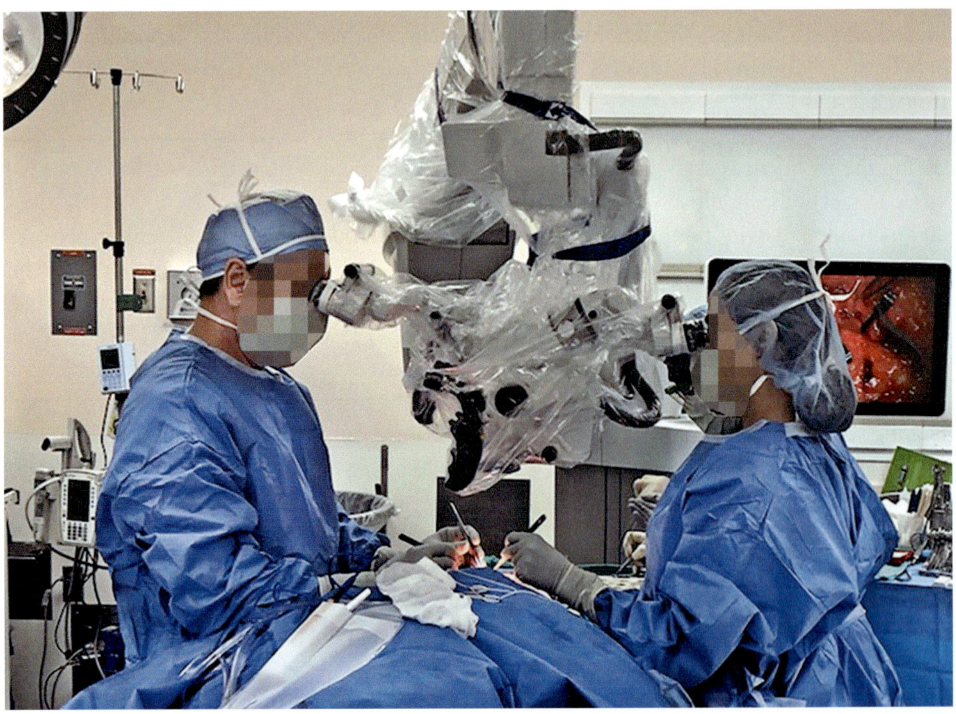

Fig. 1.4 Orientation of the team and the microscope should allow comfortable micro-anastomosis. A case of scalp reconstruction using a free anterolateral flap (ALT), the left superficial temporal vessels were used as recipient

Conclusion

Reconstructive microsurgery is an art and science that combines the knowledge of anatomy and surgical skill, both outside and under the microscope, which enables the transfer of tissue for achievement of a particular cosmetic and/or reconstructive goal.

References

1. Gurunluoglu R, Spanio S, Rainer C, Ninkovic M. Skin expansion before breast reconstruction with the superior gluteal artery perforator flap improves aesthetic outcome. Ann Plast Surg. 2003;50(5):475–9.
2. Bayramiçli M, Tetik C, Sönmez A, Gurunluoglu R, Baltaci F. Reliability of primary vein grafts in lower extremity free tissue transfers. Ann Plast Surg. 2002;48(1):21–9.
3. Schoeller T, Meirer R, Gurunluoglu R, Piza-Katzer H, Wechselberger G. Gracilis muscle split into two free flaps. J Reconstr Microsurg. 2003;19(5):295–8.
4. Schoeller T, Bauer T, Gurunluoglu R, Hussl H, Otto-Schoeller A, Piza-Katzer H, Wechselberger G. Modified free paraumbilical perforator flap: the next logical step in breast reconstruction. Plast Reconstr Surg. 2003;111(3):1093–8. discussion 1099–1101
5. Schoeller T, Huemer GM, Shafighi M, Gurunluoglu R, Wechselberger G, Piza-Katzer H. Free anteromedial thigh flap: clinical application and review of literature. Microsurgery. 2004;24(1):43–8. Review.
6. Ninkovic M, Moser-Rumer A, Ninkovic M, Spanio S, Rainer C, Gurunluoglu R. Anterior neck reconstruction with pre-expanded free groin and scapular flaps. Plast Reconstr Surg. 2004;113(1):61–8.
7. Gurunluoglu R, Shafighi M, Schwabegger A, Ninkovic M. Secondary breast reconstruction with deepithelialized free flaps from the lower abdomen for intractable capsular contracture and maintenance of breast volume. J Reconstr Microsurg. 2005;21(1):35–41.
8. Gilman K, Ipaktchi K, Moore EE, Barnett C, Gurunluoglu R. Reconstruction of an emergency thoracotomy wound with free rectus abdominis flap: anatomic and radiologic basis for the surgical technique. World J Emerg Surg. 2010;5:12.
9. Gurunluoglu R. The ascending branch of the lateral circumflex femoral vessels: review of the anatomy and its utilization as recipient vessel for free-flap reconstruction of the hip region. J Reconstr Microsurg. 2010;26(6):359–66.
10. Gurunluoglu R, Glasgow M, Williams SA, Gurunluoglu A, Antrobus J, Eusterman V. Functional reconstruction of total lower lip defects using innervated gracilis flap in the setting of high-energy ballistic injury to the lower face: preliminary report. J Plast Reconstr Aesthet Surg. 2012;65(10):1335–42.
11. Gurunluoglu R, Shah M, Kim F. Microsurgical penile replantation after self-inflicted amputation in a schizophrenic patient: 5-year follow-up. Plast Reconstr Surg Glob Open. 2015;3(3):e319.
12. Sacak B, Gurunluoglu R. The innervated gracilis muscle for microsurgical functional lip reconstruction: review of the literature. Ann Plast Surg. 2015;74(2):204–9.
13. Gurunluoglu R, Ghaznavi A, Krpata D, Zins J, Rosen MJ. Arteriovenous loop graft in abdominal wall reconstruction using free tissue transfer. J Plast Reconstr Aesthet Surg. 2016;69(11):1513–5.
14. Currie KB, Ross P, Collister P, Gurunluoglu R. Analysis of scalp and forehead injuries in a level I trauma center. J Craniofac Surg. 2017;28(5):1350–3.
15. Gurunluoglu R, Rosen MJ. Recipient vessels for microsurgical flaps to the abdomen: a systematic review. Microsurgery. 2017;37(6):707–16.
16. Knackstedt R, Aliotta R, Gatherwright J, Djohan R, Gastman B, Schwarz G, Hendrickson M, Gurunluoglu R. Single-stage versus two-stage arteriovenous loop microsurgical reconstruction: a meta-analysis of the literature. Microsurgery. 2018;38(6):706–17.
17. Gatherwright J, Knackstedt RW, Ghaznavi AM, Bernard S, Schwarz G, Moreira A, Gurunluoglu R, Djohan R. Prospective, randomized, controlled comparison of bupivacaine versus liposomal bupivacaine for pain management after unilateral delayed deep inferior epigastric perforator free flap reconstruction. Plast Reconstr Surg. 2018;141(6):1327–30.
18. Aliotta RE, Gatherwright J, Krpata D, Rosenblatt S, Rosen M, Gurunluoglu R. Complex abdominal wall reconstruction, harnessing the power of a specialized multidisciplinary team to improve pain and quality of life. Hernia. 2019;23(2):205–15.
19. Gurunluoglu R, Gatherwright J. Microsurgical reconstruction of complex maxillofacial gunshot wounds: outcomes analysis and algorithm. Microsurgery. 2019;39(5):384–94.
20. Lee YJ, Baek SE, Lee J, Oh DY, Rhie JW, Moon SH. Perforating vessel as an alternative option of a recipient selection for posterior trunk-free flap reconstruction. Microsurgery. 2018;38(7):763–71.
21. Kiil BJ, Rozen WM, Pan WR, Grinsell D, Ashton MW, Corlett RJ, Taylor GI. The lumbar artery perforators: a cadaveric and clinical anatomical study. Plast Reconstr Surg. 2009;123(4):1229–38.

Part II

Head and Neck Reconstruction

External Carotid Branches/External Jugular/Internal Jugular

2

Patrick Tassone and Joseph Scharpf

Introduction

The head and neck are extremely well vascularized in the previously unoperated patient. The external carotid system gives off several accessible and robust branches within the neck, often with helpful proximity to the defect site. Careful selection of a branch of the external carotid artery must take into consideration vessel length, caliber, blood flow, and final pedicle geometry.

Likewise, there are often many named and unnamed branches of the internal jugular vein that are surgically accessible in the neck; in most cases, the internal jugular vein itself may also be used for anastomosis. The external jugular vein can also be useful for its length, frequently large caliber, and separate drainage pathway.

Several cranial nerves and their branches will be routinely encountered when using branches of the external carotid artery and internal jugular vein, and knowledge of their anatomy helps to protect them from injury, and may also serve to optimize anastomosis geometry.

Arterial Anatomy and Selection

Access to the carotid sheath can be obtained by dissecting along the anterior border of the sternocleidomastoid muscle (SCM). As the SCM is retracted laterally and the dissection proceeds posteriorly, the internal jugular vein (IJV) is typically the first structure encountered within the carotid sheath (Video 2.1). Retraction of the IJV laterally reveals the vagus nerve and common carotid artery, which can be dissected superiorly to its bifurcation into the external and internal carotid arteries [1].

The common carotid artery bifurcates into the external and internal carotid arteries at the carotid bulb. The carotid bifurcation is typically located at approximately the superior border of the thyroid cartilage [1, 2]. In cadaveric studies, the bifurcation is located superior to this point in approximately 25% of patients [2]. In patients with a high bifurcation, the posterior belly of the digastric and the stylohyoid muscles may overlie the bifurcation; dissection of the external carotid in this area will require either retraction or division of these muscles.

The external carotid typically gives off eight branches: superior thyroid, ascending pharyngeal, lingual, facial, occipital, posterior auricular, internal maxillary, and superficial temporal [1]. The superficial temporal artery is the terminal branch. Anterior cervical branches include the superior thyroid, lingual, and facial arteries, and their relative anatomy has been described in several cadaveric studies.

Although classically described as the first branch of the external carotid artery, the superior thyroid artery (STA) is found to arise from the common carotid artery in approximately 40% of cadavers [3]. Its external caliber at its origin averages 1–3.5 mm [4, 5]. Use of the superior thyroid artery is preferred by some authors [6], while others avoid it for its often smaller caliber [4]. If the STA is to be used, careful consideration must be made for its natural orientation and final configuration in a microvascular anastomosis. The STA is caudally oriented as it descends toward the thyroid gland, and rearrangement to accommodate a more cranial anastomosis site can introduce kinking into the artery [7].

The lingual and facial arteries are frequently used for their robust caliber and length, as well as their proximity to the defect for many head and neck patients. Average caliber of

Supplementary Information The online version of this chapter (https://doi.org/10.1007/978-3-030-75389-4_2) contains supplementary material, which is available to authorized users.

P. Tassone
Department of Otolaryngology – Head & Neck Surgery, University of Missouri School of Medicine, Columbia, MO, USA
e-mail: tassonep@health.missouri.edu

J. Scharpf (✉)
Head & Neck Institute, Cleveland Clinic, Cleveland, OH, USA
e-mail: scharpj@ccf.org

R. Gurunian, R. Djohan (eds.), *Recipient Vessels in Reconstructive Microsurgery*, https://doi.org/10.1007/978-3-030-75389-4_2

both lingual and facial arteries averages 2–3.5 mm [4, 5]. Their takeoff from the external carotid is variable, with approximately 20% of cadavers having a common lingual-facial artery that gives rise to the two separate branches [2, 5, 8].

Access to the lingual, facial, and more distal branches of the external carotid artery can be achieved by superior dissection along the external carotid artery. In most cases, the posterior belly of the digastric and the stylohyoid muscles will need to be retracted superiorly to gain access to the arterial branch points [1]. In a patient with a long neck and an inferiorly positioned hyoid bone, the branch point of the facial artery may be accessible by inferior retraction of the same muscles.

The facial artery ascends deep to the posterior belly of the digastric muscle to supply branches to the posterior border of the submandibular gland before crossing the mandible at the facial notch [1]. The entire length can be preserved even during a thorough oncologic neck dissection, though it is often injured during dissection in level 1B (Fig. 2.1, Video 2.1). In cases where a neck dissection is not performed, the facial artery can be accessed through a small incision over the facial notch [9].

The lingual artery courses anteriorly, in close proximity to the hypoglossal nerve, to pierce the hyoglossus muscle [1]. Dissection of the lingual artery beyond this muscle may lead to inadvertent entry into the pharynx. The lingual artery may be inadvertently injured in neck dissection or in primary tumor resection, especially total laryngectomy.

The external carotid artery (ECA) can be also be used, in either an end-to-end or end-to-side fashion, for microvascular anastomosis [4, 7]. Its average 4 mm diameter may require mitigation of vessel mismatch by the use of carefully placed microvascular sutures [4]. It is often necessary to ligate the distal ECA in order to mobilize it into the neck for visualization of anastomosis under the mandible [10]. Use of the ECA as a recipient vessel has been reported to produce reliable arterial flow with low risk of arterial thrombosis, even in the vessel-depleted neck [10, 11].

Preoperative planning and intraoperative dissection are paramount to successful arterial selection. In previously operated patients, preoperative computed tomography angiography (CTA) of the neck can identify the presence or absence of patent arterial branches of the external carotid artery [12, 13]. In tumor cases, a preoperative conversation between ablative and reconstructive surgeon helps identify planned arterial selection.

After tumor ablation and neck dissection have been performed, the reconstructive surgeon must evaluate the potential recipient arteries carefully. This should be done before a flap is ischemic. The entire length of the dissected artery should be examined, and adequate blood flow should be confirmed. If the lingual or facial artery is to be used, it is often helpful to circumferentially dissect the vessel to its takeoff from the external carotid artery, to allow for maximal mobility of the vessel. It may be necessary to divide the posterior belly of the digastric and stylohyoid muscles to optimize arterial pedicle geometry.

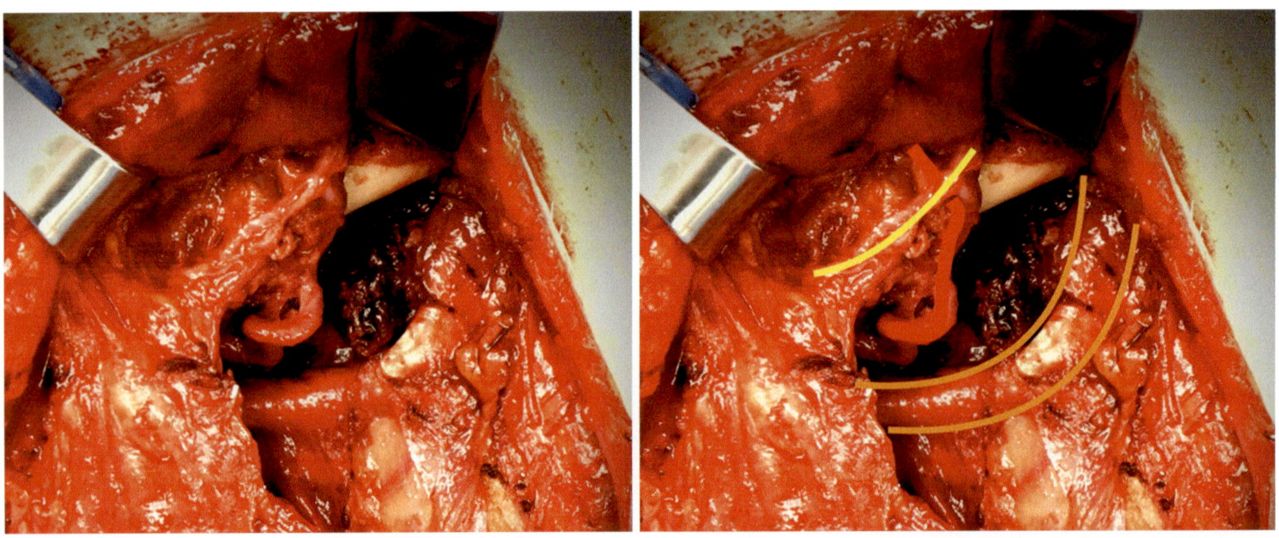

Fig. 2.1 The facial artery (highlighted in red, right panel) crosses the inferior border of the mandible at the facial notch, where the marginal mandibular branch of the facial nerve (highlighted in yellow, right panel) travels superficial to the artery. The artery can be dissected proximally to its takeoff from the external carotid artery deep to the posterior belly of the digastric muscle (highlighted in orange, right panel)

Venous Anatomy and Selection

External Jugular Vein

The external jugular vein (EJV) arises from the retromandibular and postauricular veins, descends postero-inferiorly over the sternocleidomastoid muscle, and drains into the subclavian or low internal jugular veins [1]. The EJV may be anatomically diminutive or may be surgically absent following prior neck dissection; the patency and presence of the EJV can often be assessed on contrasted computed tomography scan (Fig. 2.2). In a cadaveric study of EJVs, 83% of EJVs were found to be singular, with the remaining 17% having two parallel branches [8].

EJV is at particular risk during raising of subplatysmal flaps for neck dissection, and preoperative discussion with the ablative surgeon can help to preserve an intact EJV (Video 2.1). In lateral neck level 4, the EJV is often visualized as it drains into the subclavian or internal jugular vein. Injury to the EJV in this area may not be recognized by the surgeon performing the neck dissection, and so thorough inspection of the EJV before using it as a recipient vein is mandatory.

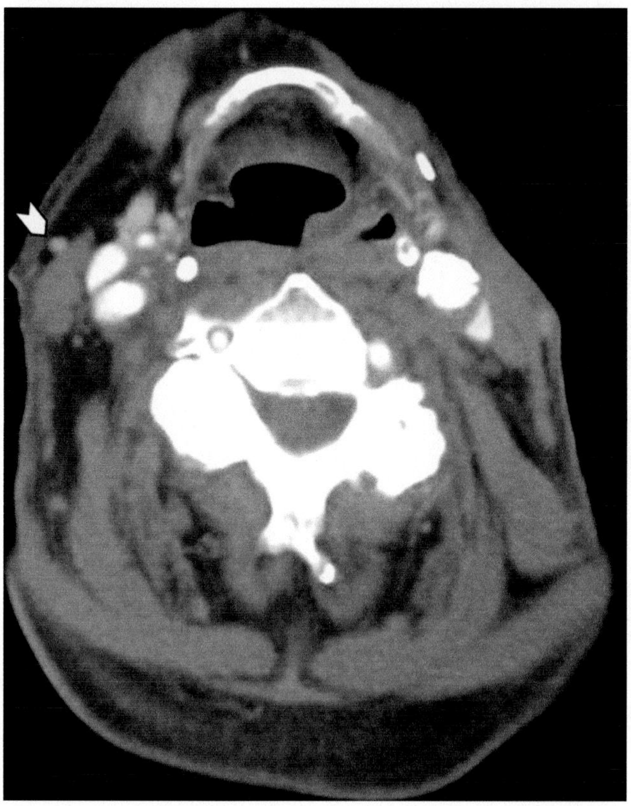

Fig. 2.2 Axial cut contrasted computed tomography scan showing patent right external jugular vein (arrowhead) with venous contrast filling. Note the absence of left external jugular vein after previous neck dissection

If dissected both distally and proximally, the EJV affords excellent mobility for microvascular anastomosis. Its longitudinal orientation and frequently robust size have led some authors to advocate for its routine use in flaps [7]. An end-to-side anastomosis with the EJV allows for multiple donor veins to be drained, and may allow for even greater control of final pedicle geometry [7].

Internal Jugular Vein

The internal jugular vein (IJV) is typically accessed within the carotid sheath by retraction of the sternocleidomastoid muscle laterally, as described above (Video 2.1). The IJV and its branches have significant anatomic variability. Facial, lingual, and superior thyroid veins are usually present, and the most common arrangement in one cadaveric study was for all three branches to drain as a single large vein off the IJV [8]. These branches can be identified by dissection along the anterior border of the IJV along its length in the neck.

When intact, facial vein branches often have excellent length and diameter, as well as multiple branches; this allows for end-to-end anastomosis of more than one donor vein into the facial vein system. However, facial vein branches are often sacrificed as part of oncologic neck dissections, leaving the reconstructive surgeon with little, if any, length of the facial vein remaining. Additionally, size mismatch may occur between often large facial vein branches and commonly small donor venae comitantes. When facial veins are left in continuity, an end-to-side anastomosis to a freely flowing facial vein may be performed to discourage venous stasis (Fig. 2.3).

Many authors advocate for the use of end-to-side anastomosis to the internal jugular vein as the preferred choice of venous anastomosis [14, 15]. End-to-side anastomosis overcomes problems of vessel mismatch, and may provide a "respiratory venous pump system" as the IJV is subject to negative intrathoracic pressure, which may encourage venous outflow through the anastomosis [14]. In the event that the IJV is sacrificed as part of a radical neck dissection, the IJV stump may still be used for end-to-side anastomosis [16].

When performing end-to-side anastomosis to the IJV, vessel loops or vascular clamps can significantly distort the anatomy of the vein during anastomosis [7]. Before loops or clamps are placed, it is helpful to mark the most anatomically advantageous position of the anastomosis to ensure excellent final pedicle geometry (Fig. 2.4).

As the internal jugular vein is usually present and patent even in operated or radiated necks, the head and neck reconstructive surgeon must be facile with its use as a recipient vessel.

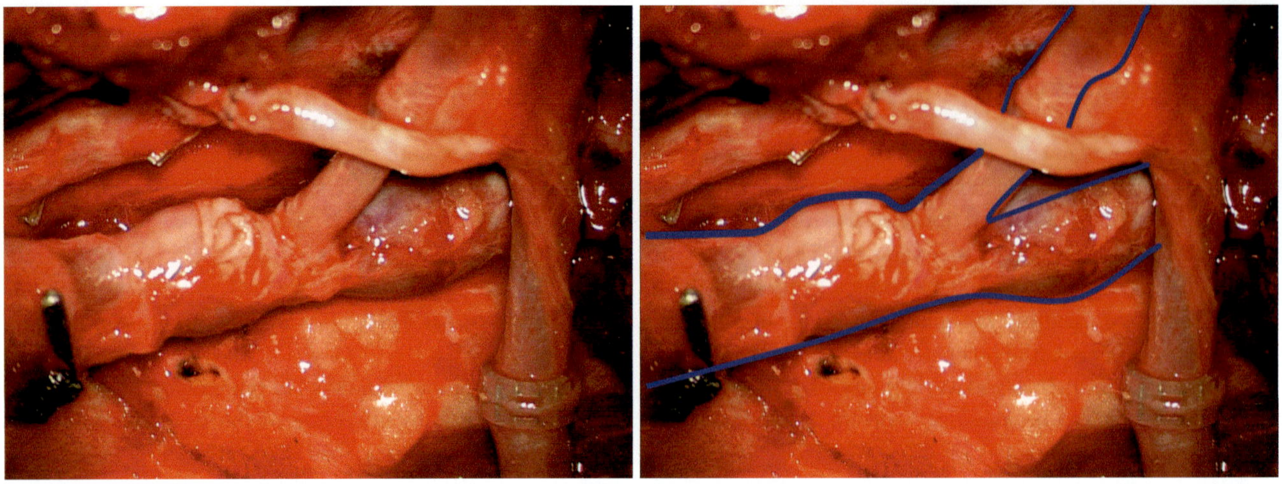

Fig. 2.3 End-to-side venous anastomosis to the right common facial vein. When the facial vein is large and has been left in continuity (highlighted in blue, right panel), end-to-side anastomosis to the facial vein may discourage venous stasis, optimize pedicle geometry, and mitigate vessel size mismatch

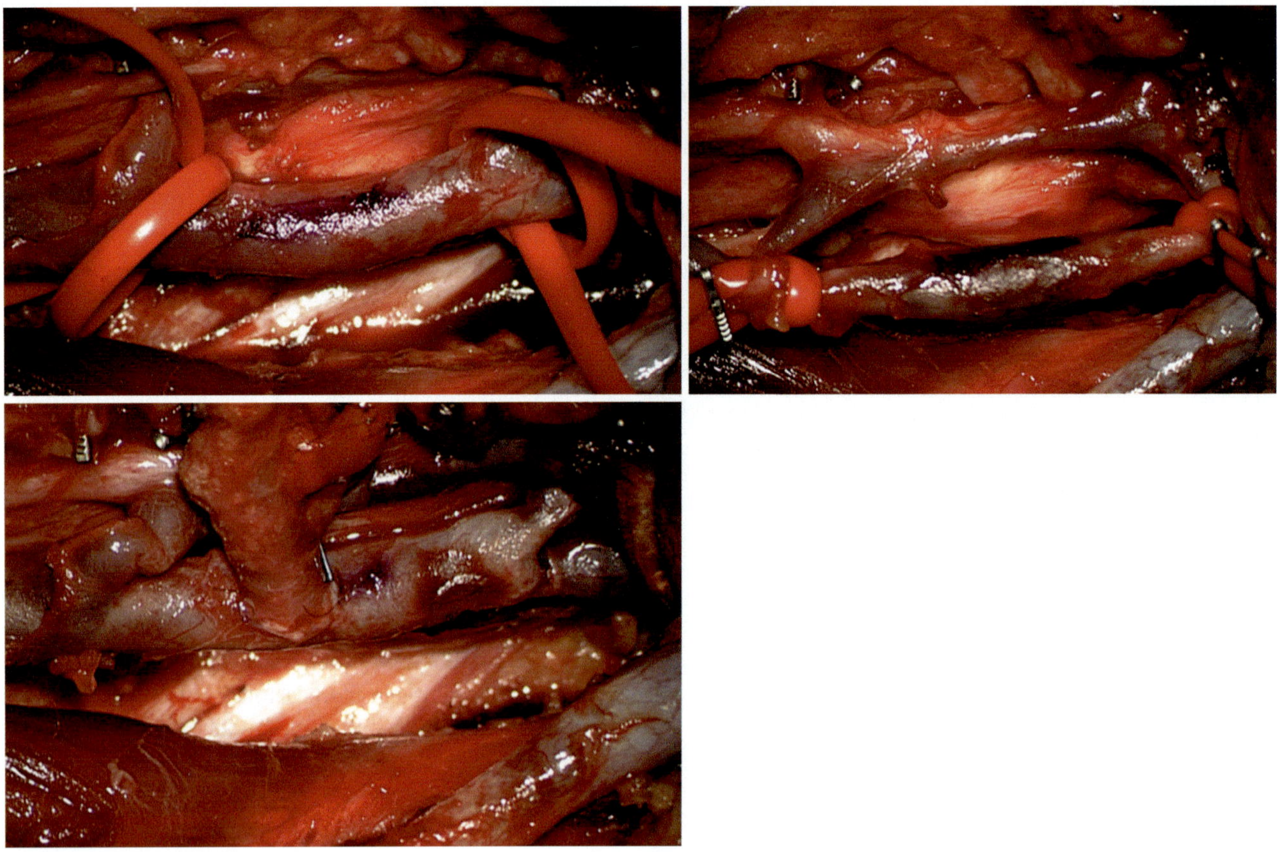

Fig. 2.4 Prior to occlusion of the internal jugular vein (IJV), the planned final position of the venous anastomosis is marked in situ (top panel). Once the IJV is occluded with vessel loops, the vein rotates (middle panel). After end-to-side anastomosis, vessel loops are removed and favorable anastomotic geometry is preserved (bottom panel)

Nerve and Lymphatic Anatomy and Considerations

Several cranial nerves or their branches are at risk of injury during neck vessel dissection or preparation. The marginal mandibular nerve branch of the facial nerve emerges from the anterior border of the parotid tail, and courses anterosuperiorly over the mandible at the facial notch [1]. Here, it lies superficial to the facial vessels (Fig. 2.1); if access to the facial vessels is obtained through an incision at the facial notch, the marginal mandibular nerve may be inadvertently injured, leading to an ipsilateral lower lip weakness.

The vagus nerve exits the jugular foramen and courses inferiorly within the carotid sheath, posterior the internal jugular vein [1]. If the IJV is to be used as a recipient vein, it is important to isolate only the vein before vessel loops or clamps are placed, to avoid crush or traction injury to the vagus nerve.

The hypoglossal nerve, after exiting the skull through the hypoglossal canal, courses anteriorly to supply the muscles of the tongue. It lies deep to the IJV and superficial to the ECA or carotid bulb [1]. Dissection of the proximal ECA and its branches requires care to protect the hypoglossal nerve. In some cases, it may be necessary to transpose ECA branches underneath the hypoglossal nerve in order to reach donor vessels lower in the neck.

While both sides of the neck contain significant lymphatic channels, the left side contains the much larger thoracic duct. The thoracic duct ascends into the inferior neck posterior to the common carotid artery and travels laterally, crossing anterior to the transverse cervical vessels before emptying into the left subclavian vein [1]. The right-sided lymphatic duct, whose anatomy is more variable, empties into the right subclavian vein or inferior internal jugular vein. While the lymphatic channels themselves are not of consequence to vessel selection or pedicle geometry, the reconstructive surgeon should assess this anatomic area for evidence of chyle leak. Chyle leak should be controlled intraoperatively, and if a high-flow leak was seen at the time of neck dissection, the reconstructive surgeon may select a recipient vessel from the contralateral neck, if it is available.

Conclusion

The microvascular reconstructive surgeon is well-served by a frequent abundance of recipient vessels as part of the external carotid artery, external jugular vein, and internal jugular vein systems. Intimate knowledge of the anatomy of these systems allows for their successful use in free tissue transfer; the surgeon often has several options, and may select from them based on length, size, flow, and anticipated final pedicle geometry. In cases of prior surgery or radiation treatment, these systems often still allow for excellent vessel options, as long as the reconstructive surgeon has adequate experience in the many ways in which they may be used.

References

1. Janfaza P, Fabian R. Anatomy of the neck: general considerations. In: Surgical anatomy of the head and neck. Cambridge, MA: Harvard University Press; 2001. p. 508–77.
2. Devadas D, Pillay M, Sukumaran TT. A cadaveric study on variations in branching pattern of external carotid artery. Anat Cell Biol. 2018;51(4):225–31.
3. Anagnostopoulou S, Mavridis I. Emerging patterns of the human superior thyroid artery and review of its clinical anatomy. Surg Radiol Anat. 2013;36(1):33–8.
4. Hiller A, Davis J, Schulz S, Henderson J, Wilhelmi BJ. Recipient vessel selection in head and neck reconstruction. Eplasty. 2017;e42.
5. Ozgur Z, Govsa F, Ozgur T. Assessment of origin characteristics of the front branches of the external carotid artery. J Craniofac Surg. 2008;19(4):1159–66.
6. Chia H-L, Wong C-H, Tan B-K, Tan K-C, Ong Y-S. An algorithm for recipient vessel selection in microsurgical head and neck reconstruction. J Reconstr Microsurg. 2010;27(01):047–56.
7. Urken ML, Vickery C, Weinberg H, Buchbinder D, Biller HF. Geometry of the vascular pedicle in free tissue transfers to the head and neck. Arch Otolaryngol Head Neck Surg. 1989;115(8):954–60.
8. Shima H, Luedinghausen MV, Ohno K, Michi K-I. Anatomy of microvascular anastomosis in the neck. Plast Reconstr Surg. 1998;101(1):33–41.
9. Revenaugh PC, Fritz MA, Haffey TM, Seth R, Markey J, Knott PD. Minimizing morbidity in microvascular surgery. JAMA Facial Plastic Surg. 2015;17(1):44.
10. Garg RK, Poore SO, Wieland AM, Sanchez R, Baskaya MK, Hartig GK. Recipient vessel selection in the difficult neck: outcomes of external carotid artery transposition and end-to-end microvascular anastomosis. Microsurgery. 2015;37(2):96–100.
11. Schusterman MA, Miller MJ, Reece GP, Kroll SS, Marchi M, Goepfert H. A single center's experience with 308 free flaps for repair of head and neck cancer defects. Plast Reconstr Surg. 1994;93(3):479–80.
12. Tan O, Kantarci M, Parmaksizoglu D, Uyanik U, Durur I. Determination of the recipient vessels in the head and neck using multislice spiral computed tomography angiography before free flap surgery. J Craniofacial Surg. 2007;18(6):1284–9.
13. Chen Y-W, Yen J-H, Chen W-H, Chen I-C, Lai C-S, Lu C-T, et al. Preoperative computed tomography angiography for evaluation of feasibility of free flaps in difficult reconstruction of head and neck. Ann Plast Surg. 2016;76
14. Yamamoto Y, Nohira K, Kuwahara H, Sekido M, Furukawa H, Sugihara T. Superiority of end-to-side anastomosis with the internal jugular vein: the experience of 80 cases in head and neck microsurgical reconstruction. Br J Plast Surg. 1999;52(2):88–91.
15. Halvorson EG, Cordeiro PG. Go for the jugular. Ann Plast Surg. 2007;59(1):31–5.
16. Graham BB, Varvares MA. End-to-side venous anastomosis with the internal jugular vein stump: a preliminary report. Head Neck. 2004;26(6):537–40.

Minimal Access Approach for Facial Vessels

3

Andrea Hanick, Janki Shah, and Michael Fritz

Introduction

The facial artery and vein are among the most commonly utilized vessels in microvascular head and neck reconstruction. With reliable caliber and anatomic position, these vessels are typically isolated during concomitant neck dissection or after relatively extensive level 2 neck exploration; this process requires significant tissue manipulation, relatively large incision size, and postoperative drain placement. However, when neck dissection is not required or when an anatomically superior point of vessel isolation is advantageous for pedicle reach, these vessels are easily accessed via a minimal access incision and isolated as they transition from the neck over the mandible into the face. This approach allows for focal and facile exposure via an aesthetically favorable incision and confers significantly less patient morbidity while optimizing the extent of pedicle reach in midface, nasal, and palatal reconstruction [1–3]. Isolation of vessels in this location over the mandible adds several centimeters of pedicle reach compared to vessel isolation in the adjacent level 2 neck. As a result, the minimal access exposure for facial vessel isolation provides an invaluable tool in microvascular head and neck reconstruction.

Preoperative Considerations

Microvascular reconstruction of midface, nasal, and palatal defects can be complicated by issues of pedicle reach and geometry, particularly when defects mandate high tissue reach to the skull base or extensive bone replacement and manipulation [2, 3]. In this setting, options for recipient vessels that provide adequate pedicle reach are limited. Vessel isolation in proximity to the defect may obviate vein grafting and thus provide for a more simple and reliable reconstruction. The distal facial artery and vein as they traverse the mandible are optimal recipient vessels with a consistent anatomic location and a superficial and higher position as compared to other recipient vessels. Importantly, the proximal facial artery and vein must be intact and preserved to allow for use in this setting. As a result, it is critical to ascertain preoperative vascular integrity if previous surgery or oncologic treatment has been performed. In the setting of planned concomitant neck dissection, communication with the ablative surgeon to preserve these vessels in level 2 is needed. As the marginal mandibular nerve is consistently identified and preserved during this dissection, assessment and documentation of preoperative functional status is critical (Fig. 3.1).

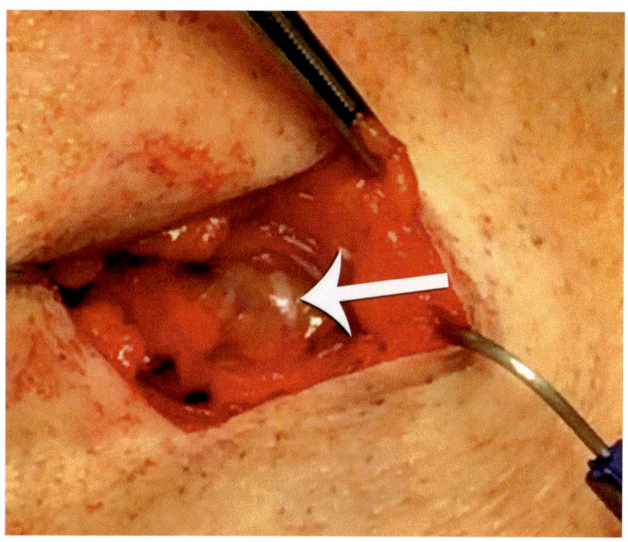

Fig. 3.1 Intraoperative dissection demonstrating the marginal mandibular branch of the facial nerve (arrow) identified in close proximity and just superficial to the level of the facial vessels

Supplementary Information The online version of this chapter (https://doi.org/10.1007/978-3-030-75389-4_3) contains supplementary material, which is available to authorized users.

A. Hanick · J. Shah · M. Fritz (✉)
Head & Neck Institute, Cleveland Clinic, Cleveland, OH, USA
e-mail: fritzm1@ccf.org

R. Gurunian, R. Djohan (eds.), *Recipient Vessels in Reconstructive Microsurgery*, https://doi.org/10.1007/978-3-030-75389-4_3

Relevant Anatomy

The facial vessels have predictable anatomy and run deep to the platysma muscle within the superficial layer of deep cervical fascia. The facial artery follows a course from its origin deep to the digastric muscle passing through the submandibular gland, and then crosses the mandibular border at the antegonial notch anterior to the medial insertion of the masseter muscle, about 3 cm anterior to the gonion [4]. It then follows a course toward the oral commissure and nasolabial fold. Notably, the artery and vein may run immediately parallel to one another (Fig. 3.2); however, they are frequently separate and must be carefully identified individually. The facial vein lies consistently posterior to the artery and runs over the mandible within the confluence of parotidomasseteric fascia at the anterior margin of the masseter muscle [5]. The marginal mandibular branch of the facial nerve is intimately related to the facial vessels at this point of isolation. While its branching pattern and relationship to the facial artery are varied, the nerve is most commonly superficial to the facial artery and always located deep to the facial vein [5, 6]. With meticulous technique, the nerve is easily identified and preserved during vessel isolation [1].

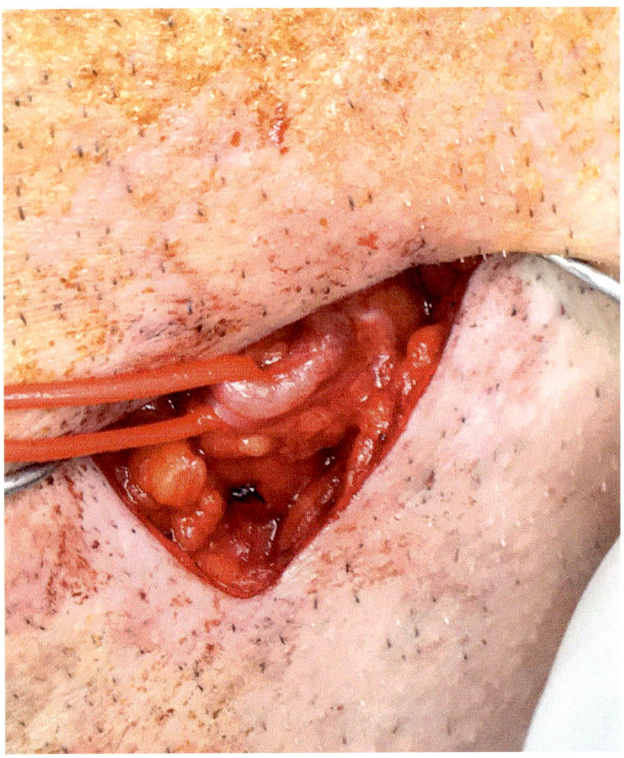

Fig. 3.2 Intraoperative dissection of the facial artery and vein via a minimal access incision for microvascular anastomosis. The vein in consistently identified posterior to the artery

Operative Technique

The location of the facial artery is identified in the area of the antegonial notch by palpation or Doppler probe evaluation. A 2.5–3 cm incision is then demarcated just below the inferior mandibular border and centered posterior to the facial artery (allowing easier access to the facial vein) (Fig. 3.3). The skin and subcutaneous tissue are incised and the platysma muscle is identified and precisely and completely divided. Subplatysmal flaps are elevated superiorly and inferiorly, giving broad exposure of the underlying fascia (superficial or investing layer of deep cervical fascia). Commonly, the location of the facial artery is revealed by visible pulsations in this layer. Also, traveling within this layer, the marginal mandibular nerve can often be directly visualized without dissection (Fig. 3.1).

Fascia is then carefully elevated and divided in translucent layers after confirming the absence of neural structures. As the fascia is thinned, the facial artery becomes readily identifiable and is exposed with parallel blunt spreading and then retracted with a vessel loop. As it is followed distally and proximally to isolate sufficient length for anastomosis, care is taken to avoid traction or injury to the marginal nerve, which is commonly (but not exclusively) located superficial to the artery. Attention is then focused on isolation of the facial vein, and identification and isolation proceeds similarly with meticulous technique. The vein always lies posterior to the artery and superficial to the marginal mandibular nerve; as previously mentioned, the vein can also lie immediately parallel and posterior to the artery and can (less commonly) be isolated conjoined with the artery (Fig. 3.2, Video 3.1).

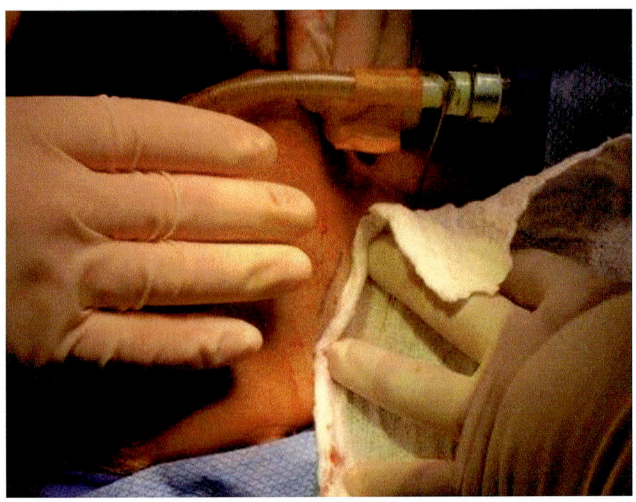

Fig. 3.3 Minimal access incision for isolation of facial vessels for free tissue transfer. A 2.5–3 cm incision is made just below the inferior mandibular border and centered posterior to the facial artery (allowing easier access to the facial vein)

In order to pass the pedicle from the flap location to the site of the recipient facial vessels, a tunnel needs to be created. This may be performed in a subcutaneous or subplatysmal plane, with the extent and technique of the latter limited and performed to avoid nerve injury more superiorly. Passage of the pedicle through this tunnel is facilitated with use of a 5/8 inch Penrose drain. In order to employ this technique without pedicle compression or facial distortion, the free flap must be harvested as a perforator flap without perivascular soft tissue bulk [1, 7, 8].

Discussion

Isolation of distal facial vessels via a minimal access approach allows for facile exposure of reliable recipient vessels with low morbidity and excellent cosmesis [1, 9]. Given their significantly higher location as compared to facial vessels isolated via traditional mid-neck incisions, these vessels confer a substantial advantage in pedicle reach for midface, nasal, and skull base reconstruction [2, 3, 9]. Using this minimal access approach, vascular pedicles can be tunneled superiorly, laterally, or inferiorly, simplifying mandibular and contralateral neck reconstruction as well. Furthermore, in patients undergoing salvage oncologic surgery or revision reconstruction, this approach allows the surgeon to avoid the most heavily irradiated or scarred portions of the neck and potential surgical and wound healing challenges conferred by tissue distortion and fibrosis. Obviously, it is of paramount importance to ensure that these vessels remain in proximal continuity with their sources.

While the presence of the marginal mandibular nerve in the vicinity of dissection must be at all times considered, consistent anatomy, easy visualization, and protection with meticulous technique allow for reliable identification and preservation of nerve function. This has been corroborated by published series with no incidence of marginal nerve weakness using this approach [1, 7, 8].

In our practice, use of this site as well as angular and superficial temporal vessel isolation has become commonplace. Utilization of minimal access incisions and tunneled pedicles allows for either complete wound closure or short-term (1–2 day) passive (Penrose) drain placement. Postoperative edema and patient discomfort are also minimized. These factors have lowered the complexity of postoperative care and contributed to dramatically shorter hospital stays without compromising flap success rates [7, 8, 10]. As a result, overall indications for vascularized free tissue transfer in facial reconstruction have continued to expand.

Conclusion

Isolation of distal facial vessels using a minimal access approach at the lower border of the mandible provides a reliable source of free flap revascularization with improved pedicle reach and minimal morbidity. As a result, this technique serves as an invaluable tool in the armamentarium for complex head and neck reconstruction.

References

1. Revenaugh PC, Fritz MA, Haffey TM, Seth R, Markey J, Knott PD. Minimizing morbidity in microvascular surgery: small-caliber anastomotic vessels and minimal access approaches. JAMA Facial Plast Surg. 2015;17(1):44–8.
2. Shipchandler TZ, Waters HH, Knott PD, Fritz MA. Orbitomaxillary reconstruction using the layered fibula osteocutaneous flap. Arch Facial Plas Surg. 2012;14(2):110–5.
3. Trosman SJ, Haffey TM, Couto RA, Fritz MA. Large orbital defect reconstruction in the setting of globe-sparing maxillectomy: the titanium hammock and layered fibula technique. Microsurgery. 2018;38(4):354–61.
4. Lee HJ, Won SY, Jehoon O, Hu KS, Mun SY, Yang HM, Kim HJ. The facial artery: a comprehensive anatomical review. Clin Anat. 2018;31(1):99–108.
5. Cotofana S, Steinke H, Schlattau A, Schlager M, Sykes JM, Roth MZ, Gaggl A, Giunta RE, Gotkin RH, Schenck TL. The anatomy of the facial vein: implications for plastic, reconstructive, and aesthetic procedures. Plast Reconstr Surg. 2017;139(6):1336–53.
6. Toure G, Tran de Fremicort MK, Randriamanantena T, Vlavonou S, Priano V, Vacher C, et al. Vascular and nerve relations of the marginal mandibular nerve of the face: anatomy and clinical relevance. Plas Reconstr Surg. 2019;143(3):888–99.
7. Hanick A, Meleca JB, Fritz MA. Early discharge after free tissue transfer does not increase adverse events. Am J Otolaryngol. 2020;41(2):1–4.
8. Devine CM, Haffey TM, Trosman S, Fritz MA. Short-stay hospital admission after free tissue transfer for head and neck reconstruction. Laryngoscope. 2016;126(2):2679–83.
9. Kerr RP, Hanick A, Fritz MA. Fascia lata free flap reconstruction of limited hard palate defects. Cureus. 2018;10(3):e2356.
10. Hanick AL, Ciolek PJ, Fritz MA. Angular vessels for free-tissue transfer in head and neck reconstruction: clinical outcomes. Laryngoscope. 2020;00:1–4.

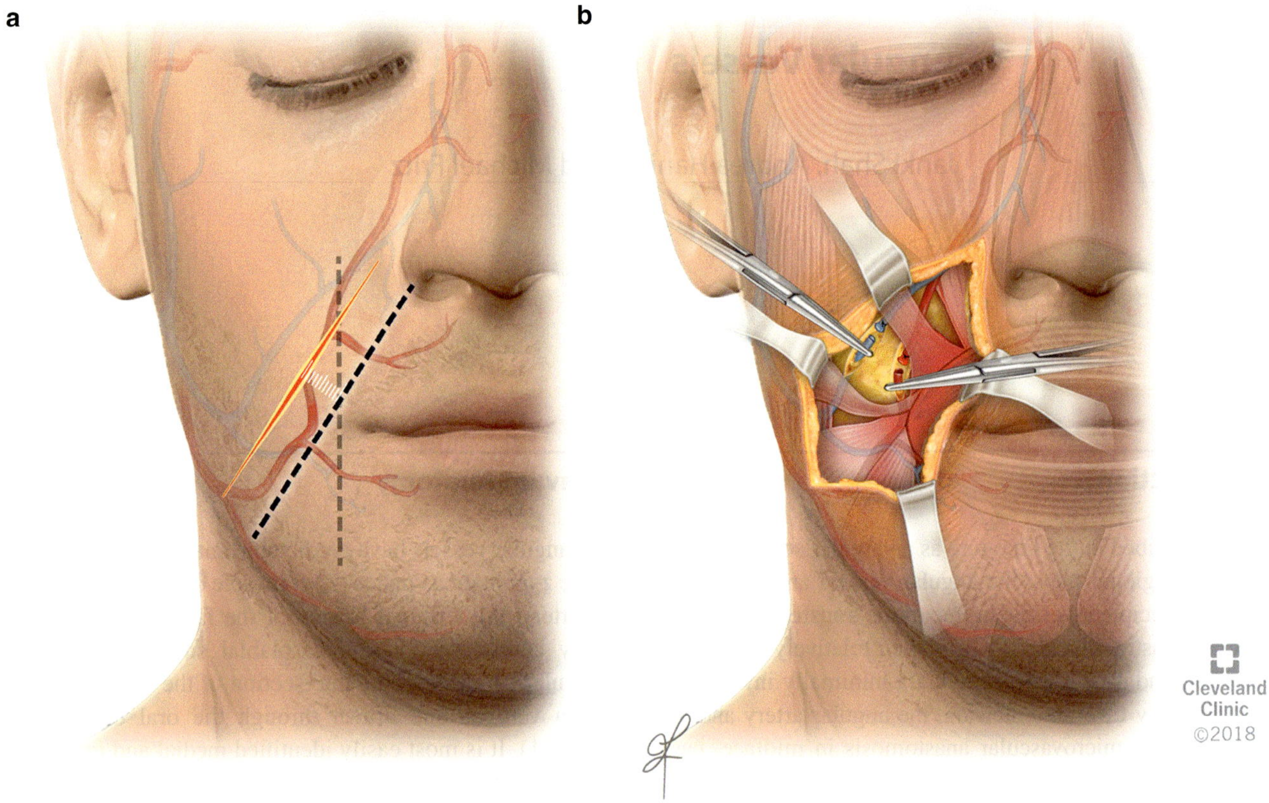

Fig. 4.1 Illustration of the course of the angular artery in relation to external landmarks. The angular artery consistently runs within the nasolabial sulcus toward the nasofacial sulcus and is found deep to the intersection point of the nasolabial fold and a vertical line drawn through the oral commissure. (Reprinted with permission, Cleveland Clinic Center for Medical Art & Photography ©2020. All Rights Reserved)

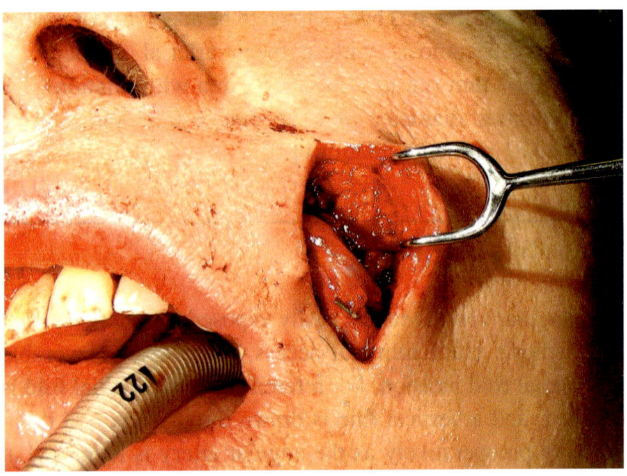

Fig. 4.2 Intraoperative dissection depicting the anatomic location and relationship of the angular artery and vein through a nasolabial fold incision. Both the angular artery and vein course deep to the zygomaticus muscle (ZM) complex. The angular artery is identified medial and inferior to the zygomaticus insertion, while the vein dependably runs in a plane deeper and superolateral to the artery along the lateral border of the ZM complex

vein is dissected free from surrounding tissue and a vessel loop is placed. Attention is then turned to identification of the angular artery. Blunt dissection is continued until the angular artery is identified medial and inferior to the zygomaticus insertion or just deep to the orbicularis oris muscle at the level of the commissure. Once identified, the artery is dissected free from surrounding tissue and followed along its course to ensure adequate mobilization and length for reconstruction; a vessel loop is placed around the artery. It should be noted that the vein lies more lateral (2–3 cm) and superior (1.5 cm) and in a deeper plane than the artery. The artery and vein are then circumferentially dissected and mobilized as needed for microvascular anastomosis. Of note, the superior labial artery is often encountered during dissection of the artery branching off of the distal facial artery at or underneath the zygomaticus major. In addition, the midface branches of the facial nerve that innervate the lip elevators and orbicularis oris lie deep to the nasolabial fold and should be protected (Video 4.1).

Discussion

Often challenging due to limitations on pedicle length and geometry, microvascular reconstruction of skull base and midface defects can be successfully achieved using smaller-caliber vessels when careful attention is devoted to vessel exposure and pedicle orientation [2–4]. While the facial and superficial temporal vessels have sufficient caliber and can be utilized for microvascular anastomosis, they require substantial pedicle length, which is often limiting in certain cases such as palatomaxillary and nasal reconstruction. Easily accessed via a minimally invasive, camouflaged incision with consistent anatomic relationships and adequate caliber, the angular vessels have been proven to be reliable recipient vessels for free flap reconstruction [3–6]. In a retrospective study, Hanick et al. reported successful use of angular vessels for microvascular anastomosis for reconstruction of 31 patients with 97% success rate [3].

Given their close proximity, these vessels are ideal for free flap reconstruction of defects involving the nose/nasal lining, central skull base, midface, palate, and upper oral cavity [2–4, 7–9]. Best suited for use when pedicle length is limited and ipsilateral facial vessels are intact, the angular vessels obviate the need for extensive neck exploration and use of vein grafts for reconstruction and consequently decrease surgical complexity, operative time as well as the length of hospital stay [3, 7]. Accessed with excellent cosmesis and minimal morbidity, the angular vessels are a valuable option in head and neck microvascular reconstruction.

Conclusion

The angular vessels can be easily and reliably identified via a minimal access approach with low morbidity and excellent cosmesis. Given their predictable anatomic relationships, ease of exposure, adequate caliber, and close proximity with improved pedicle reach for microvascular anastomosis, these vessels are valuable for midface, nasal, and skull base free flap reconstruction.

References

1. Kim SW, Kim YH, Kim JT. Angular artery perforator-based transposition flap for the reconstruction of midface defect. Int J Dermatol. 2012;51:1366–70.
2. Haffey TM, McBride JM, Fritz MA. Use of angular vessels in head and neck free-tissue transfer: a comprehensive preclinical evaluation. JAMA Facial Plast Surg. 2014;16:348–51.
3. Hanick AL, Ciolek PJ, Fritz MA. Angular vessels for free-tissue transfer in head and neck reconstruction: clinical outcomes. Laryngoscope. 2020;130:2589–92.
4. Revenaugh PC, Fritz MA, Haffey TM, Seth R, Markey J, Knott PD. Minimizing morbidity in microvascular surgery: small-caliber anastomotic vessels and minimal access approaches. JAMA Facial Plast Surg. 2015;17:44–8.
5. Shimizu F, Oatari M, Uehara M. Choice of recipient vessels for nasal ala reconstruction using a free auricular flap. J Plast Reconstr Aesthet Surg. 2015;68:907–13.
6. Oh SJ, Jeon MK, Koh SH. Nasolabial facial artery and vein as recipient vessels for midface microsurgical reconstruction. J Craniofac Surg. 2011;22:789–91.
7. Devine CM, Haffey TM, Trosman S, Fritz MA. Short-stay hospital admis- Sion after free tissue transfer for head and neck reconstruction. Laryngoscope. 2016;126:2679–83.
8. Seth R, Revenaugh PC, Scharpf J, Shipchandler TZ, Fritz MA. Free anterolateral thigh fascia lata flap for complex nasal lining defects. JAMA Facial Plast Surg. 2013;15(1):21–8.
9. Shipchandler TZ, Waters HH, Knott PD, Fritz MA. Orbitomaxillary reconstruction using the layered fibula osteocutaneous flap. Arch Facial Plast Surg. 2012;14(2):110–5.

5 Superficial Temporal Vessels

Fatma Betul Tuncer, Michelle Djohan, Raffi Gurunian, and Risal Djohan

Introduction

The superficial temporal artery and vein are one of the most preferred recipient vessels in the head and neck region. Other vessels that are commonly used in head and neck reconstruction are the facial artery, superior thyroid artery, external carotid artery, and transverse cervical artery (Chaps. 2, 3, 4, and 6). The superficial temporal artery (STA) and superficial temporal vein (STV) have many advantages over other recipient vessels in upper two-thirds of the face and/or scalp reconstruction due their proximity to the defect site [1, 2]. This proximity often obviates the need for vein grafting or flaps with extra-long vascular pedicle. STA and STV are particularly preferred in the nasal reconstruction and facial reanimation because of their proximity to the reconstruction site and the advantage of concealing the incision scars in the preauricular area and the temple.

Supplementary Information The online version of this chapter (https://doi.org/10.1007/978-3-030-75389-4_5) contains supplementary material, which is available to authorized users.

F. B. Tuncer
Department of Plastic Surgery, Cleveland Clinic, Cleveland, OH, USA

Division of Plastic Surgery, University of Utah, Salt Lake City, UT, USA
e-mail: fatma.tuncer@hsc.utah.edu

M. Djohan
Case Western Reserve University/MetroHealth Hospitals, Cleveland, OH, USA

R. Gurunian · R. Djohan (✉)
Department of Plastic Surgery, Cleveland Clinic, Cleveland, OH, USA

Cleveland Clinic Lerner College of Medicine, Case Western Reserve University, Cleveland, OH, USA
e-mail: gurunir@ccf.org; djohanr@ccf.org

Preoperative Assessment

The superficial temporal artery has a reliable anatomy. Absent or atrophic STA has rarely been described. Preoperative imaging studies such as computed tomography angiography are usually not warranted. STA can be examined by palpation or handheld Doppler before the surgery. One should also examine the skin over the course of the artery for any scars as these vessels can easily be injured during skin biopsies or previous surgeries. History of radiation should be noted as vessel damage is likely to occur, which requires bailout plan for alternative recipient vessel selection. Also, possibility of vein grafts or arteriovenous loop grafts may be considered.

Applied Anatomy

The superficial temporal artery is one of the two terminal branches of the external carotid artery (ECA). ECA continues as the superficial temporal artery after the internal maxillary artery branches off. The course of STA begins in the substance of the parotid gland and becomes more superficial as it travels cranially. STA crosses the zygomatic arch anteriorly, while it is covered by anterior auricular muscles and a dense fascia given off by the parotid gland [3]. Auriculotemporal nerve lies behind the STA at this level. Facial nerve branches to the frontalis and orbicularis oculi muscles lie in proximity to the STA at the level of the zygomatic arch but they cross it more anteriorly than the STA does [4]. The most posterior branch of the facial nerve is 24 mm to the tragus at this level [5]. Hence, STA can be safely dissected at its course.

STA bifurcates into frontal and parietal branches 2–3 cm above the zygomatic arch in the temporoparietal fascia. The STA bifurcation point is located above the zygomatic arch in 65–80% of people, below in 10–15%, and on the arch in the remaining 5–10% [6]. During its

R. Gurunian, R. Djohan (eds.), *Recipient Vessels in Reconstructive Microsurgery*, https://doi.org/10.1007/978-3-030-75389-4_5

course, it gives off the transverse facial artery, zygomatico-orbital artery, and small arterial branches to the tragus and helix of the ear. A caliber of 2 to 2.7 mm and 1.1 to 3 mm was reported at the zygomatic arch level for STA and STV, respectively [5, 7, 8].

The superficial temporal vein runs lateral and superficial to the artery. It shows more anatomic variation and branching patterns than the STA does. Cranially, anterior and posterior branches of the superficial temporal vein unite above the zygoma to form the main trunk. The middle temporal vein, which receives blood from the temporalis muscle, drains into the main trunk at the upper border of the zygoma. STV descends between the external auditory meatus and the mandibular condyle, enters the substance of the parotid gland, and unites with the maxillary vein to form the temporo-maxillary vein (the retromandibular vein). The temporo-maxillary vein descends between the ramus of the mandible and the sternocleidomastoid muscle, on the outer surface of the external carotid artery, and below the facial nerve. The temporo-maxillary vein divides into two branches. The anterior branch forms the common facial vein by uniting with the facial vein and drains into the internal jugular vein. The posterior branch (also called the posterior facial vein) unites with the posterior auricular vein and forms the external jugular vein [3].

Surgical Site Exposure

The location of STA is marked on the skin preoperatively using handheld Doppler or by simply palpating the artery. The head is turned to the opposite side for an easier dissection. Muscle relaxants should be avoided to monitor and protect branches of the facial nerve. A preauricular skin incision following the anatomical boundaries of hairline, preauricular crease, and ear lobule is made from 3–4 cm above the zygomatic arch to the ear lobule. An incision slightly medial to the markings are preferred to avoid any injury at the initial part of the dissection. Local anesthetics with epinephrine are avoided because of their vasospastic effect. Dissection of the superficial temporal vessels starts cranially superior to the level of the superior border of the helix in the temporal area. STA and STV are identified in the subcutaneous plane at this location. Extra caution should be exercised at the initial part of dissection as these vessels run very superficially. After the vessels are located, an operating microscope can be used for further dissection from cranial to caudal dissection. Small branches of the STA and STV are easily dissected and ligated under the operating microscope. STV runs lateral and superficial to the artery. The superficial temporal vein has a very thin wall and it needs to be handled gently.

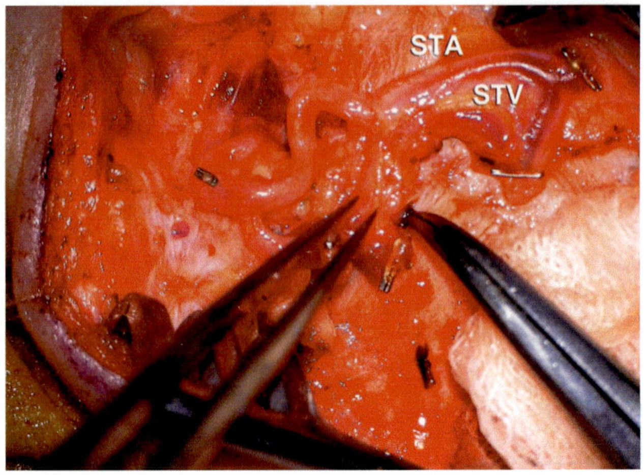

Fig. 5.1 Superficial temporal artery (STA) and superficial temporal vein (STV). Please note that the artery has a tortuous configuration; peri-adventitial tissues need to be released and removed during vessel preparation

When superficial temporal vessels with an appropriate size match to the target artery and vein are found, they are prepared for microvascular anastomosis using the operating microscope (Video 5.1).

However, if necessary, the vessel dissection can be carried out further caudally to obtain vessels with a larger caliber. The diameter of the artery and the vein enlarges progressively as the dissection proceeds into the parotid gland. The superficial part of the parotid gland is divided with bipolar cautery for a better exposure. Both artery and vein dive deep into the parotid gland proximally. STA gets closer to the facial nerve below the ear lobe. But the dissection is usually not necessary beyond the tragus, where the caliber of artery and vein is large enough for microsurgical anastomosis. The surficial temporal artery has a tortuous configuration; peri-adventitial tissues need to be released and removed during vessel preparation (Figs. 5.1 and 5.2). Neuro-patties soaked with 2% lidocaine or papaverine can be placed over the STA and STV for vasodilation as they rest until the microsurgical anastomosis. A case of microsurgical scalp reconstruction using left-sided superficial temporal vessels is presented in Figs. 5.3 and 5.4.

Discussion

Several surgeons have anecdotally noted that superficial temporal vessels are unreliable in microsurgical reconstruction because of their size and tendency to spasm. However, many studies showed no difference in the success of free flaps when the STA and STV are used as recipient vessels [9–12]. Halvarson et al. reported the use of STA and STV for perior-

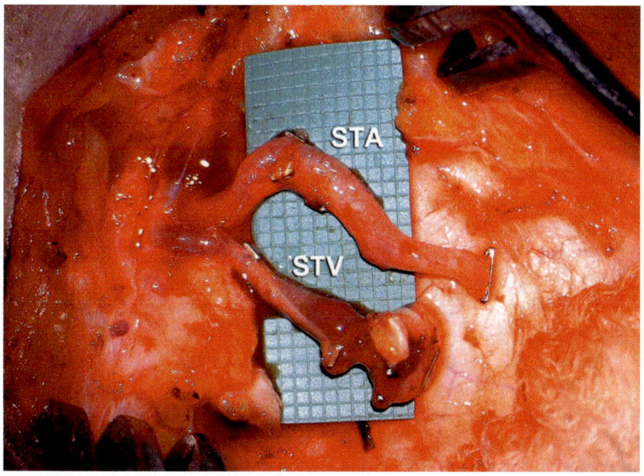

Fig. 5.2 The authors recommend the vessel dissection be performed under the microscope to prepare STA and STV for microvascular anastomosis. Close-up of STA and STV ready for use

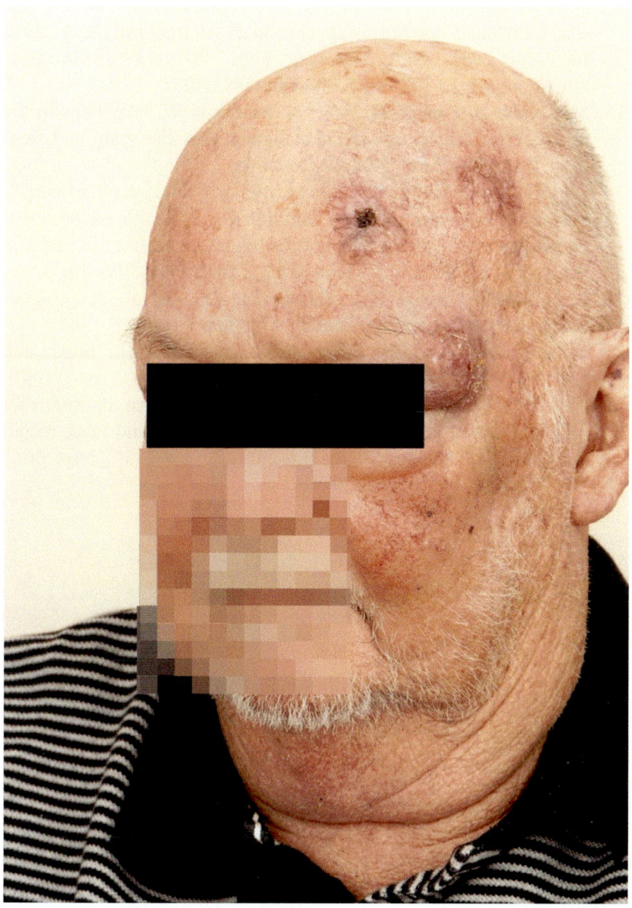

Fig. 5.3 A 72-year old-male with multicentric invasive and moderately differentiated squamous cell carcinoma of the left periorbital region, left temple, and parietal area. Patient underwent wide local excision of all areas en bloc including the pericranium. Cadaveric skin was applied until confirmation of margin clearance

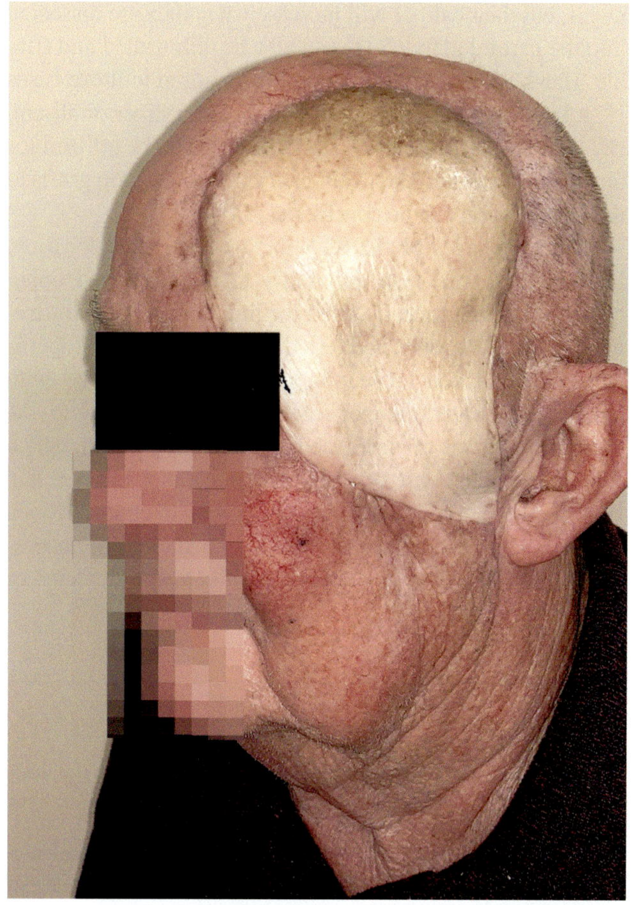

Fig. 5.4 Patient then received microsurgical reconstruction of the parietotemporal scalp/forehead and upper cheek defect using anterolateral thigh flap harvested from the left thigh. Arterial anastomosis was performed using 9–0 Ethilon sutures between the recipient superficial temporal artery and the descending branch of the lateral circumflex femoral artery. Venous anastomosis was performed using 2.5 mm coupler device between the superficial temporal vein and vena comitantes of the flap

bital and scalp reconstruction in 28 patients [11]. The rates of partial or total flap loss in these 28 patients were not different than those of 282 flaps anastomosed to other head and neck vessels [11]. In the same study, 2 out of 28 patients (7%) developed a partial flap loss, and they both had a history of radiotherapy, similar to the reports by McCombe et al. [11, 13]. They suggested to exercise caution and have an alternative recipient vessel available when attempting anastomosis to the STA/V in patients with a history of radiotherapy [11].

Hansen et al. and Siebert et al. reported safe and reliable use of STA/V in a series of 45 and 35 patients, respectively [9, 10]. Siebert et al. underscored the favorable location of the STA and STV as recipient vessels in microsurgical reconstruction of the facial asymmetry [10].

Superficial temporal vessels may be susceptible to spasm and may have inadequate diameter for microsurgical anastomosis, but their caliber will increase when they are dissected into the parotid gland. STV can also be thin walled and friable. Hand-sewn anastomosis may be required in those cases [12]. In cases where STV is of insufficient caliber or absent, IJV or transposed posterior auricular vein can be utilized for the venous outflow. Also, vein or arteriovenous loop grafts to the neck vessels can be considered [14].

The advantages of the STA include consistent location, few anatomic variation, proximity to the scalp and upper two-thirds of the face, no need for limitation of neck movements postoperatively, and less dissection due to its superficial course. It can be readily palpated or examined with handheld Doppler preoperatively. Their proximity to the scalp and midface obviates the need for vein grafting, which was shown to increase thrombotic complications in free flap [15]. It also enables reconstructive surgeon to choose from a wider variety of free flaps as extra-long pedicle is not necessarily required. STA may also be used in vessel depleted or irradiated necks [16].

References

1. Currie KB, Ross P, Collister P, Gurunluoglu R. Analysis of scalp and forehead injuries in a Level I Trauma Center. J Craniofac Surg. 2017;28(5):1350–3.
2. Gurunluoglu R, Gatherwright J. Microsurgical reconstruction of complex maxillofacial gunshot wounds: outcomes analysis and algorithm. Microsurgery. 2019;39(5):384–94.
3. Gray H. Blood-vascular system. In: Pick TP, Howden R, editors. Gray's anatomy. New York: Barnes & Noble; 2010. p. 470–1 and p. 574–5.
4. Djohan R, Afifi A. Chapter 1: Anatomy of the head and neck. In: Plastic surgery volume three: craniofacial, head and neck surgery, pediatric plastic surgery. 3rd ed. London, New York: Elsevier; 2013. p. 11.
5. Tayfur V, Edizer M, Magden O. Anatomic bases of superficial temporal artery and temporal branch of facial nerve. J Craniofac Surg. 2010;21(6):1945–7. https://doi.org/10.1097/SCS.0b013e3181f4ee6a.
6. Koziej M, Trybus M, Hołda M, et al. The superficial temporal artery: anatomical map for facial reconstruction and aesthetic procedures. Aesthet Surg J. 2019;39(8):815–23. https://doi.org/10.1093/asj/sjy287.
7. Pinar YA, Govsa F. Anatomy of the superficial temporal artery and its branches: its importance for surgery. Surg Radiol Anat. 2006;28(3):248–53. https://doi.org/10.1007/s00276-006-0094-z.
8. Delgove L, Lebeau J, Raphaël B, Champetier J. Drainage of the scalp by the superficial temporal vein: surgical implications. Surg Radiol Anat. 1991;13(4):277–82. https://doi.org/10.1007/bf01627758.
9. Hansen SL, Foster RD, Dosanjh AS, Mathes SJ, Hoffman WY, Leon P. Superficial temporal artery and vein as recipient vessels for facial and scalp microsurgical reconstruction. Plast Reconstr Surg. 2007;120:1879–84.
10. Siebert JW, Anson G, Longaker MT. Microsurgical correction of facial asymmetry in 60 consecutive cases. Plast Reconstr Surg. 1996;97:354–63.
11. Halvorson EG, Cordeiro PG, Disa JJ, Wallin EF, Mehrara BJ. Superficial temporal recipient vessels in microvascular orbit and scalp reconstruction of oncologic defects. J Reconstr Microsurg. 2009 Jul;25(6):383–7.
12. Chen JT, Sanchez R, Garg R, Poore SO, Siebert JW. Helpful hints for the superficial temporal artery and vein as recipient vessels [published correction appears in Plast Reconstr Surg. 2018 Jul;142(1):295]. Plast Reconstr Surg. 2017;139(3):818e–20e. https://doi.org/10.1097/PRS.0000000000003081
13. McCombe D, Donato R, Hofer S, Morrison W. Free flaps in the treatment of locally advanced malignancy of the scalp and forehead. Ann Plast Surg. 2002;48(6):600–6.
14. Knackstedt R, Aliotta R, Gatherwright J, Djohan R, Gastman B, Schwarz G, Hendrickson M, Gurunluoglu R. Single-stage versus two-stage arteriovenous loop microsurgical reconstruction: a meta-analysis of the literature. Microsurgery. 2018;38(6):706–17.
15. Khouri RK, Cooley BC, Kunselman AR, et al. A prospective study of microvascular free-flap surgery and outcome. Plast Reconstr Surg. 1998;102(3):711–21. https://doi.org/10.1097/00006534-199809030-00015.
16. Chia HL, Wong CH, Tan BK, Tan KC, Ong YS. An algorithm for recipient vessel selection in microsurgical head and neck reconstruction. J Reconstr Microsurg. 2011;27(1):47–56. https://doi.org/10.1055/s-0030-1267829.

6 Transverse Cervical Vessels

Andrea Sisti, Lynn M. Orfahli, Bahar Bassiri Gharb, Raffi Gurunian, and Antonio Rampazzo

Introduction

Branches of the external carotid artery (ECA) are commonly selected as recipient sites in reconstructive surgery of the head and neck. However, these vessels, which include the facial, superior thyroid, lingual, and superficial temporal arteries, are prone to significant scarring from irradiation or previous surgery [1]. This can render them unavailable, resulting in what is known as a "frozen" or "vessel-depleted" neck [2, 3]. In these patients, the transverse cervical vessels (TCVs) can be used as alternative recipient sites for free flap reconstruction of the head and neck [1, 4, 5]. TCVs have been used as "second-line" recipient vessels in thoracic and upper arm reconstructions as well [6, 7].

As early as 1989, Urken et al. [8] expressed their preference for the TCVs because they are less prone to damage by previous radiotherapy, tumor, or atherosclerosis compared to the branches of ECA [1]. Even when other vessels are available, the geometry of the TCVs may be more favorable—the axis of the vascular pedicle runs in a longitudinal direction, providing ideal flow and blood pressure conditions and reducing the risk of kinking [1, 5, 8]. Furthermore, their dissection does not involve the risk of damaging the carotid artery system.

Supplementary Information The online version of this chapter (https://doi.org/10.1007/978-3-030-75389-4_6) contains supplementary material, which is available to authorized users.

A. Sisti · L. M. Orfahli
Department of Plastic Surgery, Cleveland Clinic, Cleveland, OH, USA
e-mail: lmo28@case.edu

R. Gurunian
Department of Plastic Surgery, Cleveland Clinic, Cleveland, OH, USA

Cleveland Clinic Lerner College of Medicine, Case Western Reserve University, Cleveland, OH, USA
e-mail: gurunir@ccf.org

B. B. Gharb · A. Rampazzo (✉)
Department of Plastic Surgery, Cleveland Clinic, Cleveland, OH, USA

Cleveland Clinic Lerner College of Medicine, Case Western Reserve University, Cleveland, OH, USA
e-mail: bassirb@ccf.org; rampaza@ccf.org

Applied Anatomy

The transverse cervical artery (TCA) has been known by several names including the arteria transversa colli, the transverse artery of the neck, and the arteria transversa cervicis [9]. Currently, the TCA is defined as a branch of the thyrocervical trunk that courses superficially across the posterior cervical triangle, placing it lateral to the sternocleidomastoid muscle (SCM) and superior to the clavicle (Figs. 6.1 and 6.2) [10].

Variations in the origin of the TCA in humans are numerous and have been widely discussed by anatomists and surgeons [11]. Most commonly, it arises from the thyrocervical trunk (77%); other reported origins include the subclavian or internal mammary arteries. Classically, the thyrocervical trunk also gives rise to the suprascapular artery (SSA), which runs inferior to the TCA (Fig. 6.1). It can be distinguished from the TCA by its smaller diameter and its more protected course lower in the neck, deep to the clavicle [1, 5, 8–10, 12–18]. The TCA is considered distinct from the dorsal scapular artery (also known as the descending scapular artery), a deep vessel that variably originates from the TCA (25% of cases), the thyrocervical trunk, or directly from the subclavian artery [9, 10]. When the dorsal scapular artery does arise from the TCA, it is also called the deep branch of the TCA [11]; their junction is named the cervicodorsal trunk. The transverse cervical vein drains into the external jugular vein (EJV) or subclavian vein [16].

The TCVs are located in an anatomical region delineated medially by the dorsal edge of the SCM, inferiorly by the superior edge of the clavicle forming the inferior border, and laterally by the EJV [1, 12, 15]. During dissection, care should be taken in order to prevent injury to the brachial plexus, which was demonstrated to lie deep to the proximal third of the vessel by Cordova et al. in a cadaver study [13] (Figs. 6.3 and 6.4).

R. Gurunian, R. Djohan (eds.), *Recipient Vessels in Reconstructive Microsurgery*, https://doi.org/10.1007/978-3-030-75389-4_6

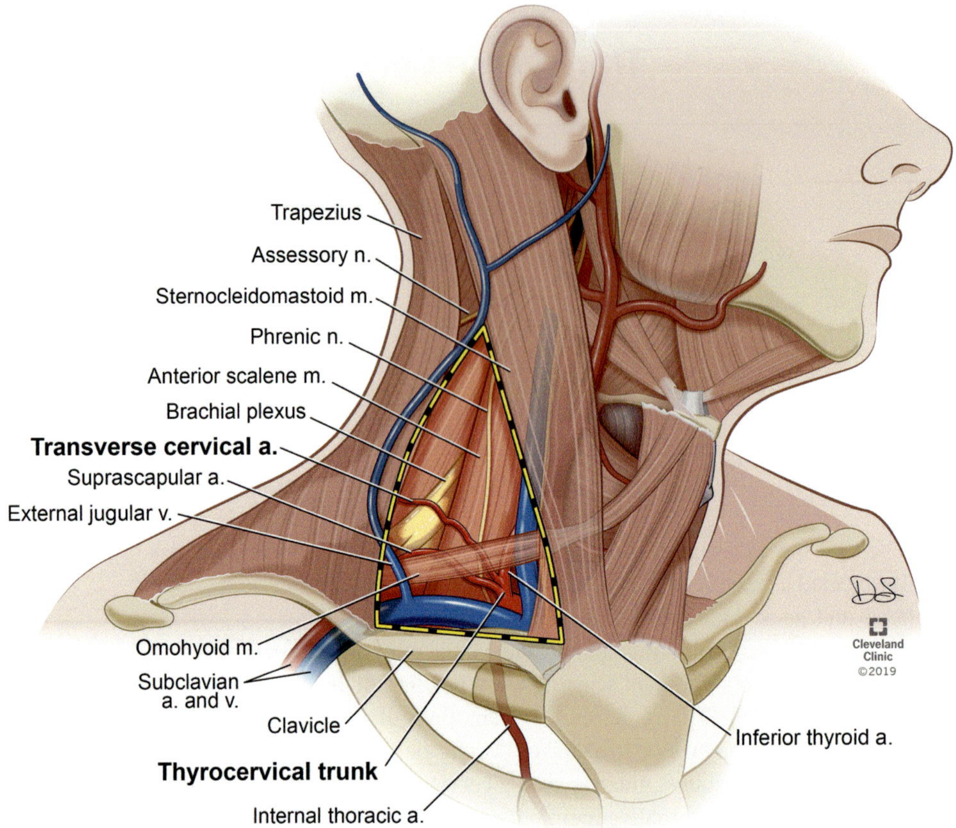

Fig. 6.1 Illustration of the transverse cervical vessels after dissection. Anatomical landmarks are highlighted with a dotted yellow line. (Reprinted with permission, Cleveland Clinic Center for Medical Art & Photography ©2020. All Rights Reserved)

A recent study from Reissis et al. [9] defines the mean distances from the origin of the TCA to the angle of the mandible, floor of the mouth, and mandibular symphysis as 10.0, 9.2, and 12.6 cm, respectively. The mean diameter of the TCA measuring 2 cm from its origin was 2.2 mm [9]. Tessler et al. [1] report that the length of the TCA ranges from 4.0 to 7.0 cm with a mean diameter of 2.65 mm; the origin of the TCA was a mean of 33 mm from the midline of the neck and 17 mm cranial to the clavicle at the anterior border of the SCM [1].

The transverse cervical vein can be much smaller than the artery, sometimes rendering it unsuitable for anastomosis. In these instances, the EJV or branches of the internal jugular vein have been used as recipient vessels without necessitating vein grafts [5]. The use of cephalic vein transposition or contralateral neck veins has also been reported [3, 19, 20]. Other veins that have been suggested for consideration include the superficial temporal vein, superior thyroid vein, facial vein, internal mammary vein, and thoracoacromial vein; however, they are located far from the transverse cervical artery and they require vein grafts during the anastomosis [21, 22].

Surgical Site Exposure

Turning the head to the contralateral direction prior to dissection is suggested. The borders of the posterior triangle of the neck are demarcated, starting with the medial and lateral borders of the SCM muscle, the key landmark, followed by the clavicle and the position of the EJV. A skin incision is marked just posterior to the SCM muscle. The skin and adipose tissue of the neck are divided, including the platysma muscle. The posterior triangle's landmarks are identified: the EJV, the clavicle, and the SCM muscle. The omohyoid muscle, which crosses the surgical field from lateral to medial, is then identified and divided in order to expose the deeper anatomic structures (Video 6.1).

The TCVs can be easily identified by following the superficial branches to the skin. The vein can be very small and not suitable for microsurgical anastomosis. In these instances, an alternative vein, as described in the previous section, should be identified. The TCA is dissected up to the thyrocervical trunk, which is its origin in most instances; attention should be paid to the lymph nodes and adipose tissue coming off of the vessel. The dissection of the TCA should be continued until satisfactory length and caliber is obtained for microvascular anastomosis.

Discussion

TCVs have been demonstrated to be a suitable and reliable option for secondary microvascular free flap reconstruction of the head and neck when branches of the ECA are damaged by previous surgery or radiotherapy [3, 20, 23, 24]. It is offered as a first choice in Hanasono [2] and colleagues' proposed algorithm for choosing recipient vessels in microvas-

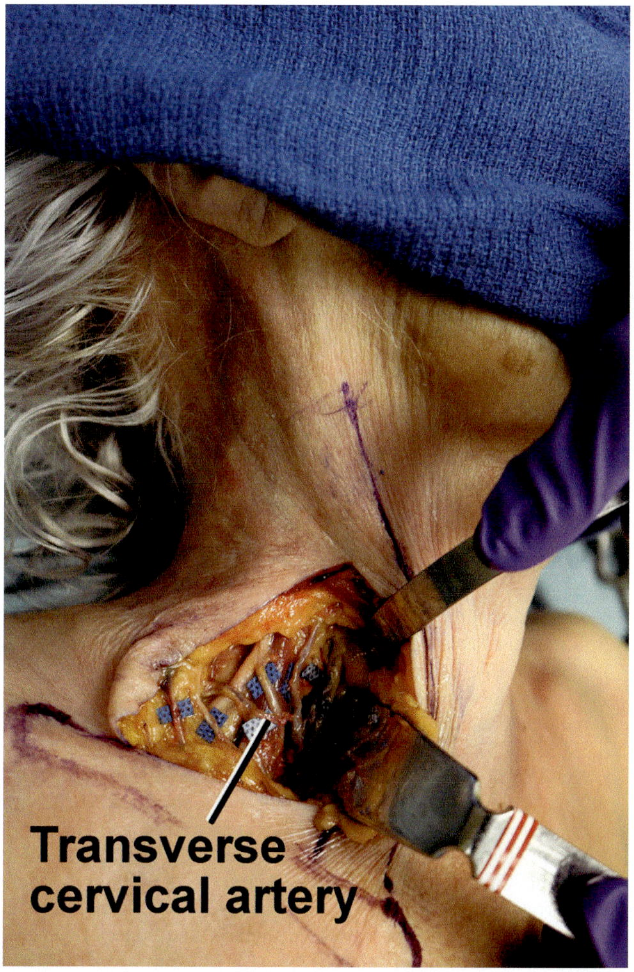

Fig. 6.2 This zoomed out photograph depicts the posterior cervical triangle with additional anatomical landmarks outside of the field of dissection

cular reconstruction of head and neck defects when the ipsilateral ECA system is unavailable.

A recent literature review [21] on microsurgical reconstruction of the vessel-depleted neck found that the arteries most frequently chosen for anastomosis were the internal mammary artery ($n = 81$; 28%), the transverse cervical artery ($n = 46$; 15.9%), and the superficial temporal artery ($n = 43$; 14.9%). The cephalic vein ($n = 84$; 25.9%), the internal mammary vein ($n = 79$; 24.4%), and the superficial temporal vein ($n = 50$; 15.4%) were the most successfully applied veins [21].

Yu [20] reported a series of 26 patients requiring head and neck reconstruction who underwent exploration of the neck for the TCVs. Seventeen patients had previous surgery, radiotherapy, or both; 13 were found to have frozen necks. One patient underwent reconstruction with a free radial forearm flap, while

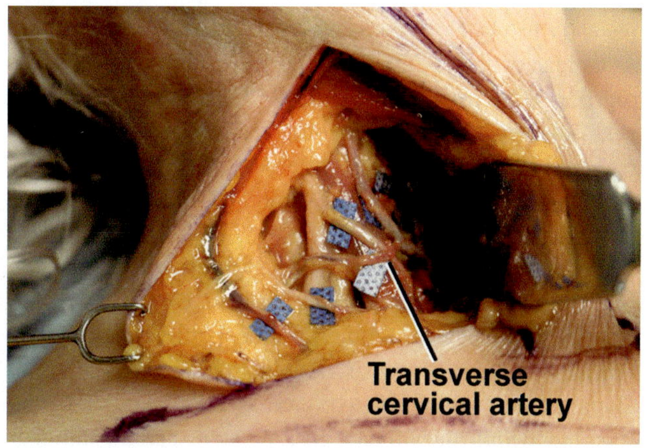

Fig. 6.4 Photograph depicting the vascular anatomy of the posterior cervical triangle, including the transverse cervical artery (labeled)

Fig. 6.3 Illustration of the origin of the transverse cervical vessels from the thyrocervical trunk. (Reprinted with permission, Cleveland Clinic Center for Medical Art & Photography ©2020. All Rights Reserved)

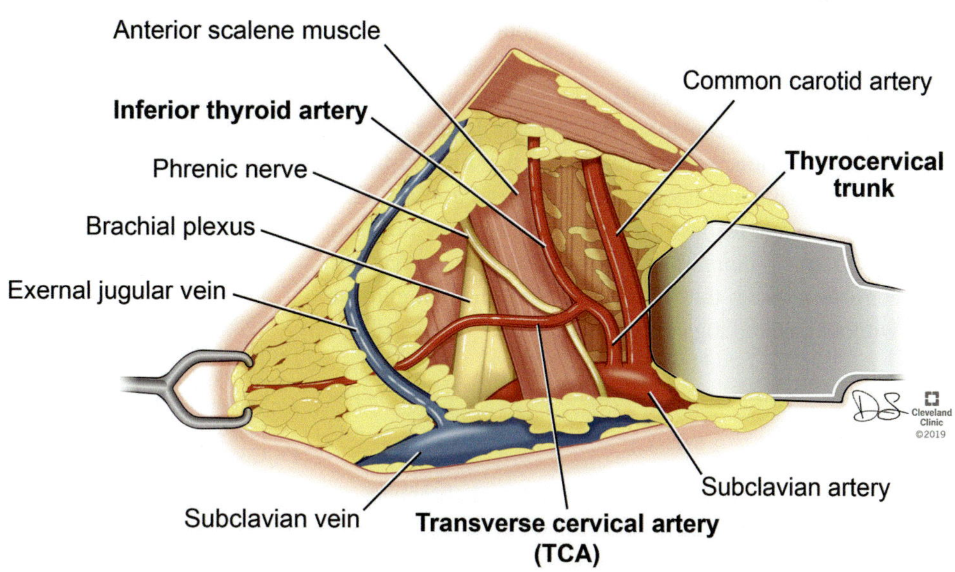

the remaining surgeries were performed with an anterolateral thigh (ALT) flap. Six patients required exploration of the contralateral side due to absence or inadequate size of the ipsilateral TCVs; they were found to be absent or unsuitable bilaterally in two patients. Two patients early in the series suffered an injury of the thoracic duct during exploration of the left neck; to avoid this, gentle blunt dissection should be started well above the clavicle, and any oozing must be investigated and the injured lymphatic vessel either ligated or repaired.

Xu et al. [5] described their use of TCVs in secondary reconstruction of the head and neck in eight previously operated patients, five of whom also had radiotherapy. The TCVs were preferred over branches of the ECA and jugular veins because these were generally found to be compromised from the previous treatments. Flaps used included the fibular flap, anteromedial thigh (AMT) flap, and ALT flap. Complications, reported in two out of the eight patients, consisted of delayed wound healing and a fistula. No flap loss was reported in any patient.

Ciudad et al. [25] reported their experience using the retrograde TCA as a recipient vessel in nine patients with vessel-depleted necks undergoing secondary head and neck reconstruction. Flap survival rate was 100% with no partial flap loss. No re-exploration was required and no postoperative complications were reported.

In 2019, Lin et al. [23] published a series of 15 patients who underwent reconstruction with the ALT flap and TCA, all of whom had a vessel-depleted neck due to severe scarring and radiation fibrosis. All TCAs were found to be damage-free. No immediate mortalities or flap failures were reported within the 30-day postoperative period, although two patients developed oro-cutaneous fistulae and were further managed with wound care [23].

Because the TCVs are located near the base of the neck, they can also be considered for use as second-line recipient vessels in thoracic or upper arm reconstruction. In their 2018 series on reconstructions with the TCA, Muppireddy et al. reported five such cases: fibular osteocutaneous flaps for sternal and humeral reconstruction, a gracilis flap for restoration of elbow flexion, a tensor fascia lata flap for soft tissue defect of the axilla and lateral chest wall, and a tubed ALT flap for esophageal reconstruction. Some degree of pivoting of the TCA was required to provide the requisite length for the recipient pedicle; the vessels tolerated this realignment well without any kinking or redundancy [6].

Conclusion

In reconstructive surgery of the head and neck, branches of the ECA such as the facial, superior thyroid, lingual, and superficial temporal arteries are often selected as recipient vessels. However, these vessels are vulnerable to significant damage from radiotherapy or previous surgery, resulting in vessel-depleted necks. In these patients, the transverse cervical vessels should be taken into consideration as alternative recipient vessels for microsurgical flap reconstruction.

Acknowledgment We would like to acknowledge Carlos Ordeñana, MD, for his time and assistance in editing the dissection video.

References

1. Tessler O, Gilardino MS, Bartow MJ, St Hilaire H, Womac D, Dionisopoulos T, et al. Transverse cervical artery: consistent anatomical landmarks and clinical experience with its use as a recipient artery in complex head and neck reconstruction. Plast Reconstr Surg. 2017;139(3):745e–51e.
2. Hanasono MM, Barnea Y, Skoracki RJ. Microvascular surgery in the previously operated and irradiated neck. Microsurgery. 2009;29(1):1–7.
3. Jacobson AS, Eloy JA, Park E, Roman B, Genden EM. Vessel-depleted neck: techniques for achieving microvascular reconstruction. Head Neck. 2008;30(2):201–7.
4. Mizerny BR, Lessard ML, Black MJ. Transverse cervical artery fasciocutaneous free flap for head and neck reconstruction: initial anatomic and dye studies. Otolaryngol Head Neck Surg. 1995;113(5):564–8.
5. Xu ZF, Duan WY, Zhang EJ, Bai S, Tian Y, Tan XX, et al. Transverse cervical vessels as recipient vessels in oral and maxillofacial microsurgical reconstruction after former operations with or without radiotherapy. World J Surg Oncol. 2015;13:183.
6. Muppireddy S, Ravula P, Rangachari S, Shaik N, Maaturu S. Transverse cervical vascular pedicle: It's extended use as 'second-line' recipient vessels in thoracic and upper arm reconstructions in addition to head-and-neck reconstructions. Indian J Plast Surg. 2018;51(2):182–9.
7. Yagi S, Suyama Y, Fukuoka K, Takeuchi H, Kitano H. Recipient vessel selection in head and neck reconstruction based on the type of neck dissection. Yonago Acta Med. 2016;59(2):159–62.
8. Urken ML, Vickery C, Weinberg H, Buchbinder D, Biller HF. Geometry of the vascular pedicle in free tissue transfers to the head and neck. Arch Otolaryngol Head Neck Surg. 1989;115(8):954–60.
9. Reissis M, Reissis D, Bottini GB, Messiha A, Davies DC. A morphometric analysis of the suitability of the transverse cervical artery as a recipient artery in head and neck free flap microvascular reconstruction. Surg Radiol Anat. 2018;40(8):891–7.
10. Huelke DF. A study of the transverse cervical and dorsal scapular arteries. Anat Rec. 1958;132(3):233–45.
11. Koizumi M, Sekiya S, Horiguchi M, Harada M. A study of the deep ascending cervical artery (new definition) and its relation to some other arteries in the human cervical region. Ann Anat. 1994;176(3):233–42.
12. Alves HR, Ishida LC, Ishida LH, Besteiro JM, Gemperli R, Faria JC, et al. A clinical experience of the supraclavicular flap used to reconstruct head and neck defects in late-stage cancer patients. J Plast Reconstr Aesthet Surg. 2012;65(10):1350–6.
13. Cordova A, D'Arpa S, Pirrello R, Brenner E, Jeschke J, Moschella F. Anatomic study on the transverse cervical vessels perforators in the lateral triangle of the neck and harvest of a new flap: the free supraclavicular transverse cervical artery perforator flap. Surg Radiol Anat. 2009;31(2):93–100.
14. Kruse AL, Luebbers HT, Gratz KW, Obwegeser JA. Factors influencing survival of free-flap in reconstruction for can-

cer of the head and neck: a literature review. Microsurgery. 2010;30(3):242–8.
15. Weiglein AH, Moriggl B, Schalk C, Kunzel KH, Muller U. Arteries in the posterior cervical triangle in man. Clin Anat. 2005;18(8):553–7.
16. Wong KK, Higgins KM, Enepekides DJ. Microvascular reconstruction in the vessel-depleted neck. Curr Opin Otolaryngol Head Neck Surg. 2010;18(4):223–6.
17. Lloyd G, Phillips J. The transverse cervical artery: new origins and pathways. Clin Anat. 1989;2(2):93–102.
18. Naidoo N, Lazarus L, De Gama BZ, Satyapal KS. The variant course of the suprascapular artery. Folia Morphol (Warsz). 2014;73(2):206–9.
19. Vasilakis V, Patel HD, Chen HC. Head and neck reconstruction using cephalic vein transposition in the vessel-depleted neck. Microsurgery. 2009;29(8):598–602.
20. Yu P. The transverse cervical vessels as recipient vessels for previously treated head and neck cancer patients. Plast Reconstr Surg. 2005;115(5):1253–8.
21. Frohwitter G, Rau A, Kesting MR, Fichter A. Microvascular reconstruction in the vessel depleted neck – a systematic review. J Craniomaxillofac Surg. 2018;46(9):1652–8.
22. Offodile AC 2nd, Chang KP, Chen HH, Loesch E, Hung SY, Kao HK. Feasibility and outcomes of the third or more episodes of sequential microvascular reconstruction for recurrent or second primary oral cancer. Ann Surg Oncol. 2016;23(11):3765–72.
23. Lin KW, Huang TC, Cheng HT. Utilization of anterolateral thigh flap and transverse cervical recipient vessels for head and neck cancer patients with former neck dissection and irradiation: a case series study. Ann Plast Surg. 2019;82(4):415–9.
24. Yazar S. Selection of recipient vessels in microsurgical free tissue reconstruction of head and neck defects. Microsurgery. 2007;27(7):588–94.
25. Ciudad P, Agko M, Manrique OJ, Date S, Kiranantawat K, Chang WL, et al. The retrograde transverse cervical artery as a recipient vessel for free tissue transfer in complex head and neck reconstruction with a vessel-depleted neck. Microsurgery. 2017;37(8):902–9.

Recipient Vessels: Laryngopharynx Reconstruction

7

Stefanos Boukovalas and Matthew M. Hanasono

Introduction

Defects of the larynx and pharynx after surgical resection cause significant functional impairment, given the critical role of this anatomical region in breathing, speech, and swallowing. Reconstruction can be challenging given the anatomical relationship with vital neurovascular structures and the limited options for locoregional reconstruction. Previously described methods with pedicled flaps, such as the pectoralis muscle, are now considered second- or third-line options. Free tissue transfer is considered standard of care for the majority of patients, with the free anterolateral thigh (ALT), radial forearm (RFF), and jejunum flaps being the most commonly used [1, 2].

The choice of the optimal reconstructive method is often dependent on the surgeon's experience and training. All flaps possess advantages and disadvantages [2–8]. The jejunum flap has been widely used for pharyngoesophageal reconstruction. It provides a tubular conduit with favorable diameter and has been associated with relatively low rates of fistula formation. On the other hand, it requires intraabdominal surgery, which is associated with potential complications, such as postoperative ileus, small bowel obstruction, and ventral hernia, as well as prolonged hospital stay. Additionally, patients undergoing reconstruction with free jejunum flap demonstrate wet, cavernous speech with tracheoesophageal puncture (TEP), and an impaired swallowing mechanism, likely due to mucosal secretions and smooth muscle dysmotility [2, 4, 5, 8–11]. The RFF is a thin fasciocutaneous flap that may provide improved speech but has been shown to have a higher fistula rate in some studies. It is more commonly utilized in reconstruction of partial defects as a patch, when reinforcement with additional soft tissue is not necessary. Furthermore, the RFF results in significant donor site morbidity, especially in circumferential or near-circumferential defects that require a large skin paddle for creation of the neo-pharynx [7].

The use of the ALT flap has been popularized in the last 2 decades and is the preferred reconstruction option in our institution, especially for circumferential defects. It is a fasciocutaneous flap, which offers the advantages of superior speech quality with TEP and superior swallowing function compared to the jejunum flap. Its versatile design can provide additional soft tissue coverage for closure of the neck skin and/or obliteration of dead space with well-vascularized tissue, by incorporating additional skin paddles or vastus lateralis muscle, leading to favorable results in terms of fistula and anastomotic leak rates compared to the RFF [6, 12]. Finally, it is associated with minimal donor site morbidity and shorter hospital stay [3–6].

In patients with advanced cancer of the larynx and hypopharynx, treatment with combined radiation and chemotherapy, or with surgery reserved for residual or recurrent disease, preserves the larynx and has been shown to provide comparable survival rates compared to traditional treatment with surgical resection and postoperative radiation treatment [13]. Unfortunately, this treatment modality is not always effective, and patients may require salvage laryngopharyngectomy, which in this situation takes place in an irradiated field making dissection of recipient blood vessels for free flap reconstruction more challenging (Fig. 7.1). Prior or concurrent neck dissection may also result in a paucity of potential recipient blood vessels. Due to these factors, laryngopharyngectomy reconstruction with microvascular free flaps is often a more challenging procedure than other head and neck reconstructions. This chapter provides a comprehensive analysis of available recipient vessels and special considerations in the vessel-depleted neck.

S. Boukovalas · M. M. Hanasono (✉)
Department of Plastic Surgery, The University of Texas MD Anderson Cancer Center, Houston, TX, USA
e-mail: sboukovalas@mdanderson.org; mhanasono@mdanderson.org

R. Gurunian, R. Djohan (eds.), *Recipient Vessels in Reconstructive Microsurgery*,
https://doi.org/10.1007/978-3-030-75389-4_7

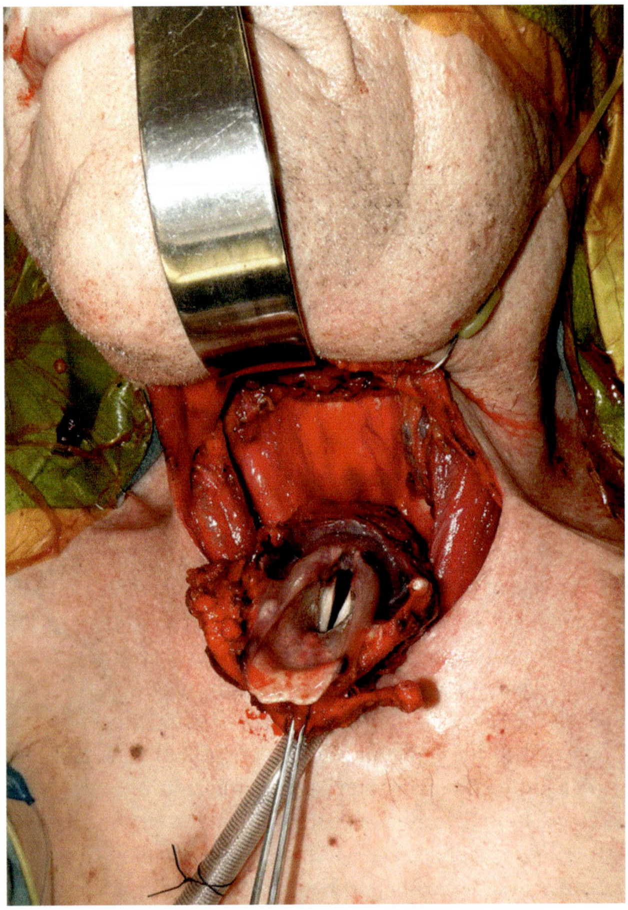

Fig. 7.1 Laryngopharyngectomy dissection including circumferential pharynx for recurrent hypopharyngeal cancer

Upper Cervical Vessels

Carotid and Jugular Systems

The carotid arterial system and the jugular venous system are the most common recipient vessels in free flap reconstruction of the head and neck region. The common carotid artery bifurcates to the internal and external carotid artery (ECA) at the level of the fourth cervical vertebra [14, 15]. The ECA is anterior to the ICA. Given its location, the branches of the ECA, or the ECA itself, are most commonly used as recipient arteries in the majority of head and neck reconstructions. In the neck, the ECA provides the following branches in order from proximal to distal: superior thyroid artery, ascending pharyngeal artery, lingual artery (LA), facial artery (FA), occipital artery, and posterior auricular artery (Fig. 7.2). At the level of the parotid and the area where the mandibular ramus and condyle join, the ECA bifurcates to the superficial temporal artery (STA) and the maxillary artery (MA).

Branches of the ECA in the neck that originate at the anterior surface of the vessel are optimal for microsurgical anastomosis since they have a favorable orientation (Fig. 7.3). These include the superior thyroid, lingual, and facial arteries. Their diameter is usually adequate for anastomosis, and unless there is atherosclerotic disease in the carotid system, or there is history of radiation or previous neck surgery, blood flow is excellent to supply free flap reconstruction. It is usually necessary to extend the patient's neck and turn it toward the opposite side for optimal exposure of the LA and FA. Otherwise, they will tend to sit very high in the neck, under the mandible, making microvascular anastomosis difficult, even if they are transposed under the digastric muscle and hypoglossal nerve.

Several variations have been described in the anatomy of the ECA system [14–16]. The superior thyroid artery is commonly preserved in neck dissection and it's a commonly used recipient vessel. Before reaching the thyroid gland, it provides multiple muscular branches. Occasionally, one of the proximal branches may originate directly from the ECA, in which case the superior thyroid may be smaller in caliber. The FA is often ligated in neck dissection below the submandibular gland and above the posterior belly of the digastric muscle. It usually arises from the ECA (about 80% of the time). However, it may arise with the lingual artery as a common trunk and then bifurcate with a high or low takeoff (about 20% of the time). Regardless of the exact branching pattern, it has been described that the FA is hypoplastic in approximately 10% of the population and can even be vestigial (1%). In these cases, the arterial supply of its territory is supplied by the contralateral FA or the transverse facial artery, which is a branch of the STA. In case the LA is utilized as a recipient vessel, care must be taken to confirm that the contralateral LA is patent to avoid tongue ischemia or necrosis.

The neck venous system is comprised mainly of the internal and external jugular veins (Fig. 7.4) [14–16]. The internal jugular vein (IJV) provides venous drainage of the brain, as well as parts of the face and neck. One on each side, they travel posterior and lateral to the common carotid arteries in the carotid sheath and merge with the subclavian veins to form the brachiocephalic veins at the base of the neck. Many smaller veins drain in the IJV as it courses from the base of the skull caudally, including the occipital, facial, lingual, pharyngeal, superior, and middle thyroid veins. Anomalous size and course of the IJ has been calculated to be found in approximately 10% of the population.

The external jugular vein (EJV) provides drainage for greater part of the cranium and face, and it is formed by the merging of the retromandibular and posterior auricular veins. In the neck, it courses lateral and superficial to the IJV, approximately from the angle of the mandible to the middle of the clavicle, and it crosses superficial to the sternocleidomastoid muscle (SCM) but deep to the platysma muscle and drains to the subclavian vein on each side. Branches that contribute to the formation of the EJV include the maxillary, superficial temporal, transverse cervical,

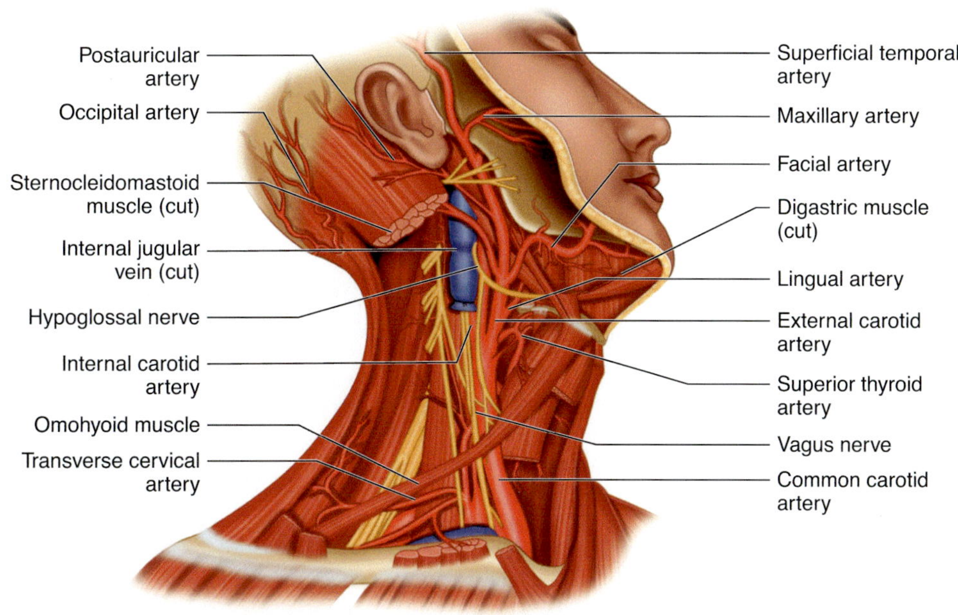

Fig. 7.2 External carotid artery system and its branches

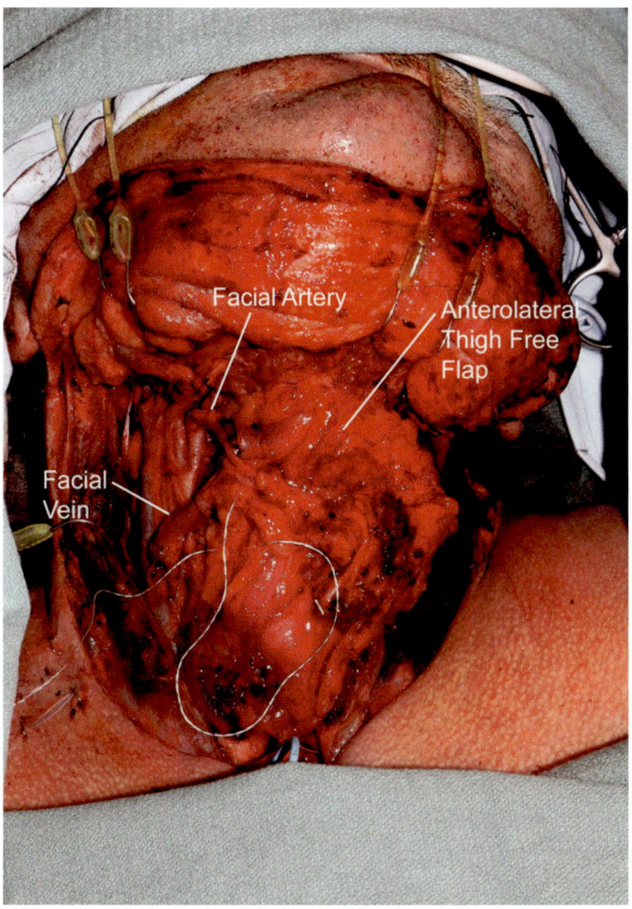

Fig. 7.3 Pharyngoesophageal reconstruction with a tubed anterolateral thigh free flap. The microvascular anastomoses were performed to the right facial artery and vein. The right sternocleidomastoid muscle is retracted lateral and the external carotid artery and internal jugular vein are visible

suprascapular, and anterior jugular veins. Significant variation of the superficial veins has been described. Both the IJV and the EJV have been shown to be excellent recipient vessels for venous outflow, and both provide a reliable option in head and neck reconstruction when available [17]. When both jugular veins are unavailable after radical neck dissection, the IJV stump is usually available and sufficient for microvascular anastomosis.

Applied Anatomy

Transverse Cervical Vessels

In patients that have a history of radiation to the neck or previous surgery, the external carotid and jugular vessels may be absent or not suitable for microvascular anastomosis. Even when present and patent, scarring and radiation fibrosis may render dissection of these vessels perilous. In these cases, we prefer using the transverse cervical vessels (Fig. 7.5). The transverse cervical artery (TCA) is one of the three branches of the thyrocervical trunk, along with the suprascapular and the inferior thyroid artery. It courses from medial to lateral in a more or less horizontal orientation deep and inferior to the inferior belly of the omohyoid muscle toward the anterior margin of the trapezius muscle. It lies superficial to the brachial plexus and then divides into a superficial branch, which supplies mainly the trapezius, and a deep branch, which supplies the trapezius, levator scapulae, and rhomboid muscles. Variations of the TCA have been described in several previously published studies [18–21]. The artery has been found to originate from the thyrocervical

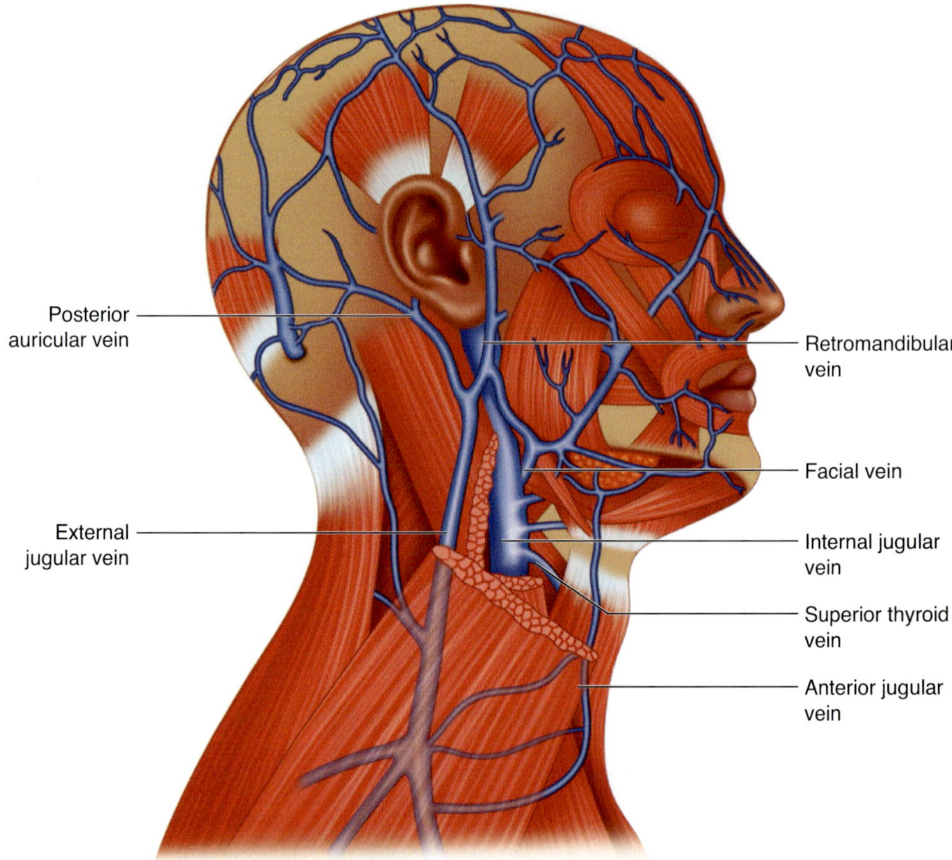

Fig. 7.4 Internal and external jugular veins and branches

trunk in approximately 80% of dissections [18–21]. Alternatively, it may arise directly from the subclavian artery, in which case the TCA tends to be of smaller caliber.

The transverse cervical vein (TCV) runs in close proximity with the artery (usually more superficial) and drains in the EJV or directly into the subclavian vein in the posterior neck triangle lateral to the lateral border of the SCM muscle. Even though the course of the artery is in general consistent, the vein may course deep (75%) or superficial (25%) to the omohyoid muscle.

In a cadaveric study performed by Yu [18], there were no absent arteries and only 2 veins were missing out of 33 dissections (6%). The artery had a diameter greater than 2 mm in 74% of dissections, and the vein was greater than 2 mm in diameter in 87% of dissections. All the identified vessels were free of disease and in excellent condition, even though 13 out of 26 patients had "frozen necks." In a different study by Tessler et al., the TCA was present in all 72 specimens (100%), and the TCV was present in 85% of specimens [19]. The pedicle length ranged from 4 to 7 cm, the mean caliber of the artery was 2.65 mm, and the mean caliber of the vein was 2.90 mm. These findings, along with the clinical data presented in these studies, suggest that the TC vessels have relatively consistent anatomy and provide a reliable alternative to the carotid and jugular vessels or their branches.

Surgical Site Exposure

The right side of the neck is preferred when all other factors are equal, to avoid injury to the thoracic duct that drains into the left brachiocephalic vein where the left IJ and subclavian veins merge. There is a smaller in caliber accessory lymphatic duct that drains into the right subclavian vein or the right IJV, or, rarely, at the junction of the two, and care must be taken to avoid its injury, even in the right neck [18, 19]. The transverse cervical vessels are found 1–2 cm cephalad to the clavicle and lateral to the SCM. If there is a visor neck incision already made for the laryngopharyngectomy, then a perpendicular incision is made toward the middle of the clavicle. If there are no prior incisions in the lower neck, a new transverse incision is made approximately 2 cm superior and parallel to the clavicle and lateral to the SCM. If the EJV is encountered before it merges to the subclavian vein, it is preserved and carefully dissected out as it may be used as a recipient vein rather than the TCV. The omohyoid muscle is identified right above the clavicle and lateral to the SCM. Deep to this muscle, fatty tissue is bluntly dissected in order to locate the TCV. The TCA is usually located deep and slightly cephalad to the vein. A handheld Doppler can be utilized to facilitate locating the vessels within the submuscular fat.

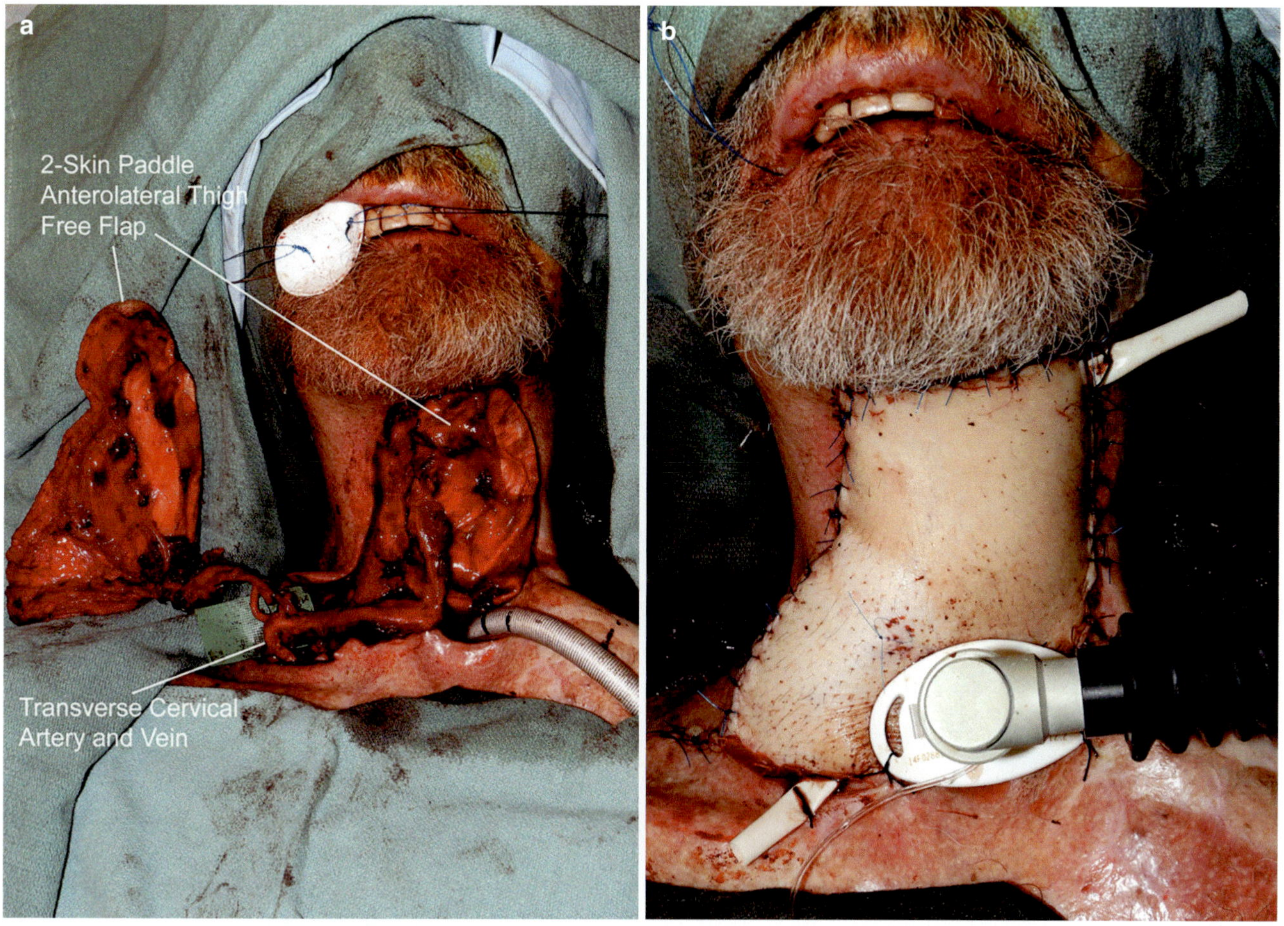

Fig. 7.5 Circumferential pharyngoesophageal and large neck skin defect reconstructed with a two-skin paddle anterolateral thigh free flap (**a**). The microvascular anastomoses were performed to the right transverse cervical artery and vein. Completed reconstruction (**b**)

Vessels Outside the Head and Neck Region

When there are no available recipient vessels in the neck area, alternative options need to be considered outside the neck region in order to identify appropriate blood supply for the flap. Several vessels have been described, including the internal mammary, thoracoacromial, and cephalic vein (Fig. 7.6) [16, 22–29].

The internal mammary artery and vein (IMA and IMV, respectively), also known as the internal thoracic artery and vein, are branches of the subclavian vessels. They are more commonly used as recipient vessels in breast reconstruction but can be used as a second- or third-line option in head and neck reconstruction [16, 22–29]. Beneath the second or third costal cartilage is the most consistent and reliable area to identify vessels of adequate caliber (Fig. 7.7). The pectoralis major muscle is divided over this region to expose the costal cartilages, which are removed being cautious not to injure the pleura or lung beneath the vessels. The location of the internal mammary vessels may require interposition vein grafting to reach.

The thoracoacromial artery is a branch of the axillary artery and gives off four branches: pectoral, deltoid, clavicular, and acromial. The pectoral branch of the thoracoacromial artery is the main pedicle for the pectoralis muscle flap, so if this artery is used as recipient vessel, the ipsilateral pectoralis muscle flap cannot be used anymore for future reconstruction. The thoracoacromial trunk can be identified through a muscle-splitting incision right below the clavicle and usually provides reliable quality of vessels for microvascular anastomosis [22, 23, 27, 28]. The artery and vein tend to be of small caliber, which can result in a size mismatch with the free flap pedicle vessels and make microvascular anastomosis troublesome.

For the vein only, the cephalic vein can be transposed into the neck to serve as a recipient vein. The cephalic vein is usually divided just above the elbow flexion crease and is elevated off of the anterolateral surface of the biceps muscle. It is dissected to its origin at the axillary vein in between the deltoid and pectoralis major muscles, within the deltopectoral groove. This vein will reach quite high into the neck if dissected for this length. Care should be taken to make sure

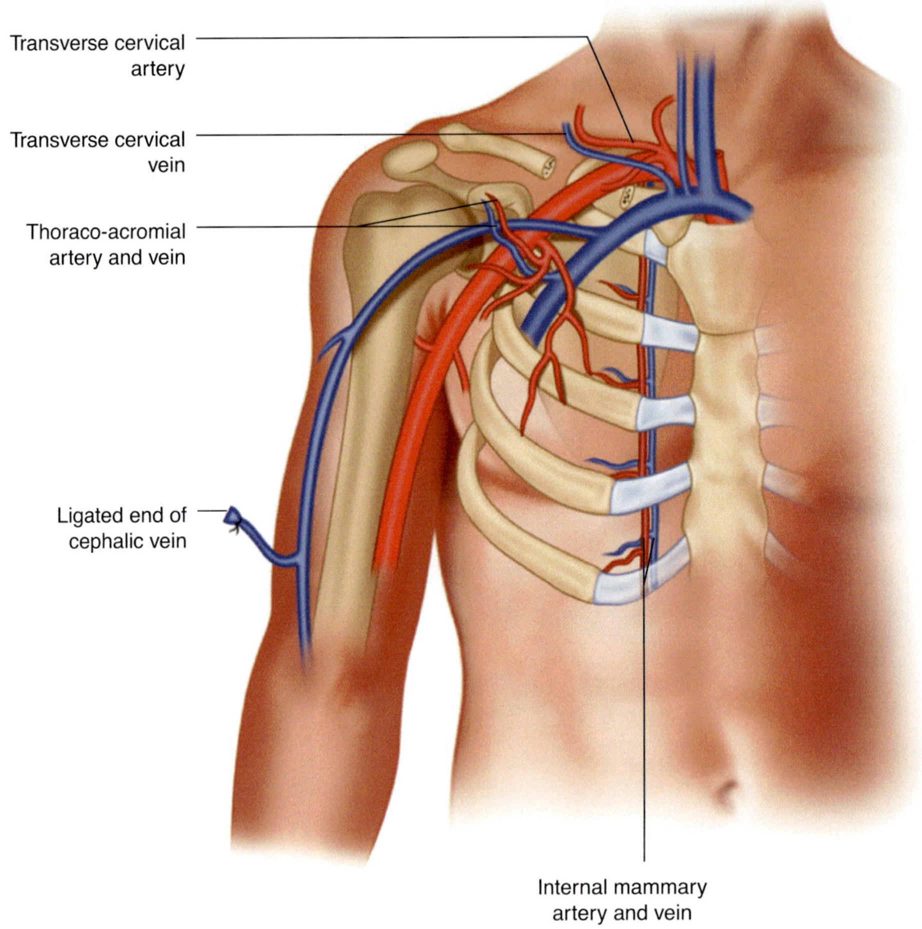

Fig. 7.6 Recipient vessels outside the neck region as well as the transverse cervical vessels

the vein is not kinked near its origin, instead taking a gentle curve as it is transposed superiorly into the neck region.

In the vessel-depleted neck and when the vascular pedicle of the flap is not long enough for a tension-free anastomosis with the recipient vessels, use of interposition vein grafts may be necessary. Various donor sites have been described for the vein graft, including in frequency order the greater saphenous, external jugular, cephalic, lesser saphenous, and anterior jugular veins [30]. Maricevich et al. performed a retrospective study examining patients that underwent head and neck reconstruction in a 10-year period at our institution. This cohort was found to have higher rate of flap compromise and loss (14.5% and 6.4%, respectively) compared to no vein graft controls (3.4% and 1.1%, respectively). However, this still meant that a 94.6% success rate was achieved in a cohort of patients with a significantly higher rate of preoperative radiation, chemotherapy, prior neck dissection, prior free flap reconstruction, osteoradionecrosis, and multiple free flap reconstruction. The authors concluded that interposition vein grafting was, therefore, associated with an acceptable success rate in a particularly challenging subset of patient such as those undergoing salvage laryngopharyngectomy [31].

Discussion

Algorithm for Recipient Vessel Selection

Hanasono et al. [22] retrospectively analyzed the incidence of inadequate recipient vessels in patients that had undergone preoperative radiation therapy and/or previous neck surgery. Among 226 patients, 35% had history of radiation in the neck, 2.1% isolated prior neck dissection, and 15.2% had both; 47.7% of patient had no history of radiation or neck dissection. Not surprisingly, the ECA or one of its branches was not satisfactory more commonly in patients that had previous radiation, surgery, or both, compared to no history of the above (19.3%, 20%, 36.1% vs 11.5%, respectively, $P = 0.03$). Similarly, the EJV/IJV systems were not adequate

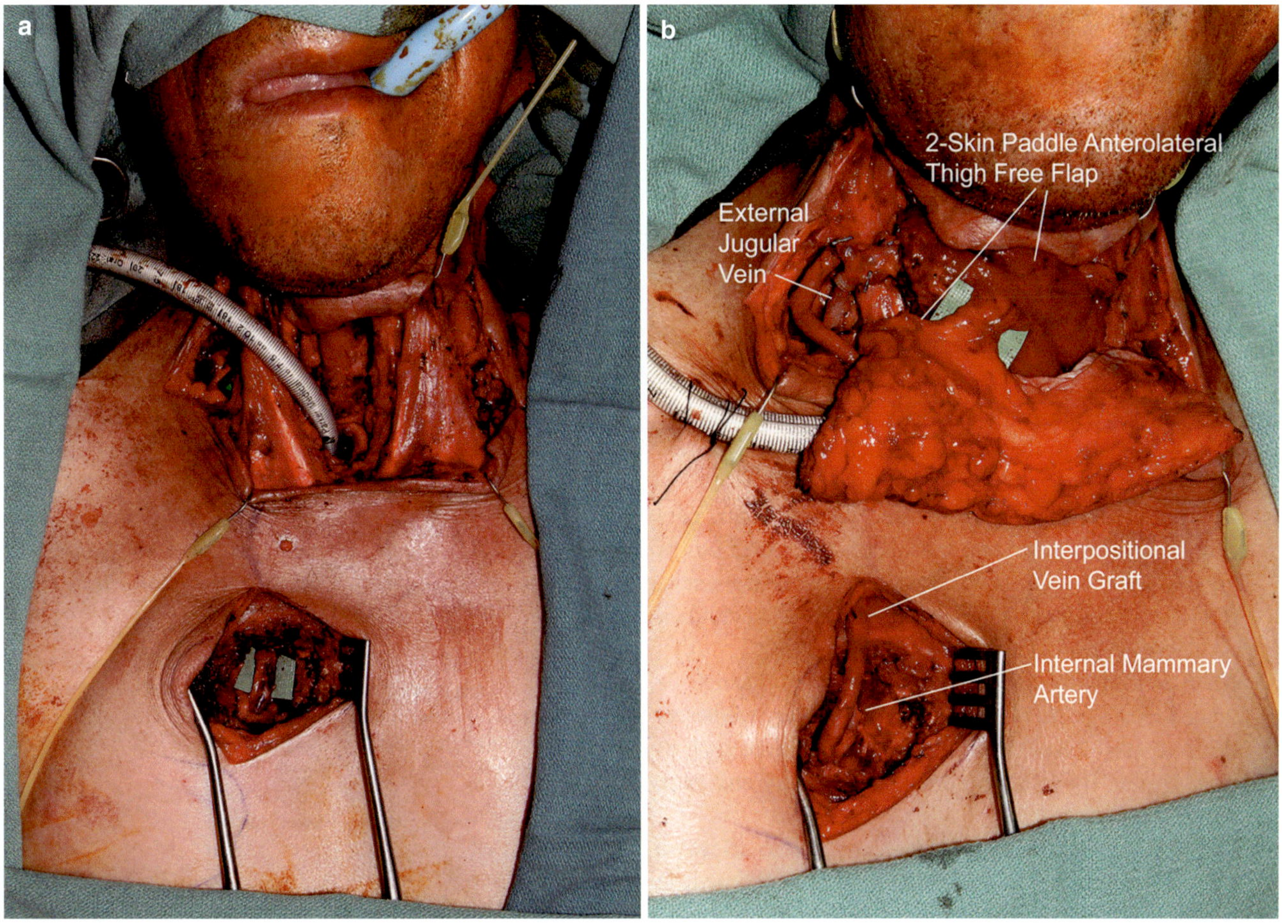

Fig. 7.7 Exposure of the right internal mammary artery and vein after removal of the second costal cartilage (**a**). Pharyngoesophageal and neck reconstruction with a two-skin paddle anterolateral thigh free flap including the vastus lateralis muscle to eliminate dead space (**b**). The microvascular anastomoses were performed to the right internal mammary artery via a greater saphenous vein interposition graft and the right external jugular vein

for anastomosis more commonly in patients that had previous radiation or surgery or both, compared to no history of the above (13.2%, 20%, 38.9% vs 9.7%, respectively, $P = 0.002$). The authors of the study recommended an algorithmic approach to facilitate recipient vessel selection [22]. With regard to the arterial anastomosis, if the ipsilateral ECA, or branches of it, are not available, the transverse cervical artery or the contralateral neck branches are selected, depending on which vessels were closer in proximity and had better flow. Interposition vein grafts were used as needed to achieve a tension-free anastomosis. The arterial anastomosis can be performed to the internal mammary artery or to a side branch of another free flap, in case of a two-flap reconstruction. Similarly, with regard to the venous anastomosis, in case the ipsilateral IJV and EJV are not available, the transverse cervical vein or the contralateral neck veins are selected, using vein grafting if necessary. If these are not adequate, other options include a cephalic vein turndown or anastomosis to a side branch of another flap if a second flap is present. Finally, similar to the recipient artery algorithm, the internal mammary vein can be used as a recipient vein.

Preoperative Assessment Tools

Preoperative studies are not routinely obtained for recipient vessel selection or flap planning in patients undergoing pharyngolaryngectomy and reconstruction. In patients with history of radiation or previous surgery when vessel-depleted neck is suspected or anticipated, CT angiography can be considered to identify possible recipient blood vessels, especially when a prior free flap has been performed at an outside institution. Regarding flap selection and planning, CT angiography of the thigh can be obtained to better assess the blood supply of the soft tissues in the region and examine the presence and location of perforators, especially when a second skin paddle is required [32, 33]. However, we routinely rely on anatomic landmarks instead, since the anatomy of the aforementioned flaps is typically reliable and consistent.

Technical Pearls

- We recommend turning the head to the contralateral side for maximum exposure when dissecting the upper neck to dissect branches of the ECA and IJV as recipient vessels and perform microvascular anastomosis.
- When the TCA and TCV are used for recipients, care must be taken to avoid injury of the thoracic duct on the left side and the accessory thoracic duct on the right side.
- The inferior belly of the omohyoid muscle is a landmark for identifying the TCA and TCV.
- When satisfactory recipient blood vessels cannot be located in the neck, it is sometimes necessary to dissect blood vessels outside the head and neck region, such as the IMA and IMV, the thoracoacromial artery and vein, and the cephalic vein.
- Interposition vein grafting is used as needed to achieve a tension-free anastomosis without kinking of the pedicle or recipient blood vessels.
- In case there is a need for two-skin paddle reconstruction and the ALT flap is used, the orientation of the inset of the flap depends on the recipient vessel selection. If the flap is anastomosed to the ECA and IJV, or branches of those vessels, we recommend orienting the ALT flap in such way that the proximal part is used for the pharyngeal reconstruction and the distal part for the external neck skin. In case the TC vessels are used as recipient vessels, then the ALT flap is oriented and inset in a way that the proximal part of the ALT is used for the neck skin and the distal for the pharynx. This allows for optimal positioning of the pedicle close to the recipient vessels, thus minimizing the need for vein graft.

Conclusion

Identifying adequate recipient vessels in free flap reconstruction after laryngopharyngectomy is critical for flap survival and successful reconstruction. Knowledge of the neck anatomy in addition to implementation of an algorithmic approach in recipient vessel selection will assist the surgeon in decreasing complication rates and associated morbidity, even in challenging patients with vessel-depleted neck.

References

1. Krespi YP, Wurster CF, Sisson GA. Immediate reconstruction after total laryngopharyngoesophagectomy and mediastinal dissection. Laryngoscope. 1985;95(2):156–61.
2. Wong C-H, Wei F-C. Microsurgical free flap in head and neck reconstruction. Head Neck. 2010;32(9):1236–45.
3. Yu P, Robb GL. Pharyngoesophageal reconstruction with the anterolateral thigh flap: a clinical and functional outcomes study. Plast Reconstr Surg. 2005;116(7):1845–55.
4. Lewin JS, Barringer DA, May AH, Gillenwater AM, Arnold KA, Roberts DB, et al. Functional outcomes after circumferential pharyngoesophageal reconstruction. Laryngoscope. 2005;115(7):1266–71.
5. Yu P, Hanasono MM, Skoracki RJ, Baumann DP, Lewin JS, Weber RS, et al. Pharyngoesophageal reconstruction with the anterolateral thigh flap after total laryngopharyngectomy. Cancer. 2010;116(7):1718–24.
6. Selber JC, Xue A, Liu J, Hanasono MM, Skoracki RJ, Chang EI, et al. Pharyngoesophageal reconstruction outcomes following 349 cases. J Reconstr Microsurg. 2014;30(9):641–54.
7. Anthony JP, Singer MI, Mathes SJ. Pharyngoesophageal reconstruction using the tubed free radial forearm flap. Clin Plast Surg. 1994;21(1):137–47.
8. Disa JJ, Pusic AL, Hidalgo DA, Cordeiro PG. Microvascular reconstruction of the hypopharynx: defect classification, treatment algorithm, and functional outcome based on 165 consecutive cases. Plast Reconstr Surg. 2003;111(2):652–3.
9. Schusterman MA, Shestak K, de Vries EJ, Swartz W, Jones N, Johnson J, et al. Reconstruction of the cervical esophagus: free jejunal transfer versus gastric pull-up. Plast Reconstr Surg. 1990;85(1):16–21.
10. Reece GP, Schusterman MA, Miller MJ, Kroll SS, Robb GL, Baldwin BJ, et al. Morbidity and functional outcome of free jejunal transfer reconstruction for circumferential defects of the pharynx and cervical esophagus. Plast Reconstr Surg. 1995;96(6):1307–16.
11. Cordeiro PG, Shah K, Santamaria E, Gollub MJ, Singh B, Shah JP. Barium swallows after free jejunal transfer: should they be performed routinely? Plast Reconstr Surg. 1999;103(4):1167–75.
12. Clemens MW, Yu P. Nearly circumferential pharyngoesophagectomy reconstruction with a double-skin paddle anteromedial thigh and sartorius muscle free flap. Plastic Reconstr Surg. 2012;129:594e–5e.
13. Wolf GT, Fisher SG, Hong WK, Hillman R, Spaulding M, Laramore GE, et al. Induction chemotherapy plus radiation compared with surgery plus radiation in patients with advanced laryngeal cancer. N Engl J Med. 1991;324(24):1685–90.
14. Nahum AM. Grant's atlas of anatomy. 7th ed. Edited by James E. Anderson, 608 pp, illus, Baltimore: Williams & Wilkins; 1978. $30.00. Head Neck Surg. 2007.
15. Molloy RG, Crowley B. The arterial anatomy of skin flaps. 2nd ed. Cormack GC, George B, Lamberty BGH. 282 × 222 mm. Pp. 538. Illustrated. 1994. Edinburgh: Churchill Livingstone. £179. Br J Surg. 2007.
16. Tan B-K, Wong C-H, Chen H-C. Anatomic variations in head and neck reconstruction. Semin Plast Surg. 2010;24(2):155–70.
17. Ibrahim AE, Adelman DM, Parham C, Hong Z, Villa M, Chahine FM, et al. The external jugular vein used as recipient vessel in head and neck free flap reconstruction: outcomes compared to the internal jugular vein. J Craniofac Surg. 2019;30(1):178–83.
18. Yu P. The transverse cervical vessels as recipient vessels for previously treated head and neck cancer patients. Plast Reconstr Surg. 2005;115(5):1253–8.
19. Tessler O, Gilardino MS, Bartow MJ, St Hilaire H, Womac D, Dionisopoulos T, et al. Transverse cervical artery: consistent ana-

tomical landmarks and clinical experience with its use as a recipient artery in complex head and neck reconstruction. Plast Reconstr Surg. 2017;139(3):745e–51e.
20. Huelke DF. A study of the transverse cervical and dorsal scapular arteries. Anat Rec. 1958;132(3):233–45.
21. Daseler EH, Anson BJ. Surgical anatomy of the subclavian artery and its branches. Surg Gynecol Obstet. 1959;108(2):149–74.
22. Hanasono MM, Barnea Y, Skoracki RJ. Microvascular surgery in the previously operated and irradiated neck. Microsurgery. 2009;29(1):1–7.
23. Shimizu F, Lin MP, Ellabban M, Evans GRD, Cheng M-H. Superficial temporal vessels as a reserve recipient site for microvascular head and neck reconstruction in vessel-depleted neck. Ann Plast Surg. 2009;62(2):134–8.
24. Jacobson AS, Eloy JA, Park E, Roman B, Genden EM. Vessel-depleted neck: techniques for achieving microvascular reconstruction. Head Neck. 2008;30(2):201–7.
25. Buck PM, Wax MK, Petrisor DI. Internal mammary vessels: alternate recipient vessels in microvascular head and neck reconstruction. J Oral Maxillofac Surg. 2016;74(9):1896.e1–6.
26. Roche NA, Houtmeyers P, Vermeersch HF, Stillaert FB, Blondeel PN. The role of the internal mammary vessels as recipient vessels in secondary and tertiary head and neck reconstruction. J Plast Reconstr Aesthet Surg. 2012;65(7):885–92.
27. Urban V, Fritsche E. Internal thoracic vessels as recipient vessels for freze flap reconstruction in head and neck surgery. J Plast Reconstr Aesthet Surg. 2006;59(12):1348–9.
28. Urken ML, Higgins KM, Lee B, Vickery C. Internal mammary artery and vein: recipient vessels for free tissue transfer to the head and neck in the vessel-depleted neck. Head Neck. 2006;28(9):797–801.
29. Onoda S, Sakuraba M, Asano T, Miyamoto S, Hayashi R, Asai M, et al. Thoracoacromial cvessels as recipients for head and neck reconstruction and cause of vascular complications. Microsurgery. 2011;31(8):628–31.
30. Aycock JK, Stenson KM, Gottlieb LJ. The thoracoacromial trunk: alternative recipient vessels in reoperative head and neck reconstructive microsurgery. Plast Reconstr Surg. 2008;121(1):88–94.
31. Maricevich M, Lin LO, Liu J, Chang EI, Hanasono MM. Interposition vein grafting in head and neck free flap reconstruction. Plast Reconstr Surg. 2018;142(4):1025–34.
32. Chen SY, Lin WC, Deng SC, Chang SC, Fu JP, Dai NT, et al. Assessment of the perforators of anterolateral thigh flaps using 64-section multidetector computed tomographic angiography in head and neck cancer reconstruction. Eur J Surg Oncol. 2010;36(10):1004–1011.
33. Garvey PB, Selber JC, Madewell JE, Bidaut L, Feng L, Yu P. A prospective study of preoperative computed tomographic angiography for head and neck reconstruction with anterolateral thigh flaps. Plast Reconstr Surg. 2011;127(4):1505–14.

Recipient Vessels: Voice Reconstruction

8

Alberto Bolletta, Samir Mardini, and Hung-Chi Chen

Introduction

The major cause for voice reconstruction is determined by oncological resections. While hypopharyngeal cancer is considered a rare occurrence, responsible for nearly 3% of malignancies affecting the head and neck region, laryngeal cancer is the second most common tumor affecting this region [1, 2]. Determinants of treatments are tumor size and characteristics, together with infiltration of nearby structures or extension to lymph node stations or metastasis. The treatment of these tumors is frequently challenging, since they are often found at advanced stage. This is mainly a consequence of their location which makes early detection very difficult. In recent years, larynx preservation strategies have become available and may be indicated in selected patients. Often though, the surgical approach is still the main option for patients to achieve locoregional control of the disease and to improve long-term survival. In these cases, a total laryngopharyngectomy is performed, along with neck dissection and adjuvant radiotherapy, when adverse pathologic factors are present [3]. As a result of this surgical approach, the patient sustains a circumferential defect of the upper digestive tract, together with voice loss. In order to restore the voice mechanism, a voice reconstruction strategy must be included in the reconstructive approach aimed at restoring the continuity of the digestive tract. Up to date there is still no consensus on the gold standard for reconstruction after total laryngopharyngectomy. One of the strategies suggested involves the use of free flaps in order to create a structure called "voice tube." The concept implements restoring voice production by creating a conduit allowing air to flow from the trachea to the upper digestive tract. This airflow is hence responsible for sound production by vibration of the walls of the pharynx (or neopharynx in case of concomitant hypopharyngeal reconstruction). Potential free flaps include fasciocutaneous flaps, like radial forearm and anterolateral thigh flap, but also enteric flaps can be used for this purpose. The latter, and in particular the ileocolon flap, is considered a better choice for reconstruction by the authors of this chapter. If a hypopharyngeal-esophageal defect has to be reconstructed together with a voice tube, a portion of the ascending colon, together with the ileocecal valve and a segment of terminal ileum, is harvested based on the ileocolic vessels. This flap pattern therefore includes a segment of the ascending colon to restore digestive tract continuity and the ileum for the voice tube. The ileocecal valve is then used as a one-way valve mechanism. In fact it allows airflow from the trachea to the pharynx, but it prevents food and liquid leakage. Since the inset of these flaps involves the anterior aspect of the neck, there are several recipients that can be chosen for microvascular anastomosis. The first branches of the external carotid artery are located in an advantageous position, and they offer good caliber and flow, allowing for end-to-end anastomosis. They are often in close proximity with the corresponding veins, but also the external and internal jugular veins may be considered as they are close to the defect (also see Chap. 2). Many factors should be considered in selecting proper recipient vessels based on the specifics of each individual case. These patients often have history of major procedures such as prior neck dissection, and radiotherapy, which may jeopardize availability of healthy vessels in the neck. Previous surgery combined with radiation therapy results in significant scarring, hence making it very challenging to dissect the potential recipients, which may have also been injured before. Wound complications are increased in such circumstances [4–6], Thus, it might be necessary to consider other vessels, such as those of the supraclavicular

A. Bolletta · H-C. Chen (✉)
Department of Plastic Surgery, International Medical Service Center of China Medical University Hospital, China Medical University, Taichung, Taiwan
e-mail: D19722@mail.cmuh.org.tw

S. Mardini
Division of Plastic Surgery, Department of Surgery, Mayo Clinic, Rochester, MN, USA
e-mail: mardini.samir@mayo.edu

R. Gurunian, R. Djohan (eds.), *Recipient Vessels in Reconstructive Microsurgery*,
https://doi.org/10.1007/978-3-030-75389-4_8

area, like the transverse cervical artery (also see Chap. 6), and those further away, like the thoracoacromial vessels (also see Chap. 14) and the cephalic vein (also see Chap. 13). Another important aspect to keep in mind is that, in order to obtain satisfactory sound production and speech, the inset of the voice tube has to be carefully planned in terms of both length of the flap and its course. This may affect the pedicle location, hence vessel selection. This chapter focuses on the selection of recipient vessels in microsurgical strategies for voice reconstruction, in particular with enteric free flaps.

Anatomy of the Larynx and Phonatory Physiology

The larynx is composed of nine cartilages and one bone, which is the hyoid bone.

The cartilages consist of the three solitary ones, the thyroid, cricoid, and epiglottis, and three bilateral ones, the arytenoids, corniculates, and cuneiforms. The hyoid bone suspends the rest of the larynx, and the whole structure is connected by joints and ligaments. The larynx is divided into three sections, called the supraglottis, glottis, and subglottis. The most cranial aspect of the larynx, the supraglottis, comprises the area between the superior aspect of the hyoid bone and the glottis. The glottis is crucial as it includes the vocal folds. The vocal cords are determined by the free upper edges of the cricothyroid membrane, where they become the cricovocal ligament and are covered with mucosa. Their position, tension, and length are determined by the action of the intrinsic and extrinsic muscles of the larynx. The caudal aspect of the larynx is the subglottis and it extends to the lower border of the cricoid cartilage. The larynx is responsible for originating the fundamental tone for sound production. This tone is generated by the airflow expelled from the lungs through the adducting vocal folds. The airflow is turned in periodic sound waves by rapid cycles of opening and closing of the vocal folds. This vibrating movement of the vocal folds is explained by the aerodynamic myoelastic theory, and it is majorly responsible for phonation [7].

Histologic characteristics and composition of the vocal fold affect its vibration, hence phonation [8]. In particular, the vocal fold is composed of three layers, the outer cover, a transition layer, and a proper body. The histological characteristics of each layer affect its overall mechanics, and for this reason, the vocal folds are able to create a variety of sounds in terms of frequency, intensity, and quality. Phonation is the result of the interaction between airflow, air pressure, and extrinsic and intrinsic muscular activity determining length, tension, and mass of the vocal folds. This sound is then altered by the resonating chambers above and below the larynx and converted to speech in the mouth through the interaction between the tongue, palate, teeth, and lips.

Vascular Anatomy of the Neck

Knowledge of the vascular anatomy of the neck and nearby regions is essential in order to identify and preserve the vessels located in this area suitable for microvascular anastomosis.

Branches of the Carotid System

The *common carotid artery* is located in the anterior triangle (carotid triangle) of the neck in a deeper and medial position compared to the *internal jugular vein*, and at the level of the thyroid cartilage, it divides into the *external carotid artery* and *internal carotid artery*.

The *external carotid artery* is largely responsible for the vascular supply of the neck and facial region, by giving off many branches along its course (also see Chap. 2 and Video 2.1).

The *superior thyroid artery* is the most proximal branch of the external carotid artery, although, in a minor number of cases, it may originate from the bifurcation, the common carotid artery, or even the internal carotid artery. Ozgur et al. measured the diameter of the superior thyroid artery at its origin in a cadaveric study, finding it to be 3.53 mm ± 1.17 mm in diameter [9]. This artery usually arises from the anterior surface of the external carotid artery, just below the level of the greater horn of the hyoid bone, and then travels anteriorly and medially, and it then turns inferiorly, descending adjacent to the thyroid cartilage toward the thyroid gland where it divides into multiple branches [10].

The following branch of the external carotid artery is the *lingual artery*, arising medially, approximately 1.2 cm from the carotid bifurcation with an average diameter of 3.06 mm ± 0.65 mm [9]. Even though it usually originates individually, sometimes it shares a common trunk with the superior thyroid or facial artery. The course of the lingual artery starts cranially, before turning inferiorly and medially toward the greater horn of the hyoid bone, forming a loop which is crossed by the hypoglossal nerve. Then it enters deep to the hyoglossus at its posterior border, just above the greater horn of the hyoid bone, reappearing at the anterior border of the muscle, and finally, continuing on the inferior surface of the tongue till its tip as the deep lingual artery [11, 12].

The *facial artery* arises from the external carotid artery, around 2 cm cranially to the bifurcation, posterior to the mandibular angle. At its origin, its caliber has been measured at 3.35 mm ± 0.68 mm [9]. Its course is then through the submandibular triangle, deep to the posterior belly of the digastric and medial to the submandibular gland. It crosses the inferior border of the mandible at the anterior edge of the masseter muscle in a tortuous fashion in order to allow the movements of the head. The artery then travels on the lateral surface of the mandible toward the buccal region, crossing the buccinator muscle toward the angle of the mouth, branching into the labial arteries and the angular artery [13] (also see Chaps. 3 and 4).

Venous Anatomy of the Neck

As usual, the venous network is characterized by great variability, in terms of both number and location of veins, as well as drainage patterns.

The *external jugular vein* is one of the main and most reliable veins of the neck, originating posterior to the angle of the mandible, from the confluence of the posterior division of the retromandibular vein with the posterior auricular vein. Even though usually there is one external jugular vein, sometimes multiple external jugular veins are present or it may be absent. Its course is directed caudally, running superficial to the sternocleidomastoid muscle. Being so superficial, it is easily detected through inspection and rapidly encountered during neck dissection. The average diameter of the external jugular vein midway through its course is reported to be about 4.6 mm ± 1.5 mm [14]. It usually drains into the convergence of the subclavian vein with the internal jugular vein. It may also drain directly into the subclavian vein or, more rarely, into the internal jugular vein.

The *internal jugular vein* is the largest vein of the neck, with a mean diameter of 7.9 mm ± 1.9 mm, and is responsible for the major venous return from the brain, upper face, and neck [14]. It exits from the jugular foramen, and, in the neck, its course is deep to the sternocleidomastoid muscle, lateral to the internal carotid artery first, and common carotid artery in the lower neck. Even though posterior and lateral branches of the internal jugular vein have been described, the main branches usually originate from the anterior aspect of the vein. These include the *superior thyroid vein*, *lingual vein*, and *facial vein*. Their main diameters at origin have been reported as 2.7 mm ± 0.8 mm, 2.7 mm ± 0.9 mm, and 3.6 mm ± 1.2 mm, respectively [14]. The internal jugular vein then drains into the brachiocephalic vein. As previously described for the external jugular vein, even the internal jugular vein may be absent or duplicated in rare cases [15].

The Transverse Cervical Vessels

In the last decades, various definitions have been used to address the *transverse cervical artery* (also see Chap. 6 and Video 6.1). In this chapter, we refer to the *transverse cervical artery* as a branch of the thyrocervical trunk, continuing through the posterior cervical triangle superficially, and differentiated from the dorsal scapular artery, which is a deep branch of the thyrocervical trunk [16]. Most frequently, the *transverse cervical artery* originates from the thyrocervical trunk, but it can also be a branch of the subclavian artery. The anatomical course of the *transverse cervical artery* is usually constant, starting deep to the inferior belly of the omohyoid muscle and then proceeding with a posterolateral course through the posterior cervical triangle above the anterior scalene muscles toward the anterior border of the trapezius muscle. The mean diameter of this artery at 2 cm from its origin is 2.2 mm ± 0.47 mm [16]. Compared to the artery, the course of the *transverse cervical vein* is more inconstant [17]. This vein may be found deeper than the omohyoid muscle in the majority of cases, but also superficially, in approximately 25% of cases. The reported mean diameter of the transverse cervical vein is 2.90 mm [18]. It drains into the external jugular vein or the subclavian vein [19].

The Thoracoacromial Vessels

The *thoracoacromial artery* originates from the second part of the axillary artery located posterior to the pectoralis minor muscle (also see Chap. 14 and Video 14.1). The reported average diameter of the artery at its origin is 2.5 ± 0.5 mm [20]. The thoracoacromial artery courses for a short tract deep to the medial border of the pectoralis minor muscle and then passes through the clavipectoral fascia 6 to 10 cm lateral to the sternoclavicular joint. It then divides into four branches including the clavicular, acromial, pectoral, and deltoid branches. The pectoral branch, supplying the pectoralis major muscle, courses along the undersurface of the pectoralis major muscle and is enclosed in protective perivascular sheath [21]. The concomitant veins run along the pectoral branch, and at the level of the clavicle, they merge into a single vein, with a reported diameter at this level of 2.8 mm, and drain into the axillary vein 1 to 2 cm away from the origin of the thoracoacromial arterial trunk from the axillary artery [22, 23].

The Cephalic Vein

At the arm level, the *cephalic vein* enters the deltopectoral groove by following the lateral bicipital groove, and it usually runs along the deltoid branch of the thoracoacromial artery (also see Chap. 24 and Video 24.1, Chap. 13 and Video 13.1). At the level of the deltopectoral triangle, it pierces the costocoracoid membrane (clavipectoral fascia) at the upper edge of the pectoralis minor muscle to drain into the axillary vein (also see Chap. 24). At the lateral edge of the pectoralis major muscle, it has a reported diameter of 3.7 ± 1.30 mm [24]. In a minority of cases, the cephalic vein crosses anterior to the clavicle and perforates the cervical fascia, ending in the external jugular vein [25].

Surgical Options for Voice Reconstruction

Microsurgical strategies for voice reconstruction usually involve using free flap transfer in order to create a structure known as "voice tube," which is a conduit that allows air to flow from the trachea to the pharynx, to the esophagus, or to the newly reconstructed homologous structures in case of contextual pharyngoesophageal reconstruction. The airflow is responsible for sound production by inducing the vibration of the walls of the structures encountered, and it is then articulated into speech in the mouth by the tongue, lips, and teeth. In order to function properly, the inlet of the voice tube is connected to the trachea, and, for voice production, the tracheostoma is occluded by the patient using his or her thumb or finger. It is sometimes useful to devise a "voice hood" by using a local fasciocutaneous flap to create a bulging mass near the tracheostoma, facilitating the patient when occluding it to talk. The outlet of the voice tube, which connects to the upper digestive tract, must present or be conformed in such way to create a valve-like mechanism. This is to allow the airflow while impeding the retrograde leakage of food and fluids into the trachea. According to the reconstructive choice, the voice tube can be shaped out of different tissue transfers. It can be made of skin in case fasciocutaneous flaps are used, such as the radial forearm flap or the anterolateral thigh flap. However, according to the authors' experience, enteric tissues like jejunum, ileocolon, and appendix free flaps are better suited for this use. An important advantage of using intestinal flaps is represented by the fact that they already present in a tubular shape, hence reducing the risk of leakage and fistula formation from the otherwise necessary long suture lines indispensable to create a tube out of a flat skin surface. Moreover, intestinal flaps present with a mucosal lining, able of secretion and self-cleansing function, important to prevent stagnation of food and obstructions. A disadvantage may be represented by the fact that the harvesting of these flaps is challenging, in particular for those surgeons not familiar with abdominal surgery [26]. The authors of this chapter, along with many others, prefer the ileocolic region as donor site for these reconstructions, since it presents with unique characteristics and allows selecting and harvesting different segments of the ileum and colon, supplied by the ileocolic artery. After total laryngopharyngectomy, leaving a hypopharyngeal-esophageal defect to be reconstructed together with a voice tube, a segment of the ascending colon, together with the ileocecal valve and a tract of terminal ileum, can be harvested based on the ileocolic vessels. The reconstructive strategy then includes the segment of the ascending colon to restore digestive tract continuity and a segment of the ileum to be used for the voice tube. The presence of the ileocecal valve is valuable since it provides a natural one-way valve mechanism, but, in order to improve its function in this setting, it is usually necessary to perform an internal and external plication of the valve tissue to reduce its opening to 0.5 cm of diameter. It is possible to inset the colon flap in both isoperistaltic and antiperistaltic directions. Even though the direction of inset may vary in different patients, the authors prefer to place the flap in an antiperistaltic way. The antiperistalsis does not affect swallowing due to the fact that usually relatively short portions of the colon are used. In addition, this inset presents numerous advantages, for example, it allows harvesting a shorter section of the ileum to reach the tracheostoma. Moreover, this inset favors sound production, as the ileocecal valve is located in the caudal aspect of the neopharynx, determining a wider involvement of its walls for vibration. Due to its wide diameter, the colon flap is adequate for reconstructing defects reaching cranially up to the oropharynx. Caudally though, its caliber might be too large to match with the esophagus. In that case, surgical tapering of the colon flap might be performed by removing a wedge of tissue from its caudal edge, in order to obtain a proper match to the native esophagus. The ileum segment, in this reconstructive approach, forms the voice tube and its optimal length is 10–12 cm. It is gently positioned in the neck, paying attention not to make a steep curve, and it is anastomosed at the level of the tracheostoma. To cover the exposed area in the neck and the flap, usually the local skin is not sufficient; moreover, it may have been damaged by radiation therapy. In this case, a deltopectoral flap may be elevated to cover the flap and anastomotic sites. The preferential recipient vessels for this reconstructive approach will be described in detail in the next section of this chapter. The ileocolon free flap represents a valuable tool for voice reconstruction, with studies reporting satisfying swallowing function in 78% of patients treated and a good to moderate speech outcome in 85% of patients [26]. In order to achieve good results in terms of voice production, speech training is essential, and it usually takes from 3 months to 1 year after surgery. Also the free jejunum flap finds its indication in either voice reconstruction alone or combination with reconstruction of the pharynx and cervical esophagus. In the first case, a shorter segment of the jejunum is necessary, and, once harvested and vascular anastomoses are performed, it is inset as a voice tube by placing it between the cervical esophagus and the trachea. Since this flap does not present a natural valve, a mechanism of valve has to be created at the junction between the voice tube and the pharynx/esophagus [27]. In order to achieve a valve-like mechanism, the stump of the jejunum flap can be tapered and its diameter reduced to 0.5 cm by removing a wedge of full-thickness tissue, and the inset can be made into an antigravity fashion to prevent food leakage into the voice tube. As stated above, the jejunum flap may also be used for concomitant reconstruction of the pharynx/cervical esophagus; in this case, a longer segment of the jejunum must be harvested based on the same vascular pedicle. The jejunum flap is divided into two parts after vessel anastomoses, making sure not to damage the blood supply to either part. One segment of the flap is used as voice tube and the other to restore digestive tract continuity. The appendix free flap can also be used in voice reconstruction, usually when there is isolated defect of the larynx and not related with pharyngoesophageal defect. It has to be stated though that this option is thought to be inferior in terms of phonation quality and loudness compared to the other methods described above, as well as requiring longer training [26]. Other options for voice reconstruction are skin free flaps like the radial forearm flap and the anterolateral thigh flap [28]. A major disadvantage of these flaps is that they have to be fashioned into a tube shape, increasing the risk of fistula formation. A way of overcoming this problem is by performing a two-stage procedure with prefabrication of the flap in the first stage and transferring it in the second stage. These flaps also lack a valve-like mechanism, which needs to be created by tapering the proximal stump of the flap in order to reduce its caliber to 0.5 cm and by insetting the flap in an antigravity fashion. Another important aspect to consider is that these flaps are not provided with mucosal lining. Healing between the mucosa and skin may result in a higher risk of strictures or fistulas. The junction between the cutaneous voice tube and the reconstructed esophagus may be obstructed by sebaceous material, sweat, saliva, or food due to the secretion of the skin and lack of peristalsis of the skin voice tube. For these reasons, skin flaps are considered by the authors as a second choice and indicated in patients in which abdominal surgery is contraindicated.

Recipient Vessels for Voice Reconstruction: Selection and Surgical Exposure

Tables 8.1 and 8.2 present potential recipients and their characteristics. As stated in the previous section, voice reconstruction in the authors' experience is now routinely performed with intestinal flaps. Their pedicle is usually composed of one artery and one vein. For this reason, usually only one vein anastomosis is performed in these reconstructions. Even though the selection of recipient vessels for voice reconstruction varies according to factors related to each individual case, the authors usually prefer, as first choice, the *transverse cervical artery and external jugular vein* (also see Chaps. 2 and 6). Reasons for this are that the caliber and flow of these vessels are usually adequate and their location on the lower aspect of the neck allows for reaching with the flap pedicle, but it is also slightly distant from the area where ablative surgery and radiation therapy take place. Usually, when starting the reconstructive surgery, the incisions on the neck have already been performed by the tumor ablation team. Most of the times though, these incisions do not extend to the clavicular region; therefore, they need to be extended toward the mid-clavicle, in order to expose the supraclavicular region. If the neck exposure during ablative surgery is bilateral, it is advisable to select the vessels on the right side of the neck, in order to avoid risking the injury of the thoracic duct, which is located in the left neck. The pulsation of the transverse cervical artery may be searched preoperatively in the supraclavicular area using palpation and a handheld pencil Doppler. The first step for the dissection is the location of the omohyoid muscle, which can be found laterally to the sternocleidomastoid muscle, just above the clavicle. Attention must be paid during blunt dissection of the fatty tissue located in the triangular area between the inferior belly of the omohyoid muscle and the sternocleidomastoid muscle, as the transverse cervical vein may be found at this level either superficial or with a deeper course (also see Video 6.1). Usually, the transverse cervical artery is found at a deeper level compared to the vein, and its course is traced proximally, behind the inferior belly of the omohyoid muscle, to gain at least 2–3 cm of vessel length and greater caliber to facilitate microsurgical anastomosis. In order for the pedicle to reach, it can be passed either to superficial position or under the sternocleidomastoid muscle, but, in the latter case, it is imperative to release part of the muscle if tension

Table 8.1 Diameter of arteries

Artery	Diameter
Superior thyroid artery (at origin)	3.53 mm ± 1.17 mm
Lingual artery (at origin)	3.06 mm ± 0.65 mm
Facial artery (at origin)	3.35 mm ± 0.68 mm
Transverse cervical artery (at 2 cm from origin)	2.2 mm ± 0.47 mm
Thoracoacromial artery (at origin)	2.5 mm ± 0.5 mm

The values of diameter for each vessel are reported according to literature and references are cited in the corresponding part of the chapter

Table 8.2 Diameter of veins

Vein	Diameter
Superior thyroid vein (at origin)	2.7 mm ± 0.8 mm
Lingual vein (at origin)	2.7 mm ± 0.9 mm
Facial vein (at origin)	3.6 mm ± 1.2 mm
External jugular vein (midway through its course)	4.6 mm ± 1.5 mm
Internal jugular vein (mean value)	7.9 mm ± 1.9 mm
Transverse cervical vein (mean value)	2.90 mm
Thoracoacromial vein (at origin)	2.8 mm
Cephalic vein (at lateral edge of pectoralis major muscle)	3.7 ± 1.30 mm

The values of diameter for each vessel are reported according to literature and references are cited in the corresponding part of the chapter

is present, as it may compress the pedicle [19, 29]. The arterial anastomosis is usually performed with 9-0 interrupted sutures. Even though the use of a vein coupler is widely acknowledged in modern microsurgery, the authors prefer, in these cases, to perform venous anastomosis with interrupted sutures as well, since there is usually a caliber mismatch between the transverse cervical vein and the intestinal vein in the flap pedicle, and they feel that manual anastomosis may be better to address this issue. It is important also to highlight that, in a not negligible amount of cases, the transverse cervical vein presents with a small caliber, hence making it hard to overcome the mismatch with the pedicle vein. In addition to that, it is important to ensure adequate venous drainage for intestinal flaps to avoid venous congestion. In these cases, the best solution according to the authors is to use the *external jugular vein* in an end-to-end fashion. For this reason, it is always important to preserve this superficial vein and carefully dissect it during vessel preparation. Studies have shown no increase in complication rates when using the external jugular vein for free flap anastomoses [30]. The use of the anterior jugular vein, on the other hand, is not advisable since its course is near the neck midline and it can be easily damaged during tracheostomy [31]. Another valuable option, especially in primary cases where the neck has not been exposed to radiation therapy previously, is using the main branches of the external carotid artery. In these cases, the authors generally prefer the *superior thyroid artery*. Due to its location, this branch is routinely identified and preserved during the ablative procedures. When suitable, the anastomosis is performed in an end-to-end fashion with interrupted sutures. In case this recipient artery is selected, a close-by vein may be used. The tributaries of the internal jugular vein, like the *superior thyroid vein*, if preserved during ablative surgery, represent a good option. Since these veins drain into the deep system, the negative intrathoracic pressure developed during inspiration may favor venous outflow and reduce the risk of venous thrombosis [32–34]. In the authors' experience though, in many cases, there is no feasible branch of the internal jugular vein. In these cases, the suggestion is to consider an end-to-side anastomosis directly to the *internal jugular vein*. In order to do so, the internal jugular vein should be dissected circumferentially for a segment of approximately 2 cm, paying attention not to damage it, especially in secondary surgeries. This allows for creating a comfortable setting to perform an end-to-side anastomosis. When the anastomoses are performed with these recipient vessels, which are located in close proximity to the midline of the neck and to the defect area, special care must be taken during flap inset. In particular, it is important to avoid compressions of the pedicle and anastomoses sites during the inset of the "voice tube" between the esophagus and the tracheostoma. A lesser commonly used branch of the external carotid artery used for voice reconstruction is the *facial artery*. This is due to its location more cranial in the neck; hence, it is usually a better option for reconstruction after ablative maxillofacial procedures. It is important to remind though that, despite general indications, during each surgery the integrity and quality of the selected vessels should be evaluated, together with rational and general considerations regarding pedicle positioning and handling. For these reasons sometimes, as already mentioned, multiple surgeries along with previous radiotherapy determine the need for alternative choices of recipient vessels. These include the already described transverse cervical vessels but also the *thoracoacromial system* and the *cephalic vein* [19, 35, 36]. In order to expose the *thoracoacromial vessels*, a curved incision is usually performed in such manner to preserve the deltopectoral flap while exposing the lateral aspect of the clavicle and the lateral portion of the pectoralis major muscle. At this stage, the lateral attachment of the muscle to the clavicle is divided by a horizontal incision. The main thoracoacromial trunk is then identified by meticulous dissection of the fat pad located under the pectoralis major muscle but superficial to the pectoralis minor muscle (also see Video 14.1). At this level, it is possible to identify different arterial branches for anastomosis, comprising the pectoral branch. This branch is usually spared, if possible, in order not to compromise the use of the pectoralis major flap, a very useful pedicled flap, especially for salvage procedures in head and neck reconstructions. It may be possible that the pectoralis major flap has already been used, especially in complicated cases, with multiple reconstructive attempts. In this instance, the pectoral branch of the thoracoacromial artery can be found on the surface of the elevated muscle, and, if sufficient time has passed from the flap transfer for flap autonomization, the thoracoacromial vessels may be used as recipient vessels for free tissue transfer [35]. If one branch of the thoracoacromial trunk is used for arterial anastomosis, in its proximity, it is possible to find and use the correspondent vein as recipient vein. Also the *cephalic vein*, because of its length and location in close proximity to the neck area, is now commonly used as recipient vein in head and neck reconstructive microsurgery [37]. The cephalic vein can be found in close relationship with the deltopectoral groove; hence, the skin incision for vessel exposure is usually performed slightly medial or lateral to the groove in order to avoid accidental injury to the vein, since its location is quite superficial. This incision is extended proximally to create a connection with the area of neck exposure (also see Video 13.1).

Once identified, the vein is dissected circumferentially to allow mobilization and all the side branches are divided. The distal dissection into the arm is carried on until the length of the vein is sufficient to allow transposition to the neck. Once this is achieved, the dissection proceeds proximally toward the clavicle. The vein is then turned over the clavicle into the neck and gently positioned in order to perform a tension-free anastomosis. In order to ensure a smooth curve of the vein and reduce the risk of kinking, a small cuff of fat tissue can be positioned around the vein proximally. It is important to remember that this vein is characterized by numerous valves; for this reason, backflow may not be present when the vein is cut [37].

Discussion

Since, in many cases, voice reconstruction techniques involve the use of intestinal flaps, it is import to address specific issues particularly related to these tissue transfers.

Intestinal flaps are characterized by less ischemia tolerance when compared to other flaps, due to high metabolic demand [38, 39]. For this reason, it is mandatory, in these microsurgical reconstructions, to carefully plan the inset of the flap as well as the selection and isolation of recipient vessels before detaching the flap, in order to reduce the risk of extending the ischemia time intraoperatively. These measures include making sure that the pedicle length is sufficient to reach the recipient vessels without tension, and also ensuring the quality of the recipient artery with a spurting test on division. For the arterial anastomosis, a key factor is a proper size match between the artery of the flap pedicle and the recipient artery. In case of discrepancy, in the authors' experience, an end-to-side anastomosis to the external carotid artery is not advisable as a damage of its wall may lead to severe complications. The suggestion, in this instance, is to use a vein graft of tapering size between the two vessels as a bridge, for example, a short section of the great saphenous vein from the medial aspect of the thigh. Regarding venous anastomosis, usually the pedicles of these flaps contain one main vein of relatively large caliber, and one anastomosis of a large vein is sufficient for flap survival. On the other hand, though, it is important to keep in mind that intestinal flaps are more sensible to venous congestion, and different studies have demonstrated long recovery time after even short-time venous congestion and a related higher risk of complications and flap failure [39]. For this reason, it is important, during vein selection and preparation, to make sure that the chosen vein is of adequate caliber to provide suitable outflow. In case the selected vein appears of small caliber, it is advisable to switch to a larger vein, such as the external jugular vein in an end-to-end fashion or the internal jugular vein in an end-to-side fashion [38]. Another way to address this issue is to perform the microvascular anastomosis of the vein before arterial anastomosis, or alternatively, to keep the arterial anastomosis clamped during vein anastomosis and release both clamps at the end of the microsurgical time. In fact, even the short-timed arterial perfusion during venous anastomosis may be sufficient to cause congestion and hemorrhage in the lamina propria of the intestinal flap [39]. In order to reduce ischemia time as far as possible, the authors developed the "airborne suture technique," but every surgeon should use the approach he or she is more familiar with [40]. Moreover, to ensure proper blood supply to the flap and reduce the risk of complications, it is important to make sure that the wound closure is tensionless. In order to do so, a local flap may be used to cover the pedicle and part of the flap, in particular the anastomotic sites, to prevent leakage and fistula formation. It is important to consider that a significant edema occurs during the first 48 hours postoperatively. The exposed aspect of the flap may be covered with skin grafts, but tie-over dressing should be avoided [39]. Another concern regarding the use of intestinal flaps is their bacterial content. In order to reduce the risk of postoperative infection, the intestinal lumen of the flap is extensively washed, after detachment, first with Betadine solution followed by copious amount of warm saline solution. Moreover, antibiotics may be used postoperatively if necessary. A bacterial culture study in patients treated with ileocolon transfer for voice reconstruction found, in a high percentage of cases, the presence of gram-negative aerobes and anaerobes, and provided a useful guide to antibiotics selection [41]. In order to maximize the results of voice reconstruction, postoperative physiotherapy is mandatory. Training helps improving speech fluency and articulation. Usually, satisfactory results take from 3 months up to a year. Analysis of voice after training provides information on whether a secondary procedure is necessary. This includes shortening of the voice tube, revision of tracheostomy, and revision of the junction between the voice tube and tracheal stump. Voice tube redundancy is a possible outcome, since it is hard during flap inset to assess the appropriate length of the flap. This is a consequence of size variation that occurs to intestinal flaps due to devascularization during tissue transfer. In these cases, a secondary procedure can be performed to shorten the voice tube by removing a part of the intestine. Revision of the tracheostoma or its junction with the voice tube may involve the use of local flaps to adjust the tracheostomy size or to create a voice hood to make it easier for the patient to occlude the tracheostoma and force air into the voice tube.

References

1. Cooper JS, Porter K, Mallin K, Hoffman HT, Weber RS, Ang KK, et al. National Cancer Database report on cancer of the head and neck: 10-year update. Head Neck. 2009;31(6):748–58.
2. Ferlay J, Colombet M, Soerjomataram I, Mathers C, Parkin DM, Piñeros M, et al. Estimating the global cancer incidence and mortality in 2018: GLOBOCAN sources and methods. Int J Cancer. 2019;144(8):1941–53.
3. Kwon DI, Miles BA, Education Committee of the American Head and Neck Society (AHNS). Hypopharyngeal carcinoma: do you know your guidelines? Head Neck. 2019;41(3):569–76.

4. Shih H-S, Hsieh C-H, Feng G-M, Feng W-J, Jeng S-F. An alternative option to overcome difficult venous return in head and neck free flap reconstruction. J Plast Reconstr Aesthet Surg. 2013;66(9):1243–7.
5. Koerdt S, Tanner N, Rommel N, Rohleder NH, Stoeckelhuber M, Wolff K-D, et al. An immunohistochemical study on the role of oxidative and nitrosative stress in irradiated skin. Cells Tissues Organs (Print). 2017;203(1):12–9.
6. Frohwitter G, Rau A, Kesting MR, Fichter A. Microvascular reconstruction in the vessel depleted neck – a systematic review. J Craniomaxillofac Surg. 2018;46(9):1652–8.
7. Van Den Berg J. Myoelastic-aerodynamic theory of voice production. J Speech Hear Res. 1958;1(3):227–44.
8. Hirano M. Morphological structure of the vocal cord as a vibrator and its variations. Folia Phoniatr (Basel). 1974;26(2):89–94.
9. Ozgur Z, Govsa F, Ozgur T. Assessment of origin characteristics of the front branches of the external carotid artery. J Craniofac Surg. 2008;19(4):1159–66.
10. Won S-Y. Anatomical considerations of the superior thyroid artery: its origins, variations, and position relative to the hyoid bone and thyroid cartilage. Anat Cell Biol. 2016;49(2):138–42.
11. van Es RJ, Thuau H. Pirogoff's triangle revisited: an alternative site for microvascular anastomosis to the lingual artery. A technical note. Int J Oral Maxillofac Surg. 2000;29(3):207–9.
12. Seki S, Sumida K, Yamashita K, Baba O, Kitamura S. Gross anatomical classification of the courses of the human lingual artery. Surg Radiol Anat. 2017;39(2):195–203.
13. Pilsl U, Anderhuber F, Neugebauer S. The facial artery-the main blood vessel for the anterior face? Dermatol Surg. 2016;42(2):203–8.
14. Shima H, von Luedinghausen M, Ohno K, Michi K. Anatomy of microvascular anastomosis in the neck. Plast Reconstr Surg. 1998;101(1):33–41.
15. Deepak CA, Sarvadnya JJ, Sabitha KS. Variant anatomy of internal jugular vein branching. Ann Maxillofac Surg. 2015;5(2):284–6.
16. Reissis M, Reissis D, Bottini GB, Messiha A, Davies DC. A morphometric analysis of the suitability of the transverse cervical artery as a recipient artery in head and neck free flap microvascular reconstruction. Surg Radiol Anat. 2018;40(8):891–7.
17. Goodwin WJ, Rosenberg GJ. Venous drainage of the lateral trapezius musculocutaneous island flap. Arch Otolaryngol. 1982;108(7):411–3.
18. Tessler O, Gilardino MS, Bartow MJ, St Hilaire H, Womac D, Dionisopoulos T, et al. Transverse cervical artery: consistent anatomical landmarks and clinical experience with its use as a recipient artery in complex head and neck reconstruction. Plast Reconstr Surg. 2017;139(3):745e–51e.
19. Yu P. The transverse cervical vessels as recipient vessels for previously treated head and neck cancer patients. Plast Reconstr Surg. 2005;115(5):1253–8.
20. Geddes CR, Tang M, Yang D, Morris SF. An assessment of the anatomical basis of the thoracoacromial artery perforator flap. Can J Plast Surg. 2003;11(1):23–7.
21. Friedrich W, Lierse W, Herberhold C. Myocutaneous vascular territory of the thoracoacromial artery. A topographical and morphometric study of the arterial vascularization of the pectoralis major myocutaneous flap. Acta Anat (Basel). 1988;131(4):284–91.
22. Aycock JK, Stenson KM, Gottlieb LJ. The thoracoacromial trunk: alternative recipient vessels in reoperative head and neck reconstructive microsurgery. Plast Reconstr Surg. 2008;121(1):88–94.
23. Kompatscher P, Manestar M, Schuster A, Lang A, Beer GM. The thoracoacromial vessels as recipient vessels in microsurgery and supermicrosurgery: an anatomical and sonographic study. Plast Reconstr Surg. 2005;115(1):77–83.
24. Yeri LA, Houghton EJ, Palmieri B, Flores M, Gergely M, Gómez JE. Cephalic vein. Detail of its anatomy in the deltopectoral triangle. Int J Morphol. 2009;27(4):1037–42.
25. Hallock GG. The cephalic vein in microsurgery. Microsurgery. 1993;14(8):482–6.
26. Chen H-C, Ciudad P, Chen S-H, Agko M. Thirty-five years of single surgeon experience in the reconstruction of esophagus and voice with free ileocolon flap following total pharyngolaryngectomy. J Surg Oncol. 2018;117(3):459–68.
27. Chen H-C, Kim Evans KF, Salgado CJ, Mardini S. Methods of voice reconstruction. Semin Plast Surg. 2010;24(2):227–32.
28. Murray DJ, Novak CB, Neligan PC. Fasciocutaneous free flaps in pharyngolaryngo-oesophageal reconstruction: a critical review of the literature. J Plast Reconstr Aesthet Surg. 2008;61(10):1148–56.
29. Xu Z, Duan W, Zhang E, Bai S, Tian Y, Tan X, et al. Transverse cervical vessels as recipient vessels in oral and maxillofacial microsurgical reconstruction after former operations with or without radiotherapy. World J Surg Oncol. 2015;13:183.
30. Hong P, Taylor SM, Trites JR, Maclean J, Hart RD. Use of the external jugular vein as the sole recipient vein in head and neck free flap reconstruction. J Otolaryngol. 2006;35(6):361–5.
31. Shum JW, Melville JC, Couey M. Preparation of the neck for advanced flap reconstruction. Oral Maxillofac Surg Clin North Am. 2019;31(4):637–46.
32. Asouhidou I, Natsis K, Asteri T, Sountoulides P, Vlasis K, Tsikaras P. Anatomical variation of left internal jugular vein: clinical significance for an anaesthesiologist. Eur J Anaesthesiol. 2008;25(4):314–8.
33. Wax MK, Quraishi H, Rodman S, Granke K. Internal jugular vein patency in patients undergoing microvascular reconstruction. Laryngoscope. 1997;107(9):1245–8.
34. Chia H-L, Wong C-H, Tan B-K, Tan K-C, Ong Y-S. An algorithm for recipient vessel selection in microsurgical head and neck reconstruction. J Reconstr Microsurg. 2011;27(1):47–56.
35. Harris JR, Lueg E, Genden E, Urken ML. The thoracoacromial/cephalic vascular system for microvascular anastomoses in the vessel-depleted neck. Arch Otolaryngol Head Neck Surg. 2002;128(3):319–23.
36. Buck PM, Wax MK, Petrisor DI. Internal mammary vessels: alternate recipient vessels in microvascular head and neck reconstruction. J Oral Maxillofac Surg. 2016;74(9):1896.e1–6.
37. Chan D, Rabbani CC, Inman JC, Ducic Y. Cephalic vein transposition in the vessel-depleted neck. Otolaryngol Head Neck Surg. 2016;155(2):367–8.
38. Chen S-H, Tang Y-B, Chen H-C. Survival of transferred ileum after ischemia time longer than 1 hour: a clinical result different from animal studies. J Am Coll Surg. 2013;217(2):300–5.
39. Tsao C-K, Chen H-C, Chuang C-C, Chen H-T, Mardini S, Coskunfirat K. Adequate venous drainage: the most critical factor for a successful free jejunal transfer. Ann Plast Surg. 2004;53(3):229–34.
40. Chen H-C, Mardini S, Tsai F-C. "Airborne" suture tying technique for the microvascular anastomosis. Plast Reconstr Surg. 2004;113(4):1225–8.
41. Rampazzo A, Gharb BB, Spanio di Spilimbergo S, Chung K-P, Chen H-C. Voice reconstruction with free ileocolon flap transfer: implications for the lower respiratory tract. Plast Reconstr Surg. 2011;127(5):1916–24.

9 Recipient Vessels: Esophagus Reconstruction

Jennifer E. Fligor and Gregory R. D. Evans

Introduction

Defects involving the esophagus represent a uniquely complex challenge to the reconstructive surgeon. The planned operation must accomplish several aims: coverage of the defect, protection of vital structures of the neck, maintenance of continuity of the alimentary canal, and restoration of swallowing [1].

Most frequently resulting from removal of squamous cell carcinoma of the hypopharynx or larynx region, pathologies which commonly lead to defects of the cervical esophagus include isolated tumors of the esophagus, thyroid cancer, anastomotic or radiation-induced strictures, or tracheoesophageal or pharyngoesophageal fistulas [1]. Free tissue transfer has surpassed older methods of reconstruction—namely, local and regional flaps and pedicled jejunum and colon flaps [1]—and offers the benefit of immediate reconstruction, expediting the patient's transition to swallowing and aiding in oral nutrition intake [2]. While there are several options for free tissue transfer, and a number of possible recipient vessels, these cases often involve a "vessel-depleted" or "frozen" neck secondary to resection and treatment of malignancy. It is therefore vital that the surgeon be equipped with knowledge of various possible recipient vessels for esophageal reconstruction in the neck, as well as ways to optimize surgical technique, postoperative management, and—if necessary—reoperation in order to maximize outcomes for these patients.

The bulk of this chapter focuses on the recipient vessels available in esophagus reconstruction, and the pertinent anatomy, benefits, and downsides associated with each vessel option. In free tissue transfer-based esophageal reconstruction, as with all microsurgery, recipient vessel selection is one of the greatest keys to success: selection of the largest available vessels with the best flow and pedicle geometry helps to optimize the operation [2].

J. E. Fligor · G. R. D. Evans (✉)
Department of Plastic Surgery, University of California, Irvine, Irvine, CA, USA
e-mail: jfligor@hs.uci.edu; gevans@hs.uci.edu

Overview of Free Tissue Transfer Options

Several flaps can be considered for free tissue transfer to reconstruct esophageal defects. As the focus of this chapter is recipient vessels, we do not go into extensive detail on choice of flap or surgical technique. However, we broadly describe three of the most common flaps used for this type of reconstruction: the free jejunal flap, radial forearm flap, and anterolateral thigh flap.

The free jejunal flap is one commonly utilized free flap for esophageal reconstruction. The flap was first described by Seidenberg and colleagues in 1958, as a technique for single-stage immediate esophageal reconstruction. This flap provided a number of advantages over earlier techniques of reconstruction, such as split-thickness skin graft. Besides allowing for reconstruction in a single stage, use of the jejunal free flap did not involve a pharyngostome, allowed for wider excision, and eliminated the issue of early strictures and frequent pharyngeal leaks [3]. The jejunum is supplied by five jejunal branches off the superior mesenteric artery, and can supply sufficient donor tissue to reconstruct large defects [4]. Typically, the flap is harvested 40 to 70 cm from the ligament of Treitz, with either the second or third jejunal branch of the superior mesenteric vessels serving as the vascular pedicle, and aligned such that it is isoperistaltic [1, 4, 5]. Morbidity associated with the flap can include difficulty swallowing if redundancy develops in the flap over time, poor tracheoesophageal puncture voice quality, excessive mucosal secretions, and high stricture rates [1, 4, 5]. Entry into the abdomen represents another downside [1, 4]. Rates of fistula associated with this flap are low [1].

R. Gurunian, R. Djohan (eds.), *Recipient Vessels in Reconstructive Microsurgery*,
https://doi.org/10.1007/978-3-030-75389-4_9

Another option for free tissue transfer is the radial forearm flap. The radial forearm flap has a long pedicle (up to 20 cm), and is thin and flexible, allowing for tubing [4, 6]. Other advantages include association with good tracheoesophageal puncture voice following vocal rehabilitation and good swallowing [1]. This flap has moderate rates of stricture and fistula formation [1]. The major disadvantage of the radial forearm flap is donor site morbidity, which can be lessened by designing the flap along the longitudinal axis of the arm, such that the proximal-to-distal axis of the flap will become the circumferential axis of the tubed flap [1]. The flap's multiple perforators have been described as permitting design of two or more skin paddles, with one skin paddle used to reconstruct the anterior esophagus defect, while the other(s) serve to reconstruct neck skin and allow for external monitoring of the flap [1]. However, in the experience of the senior author, a skin bridge is typically necessary between skin paddles, limiting reconstruction of both the circumferential esophageal and skin defects with this single flap. Vascular compromise of the extremity can be avoided by performing an Allen test to confirm adequate ulnar blood supply to the hand prior to harvest of the flap on the radial artery pedicle [4]. The donor site may require a skin graft, particularly if a large flap is harvested [4].

A third source of donor tissue is the anterolateral thigh (ALT) flap. This flap is supplied by the descending branch of the lateral circumflex femoral artery, which can be quickly dissected from along the medial edge of the vastus lateralis. It is typically a thin and flexible flap amenable to reconstruction of the upper esophagus, though it can have bulkier subcutaneous tissue in obese individuals [4]. The upsides of this flap include low donor site morbidity, fast recovery time, low rates of stricture and fistula, and association with good swallowing and tracheoesophageal puncture voice quality [1]. It is possible to utilize more than one of the available ALT perforators to supply two skin paddles for reconstruction of the esophagus and neck skin, respectively [1]. However, in the senior author's experience, pedicle geometry may limit the success of this sort of split-skin paddle reconstruction. The anteromedial thigh flap can be evaluated using the same incision used to access the ALT flap if adequate perforators are not found with the former [1].

Selection of the most appropriate reconstructive flap must take into account characteristics of the defect, patient factors, and the strengths and drawbacks of each option. Regardless of the flap selected, a successful operation depends on reliable vascular inflow and outflow. The remainder of this chapter discusses various recipient vessels available in the neck, as well as select operative and postoperative technique to help optimize esophagus reconstruction.

Recipient Arteries: External Carotid Arterial System

The typical recipient arteries used in esophageal reconstruction are those of the ipsilateral external carotid arterial system. Use of the internal carotid artery is precluded by several factors: its crucial role as vascular supply to the brain, unfavorable location, and lack of extracranial branches [7]. The external carotid artery, by contrast, has a number of accessible branches which may be considered as recipient vessels (Fig. 9.1).

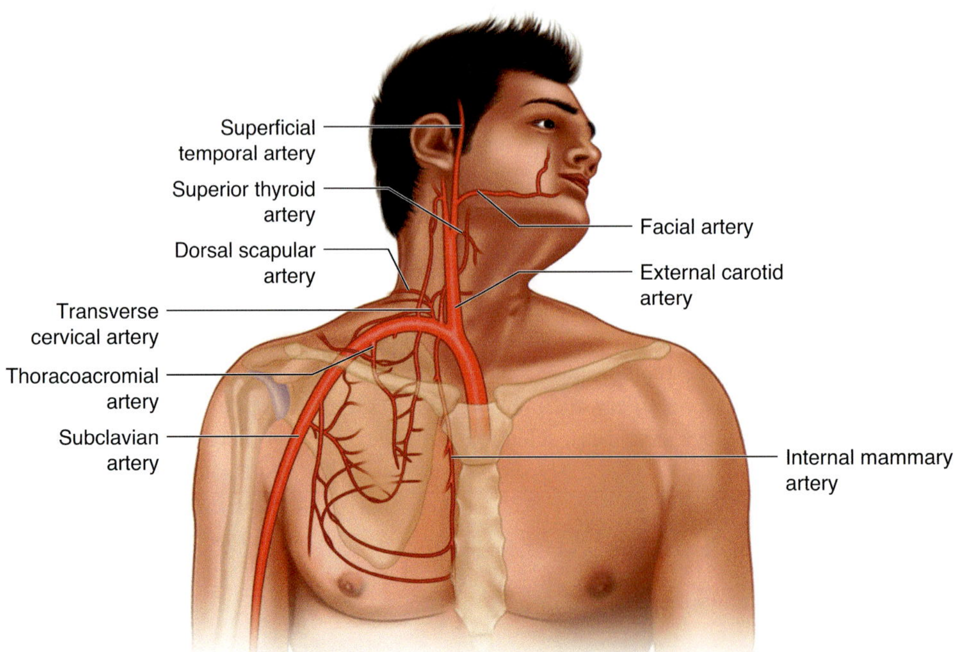

Fig. 9.1 Illustration of recipient artery options for esophagus reconstruction

At the time of reconstruction, exposure of the external carotid vessels will depend on the timing and extent of extirpative surgery. If the vessels are not yet exposed, a transverse incision is made extending from the thyroid cartilage to the mastoid process. The surgeon must incise the platysma and deep cervical fascia and locate the anterior border of the sternocleidomastoid muscle, which is then mobilized and retracted to reveal the carotid sheath, taking care to protect the marginal mandibular branch of the facial nerve. The facial vein is clipped or ligated (if not intended for use in the reconstruction). The carotid sheath is then opened and the internal jugular vein retracted. The external carotid artery will be seen branching from the common carotid artery near the superior edge of the thyroid cartilage, the superior thyroid artery slightly more superior, the lingual vessel level with the greater horn of the hyoid bone, and the facial artery superior to the lingual artery branch point [8].

The facial artery, located at the inferior border of the mandible, has an adequate diameter and flow for use as a recipient vessel. When exposing this vessel, extra care must be taken to avoid injury to the marginal mandibular branch of the facial nerve [7].

The superior thyroid artery is a common choice of recipient vessel within this system. This vessel branches from the external carotid artery 1 cm inferior to the branch point of the facial artery, and tracks toward the thyroid gland [7]. In 1980, Hester and colleagues described a series of 17 free jejunal transfers for reconstruction of the cervical esophagus and hypopharynx. They describe a two-team approach in which one team prepares the recipient vessel, typically a proximal branch of the external carotid, usually the superior thyroid artery. Their experience included a patient with carotid atherosclerosis who had undergone carotid endarterectomy on the same side as the recipient vessel, and noted that the superior thyroid artery was isolated without difficulty, and provided adequate flow to the jejunal flap. Their experience also included a number of patients treated with radiation without flap complication [9].

The superficial temporal artery has been used successfully in microsurgical reconstruction in the head and neck [10]. However, the location of this most cranial branch in the external carotid system makes it an impractical recipient vessel for esophageal reconstruction when any other recipient vessels are available for anastomosis without use of vein grafts.

The anatomic features of the maxillary artery, the ascending pharyngeal artery, and the posterior auricular artery, respectively, are generally unfavorable for microsurgical use. The occipital artery, though usable in head and neck reconstruction, is less suitably positioned for esophageal defects [7].

Though often the first choice in esophagus reconstruction, several downsides to use of the external carotid artery system should be noted. First, these vessels tend to be more affected by atherosclerosis than other vessels of the neck. Additionally, the location of the branches of the external carotid artery typically lies above the angle of the mandible, making access difficult, and possibly requiring transposition of the external carotid system for anastomosis. Anastomosis to the common carotid itself, rather than to a branch vessel, is challenging due to both intimal friability and significant wall thickness discrepancy between the donor vessel and the common carotid [11]. Finally, concern for potential cerebral injury in patients with incomplete circle of Willis should be considered.

Recipient Veins: Internal and External Jugular Venous System

The ipsilateral internal and external jugular venous systems are the primary choice for recipient veins in esophageal reconstruction (Fig. 9.2).

Recipient vein options in the internal jugular system include the facial vein, superior thyroid vein, and lingual vein, which may coalesce into a single vessel: the thyrolinguofacial trunk. The deep location of the system's other veins makes their use less favorable [7].

The more superficial external jugular vein also offers branches which can serve as recipient veins: the superficial temporal vein and anterior jugular vein. The small size of the posterior auricular vein makes it a less favorable choice [7]. Finally, the external jugular vein can serve as the recipient vein [7]. During the neck dissection, the external jugular vein can be isolated and preserved, or left intact below the platysma and raised with the skin and muscle [11]. The vein must be protected and kept moist until anastomosis, paying attention to neck positioning to avoid predisposing the vessel to thrombosis during the course of the procedure [11]. The same characteristic which makes the external jugular so easy to access—its superficial lie—also represents a susceptibility of the vessel to sacrifice during extirpation procedures [7].

While adequate venous drainage is necessary for the survival of any free tissue transfer, the jejunal free flap is particularly non-forgiving of ischemia, and venous output may represent a uniquely important aspect of flap planning if this flap is chosen [12]. Tsao and colleagues (2004) identify adequate venous drainage as "the most critical factor" in performing esophageal reconstruction with this flap [12]. The jejunal vein generally outsizes neck recipient veins, except for the internal and external jugular veins. The authors found reduced venous congestion associated with use of these recipient veins, compared to other recipient vessels [12].

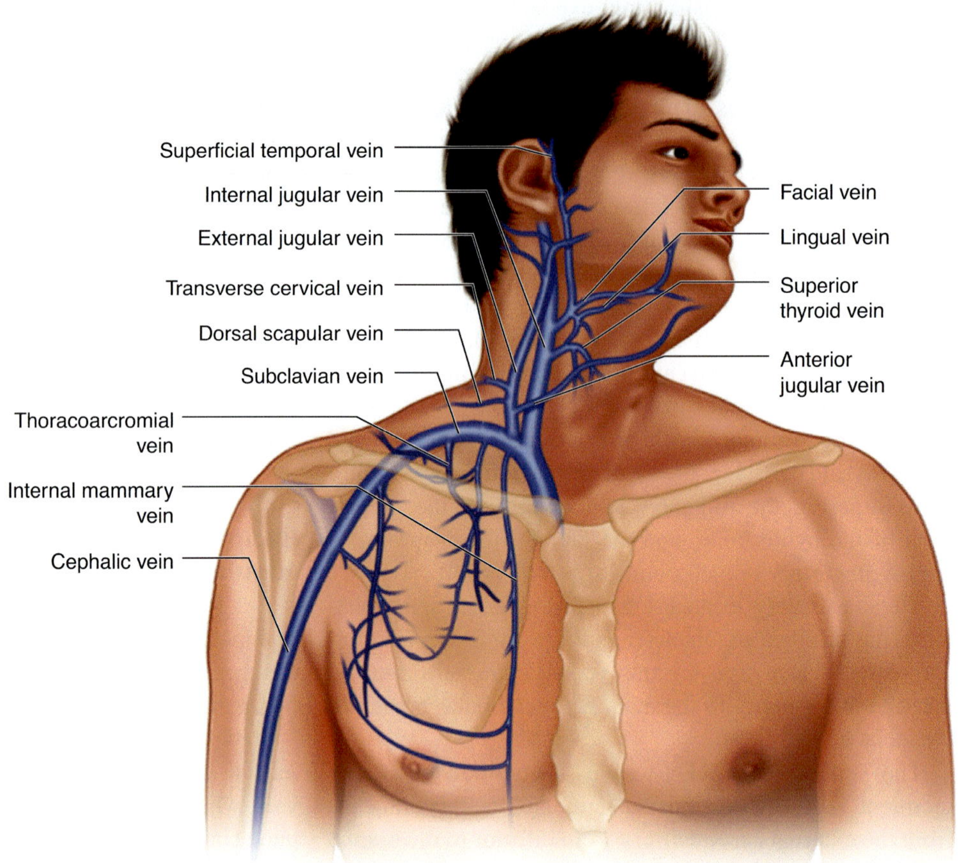

Fig. 9.2 Illustration of recipient vein options for esophagus reconstruction

Recipient Vessels in the Vessel-Depleted Neck

Head and neck reconstructive surgery is often complicated by the challenge of the vessel-depleted neck. Several factors may contribute to a lack of suitable recipient vessels in these difficult cases. Radiation-associated fibrosis can create a "frozen neck," as can scarring and disruption of tissue planes associated with prior surgeries [13]. Pharyngocutaneous fistulas can worsen the scarring and inflammation of an already fibrotic radiated neck by introducing saliva into the field [1]. The resection procedure may involve removal of or disruption—purposeful or inadvertent—of potential recipient vessels; if extirpation and reconstruction occur on the same day, as is often the case, preoperative planning around vessel availability may be complicated [13]. In their 2008 review of 261 head and neck free flaps, Hanasono and colleagues found that the ipsilateral external carotid artery or branch of this vessel was unavailable in 19% of the cases, and the ipsilateral internal and external jugular veins were unavailable in 16% of the cases. While the majority of cases in which these primary-choice vessels were not available presented in necks which had undergone prior neck dissection, irradiation, or both, a number of such situations presented in necks which had undergone neither therapy [13]. This highlights the imperative nature of approaching cases of esophageal reconstruction with an understanding of the alternative recipient vessel options available in the neck. The following sections will focus on these alternatives to the ipsilateral external carotid and internal and external jugular systems.

Contralateral Neck Vessels

One possible approach to cases in which the first-choice recipient vessels are unavailable is use of the contralateral neck. While the contralateral neck may provide vessels free of the fibrosis and disrupted tissue planes of an ipsilateral "frozen neck," use of these vessels introduces the downside of an additional donor site [13].

The surgeon has several options for reaching recipient vessels in the contralateral neck. First, reconstruction can be performed with a flap with a sufficiently long pedicle. A second option is to use vein grafts. The senior author prefers to avoid the use of vein grafts, which add additional anastomoses. Other downsides of vein grafts, particularly long grafts, include vein graft donor site morbidity and increased operative time and increased risk of thrombosis due to graft compression or kinking [13]. Vein grafts may also be associated with a lower rate of technical success [14]. A third option is transfer of a "secondary" flap. This additional free tissue can be either anastomosed to the primary reconstructive flap as a "flow-through" flap or, preferably, anastomosed to a branch of the primary flap proximal vascular pedicle [13].

Transverse Cervical Vessels

The transverse cervical artery and its accompanying vein represent alternative recipient vessel options for microsurgical reconstruction in the vessel-depleted neck.

These vessels can be accessed by extending a cervical incision inferiorly toward the ipsilateral acromial process [13]. The largest of the thyrocervical trunk branches, the transverse cervical artery, travels beneath the trapezius muscle [11] and can be found in loose fatty tissue above the clavicle and deep to the omohyoid muscle, lateral to the sternocleidomastoid [13, 15]. The vein may be deep to or, less often, superficial to the omohyoid muscle, usually caudal to the artery [15]. The vessels are typically within 10 cm of the angle of the mandible [15]. For reconstruction of the esophagus, if the sternocleidomastoid muscle has been mobilized, the pedicle of the flap can be placed beneath the muscle. Alternatively, the pedicle can be positioned over the muscle, or the sternal head of the muscle can be released to avoid tension on an underlying pedicle [15].

Use of the transverse cervical artery as a recipient vessel for esophageal reconstruction presents several benefits. One such benefit is a position more conducive to suturing [15]. Additionally, supraclavicular anastomosis typically allows for straight positioning of the pedicle with minimal kinking [15], making it less susceptible to changes in tension and redundancy [11]. These vessels are typically less atherosclerotic than the carotid vessels [11]. In a patient known to have significant neck scarring and fibrosis, planning to use the transverse cervical vessels could allow the surgeon to avoid the carotid artery system altogether [15]. These vessels are adequately sized for anastomosis. Yu and colleagues (2005) found 70% of the arteries and 55% of the veins to measure between 2 and 3 mm in diameter (24% of arteries and 6% of veins measured less than 2 mm across, and 27% of veins exceeded 3 mm in diameter) [15]. In this series, absent or small ipsilateral transverse cervical vessels were encountered in 23% of the patients, and 8% of the patients were found to have unusable transverse cervical vessels bilaterally [15]. A vein graft is not typically required to reach these vessels, and if necessary, the graft can be short [13, 15].

On the left side of the neck, the surgeon must be cognizant of the location of the thoracic duct. Lymphatic leak should be explored under the microscope and repaired with 10-0 suture, if identified [15]. On the right side of the neck, the surgery should limit exploration supraclavicularly protecting the apex of the lung and the subclavian vessels [15].

Subclavian Artery, Thoracoacromial Vessels, and Internal Mammary Vessels

Branches of the subclavian system, as well as the subclavian artery itself, can be utilized as recipient vessels [7].

The thoracoacromial artery has been described as a recipient artery in esophagus reconstruction [16, 17]. To expose the vessels, the pectoralis major muscle is divided inferior to the clavicle. Two branches, the deltoid branch and pectoral branch, can be exposed beneath the pectoralis major muscle, and either may be used for the anastomosis [16]. The thoracoacromial vessels are of good size. In their anatomic study, Kompatscher and colleagues (2005) found the average diameters of 3.1 mm for both the vein and artery [18]. Typically, the artery is paired with two veins [18]. Of note, the vessels have been noted to remain usable after both radiation and prior head and neck reconstruction with a pectoralis major myocutaneous flap [19].

The internal mammary artery and vein represent additional vessel options. The location of these vessels is particularly advantageous for thoracic esophageal defects [20]. Exposure of these vessels involves division of the pectoralis major and, if needed, removal of the costal cartilage of the second or third rib [13]. The surgeon then carefully elevates the perichondrium of the undersurface of the costal cartilage in a medial direction to reveal the vessels [13]. Downsides of these recipient vessels include increased operative time required for exposure, risk of a pneumothorax, and elimination of the vessels as an option for use in future coronary bypass surgery [13, 18]. In addition, the internal mammary veins may be fragile with unreliable anatomy [18].

Dorsal Scapular Vessels

The dorsal scapular artery and vein could be considered for use as recipient vessels in esophagus reconstruction. Though this use has not been described in the literature, use of both vessels for head and neck reconstruction with free tissue transfer has been described [21]. The dorsal scapular artery typically branches from the subclavian artery and travels with the dorsal scapular vein passing through the brachial plexus. These vessels tend to lay outside of the field of prior surgery or radiation, making them a possible choice in a vessel-depleted neck. In their CT analysis of several reconstructive cases, Rosko and colleagues (2007) found the artery to have a mean diameter of 1.8 mm, 42 mm from the subclavian artery, and 1.3 mm more distal, at 65 mm from the subclavian artery. Due to the location of these vessels, a long flap pedicle or vein graft may be needed to make the necessary anastomoses. Exposure of the vessels also requires attention to several surrounding structures—including the lung, thoracic duct, brachial plexus, and nearby vessels—to avoid related complications [21].

Cephalic Vein

In addition to the recipient veins noted, the cephalic vein can be utilized for venous drainage in reconstruction of the esophagus [17, 20].

This cephalic vein can be transposed into the cervical or thoracic region for anastomosis. A good length of vein can be freed if dissection is carried into the antecubital fossa [22] to a point a few centimeters proximal to the elbow flexion crease [13]. This allows the vein freedom to reach the necessary anastomosis point without unfavorable geometry at the pivot point of this vein, its point of entry to the costocoracoid fascia before it combines with the axillary vein [13]. This venous system is high-flow and low-pressure, permitting significant venous outflow into the cephalic vein from transferred tissue [22]. It is also adequately sized. An anatomic study by Reid and Taylor (1984) found the vein to have an average diameter of 5.4 mm, with diameters ranging from 1.0 to 12.0 mm [23]. Low functional morbidity is associated with use of this vessel [17]. Harvest of the vein can result in a long donor site incision, though an alternative approach using several short incisions, or even endoscopic guidance, can be used to avoid this type of scar [13, 22]. In the previously operated or radiated neck, the cephalic vein offers the added benefit of typically lying outside of the field of prior treatment [22].

Technique

In complement to this review of options for recipient vessels for esophagus reconstruction, we present select points of technique which may prove useful in this context. These include considerations related to preoperative assessment, the microvascular anastomosis, use of anticoagulation, and postoperative management.

Preoperative Assessment

Preparation for esophageal reconstruction should include standard preoperative evaluation, including a complete history and physical, appropriate assessment of cardiovascular health, and laboratory screening. Special attention should be paid to history of surgery on or trauma to the neck. The senior author does not routinely perform preoperative computed tomography angiography (CTA), though this step may be considered to evaluate potential recipient and donor vessel patency [24].

Anastomosis

Consideration of vessel geometry is crucial when performing any anastomosis, but anastomosis performed in the neck for reconstruction of the esophagus presents unique challenges.

To assess for adequacy or excess of pedicle length, the surgeon can clamp the vessels in an approximated position and then range the neck through a full range of motion to evaluate for tension or redundancy. This should be repeated once the anastomosis is complete. A perivascular tacking suture can be considered as a tool to improve pedicle positioning, though caution should be taken to avoid kinking the vessel with this maneuver [11].

To minimize ischemia time, the senior author recommends first creating an arteriovenous loop with the recipient artery and vein, and allowing blood to flow through the loop for a minimum of 30 min to ensure that there are no problems prior to attaching the flap to the loop.

In any microsurgical case, the type of anastomosis depends on the vessels available and the flow through those vessels. While the senior author prefers to perform end-to-end anastomosis when possible, end-to-side anastomoses can be made with the external carotid artery and internal jugular vein (Fig. 9.3). In their prospective comparison of venous end-to-side and end-to-end anastomoses in 422 patients with head and neck free tissue transfer, Piazza and colleagues (2014) took this approach—preferentially performing end-to-end anastomosis, but using end-to-side anastomosis to the internal jugular vein if necessary—and found no statistically significant difference in venous anastomosis re-exploration and failure rates [25]. When arterial end-to-side anastomosis is required, the senior author uses a size 2.5 or 2.7 aortic punch to perforate the external carotid artery (Fig. 9.3). He secures the donor artery to the recipient artery at the cranial and caudal aspects of the perforation, 180 degrees apart, and then uses running suture to secure each side of the anastomosis.

With regard to use of couplers, there are benefits and drawbacks to the use of these devices. Some literature suggests that couplers allow for much faster anastomosis: Assoumane and colleagues (2017) found in their experience with 854 venous and arterial couplers in head and neck free tissue transfer that mean time for completion of coupler-based anastomoses was 10 minutes, compared to a mean time of 43 minutes for hand-sewn anastomosis [26]. Coupler-

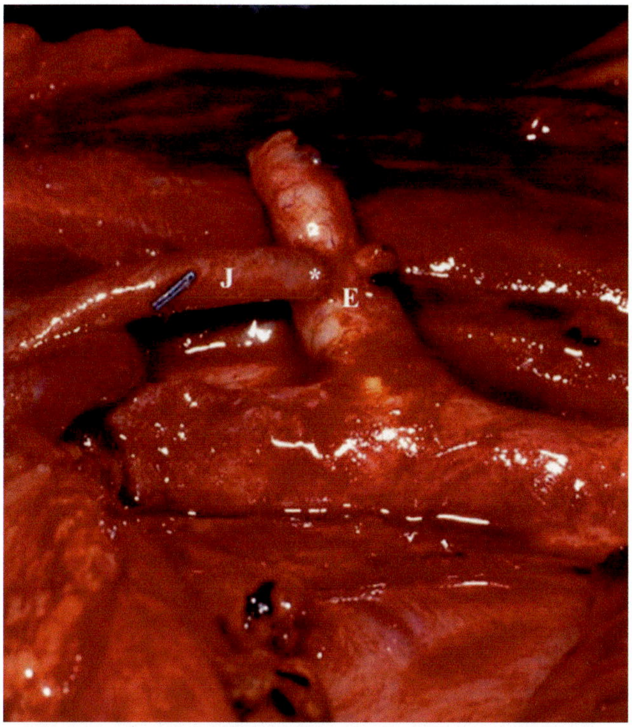

Fig. 9.3 End-to-side anastomosis in a free jejunal transfer of a jejunal branch of the superior mesenteric artery to a ligated stump of the external carotid artery. * anastomosis site, J jejunal branch of superior mesenteric artery, E ligated stump of the external carotid artery

based anastomoses may also be less thrombogenic. Wain and colleagues (2014) modeled blood through idealized sutured and coupled arterial anastomoses using computational fluid dynamics. They report a 28% increase in average wall shear stress in a sutured anastomosis compared to a coupled anastomosis. Those authors note that wall shear stress is associated with atheroma formation and platelet activation, and suggest that coupled anastomoses may, therefore, be less prone to thrombosis than their hand-sewn counterparts [27]. The senior author only uses a coupler for venous end-to-end anastomoses.

Anticoagulation

The senior author uses irrigation including 10,000 units of heparin and irrigates thoroughly locally in the area of the anastomosis. Esophageal and/or other head and neck reconstruction is unique in that the region is relatively unforgiving of small bleeds, which can quickly compress the fresh anastomosis. The senior author therefore does not routinely use systemic anticoagulation, making use of it only in cases of specific concern for hypercoagulability or if the case has required reoperation. Aspirin is not used, and DVT chemoprophylaxis is typically held for at least 24–48 hours postoperatively, again barring specific concerns for hypercoagulability. Optimization of other antithrombogenic factors—selection of appropriate recipient vessels which allow for adequate blood flow, proper operative technique during anastomosis, and assuring favorable pedicle geometry—can help the surgeon avoid the need for systemic anticoagulation [2].

Postoperative Care

The patient is typically kept intubated overnight and extubated on the morning of the first postoperative day. This approach maximizes patient safety by securing the airway during the most high-risk period of significant neck edema following a lengthy procedure. The patient should be kept well-hydrated following the procedure. As the patient begins to mobilize and ambulate, insufficient intravascular volume may result in partial vein collapse, which can be thrombogenic in irradiated vessels; adequate fluid administration can help to avoid this. The patient's head should be elevated at least 10–15 degrees at all times. While the senior author discourages immobilizing the patient's head postoperatively, the patient should be educated to minimize excessive motion of the head and neck, and no pressure should be placed over the anastomosis.

The senior author recommends obtaining a radiographic esophageal swallow study 7–10 days following reconstruction to evaluate swallow. Drains should be left in place until after this study has been performed and drain output is less than 30 cc per day. If a leak in the flap inset occurs, it will most likely present within the first 1–2 days postoperatively; drain fluid can be sent to the laboratory and evaluated for amylase content to identify formation of a spit fistula.

It is crucial to have a low threshold for intraoperative evaluation of a failing flap. The effect of edema or bleeding is amplified in head and neck anastomoses because there is no room to accommodate the extra volume—it will be transmitted as pressure onto the anastomosis. If clot is identified in an end-to-side anastomosis, it may be acceptable to redo the same anastomosis. However, in the case of clot in an end-to-end anastomosis, it is often wise to identify an alternative recipient vessel.

Conclusion

Reconstruction of the esophagus presents a number of challenges. When the defect lies in a "frozen" or vessel-depleted neck previously affected by surgery, radiation, or saliva per fistula, the task of rebuilding the alimentary conduit with free tissue transfer can seem daunting. Many factors, including choice of flap, surgical technique, and postoperative management—not to mention patient factors such as comorbidities and compliance—contribute to the likelihood of operative success or failure. However, appropriate choice of recipient vessel lays the foundation for the operation. Therefore, a command of the recipient vessels available for use proves crucial in these cases.

As discussed throughout this chapter, the anatomy, state of the operative field, and available vessels will vary from patient to patient based on their prior treatment. Therefore, rather than proposing an algorithmic approach to the choice of recipient vessel, we recommend a holistic, case-by-case assessment. Armed with the specific case characteristics, and knowledge of the anatomy, benefits, and drawbacks of different vessel options, the surgeon can formulate an operative plan that best serves the patient's needs while remaining flexible to make intraoperative adjustments.

References

1. Yu P. Pharyngoesophageal reconstruction. In: Hanasono M, Robb GL, Skoracki RJ, Yu P, editors. Reconstructive plastic surgery of the head and neck. 1st ed. New York: Thieme; 2016.
2. Evans G, Kaplan J. Principles of microsurgery. In: Evans GRD, editor. Operative plastic surgery. 2nd ed. New York: Oxford University Press; 2019.
3. Seidenberg B, Rosenak SS, Hurwitt ES, Som ML. Immediate reconstruction of the cervical esophagus by a revascularized isolated jejunal segment. Ann Surg. 1959;149(2):162–71. https://doi.org/10.1097/00000658-195902000-00002.
4. Kim EK, Evangelista M, Evans GR. Use of free tissue transfers in head and neck reconstruction. J Craniofac Surg. 2008;19(6):1577–82. https://doi.org/10.1097/SCS.0b013e3181897376.
5. Reece GP, Bengtson BP, Schusterman MA. Reconstruction of the pharynx and cervical esophagus using free jejunal transfer. Clin Plast Surg. 1994;21(1):125–36.
6. Mathes SJNF. Reconstructive surgery: principles, anatomy, and techniques. New York: Churchill Livingstone; 1997.
7. Bourget A, Wei F. Choosing recipient vessels. In: Neligan P, Wei F, editors. Microsurgical reconstruction of the head and neck. 1st ed. New York: Thieme; 2009.
8. Strauch BYH. Head and neck. In: Atlas of microvascular surgery: anatomy and operative approaches. 2nd ed. New York: Thieme; 2006.
9. Hester TR, McConnel FM, Nahal F, Jurkiewicz MJ, Brown RG. Reconstruction of cervical esophagus, hypopharynx and oral cavity using free jejunal transfer. Am J Surg. 1980;140(4):487–91. https://doi.org/10.1016/0002-9610(80)90197-x.
10. Shimizu F, Lin MP, Ellabban M, Evans GR, Cheng MH. Superficial temporal vessels as a reserve recipient site for microvascular head and neck reconstruction in vessel-depleted neck. Ann Plast Surg. 2009;62(2):134–8. https://doi.org/10.1097/SAP.0b013e318172b91d.
11. Urken ML, Vickery C, Weinberg H, Buchbinder D, Biller HF. Geometry of the vascular pedicle in free tissue transfers to the head and neck. Arch Otolaryngol Head Neck Surg. 1989;115(8):954–60.
12. Tsao CK, Chen HC, Chuang CC, Chen HT, Mardini S, Coskunfirat K. Adequate venous drainage: the most critical factor for a successful free jejunal transfer. Ann Plast Surg. 2004;53(3):229–34.
13. Hanasono MM, Barnea Y, Skoracki RJ. Microvascular surgery in the previously operated and irradiated neck. Microsurgery. 2009;29(1):1–7. https://doi.org/10.1002/micr.20560.
14. Miller MJ, Schusterman MA, Reece GP, Kroll SS. Interposition vein grafting in head and neck reconstructive microsurgery. J Reconstr Microsurg. 1993;9(3):245–51; discussion 51-2. https://doi.org/10.1055/s-2007-1006652.
15. Yu P. The transverse cervical vessels as recipient vessels for previously treated head and neck cancer patients. Plast Reconstr Surg. 2005;115(5):1253–8.
16. Numajiri T, Fujiwara T, Nishino K, Sowa Y, Uenaka M, Shimada T, et al. The thoracoacromial artery as the recipient artery for safer free jejunal transfer in patients with irradiated, extensively scarred necks. Br J Oral Maxillofac Surg. 2009;47(1):73–4. https://doi.org/10.1016/j.bjoms.2008.05.006.
17. Fujita H, Inoue Y, Kakegawa T, Yamana H, Shirozu G, Minami T, et al. Esophageal reconstruction using microvascular anastomosis to the thoracoacromial artery and cephalic vein. Jpn J Surg. 1991;21(5):512–6.
18. Kompatscher P, Manestar M, Schuster A, Lang A, Beer GM. The thoracoacromial vessels as recipient vessels in microsurgery and supermicrosurgery: an anatomical and sonographic study. Plast Reconstr Surg. 2005;115(1):77–83.
19. Aycock JK, Stenson KM, Gottlieb LJ. The thoracoacromial trunk: alternative recipient vessels in reoperative head and neck reconstructive microsurgery. Plast Reconstr Surg. 2008;121(1):88–94. https://doi.org/10.1097/01.prs.0000293858.11494.96.
20. Miyamoto S, Kayano S, Fujiki M, Sakuraba M. Combined use of the cephalic vein and pectoralis major muscle flap for secondary esophageal reconstruction. Microsurgery. 2014;34(4):319–23.
21. Rosko AJ, Ryan JT, Wizauer EJ, Ibrahim M, Srinivasan A, Stucken CL, et al. Dorsal scapular artery as a recipient vessel in the vessel-depleted neck during free tissue transfer in head and neck reconstruction. Head Neck. 2017;39(7):E72–e6. https://doi.org/10.1002/hed.24785.
22. Kim KA, Chandrasekhar BS. Cephalic vein in salvage microsurgical reconstruction in the head and neck. Br J Plast Surg. 1998;51(1):2–7.
23. Reid CD, Taylor GI. The vascular territory of the acromiothoracic axis. Br J Plast Surg. 1984;37(2):194–212.
24. Hanasono MM, Skoracki RJ. Imaging and computer modeling in head and neck reconstruction. In: Hanasono M, Robb GL, Skoracki RJ, Yu P, editors. Reconstructive plastic surgery of the head and neck: current techniques and flap atlas. 1st ed. New York: Theime; 2016.
25. Piazza C, Taglietti V, Paderno A, Nicolai P. End-to-end versus end-to-side venous microanastomoses in head and neck reconstruction. Eur Arch Otorhinolaryngol. 2014;271(1):157–62. https://doi.org/10.1007/s00405-013-2496-y.
26. Assoumane A, Wang L, Liu K, Shang ZJ. Use of couplers for vascular anastomoses in 601 free flaps for reconstruction of defects of the head and neck: technique and two-year retrospective clinical study. Br J Oral Maxillofac Surg. 2017;55(5):461–4. https://doi.org/10.1016/j.bjoms.2016.10.001.
27. Wain RA, Whitty JP, Dalal MD, Holmes MC, Ahmed W. Blood flow through sutured and coupled microvascular anastomoses: a comparative computational study. J Plast Reconstr Aesthet Surg. 2014;67(7):951–9. https://doi.org/10.1016/j.bjps.2014.03.016.

Part III

Trunk Reconstruction

Internal Mammary Vessels: Inframammary and Standard Approach

10

Christina Dami Lee, Rebecca Knackstedt, Graham Schwarz, Michelle Djohan, and Risal Djohan

Introduction

Cancer is the second leading cause of death in the United States [1]. It is predicted that 30% of newly diagnosed cancer in 2020 for female patients will be breast cancer [1]. Although the mortality rate from breast cancer has decreased, there is a rising trend in incidence of breast cancer since 2004 in the United States [1]. In 1998, the Women's Health and Cancer Right Act granted insurance coverage for breast reconstruction for breast cancer patients [2–5]. Since then, there has been a steady increase in breast reconstruction.

It is reported that autologous breast reconstruction has higher satisfaction in aesthetic results, lower rates of complications and failure, fewer required clinic visits, faster completion of reconstruction, and higher overall long-term satisfaction [2, 3, 5–10]. The current gold standard for autologous breast reconstruction is the deep inferior epigastric artery perforator (DIEP) flap [2, 6]. Muscle sparing or non-muscle sparing transverse rectus abdominis myocutaneous (TRAM) muscle flap is also commonly utilized and shares the same recipient vessels. The internal mammary artery and vein (IMA, IMV) are the most preferred recipient vessels for microsurgical breast reconstruction [11]. They are preferred over other available vessels due to their large vessel caliber, high flow rate, and consistent location [12–15].

It is known that there is a steep learning curve associated with the recipient vessel exposure. Factors contributing to the difficulty of this dissection are chest wall mobility from respiration, history of radiation, anatomical variances, and surgeon experience. Traditionally, the mastectomy incision was limited in its variety, therefore deeming dissection and the exposure process to be more predictable. Recipient vessels are exposed most commonly at the levels of the second, third, and fourth intercostal space. With advancements and innovations in surgery, we are now able to offer different types of incisions following the design of mastectomy incision. Inframammary or lower pole incisions are commonly used to provide better cosmesis in reconstructive result. However, this poses a novel challenge to prepare and expose the recipient vessels. Currently, most commonly utilized mastectomy incisions are inframammary, vertical, and lateral (radial) incisions.

In this chapter, anatomy of the internal mammary vessels and techniques to aid their dissection and exposure will be discussed. The emphasis is placed on vessel preparation using the inframammary and lateral radial incisions, and in cases of delayed immediate reconstruction where a tissue expander was previously utilized at initial phase of reconstruction followed with radiation treatment prior to DIEP reconstruction.

Supplementary Information The online version of this chapter (https://doi.org/10.1007/978-3-030-75389-4_10) contains supplementary material, which is available to authorized users.

C. D. Lee · R. Knackstedt · G. Schwarz (✉)
Department of Plastic Surgery, Cleveland Clinic, Cleveland, OH, USA
e-mail: LEEC4@ccf.org; KNACKSR@ccf.org; SCHWARG@ccf.org

M. Djohan
Case Western Reserve University/MetroHealth Hospitals, Cleveland, OH, USA

R. Djohan
Department of Plastic Surgery, Cleveland Clinic, Cleveland, OH, USA

Cleveland Clinic Lerner College of Medicine, Case Western Reserve University, Cleveland, OH, USA
e-mail: djohanr@ccf.org

Preoperative Assessment

Although immediate breast reconstruction can provide significant psychosocial benefits to the patients, the utmost priority lies with treatment of breast cancer. It is important to coordinate care with the breast surgeon regarding the appropriate treatment especially the need and timing for radiation therapy, and type of mastectomy to be performed. Preoperative discussion between other care providers and with the patient will determine the appropriate course and timing of the treatment and reconstruction.

R. Gurunian, R. Djohan (eds.), *Recipient Vessels in Reconstructive Microsurgery*, https://doi.org/10.1007/978-3-030-75389-4_10

It is important to conduct a thorough preoperative evaluation of a patient's medical and surgical history and perform a physical exam with attention to breast anatomy and chest wall morphology. In addition to a carefully designed and executed DIEP free flap dissection, recipient vessel site preparation is also critical for successful microsurgical reconstruction. Robust and un-injured recipient internal mammary vessels would provide good arterial inflow and venous outflow for flap perfusion. A few key considerations when assessing the use of internal mammary vessels and gaining their exposure are presence of chest wall deformity, prior chest wall procedures, and assessment of previous utility of the vessels.

Some tertiary or quaternary centers may obtain chest imaging in the process of evaluation of breast cancer, but it is not routinely obtained prior to microsurgical breast reconstruction. An MRI of the chest and breast may provide information regarding the internal mammary vessel caliber, anatomic relation to the chest wall, and potential internal mammary lymph node involvement in proximity to the internal mammary vessels.

Of varying treatment modalities, radiation and type of mastectomy will largely determine the course of the reconstruction. Patients requiring radiation treatment for breast cancer will present for delayed autologous reconstruction. Although effects of radiation on soft tissue are often unpredictable and inconsistent, it is well-known to decrease tissue quality. With fibrosis of surrounding soft tissue, dissection and exposure of the vessels will become more challenging. Types of mastectomies will dictate the incision pattern and require surgeons to be adaptable to different methods and approaches of dissection and exposure. The traditional skin sparing mastectomy incision is a long transverse scar which includes the removal of nipple areola complex which provides wide exposure to the chest cavity and easy access to the internal mammary vessel dissection. Nowadays, various designs of mastectomy incisions are used for strategic oncologic access for tumor removal as well as cosmetic result. This, however, can pose additional challenges in exposing and dissecting the recipient vessels.

Applied Anatomy

The internal mammary vessels supply the medial aspect of the anterior chest wall and breasts. They arise bilaterally from the subclavian vessels and travel caudally 1–2 centimeters lateral from the lateral border of the sternum. As the artery travels caudally, it gives off anterior intercostal branches which travel laterally along the caudal aspect of each rib until anastomosing with the posterior intercostal artery of that rib space. The artery also gives off perforating chest wall branches which can occasionally be utilized as recipient vessels. After passing the sixth intercostal space, the artery branches into its two terminal branches, the musculophrenic artery and the superior epigastric artery.

Anatomical studies have demonstrated that the right IMA and IMV are consistently larger than the left in all intercostal spaces. Bifurcation of the IMV typically occurs at the third intercostal space on the left, and at the fourth intercostal space on the right [12]. The IMA and IMV vessel intraluminal diameters decrease caudally, and a correlation has been found between skeletal chest width, body mass index, and vessel caliber at the third intercostal space [16–18].

The internal mammary vessels are consistently located running parallel to the sternal borders. The vessels can be found either medial or lateral to the sternal borders. The sternal borders are often the intraoperative landmark for surgeons during exposure of the IMA and IMV. A descriptive cadaveric study conducted by Lee and colleagues has estimated approximately 3% of vessels are found under the sternum, but none found laterally from the costochondral junction [12]. Therefore, using the costochondral junction as the intraoperative landmark is recommended as it is a more reliable guideline in locating the vessels.

Surgical Site Exposure

Regardless of which incision is used, recipient vessel site preparation requires adequate exposure in order to optimize the visualization of internal mammary vessels. As previously mentioned, sizable perforating vessels coming from the internal mammary vessels may also be used which then can avoid performing dissection through the chest wall intercostal muscle or rib. Safe preparation of recipient vessels in microvascular reconstruction is essential for smooth conduct of the operation. This dissection should be done using surgical loupes to ensure its precision and accuracy.

After mastectomy is completed, the chest wall cavity is then prepared with control of hemostasis. Figure 10.1 demonstrates the surgical steps in a cadaver. The medial pectoralis major muscle is then exposed, and surface anatomy can be used to locate the appropriate costal level to be dissected. Most commonly reported sites of anastomosis are at the second, third, and fourth costal levels. Pectoralis muscle can be split in the direction parallel to the muscle fibers, down to the perichondrium (Fig. 10.1a). At this level, identify the costochondral joint and plan to dissect medially from this landmark. Costochondral joints are more reliable intraoperative landmarks for this particular dissection and exposure of the internal mammary vessels than the sternal borders [12]. From the costochondral junctions, the vessels are consistently located medially. The internal mammary vessels are found approximately 1 cm, 2 cm, or 3 cm medially from the costochondral junction at the level of rib 2, 3, or 4, respectively, with the range of +/− 5 mm [12] (Fig. 10.1f). This "1-2-3 rule" can be a valuable safety tool when exposing the internal mammary vessels, especially for young surgeons

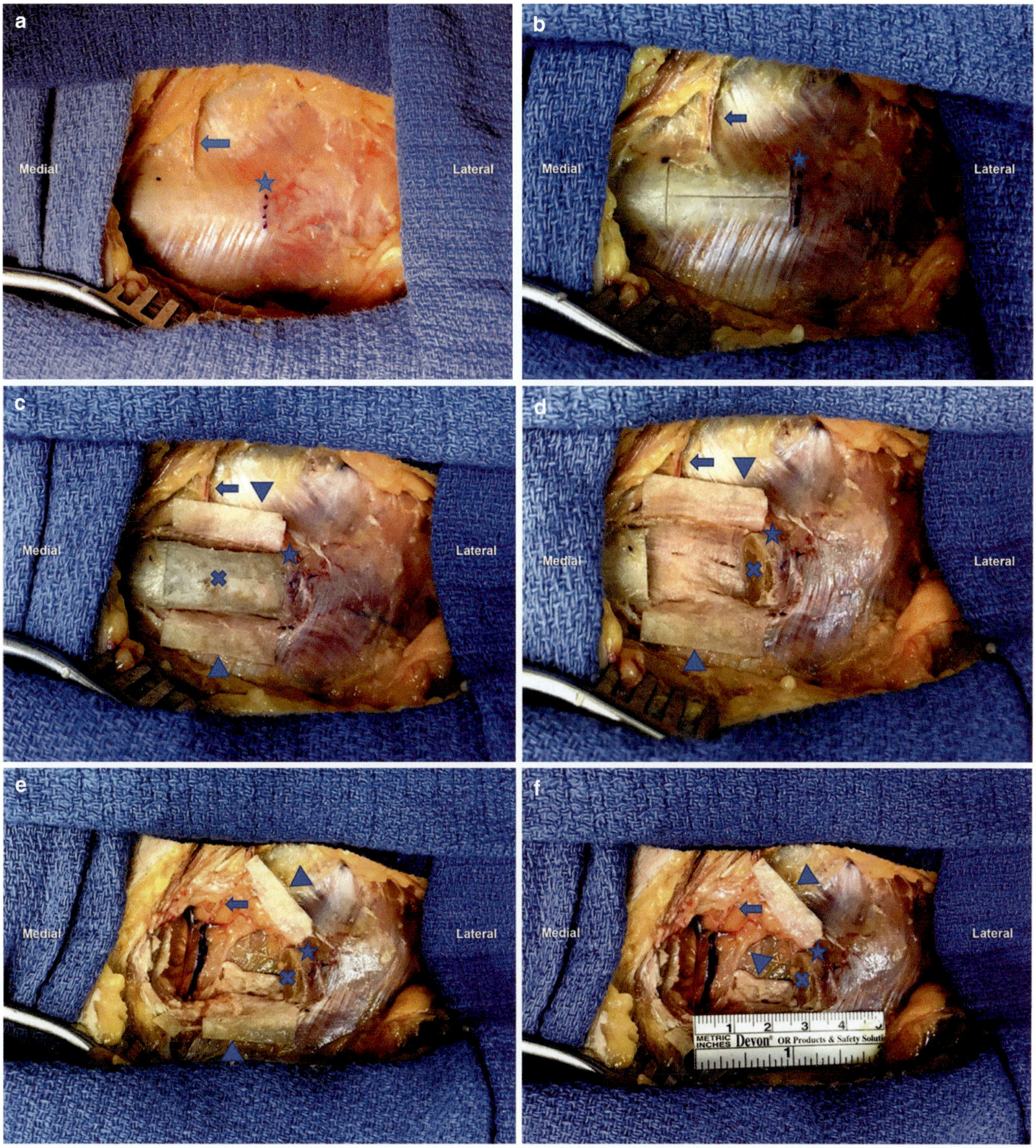

Fig. 10.1 A cadaveric step-by-step approach to exposing the internal mammary vessels on rib 4. Legends: Star = superior aspect of costochondral junction (CCJ). Arrow = perforating branch of internal mammary artery. X = cartilage. Arrowhead = pointing toward elevated perichondrium. (**a**) Rib 4 exposed after the pectoralis muscle has been retracted. (**b**) "H" incision made over the perichondrium. (**c**) Perichondrium was elevated, and rib cartilage exposed. (**d**) Partially removed rib cartilage—now posterior perichondrium exposed. (**e**) Posterior perichondrium elevated exposing loose areolar tissue (most removed) and the internal mammary vessels. The internal mammary artery was marked with surgical marker and is lateral to the internal mammary vein. No bifurcation of the vein yet at this level. (**f**) The vessel bundle was found at a distance approximately 3 cm medially from CCJ

[12]. Additionally, there is a perforating vessel through the perichondrium approximately a centimeter or two lateral from the IMA that exists in a cephalic direction (Fig. 10.1b).

Using a scalpel, a sharp cut can be made in the shape of an "H" (Fig. 10.1b). Using a freer or periosteum elevator, the perichondrium can be gently elevated from the cartilage. The perichondrium can be peeled off in a manner of "opening a book" and extended to the superior and inferior edges of the rib (Fig. 10.1c). Precautions should be taken during this dissection, especially when approaching the posterior surface of the cartilage to avoid inadvertent injury to the vessels or to the lung pleura. The goal of this dissection is to free up enough space for a doyen rib elevator to be safely inserted around the cartilage to complete the circumferential perichondral dissection. Pressure applied while using the doyen rib elevator should be toward the cartilage and never toward the vessels or the lung pleura.

There are various methods of removing the rib cartilage. It can be removed by sharply incising the medial and lateral contents of planned excisional area using the doyen rib elevator as a guard, or a rongeur may be used, or alternatively, a Vicryl suture can be used as a Gigli saw (Fig. 10.2). When approaching more inferior rib cartilages, the perichondrium may be more closely applied, and extra care is needed when approaching the posterior perichondrium. It is prudent to take extra caution while performing this dissection if the surgical field has been previously irradiated. In this instance, a rongeur may be employed to be used in a superficial to deep debridement of the cartilage to ensure the safety of dissection. Once the posterior layer of the perichondrium is exposed, it is important to identify the course of the recipient vessels. If the location is uncertain, a Doppler can be used to confirm the location. The exposed perichondrium can be picked up to ensure its posterior surface to be free of vital structures, and a small cut can be made and then used to extend this window in the perichondrium (Fig. 10.1d) [20–31].

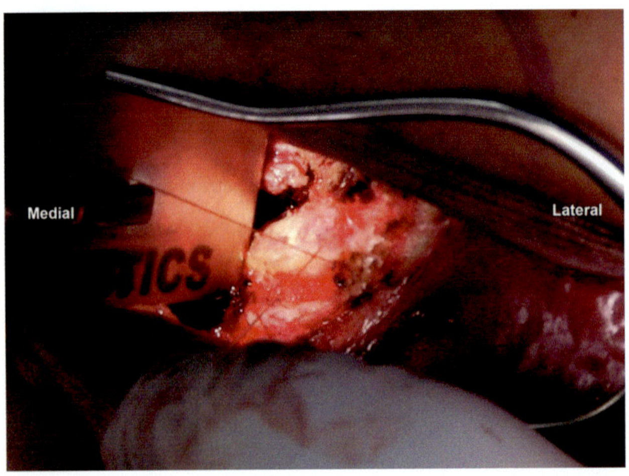

Fig. 10.2 Utilizing a Vicryl suture to incise the third rib in a controlled fashion

Once the perichondrium is exposed, loose areolar tissue can be seen encompassing the vessel bundle. Carefully confirm the vessels' location and continue the dissection (Fig. 10.1e). Here, the areolar tissue dissection near the vessels can be done using a McCabe instrument in a layer-by-layer approach, and tissue cauterization is done by using a bipolar to achieve optimal hemostasis without causing thermal spread injury to the internal mammary vessels. This dissection would be best performed when it is not directly over the vessels to avoid accidental injury to the vessels (Video 10.1).

Once adequate exposure is obtained with sufficient length of exposure of the internal mammary vessels, the remainder of preparation for microsurgery can be completed under the microscope or high-powered surgical loupes with micro instruments. Tributaries can be ligated using a bipolar electrocautery or superfine vessel clips.

Most perforators found during this dissection can be ligated. Some perforators do exhibit adequate diameter for possible additional anastomosis with the donor vessels or can be used to supercharge the flap. If the larger caliber perforator vessels are encountered during the dissection, and do not hinder the exposure of the recipient vessels, they may remain undisturbed.

Tissue quality is compromised when the surgical field has been irradiated. When the patient had previous radiation treatment, extra care has to be performed when dissecting these internal mammary vessels as the vessels can be friable and easily injured.

For advanced micro-surgeon, a rib-sparing approach to exposing the recipient vessels can be considered as an option [1, 10–17]. This method may provide adequate exposure to the internal mammary vessels by opening the intercostal muscles cephalad or caudal to the rib (also see Chap. 11). Opening to both cephalad and caudal intercostal muscles, adjacent to the rib, can also be used to maximize the exposure and length of internal mammary vessels.

Inframammary Fold Incision: Modifications in Technique

Nipple-sparing mastectomy through the inframammary fold (IMF) incision makes dissection of the internal mammary vessels challenging. To facilitate this dissection, adequate exposure is required. This may be achieved by extending the IMF incision medially to the most central extent of the fold for better exposure of the surgical field. This might lead to vascular access through more inferior costal levels (4–6). As the internal mammary vessels travel caudally, the caliber of vessels tends to decrease. In particular, anecdotally, it is described that intercostal space width may decrease and lateral convexity of the inferior sternum may impede vessel

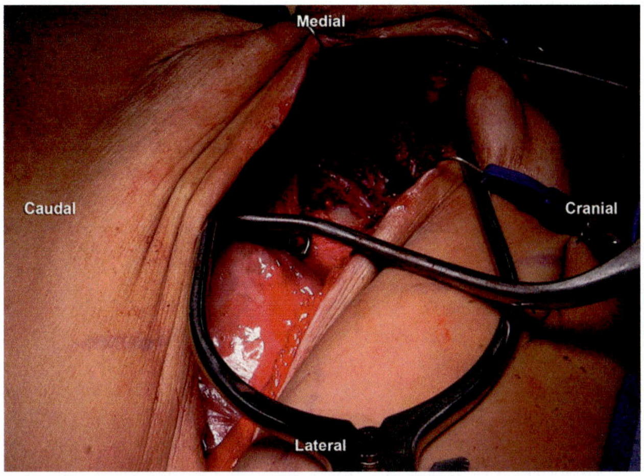

Fig. 10.3 Utilizing two retractors for ease of dissection

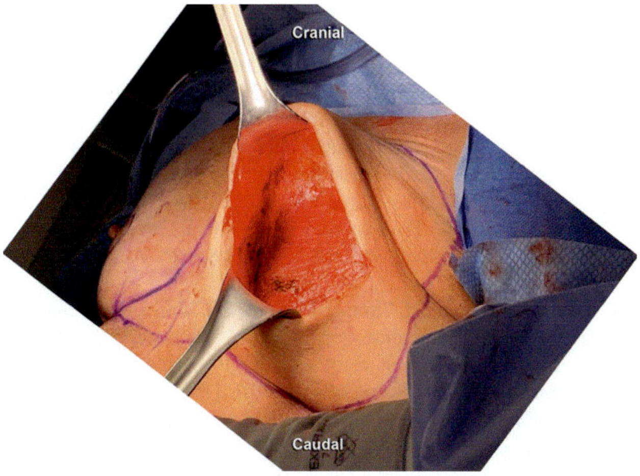

Fig. 10.4 After removal of the tissue expander, the pectoralis muscle should be sutured back to its original position to avoid window shading

access [19]. While it is possible to split the pectoralis muscle, a small triangular window can also be made with the apex laterally. Once the rib is exposed, the dissection can proceed as described previously. Two retractors can be placed perpendicular to one another to allow for ease of visualization (Fig. 10.3).

Delayed Immediate Reconstruction: Modifications in Technique

One of the most common incisions utilized in skin-sparing mastectomies is a transverse radial incision. In a delayed immediate reconstruction, even when radiation has not been employed, vessel dissection is often quite tedious. In cases where the tissue expander is placed in a subpectoral position, the preparation and recreation of the mastectomy pocket has to be completed in a structured fashion—mastectomy skin flap has to be re-elevated with care with scar tissue release above the pectoralis muscle. This can be performed if there is sufficient thickness of mastectomy skin flap. In patients who have undergone radiation therapy, adequate time should be allowed for second-stage reconstruction. In these cases, the dissection should be performed more cautiously and in a limited manner. When questions arise regarding the viability of the flap, intraoperative ICG (indocyanine green) angiography may assist. The tissue expander that was placed in the subpectoral position is removed through the lower or lateral border of the pectoralis muscle. This muscle should be sutured back in place to avoid window shading over the flap (Fig. 10.4). We have found, subjectively, that the pressure of the tissue expander on the IMA and IMV can lead to fibrosis and friability of the vessels, demanding extra care with dissection. In this condition, the internal mammary vessels can become more adherent to its surrounding tissue. Once the pectoralis muscle is split, the rib cartilage can be removed in a similar manner as described above.

Discussion

The IMA and IMV are commonly utilized recipient vessels for microsurgical breast reconstructions. Their consistent location, anatomy, and high blood flow rate make them ideal for recipient vessels. With familiarity and practice, dissection can be reproducible and efficient. However, when the breast has been exposed to radiation or when a lateral or IMF incision is employed, dissection and exposure of vessels can be difficult. Strategic retractor placement and knowledge of anatomical location of the vessels, along with the efficient and reliable techniques, can all facilitate the optimal preparation of the vessels to be set up for a successful microsurgical outcome. See video demonstration of the two techniques described above.

References

1. Siegel RL, Miller KD, Jemal A. Cancer statistics. CA Cancer J Clin. 2020; https://doi.org/10.3322/caac.21590.
2. Yueh JH, Slavin SA, Adesiyun T, et al. Patient satisfaction in postmastectomy breast reconstruction: a comparative evaluation of DIEP, TRAM, latissimus flap, and implant techniques. Plast Reconstr Surg. 2010;125(6):1585–95.
3. Albornoz CR, Bach PB, Mehrara BJ, et al. A paradigm shift in U.S. Breast reconstruction: increasing implant rates. Plast Reconstr Surg. 2013;131(1):15–23.
4. Cemal Y, Albornoz CR, Disa JJ, et al. A paradigm shift in U.S. breast reconstruction: Part 2. The influence of changing mastectomy patterns on reconstructive rate and method. Plast Reconstr Surg. 2013;131(3):320e–6e.

5. Kulkarni AR, Sears ED, Atisha DM, Alderman AK. Use of autologous and microsurgical breast reconstruction by U.S. plastic surgeons. Plast Reconstr Surg. 2013;132(3):534–41.
6. Eltahir Y, Werners LL, Dreise MM, Zeijlmans van Emmichoven IA, Werker PM, de Bock GH. Which breast is the best? Successful autologous or alloplastic breast reconstruction: patient-reported quality-of-life outcomes. Plast Reconstr Surg. 2015;135(1):43–50.
7. Kamali P, Paul MA, Ibrahim AMS, et al. National and regional differences in 32,248 Postmastectomy autologous breast reconstruction using the updated National Inpatient Survey. Ann Plast Surg. 2017;78(6):717–22.
8. Visser NJ, Damen TH, Timman R, Hofer SO, Mureau MA. Surgical results, aesthetic outcome, and patient satisfaction after microsurgical autologous breast reconstruction following failed implant reconstruction. Plast Reconstr Surg. 2010;126(1):26–36.
9. Gart MS, Smetona JT, Hanwright PJ, et al. Autologous options for Postmastectomy breast reconstruction: a comparison of outcomes based on the American College of Surgeons National Surgical Quality Improvement Program. [published correction appears in J Am Coll Surg. 2013 May;216(5):1034–5]. J Am Coll Surg. 2013;216(2):229–38.
10. Pusic AL, Matros E, Fine N, et al. Patient-reported outcomes 1 year after immediate breast reconstruction: results of the mastectomy reconstruction outcomes consortium study. J Clin Oncol. 2017;35(22):2499–506.
11. Darcy CM, Smit JM, Audolfsson T, Acosta R. Surgical technique: the intercostal space approach to the internal mammary vessels in 463 microvascular breast reconstructions. J Plast Reconstr Aesthet Surg. 2011;64(1):58–62.
12. Lee CD, Butterworth J, Stephens RE, Wright B, Surek C. Location of the internal mammary vessels for microvascular autologous breast reconstruction: the "1-2-3 rule". Plast Reconstr Surg. 2018;142(1):28–36.
13. Greer-Bayramoglu RJ, Chu MW, Fortin AJ. Feasibility of internal mammary vessel use in breast reconstruction versus coronary artery bypass surgery: an anatomic, cadaveric evaluation. Plast Reconstr Surg. 2011;127(5):1783–9.
14. Macadam SA, Bovill ES, Buchel EW, Lennox PA. Evidence-based medicine: autologous breast reconstruction. Plast Reconstr Surg. 2017;139(1):204e–29e.
15. Hamdi M, Rasheed MZ. Advances in autologous breast reconstruction with pedicled perforator flaps. Clin Plast Surg. 2012;39(4):477–90.
16. Cook JA, Tholpady SS, Momeni A, Chu MW. Predictors of internal mammary vessel diameter: a computed tomographic angiography-assisted anatomic analysis. J Plast Reconstr Aesthet Surg. 2016;69(10):1340–8.
17. Clark CP 3rd, Rohrich RJ, Copit S, Pittman CE, Robinson J. An anatomic study of the internal mammary veins: clinical implications for free-tissue-transfer breast reconstruction. Plast Reconstr Surg. 1997;99(2):400–4.
18. Tuinder S, Dikmans R, Schipper RJ, et al. Anatomical evaluation of the internal mammary vessels based on magnetic resonance imaging (MRI). J Plast Reconstr Aesthet Surg. 2012;65(10):1363–7.
19. Knackstedt R, Hashem AM, Schwarz GS. Nipple sparing mastectomy and microsurgical breast reconstruction: an approach for success. J Plast Reconstr Aesthet Surg. 2018;71(4):609–11.
20. Kitamura S, Kawachi K, Kawata T, et al. Ten-year survival and cardiac event-free rates in Japanese patients with the left anterior descending artery revascularized with internal thoracic artery or saphenous vein graft: a comparative study. Nihon Geka Gakkai Zasshi. 1996;97(3):202–9.
21. Arima M, Kanoh T, Suzuki T, et al. Serial angiographic follow-up beyond 10 years after coronary artery bypass grafting. Circ J. 2005;69(8):896–902.
22. Cohen G, Tamariz MG, Sever JY, et al. The radial artery versus the saphenous vein graft in contemporary CABG: a case-matched study. Ann Thorac Surg. 2001;71(1):180–5. discussion 185–6.
23. Haddock NT, Teotia SS. Five steps to internal mammary vessel preparation in less than 15 minutes. Plast Reconstr Surg. 2017;140(5):884–6.
24. Farid M, Gilleard O, Nikkhah D. Five steps to internal mammary vessel preparation in less than 15 minutes. Plast Reconstr Surg. 2018;141(6):961e–2e.
25. Jeevaratnam JA, Nikkhah D, Dheansa BS. The evolution of internal mammary vessel preparation in microsurgical breast reconstruction: what is the current evidence? J Plast Reconstr Aesthet Surg. 2014;67(9):e226–7.
26. Malata C, Sasaki Y, Oni G. Five steps to internal mammary vessel preparation in less than 15 minutes. Plast Reconstr Surg. 2018;142(4):581e–2e.
27. Kavouni A, Shibu M. Problems associated with the use of internal mammary vessels as recipients for free flap breast reconstruction. Br J Plast Surg. 1999;52(7):597.
28. Schwabegger AH, Gschnitzer C, Ninkovic MM. Contour deformity at the internal mammary recipient site. Br J Plast Surg. 1999;52(8):674.
29. Sasaki Y, Madada-Nyakauru RN, Samaras S, Oni G, Di Candia M, Malata CM. The ideal intercostal space for internal mammary vessel exposure during total rib-sparing microvascular breast reconstruction: a critical evaluation. J Plast Reconstr Aesthet Surg. 2019;72(6):1000–6.
30. Rosich-Medina A, Bouloumpasis S, Di Candia M, Malata CM. Total 'rib'-preservation technique of internal mammary vessel exposure for free flap breast reconstruction: a 5-year prospective cohort study and instructional video. Ann Med Surg (Lond). 2015;4(3):293–300.
31. Sacks JM, Chang DW. Rib-sparing internal mammary vessel harvest for microvascular breast reconstruction in 100 consecutive cases. Plast Reconstr Surg. 2009;123(5):1403–7.

Internal Mammary Vessels: Rib-Sparing Approach

11

Arash Momeni and David Cholok

Introduction

Autologous breast reconstruction has been demonstrated to be associated with superior long-term patient-reported outcomes when compared to prosthetic reconstruction [1]. The safety, benefits, and reliability of abdominally based free flaps including transverse rectus abdominis musculocutaneous (TRAM), muscle-sparing TRAM, and deep inferior epigastric perforator (DIEP) flaps are well-established [2]. In microvascular reconstruction, several potential recipient vessels are available to the surgeon including the thoracodorsal, thoracoacromial, lateral thoracic, and internal mammary vessels. The advantages of the internal mammary (IM) system are multiple, and accordingly the IM vessels have become the recipient vessels of choice for microvascular anastomoses. Specifically, utilization of the IM system is favored due to its constant anatomy, ease of dissection, ideal vessel size match, high arterial pressures, relatively short pedicle requirement, and favorable location, thus permitting creation of a central breast mound without the risk of lateralization. Over the previous three decades, the use of the IM system has been associated with fewer vessel conversions, a lower rate of seroma, and in the setting of pre-reconstruction radiation, an easier dissection when compared to the thoracodorsal system [3, 4]. The IM system also exhibits greater blood flow than the thoracodorsal artery prior to anastomosis [5]. Current preferences for choice of recipient vessels also reflect changes in oncologic management. The demonstrable safety and utility of sentinel lymph node biopsies has drastically reduced the need for extensive axillary surgery, and since the publication of the American College of Surgeons Oncology Group (ACOSOG) Z0011 trial, the rates of axillary lymph node dissection, a procedure which facilitates exposure of thoracodorsal vessels, have fallen precipitously over the previous decade [6].

Access to the IM system was initially conceived as a "rib-sacrificing" approach in which a segment of the third costal cartilage is excised to facilitate exposure of the IM vessels. Creation of this intercostal distance allows abundant space for the performance of microvascular anastomoses. However, resection of the rib cartilage can result in postoperative pain, and occasionally confers a visible contour depression of the chest wall. To address these deficiencies, the "rib-sparing" approach, also known as the "open-book technique," has evolved as an alternate approach to access the IM vessels. Reported advantages include a decrease in chest wall morbidity and deformation, conferring the corollary benefits of shorter hospital stays, reduced morphine requirement, and improved patient experience [7–9].

Preoperative Assessment

In the setting of breast reconstruction, the considerations of oncologic management should take precedence; the requirement of neo-/adjuvant chemotherapy or radiation, desire for prophylactic surgery, and tumor biology may all impact clinical outcome. The choice of reconstruction, timing, and potential complications should be thoroughly considered once the oncologic treatment course has been determined. Anatomically, the IM system is easily accessible and remains consistent among individuals; rarely is preoperative radiographic assessment warranted. Alternatively, flap character-

Supplementary Information The online version of this chapter (https://doi.org/10.1007/978-3-030-75389-4_11) contains supplementary material, which is available to authorized users.

A. Momeni (✉)
Division of Plastic & Reconstructive Surgery, Ryan-Upson Scholar in Plastic and Reconstructive Surgery, Director - Clinical Outcomes Research, Stanford University School of Medicine, Palo Alto, CA, USA
e-mail: amomeni@stanford.edu

D. Cholok
Division of Plastic & Reconstructive Surgery, Stanford University School of Medicine, Palo Alto, CA, USA
e-mail: dcholok@stanford.edu

R. Gurunian, R. Djohan (eds.), *Recipient Vessels in Reconstructive Microsurgery*,
https://doi.org/10.1007/978-3-030-75389-4_11

istics should also be taken into consideration, including the length and caliber of the pedicle, and operative planning may benefit from radiologic assessment including magnetic resonance angiography (MRA) or computed tomography (CTA) angiography.

Applied Anatomy

The IM vessels demonstrate a fairly consistent anatomical course. The arteries originate from the subclavian or corresponding brachiocephalic arteries and run inferiorly in a plane deep between the costal cartilage and parietal pleura; specifically the IM vessels lie anterior to the transverse intercostal muscles and deep to the intercostal muscles. Once past the sixth intercostal space and approaching the inferior border of the costal margin, the artery bifurcates; the lateral branch continues as the musculophrenic artery, and the medial branch descends as the superior epigastric artery, which forms anastomotic connections with the deep inferior epigastric arteries. As the IM artery (IMA) descends, multiple perforating branches can be found piercing the intercostal musculature at intercostal spaces 2–6. These perforating vessels may be used as recipient vessels for microsurgical anastomosis if of a sufficient caliber, potentially avoiding deeper dissection [4]. The IM vessels, unfortunately, are susceptible to trauma as they lie relatively superficial in the chest wall.

The IMA in adults ranges from 1.8 to 2.8 mm in diameter; as described in a cadaver study by Arnez et al., the arteries narrow slightly as they descend along the chest wall measuring 2.8 and 2.6 mm on average at the third and fifth intercostal spaces, respectively [10]. The arteries, typically larger on the right than on the left side, are notably resistant to atherosclerotic disease [11]. For this reason, the IMA is the preferred choice of donor graft for surgical coronary artery bypass, and yields improved long-term patency and survival [12]. Fortunately, concurrent incidence of coronary artery disease requiring surgical revascularization in women having undergone breast reconstruction is relatively rare.

The venous internal mammary system is similarly consistent regarding the vessel caliber and orientation in respect to the artery. The vein most often runs medial to the artery along the deep surface of the chest wall, on average between 2 and 18 mm from the sternal border, and bifurcates into medial and lateral branches inferior to the fourth costal cartilage [10, 11]. The medial branch is most often of a greater caliber, on average measuring 2.8, 2.6, and 2.5 mm, respectively, in the third, fourth, and fifth intercostal spaces [10]. Previous studies have reported higher rates of conversion from the IM to thoracodorsal systems due to inadequacy of the IMV, specifically on the left side [3]; this has been demonstrated anatomically by relatively diminutive size of the veins on the left, compared to the right, with a lower incidence of vessels greater than 3 mm available for anastomosis [13].

Surgical Site Exposure

The patient is placed in the supine position, with arms extended to 90 degrees, allowing surgeon and assistant access to the chest wall concurrent with flap harvest (Video 11.1).

Dissection begins with identification of the second or third intercostal space. While the second intercostal space is wider [11], it is at times challenging to access, particularly in immediate reconstruction. Hence, the authors frequently use the third intercostal space. The pectoralis muscle is split at the level of the desired intercostal space along its fibers (Fig. 11.1a, b). The ribs bordering the intercostal space are

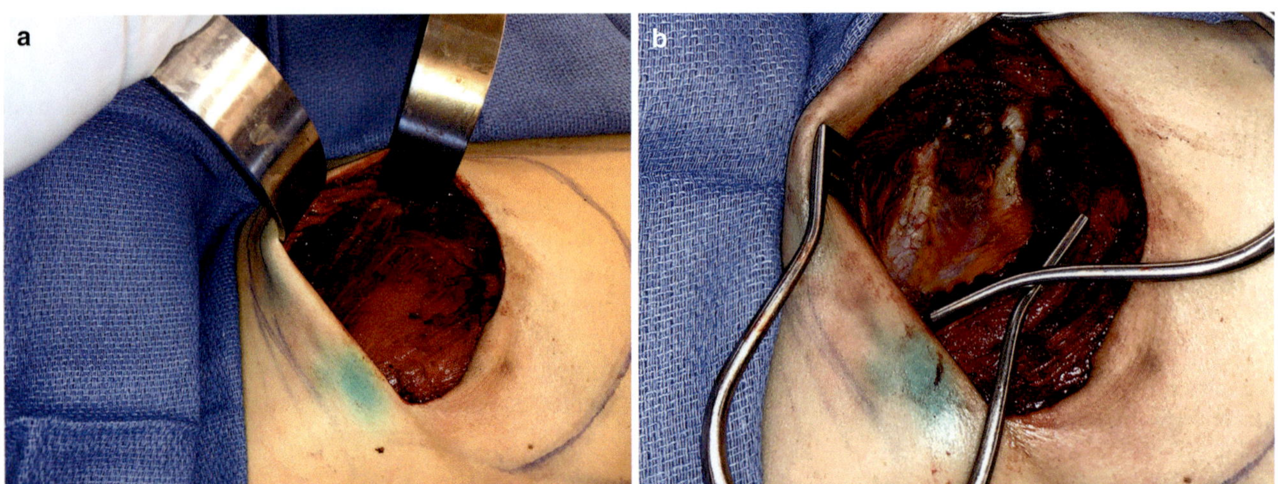

Fig. 11.1 (**a**) The third intercostal space is identified and the pectoralis major muscle split along its fibers. (**b**) Splitting the pectoralis major muscle along its fibers exposes the third intercostal space as well as the bordering third and fourth ribs

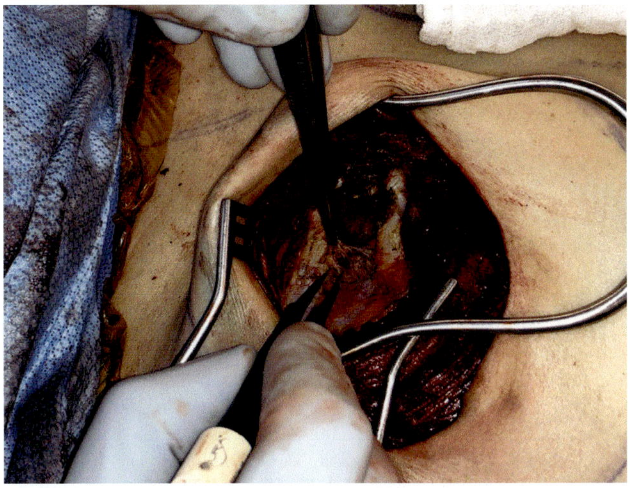

Fig. 11.2 Beginning at the level of the osseocartilaginous junction of the rib, the intercostal muscles are divided vertically with bipolar cautery until the loose areolar tissue deep to the intercostal muscles is identified

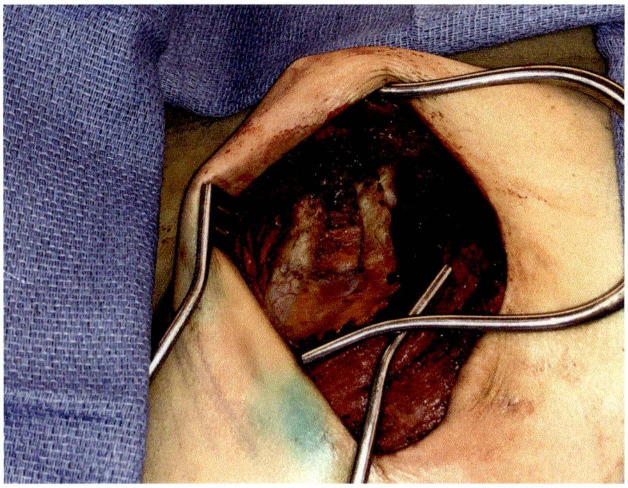

Fig. 11.3 Following medial reflection of the intercostal muscles, the internal mammary vessels come into view. Reflection of the intercostal muscles continues to the sternal border

identified. Beginning at the level of the osseocartilaginous junction of the rib, the intercostal muscles are divided vertically with bipolar cautery until the loose areolar tissue deep to the intercostal muscles is identified (Fig. 11.2). The internal mammary vessels are routinely medial to this level. Dissection then proceeds medially. Particular attention is paid to ensure that the intercostal muscles are detached from the bordering ribs. This results in exposure of the internal mammary vessels over a sufficient length to facilitate microsurgical anastomosis. Following medial reflection of the intercostal muscles, the internal mammary vessels come into view. Reflection of the intercostal muscles continues to the sternal border (Fig. 11.3). The exposed internal mammary vessels are then carefully skeletonized and prepared for microvascular anastomosis (Fig. 11.4). Of note, the rib-sparing approach to IM vessel dissection does not preclude the ability to dissect an intercostal nerve if flap neurotization is desired (Fig. 11.5).

There remains variability in surgeon preference regarding which intercostal space to utilize. On average, the second rib space provides the greatest intercostal distance; however, access may be limited in the setting of immediate reconstruction, thus, resulting in the use of the third intercostal space. Authors have previously advocated for a minimum intercostal distance of 1.5 cm to perform microvascular anastomosis safely and efficiently. But this distance is dependent on the depth of field encountered as determined by the thickness of the patient's ribs, costal cartilage, intercostal musculature, and areolar tissue. Multiple publications remark upon an initial learning curve to master the alternative approach to IM vessel harvest, but studies do not demonstrate a significantly increased rate of flap loss, or complication [7].

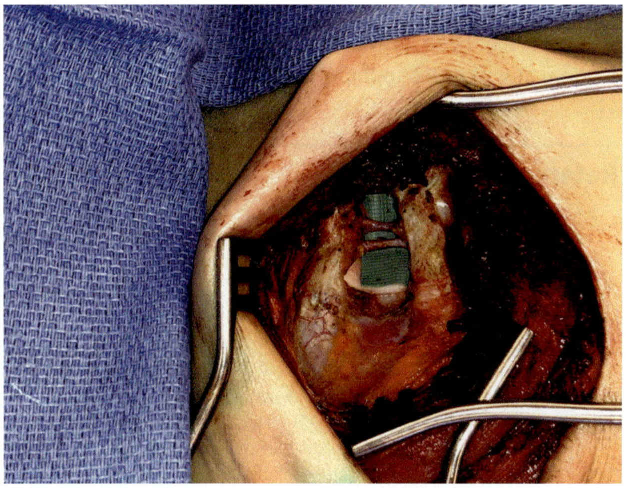

Fig. 11.4 The exposed internal mammary vessels are carefully skeletonized and prepared for microvascular anastomosis

Discussion

The chest wall contains multiple recipient vessel systems available for microvascular anastomosis, thus allowing intraoperative conversion should complications arise. The IM system, however, has been established as the preferential choice for a multitude of reasons including consistent anatomy, ease of exposure, and flap positioning. Albeit rarely, the conventional approach to IM vessel dissection, i.e., "rib-sacrificing" approach, can be associated with a visible chest wall deformity and increased postoperative pain, thus compromising the patient experience and clinical outcome. As such, the "rib-sparing" harvest of the IM vessels was introduced and seems

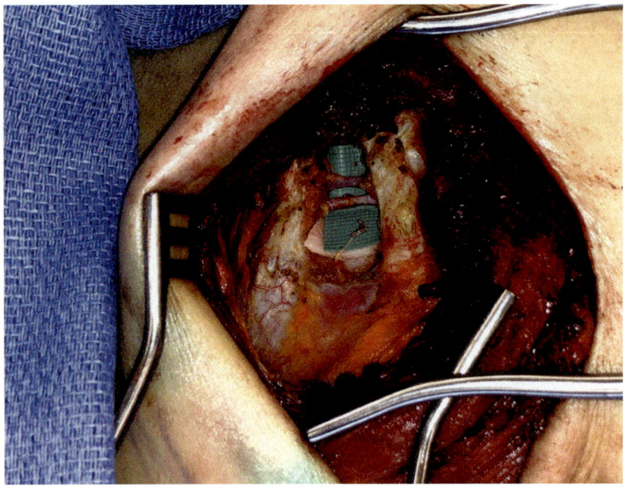

Fig. 11.5 An intercostal nerve is preserved in preparation for flap neurotization

to address these limitations. Despite the technical challenges conferred by a smaller operative field, the "rib-sparing" approach has been demonstrated to be a reliable approach without any increase in flap-related complications.

References

1. Hu ES, Pusic AL, Waljee JF, Kuhn L, Hawley ST, Wilkins E, et al. Patient-reported aesthetic satisfaction with breast reconstruction during the long-term survivorship period. Plast Reconstr Surg. 2009;124(1):1–8.
2. Tevlin R, Wan DC, Momeni A. Should free deep inferior epigastric artery perforator flaps be considered a quality indicator in breast reconstruction? J Plast Reconstr Aesthet Surg. 2019;72:1923.
3. Moran SL, Nava G, Behnam AB, Serletti JM. An outcome analysis comparing the thoracodorsal and internal mammary vessels as recipient sites for microvascular breast reconstruction: a prospective study of 100 patients. Plast Reconstr Surg. 2003;111(6):1876–82.
4. Saint-Cyr M, Chang DW, Robb GL, Chevray PM. Internal mammary perforator recipient vessels for breast reconstruction using free TRAM, DIEP, and SIEA flaps. Plast Reconstr Surg. 2007;120(7):1769–73.
5. Lorenzetti F, Kuokkanen H, von Smitten K, Asko-Seljavaara S. Intraoperative evaluation of blood flow in the internal mammary or thoracodorsal artery as a recipient vessel for a free TRAM flap. Ann Plast Surg. 2001;46(6):590–3.
6. Rosenberger LH, Thomas SM, Plichta JK, Fayanju OM, Hyslop T, Greenup RA, et al. Decreasing rates of axillary lymph node dissections over time: implications for surgical resident exposure and operative skills development. Am J Surg. 2019;218(4):786–91.
7. Sacks JM, Chang DW. Rib-sparing internal mammary vessel harvest for microvascular breast reconstruction in 100 consecutive cases. Plast Reconstr Surg. 2009;123(5):1403–7.
8. Malata CM, Moses M, Mickute Z, Di Candia M. Tips for successful microvascular abdominal flap breast reconstruction utilizing the "total rib preservation" technique for internal mammary vessel exposure. Ann Plast Surg. 2011;66(1):36–42.
9. Sasaki Y, Madada-Nyakauru RN, Samaras S, Oni G, Di Candia M, Malata CM. The ideal intercostal space for internal mammary vessel exposure during total rib-sparing microvascular breast reconstruction: a critical evaluation. J Plast Reconstr Aesthet Surg. 2019;72(6):1000–6.
10. Arnez ZM, Valdatta L, Tyler MP, Planinsek F. Anatomy of the internal mammary veins and their use in free TRAM flap breast reconstruction. Br J Plast Surg. 1995;48(8):540–5.
11. Cook JA, Tholpady SS, Momeni A, Chu MW. Predictors of internal mammary vessel diameter: a computed tomographic angiography-assisted anatomic analysis. J Plast Reconstr Aesthet Surg. 2016;69(10):1340–8.
12. Nasso G, Coppola R, Bonifazi R, Piancone F, Bozzetti G, Speziale G. Arterial revascularization in primary coronary artery bypass grafting: direct comparison of 4 strategies--results of the Stand-in-Y Mammary Study. J Thorac Cardiovasc Surg. 2009;137(5):1093–100.
13. Clark CP 3rd, Rohrich RJ, Copit S, Pittman CE, Robinson J. An anatomic study of the internal mammary veins: clinical implications for free-tissue-transfer breast reconstruction. Plast Reconstr Surg. 1997;99(2):400–4.

Subscapular-Thoracodorsal and Lateral Thoracic Vessels

12

Kavita T. Vakharia, Vahe Fahradyan, and Raffi Gurunian

Introduction

The anatomic knowledge of the branches of the axillary artery is important in trunk, extremity, breast, and head and neck reconstruction. The three segments of the axillary artery have six main branches which can be sources of recipient vessels for microvascular free tissue transfer. These arteries can also be a source for microvascular grafts in select cases.

Applied Anatomy

The relation to the pectoralis minor separates the axillary artery into three segments (Fig. 12.1). This article focuses on the second segment which is posterior to the pectoralis minor and the third segment which is inferior to the pectoralis minor. The second segment is often the location of the origin of the lateral thoracic artery (LTA).

While originally thought to arise directly from the axillary artery, the LTA most often originates as a branch from the thoracoacromial artery (see Chap. 14). Other possible origins of the artery include the axillary artery (usually the second portion but can also be the first or third), thoracodorsal artery, and subscapular artery [1]. The LTA travels along the lateral border of the pectoralis minor, and it often sends a branch into the pectoralis major muscle before becoming a cutaneous branch. It contributes to the blood supply of the axillary lymph nodes, serratus anterior, pectoralis muscles, subscapularis muscles, and breast parenchyma in females [2, 3]. The average diameter of the LTA at its origin is 1.5 mm and the pedicle length that can be harvested is on average 11 cm [4].

The third segment of the axillary artery normally provides the origin of the subscapular system. The diameter of the subscapular artery at the origin ranges from 3 mm to 7 mm. The length of the artery until its division into terminal branches is most frequently between 10 mm and 29.9 mm with an average of 18 mm [5]. Most often, the subscapular artery ends in two terminal branches, the circumflex scapular artery (scapular circumflex), which is oriented horizontally, and the thoracodorsal artery, which is oriented vertically and is a descendent branch. There are some collateral branches that go to the subscapularis muscle. There is most often one subscapular vein that forms from a confluence of the thoracodorsal vein and circumflex scapular vein [6, 7]. The subscapular artery is most often found near the axillary nerve and the radial nerve. A common pattern for the artery is to pass anterior to both of these nerves [5].

The thoracodorsal artery origin measures around 2 mm to 3.9 mm. In very few cases, the thoracodorsal artery arises as a direct branch from the axillary artery. The length of the thoracodorsal artery ranges from 5.9 cm to 18.7 cm with an average length of 13.3 cm (± 2.5 cm) [8, 9]. In most anatomic dissections, it has been observed that the thoracodorsal artery gives one and sometimes two branches to the serratus anterior muscle, and occasionally a direct cutaneous branch. On average, the first branch is 3.7 cm from the artery origin and the second branch was usually found 7.2 cm from the origin. After this branching, it goes on to supply the latissimus dorsi muscle. The thoracodorsal nerve crosses the thoracodorsal artery, mostly anteriorly, at an average of 6.1 cm from the origin [9].

Supplementary Information The online version of this chapter (https://doi.org/10.1007/978-3-030-75389-4_12) contains supplementary material, which is available to authorized users.

K. T. Vakharia (✉) · V. Fahradyan
Department of Plastic Surgery, Cleveland Clinic, Cleveland, OH, USA
e-mail: vakhark@ccf.org; FAHRADV@ccf.org

R. Gurunian
Department of Plastic Surgery, Cleveland Clinic, Cleveland, OH, USA

Cleveland Clinic Lerner College of Medicine, Case Western Reserve University, Cleveland, OH, USA
e-mail: gurunir@ccf.org

R. Gurunian, R. Djohan (eds.), *Recipient Vessels in Reconstructive Microsurgery*,
https://doi.org/10.1007/978-3-030-75389-4_12

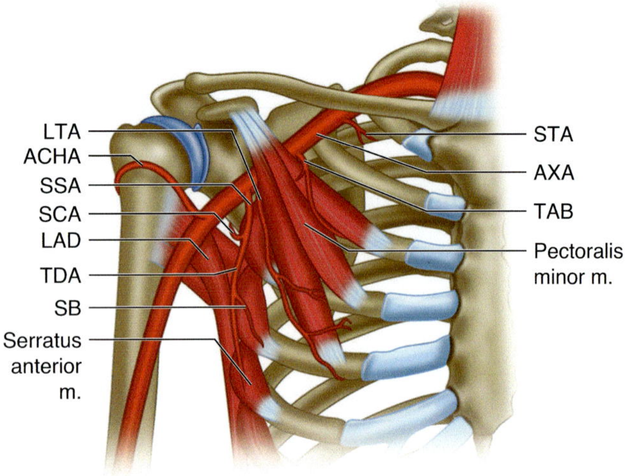

Fig. 12.1 Illustration of the axillary artery (AXA) branches: Superior thoracic artery (STA) arises from the first portion of the axillary artery. Thoracoacromial branch (TAB) and lateral thoracic (LTA) arteries usually arise from the second portion of the axillary artery. Subscapular (SSA), anterior (AHCA), and posterior humeral circumflex (not shown) arteries arise from the third portion of the axillary artery. The subscapular artery gives off the circumflex scapular (scapular circumflex: SCA) and the thoracodorsal artery (TDA). The serratus branch comes off the TDA. LAD latissimus dorsi muscle

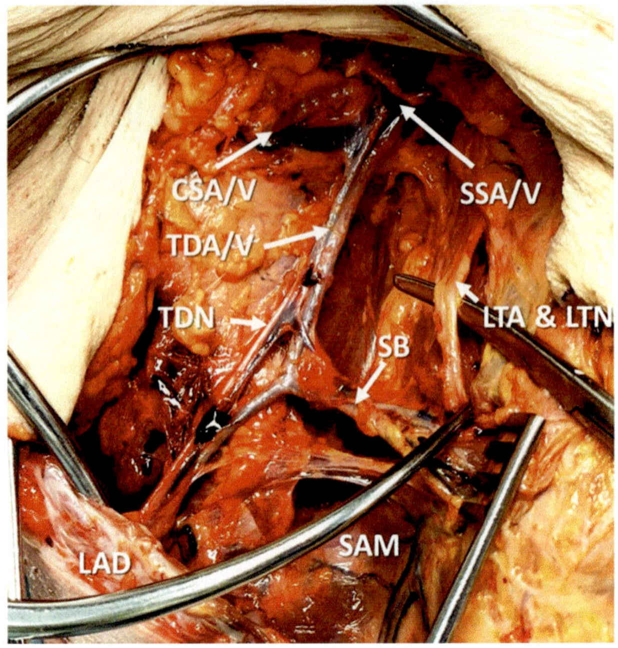

Fig. 12.2 Right axilla, cadaver dissection: Surgical exposure of the subscapular artery and vein (SSA/V), circumflex scapular (scapular circumflex) artery and vein (CSA/V), thoracodorsal artery and vein (TDA/V), and serratus branch (SB) off of the thoracodorsal artery. Also is shown the lateral thoracic artery (LTA) and long thoracic nerve (LTN). All these vessels can potentially be used as recipient for microsurgical flap reconstruction. LAD latissimus dorsi muscle, SAM serratus anterior muscle, TDN thoracodorsal nerve

Surgical Site Exposure

The subscapular vascular system and its branches can be exposed through axillary incisions that can be oriented transversely, vertically, or oblique depending on the specifics of each case (Video 12.1). However, extending the incision from the defect to be reconstructed into the axilla is often required for surgical exposure and dissection of these vessels (Fig. 12.2). Characteristics of the defect, choice of the microsurgical flap, and its pedicle length and caliber should be considered in selecting the appropriate vessels in the axilla to be used as recipient vessels.

The lateral thoracic and subscapular arteries can be exposed with the patient in the supine position and the arm abducted to 90 degrees. An incision can be made from the palpable origin of the brachial artery and then continued along the posterior and inferior margins of the hair-bearing skin of the axilla to the anterior axillary fold. Dissection is carried through the subcutaneous fat, and the clavipectoral fascia is entered. Blunt dissection is used to identify the lateral part of the pectoralis major muscle; this is reflected anteriorly and dissection is taken superiorly to identify the lateral part of the axillary vein. The axillary vein is located between the insertions of the pectoralis major anteriorly and the latissimus dorsi muscle posteriorly. Once the axillary vein is identified, the axillary artery can be found posterior to the vein. In mastectomy defects, the lateral border of the pectoralis major can be identified, and dissection can be taken superiorly into the axilla to identify the axillary vein, and then subsequently the artery as mentioned previously. However, it is often not necessary to dissect superiorly to identify the axillary artery or the vein. Once in the axilla, one can identify a branch or two and trace these vessels until sufficient length and caliber are obtained suitable for microvascular anastomosis. In posterior thoracic defects, the latissimus dorsi muscle is identified and dissected laterally to identify the anterior border. Dissection is then performed superiorly along the border to enter the apex of the axilla so that further anterior dissection can allow for finding the lateral border of the pectoralis and subsequently the axillary vein [2, 3].

Once the axillary vein and artery are identified, dissection can be taken in an anterograde fashion from the axillary artery. The lateral border of the pectoralis minor muscle may need to be reflected anteriorly to identify the second portion of the axillary artery and subsequently the lateral thoracic artery. The LTA can often be found on the axillary artery as it courses deep to the lateral border of the pectoralis major muscle and along the lateral border of the pectoralis minor muscle [10, 11]. After a mastectomy, dissection into the axilla laterally and along the lateral border of the pectoralis major may identify the LTA which courses along the anterior or middle axillary lines and further dissection can be taken retrograde to identify the origin [4].

Further dissection laterally on the axillary artery will aid in identifying the subscapular artery. The subscapular artery originates from the axillary artery at a point proximal to the medial border of the teres major muscle, and most often lateral to the pectoralis minor muscle [5]. The artery courses along the inner border of the latissimus dorsi muscle, becoming the thoracodorsal artery after giving off the circumflex scapular artery. The thoracodorsal nerve joins the vascular pedicle and supplies the latissimus dorsi muscle [10]. The thoracodorsal nerve should be identified and preserved to avoid loss of latissimus dorsi muscle function. Also, once the thoracodorsal vessels are identified, they can be traced superiorly to guide identification of the subscapular as well as circumflex scapular vessels.

Discussion

The lateral thoracic and subscapular arterial systems off of the axillary artery serve as sites of microvascular anastomosis, vascular grafts, and free or pedicled flaps. Knowledge of the anatomy of this region can significantly enhance the ability to perform reconstruction of defects of the neck, breast, trunk, and upper extremity. Although there may be variability of the branching patterns off of the axillary artery, the lateral thoracic and subscapular arteries serve as good sources of recipient vessels for reconstruction in this area. The drawbacks to the use of these arteries include close proximity to the brachial plexus and dissection through a lymph node basin which may lead to complications postoperatively related to seroma formation.

References

1. Loukas M, du Plessis M, Owens DG, Kinsella CR Jr, Litchfield CR, Nacar A, Lu O, Tubbs RS. The lateral thoracic artery revisited. Surg Radiol Anat. 2014;36(6):543–9.
2. Abrahams PH, Boon JM, Spratt JD. McMinn's clinical atlas of human anatomy. 6th ed. Edinburgh: Elsevier. 2008; p. 145.
3. Agur AMR, Lee MJ. Grant's atlas of anatomy. 10th ed. Philadelphia: Lippincott Williams and Wilkins; 1999. p. 6.
4. Yang L, Long J, Li Z, Zhou X, Peng X, Song D, Zhou B, Lv C, Wu P. The lateral thoracic vessels: a novel recipient site for breast reconstruction with DIEP flap. J Plast Reconstr Aesthet Surg. 2019;72(9):1530–6.
5. Jesus RC, Lopes MC, Demarchi GT, Ruiz CR, Wafae N, Wafae GC. The subscapular artery and the thoracodorsal branch: an anatomical study. Folia Morphol (Warsz). 2008;67(1):58–62.
6. Taylor GI, Daniel RK. The anatomy of several free flap donor sites. Plast Reconstr Surg. 1975;56(3):243–53.
7. Lhuaire M, Hivelin M, Derder M, Hunsinger V, Delmas V, Abrahams P, Sommacale D, Kianmanesh R, Fontaine C, Lantieri L. Anatomical variations of the subscapular pedicle and its terminal branches: an anatomical study and a reappraisal in the light of current surgical approaches. Surg Radiol Anat. 2019;41(4):385–92.
8. Rowsell AR, Davies DM, Eisenberg N, Taylor GI. The anatomy of the subscapular-thoracodorsal arterial system: study of 100 cadaver dissections. Br J Plast Surg. 1984;37(4):574–6.
9. Valnicek SM, Mosher M, Hopkins JK, Rockwell WB. The subscapular arterial tree as a source of microvascular arterial grafts. Plast Reconstr Surg. 2004;113(7):2001–5.
10. Harii K, Torii S, Sekiguchi J. The free lateral thoracic flap. Plast Reconstr Surg. 1978;62(2):212–22.
11. Dimovelis I, Michalinos A, Spartalis E, Athanasiadis G, Skandalakis P, Troupis T. Tetrafurcation of the subscapular artery. Anatomical and clinical implications. Folia Morphol (Warsz). 2017;76(2):312–5.

Venous Salvage Using Cephalic Vein/ External Jugular Vein

13

Steven L. Bernard

Introduction

Breast reconstruction constitutes one of the earliest uses of free flaps. In a case report from 1975, Fujino et al. described their use of a gluteal myocutaneous free flap in the reconstruction of a mastectomy defect using the thoracoacromial artery and the lateral thoracic vein as recipient vessels [1]. At that time, they recognized the limitations of these vessels. They described the potential use of the thoracodorsal (TD) system to gain extra length and make the procedure both more aesthetic and technically less demanding. Early follow-up studies to this paper also describe the use of the TD artery due to its consistent exposure following axillary dissection. This artery and vein system, however, presented other limitations including difficulty with aesthetic positioning of the flap, vascular size mismatch, difficult dissection in an irradiated field, as well as difficult microsurgical setup due to the relative depth of the axilla [2, 3]. These difficulties prompted other researchers to look for a viable alternative. Multiple authors began to report success with the internal mammary (IM) vessels as recipients for breast reconstruction [4–8]. The IM vessels are not without their issues. One concern expressed was that use of these vessels may affect the ability of cardiac surgeons to perform bypass surgery [9–11]. In addition, multiple reports mentioned the difficulty of using the *left* IM vein as a recipient due to inadequate size. Hefel found that the mean diameter of the IM vein at the cranial border of the fourth rib was 2.34 mm on the right (range of 1.27–4.45 mm) and 1.68 mm on the left (range of 0.64–1.68 mm) [2]. Clark et al. examined the veins in more detail finding that they became smaller with each caudal rib space. Sixty percent of the veins were less than 3 mm on the left below the level of the third rib, and 10% of specimens were less than 1 mm in diameter. The authors found that 90% of veins bifurcated on the left by the fourth rib [12]. Muto et al. found a complete absence of the left internal mammary vein in two cases [13]. Although the literature is mixed on the outcomes due to a small vein, the consensus of microsurgeons is that anastomosis to one vein of less than 1 millimeter in size is likely to be inadequate for venous outflow for free flap breast reconstruction [14, 15]. This belief is re-enforced by two studies where 3M venous couplers were used. Applying the couplers to veins smaller than 2 mm (as well as a history of radiation therapy) resulted in higher venous thrombosis rates [16, 17].

The findings of small IM veins on the left side of the chest and the limitations of the thoracodorsal system have motivated microsurgeons to find alternatives. All surgeons attempting to perform free flap breast reconstruction should have a backup plan for their primary choice. The chest has a number of named veins available as recipients and most have been described for use with free flaps. The remainder of this chapter is dedicated to elucidating these alternatives.

Anatomy

Figure 13.1 demonstrates the anatomy of the vessels of the thorax needed to understand the remainder of the chapter. After giving off the coronary arteries, the aorta branches into the right brachiocephalic artery, which continues to the right subclavian artery, left common carotid artery, and finally the left subclavian artery before culminating in the descending aorta. It is the subclavian artery branches and their accompanying veins that give off most of the branches of interest. Those vessels with veins large enough to reliably be used as recipients are labeled. The choice will be influenced by the

Supplementary Information The online version of this chapter (https://doi.org/10.1007/978-3-030-75389-4_13) contains supplementary material, which is available to authorized users.

S. L. Bernard (✉)
Department of Plastic Surgery, Cleveland Clinic, Cleveland, OH, USA

Cleveland Clinic Lerner College of Medicine, Case Western Reserve University, Cleveland, OH, USA
e-mail: bernars2@ccf.org

R. Gurunian, R. Djohan (eds.), *Recipient Vessels in Reconstructive Microsurgery*, https://doi.org/10.1007/978-3-030-75389-4_13

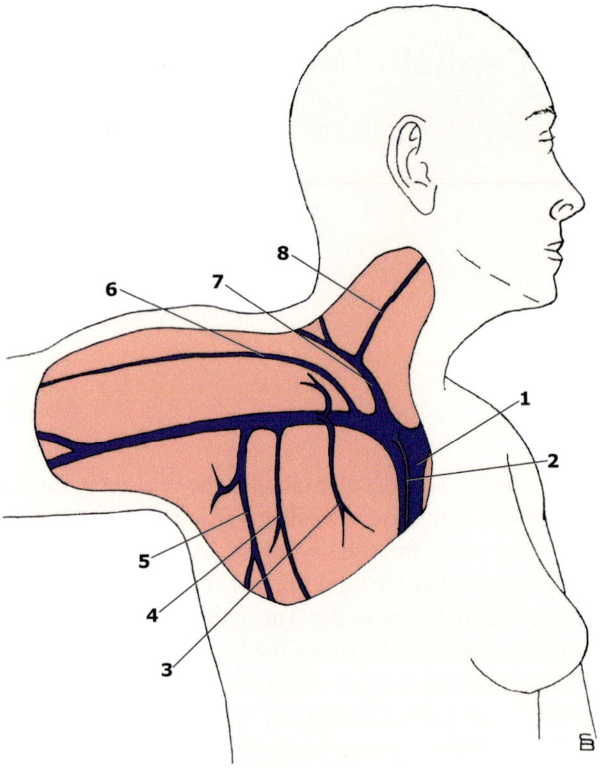

Fig. 13.1 Illustration of the key veins described in this chapter. (1) Superior vena cava, (2) internal mammary vein, (3) pectoral branch of the thoracoacromial trunk, (4) lateral thoracic vein, (5) thoracodorsal branch of the subscapular vein, (6) cephalic vein, (7) superficial cervical vein, (8) external jugular vein

length of donor vessels and the aesthetic positioning of the flap. For instance, the superior gluteal artery perforator flap has relatively short vessels and would therefore favor the IM vessels over the subscapular system which is deep in the axilla.

General rules to follow for all free flap surgery include palpation for a pulse to guide when dissecting the vessels one cannot see. When practical, dissection of donor vessels to their full length is key. When using the abdomen as a donor, the superficial inferior epigastric vein should be dissected as an alternate or additional venous outflow in case of flap congestion.

Following these guidelines, microsurgeons have reached consensus algorithm vessels to use as recipients in breast reconstruction free tissue transfer [18–24]. The recipient vessels of choice are the right and left IM artery and vein and their variants. When IM vessels are inadequate, most surgeons go to the thoracodorsal (TD) artery and vein of the subscapular system. When neither the standard IM nor TD vessels are adequate, the options are more limited and the backup plan is critical.

Internal Mammary System

As the vessels of choice for most plastic surgeons, the IM artery and vein provide significant benefits including good size match, excellent position for performing anastomosis, and adequate inflow and outflow (also see Chaps. 10 and 11). O'Neill reported being able to use the internal mammary system without modification in 99.6% of cases [25]. As stated previously, in those rare circumstances where problems do arise, it is usually due to an inadequate venous recipient and statistically, the left IM vein being too small for either anastomosis or adequate outflow. On the donor side, the deep inferior epigastric vein is approximately 3 mm when dissected out to its confluence with the external iliac vein. When the recipient vein is more than 25% smaller, maneuvers such as end-to-side anastomosis or splaying the end of the recipient vein can be attempted; however, when the mismatch becomes too large such as going from 3 mm down to 1.5 mm, the risk for failure increases. A vein of less than 1.5 mm increases the risk for venous congestion in the flap. Such a vein will be more delicate, especially with radiation therapy, increasing risk for damage and an unusable vein. When faced with these situations, alternative venous outflow must be found to ensure surgical success.

The first alternative to consider avoids dissection of the IM vein entirely by utilizing the IM perforators which emerge from the intercostal spaces. Because the perforator can be used without removing the rib cartilage, time can be saved, pain decreased, and the risk of pneumothorax eliminated. This has been proposed as an alternative to the standard dissection by several authors who use the perforators as a first choice [18, 26–28]. Proponents evaluate the size and quality of the perforator vein prior to removal of the rib cartilage. As with the IM vein proper, the size of the perforators decrease with each caudal step in ribs with the largest found at the level of the second intercostal space [29]. The perforator is usually found just lateral to the sternum on the cranial aspect of the intercostal space. Of interest, the author has, on occasion, found the perforator vein diameter larger than the IM vein proper at the same intercostal level. The significance of this finding is unknown beyond making the anastomosis easier, but those reporting regular use of this option have excellent success.

A drawback of using the IM perforator is the reliance on a breast surgeon that does not dissect their specimen so medially that they clip the vessels during mastectomy. In addition, when used as a backup option after rib removal, the perforators are often damaged necessitating dissection of more cranial veins.

As eluded to, taking into consideration the cranial-caudal size difference, one option for dealing with an inadequate IM vein is to remove a more proximal rib. The size of the vein increases more cranially and the vein is less likely to branch [14]. The downside of this technique includes the loss of a second rib cartilage which can be visible as a concavity of the chest wall, particularly in thin women. Furthermore, the more cranial anastomosis limits the ability to position the flap due to vessel length.

If the above options have been exhausted, it is still possible to use the ipsilateral IM system by utilizing the distal IM vein in retrograde fashion. This option has been used alone, as a salvage procedure, and in addition to using the proximal vein to improve outflow or to connect a second flap [30–38]. The difficulty with this technique is the valve direction and decreasing the size of the vessels, but when the proximal vein is not suitable, the distal vein will, on occasion, be usable. Its viability can only be determined at the time of the surgery.

When the ipsilateral IM vein options are depleted, it is possible to use the opposite IM system [39]. With this arrangement, two DIEP flaps would be combined into one internal mammary vascular system. With a long enough donor pedicle, the flap can be used without grafting. A scenario for this option would be a right system with large vessels, both antegrade and retrograde, while the left-sided vessels are small. The left donor flap is tunneled to the right side of the chest and anastomosed to the retrograde IM vascular system. If the donor vessels are not long enough to support this concept, vein graft utilizing saphenous vein could extend this idea [40].

Axillary System

As the system of second choice, there is a lot to like about the axillary system distal to the IM take off from the subclavian system. When an axillary dissection is completed during a mastectomy and an immediate breast reconstruction is performed, the TD vessels are readily available as a terminal branch of the subscapular artery and vein (also see Chap. 12). The diameters of the artery and vein match the deep inferior epigastric vessels well and can be dissected out to the level of the latissimus dorsi muscle for maximal length. In addition, there are many vein options of adequate size in the vicinity of the TD vessels, including the lateral thoracic vein, the branch to the serratus anterior muscle, and the circumflex scapular vein (Fig. 13.1) [41].

Another option exists proximal to the subscapular vessels: the thoracoacromial vessels (also see Chap. 14). These vessels take off just distal to the internal mammary vessels and can be accessed from within the mastectomy defect (Fig. 13.1). The vessels supply the pectoralis major muscle. As a Mathes and Nahai type V muscle, the pectoralis also gets adequate blood flow from the internal mammary perforators; therefore, using the thoracoacromial vessels as recipient for a free flap will not affect the function or viability of the muscle. This holds true even if the IM artery has been disrupted below the level of the third rib as the more proximal perforators will keep the muscle viable. As described by Singh et al., a pedicle length of approximately 5 cm can be obtained [42]. Previous research found an average artery diameter of 2.0 mm and vein diameter of 1.7 mm [43]. Their dissection time was approximately 10–15 minutes and was accomplished via a combination of elevating the pectoralis muscle from the mastectomy incision and making an infraclavicular counter incision to find the origin of the vessels.

Finally, while still in the axillary system, one could consider forming a Corlett loop with the cephalic vein into the axillary artery (or any other artery adjacent to the vein of sufficient size) to extend the reach of donor vessels if the thoracodorsal system reach proves inadequate. This maneuver would be performed by dissecting out the cephalic vein from the antecubital fossa and looping the distal end of the vessel back to the axillary or brachial artery to create an arteriovenous fistula. Once flowing, the loop can be divided yielding a vein graft to the artery and direct venous flow through the remaining cephalic vein. Of note, the vein graft will gain length once under arterial flow and therefore should be shorter than the venous side when dividing the loop [44].

Each of the above options from the axillary system can suffer from drawbacks. Poor ergonomics of working in the axilla, a history of radiation therapy to the axilla, and the distal location limiting the flap placement all detract from their use. In addition, if the IM artery has already been used successfully for inflow to the free flap but the veins are discovered to be inadequate, the TD vessels will no longer reach the flap vein which is tethered to the central chest by the arterial anastomosis to the IM artery. Overall, the IM system cannot be used 0.4–2% of the time and the thoracodorsal system 15% of the time [7, 20].

Venous Outflow Options Other Than the Internal Mammary and Axillary Systems

When both IM and axillary systems prove inadequate, an option external to these vessels will be needed. Mehrara et al. reported the use of the external jugular vein and cephalic vein finding that either can provide just such an alternative [45]. The expected scenario, as previously described, would be a successful anastomosis of the deep inferior epigastric artery to the IM artery but a failed venous coupling with either inadequate flow or too great a size mismatch. Time is of the essence in this scenario. There are two basic options to move forward with the operation. One method requires reapplication of the vascular clamps to the vessels going into the flap increasing the ischemia time and possibly risk for thrombosis. A second option is to allow the arterial anastomosis to flow but to minimize congestion, allowing a peripheral vein in the flap to bleed freely or clamp and release intermittently. This option will still cause congestion and excessive blood loss. It is the author's opinion that reapplication of clamp cutting off the blood flow is the better of the two options; however, minimizing the clamp time is critical. As such, one needs to be prepared to use either the external jugular vein or the cephalic vein to salvage the flap.

External Jugular Vein

To gain access in the external jugular vein (also see Chap. 2), a series of transverse 1–2 cm incisions are made in the neck in natural skin creases following the course the vein. As described by Mehrara, the inferior most incision is marked 1–2 cm above the clavicle and should be longer than the remaining access incisions to accommodate the deeper dissection (Fig. 13.2). Care is taken to avoid twisting when the vein is then turned down toward the recipient vessels. Some surgeons find it useful to mark the outer surface of the vein to monitor the degree of twisting. When dissected to within 2 cm of the angle of the mandible, the vein should reach to the level of the fourth rib. The length will be approximately 9 cm at this level, and care should be exercised if more length is needed as dissecting further toward and under the mandible risks damage to the marginal mandibular nerve. The diameter of the vein at this level is 3.5–5 mm, making it a good match to the deep inferior epigastric vein.

The main disadvantage of using the external jugular vein is the visible donor scarring. Fortunately, transverse scars in the neck heal well, but the patient should always be warned about the possible need of additional scars.

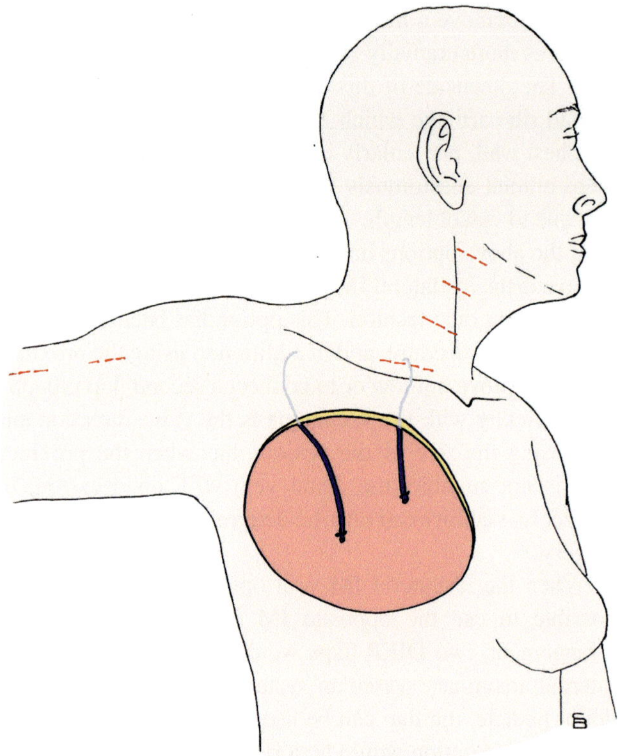

Fig. 13.2 Incisions to access the cephalic and external jugular veins

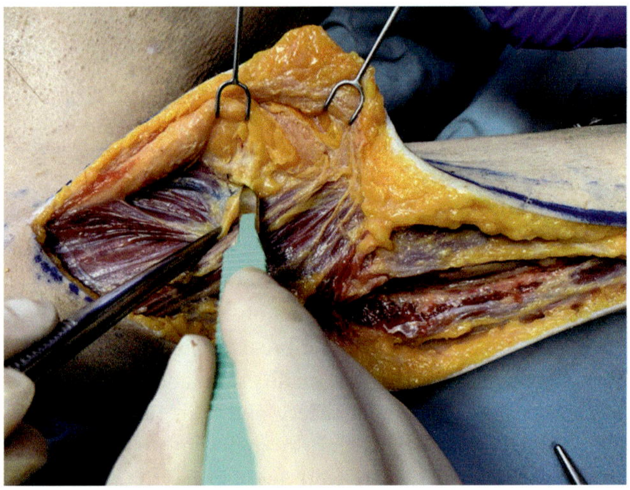

Fig. 13.3 Cadaver dissection of the cephalic vein in the deltopectoral groove

Cephalic Vein

The other readily available vein for emergency flap salvage is the cephalic vein (also see Chap. 24). Its location is consistent, and position can be fixed both proximally (deltopectoral groove) and distally (antecubital fossa). Each of the anatomic landmarks can be palpated and marked intraoperatively, even in heavier patients (Fig. 13.2). Once marked, the spots are connected by a straight line and multiple 2–3 cm incisions are made over the vein. The incisions should be close enough to each other (approximately 2 cm apart) to allow clipping of the branches in the obscured portions of the vein. In those areas not exposed by the incision, gentle blunt dissection is performed in the avascular plane superficial to the vein connecting the dissections of the disparate incisions. Dissection is carried out distally enough to accommodate the needed length to reach the recipient vessels and can be extended into the forearm if necessary (Figs. 13.2, 13.3, and 13.4). Proximally, the vein is dissected to the junction with the subclavian vein to allow for positioning without kinking the vessel (Fig. 13.5) (Video 13.1). The vessel can easily reach the midline of the chest and the diameter is typically 3–5 mm, making it an excellent match to the deep inferior epigastric vein. As with the external jugular vein, the main drawback of this procedure is the visible scarring on the cra-

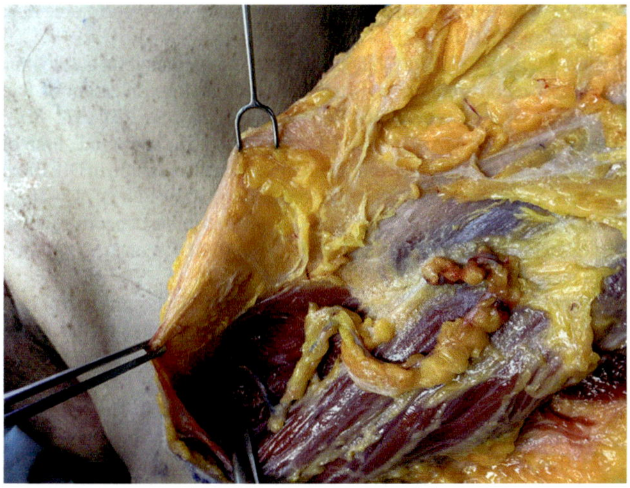

Fig. 13.4 The cephalic vein is transected distally and is ready to be transposed

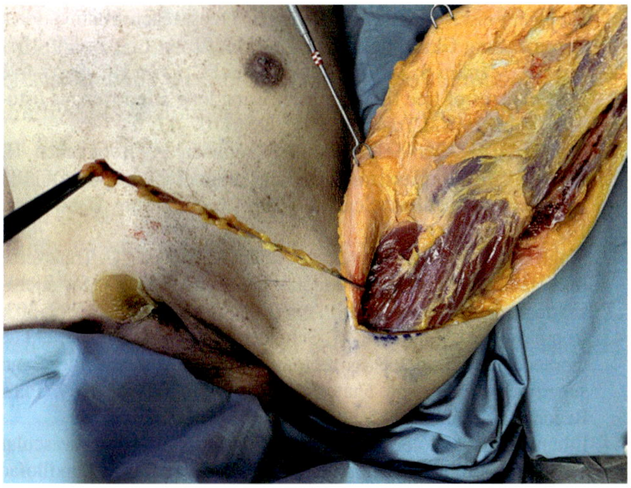

Fig. 13.5 Transposition of the cephalic vein to the chest for venous salvage

nial aspect of the upper arm. Wherein as the neck tends to scar well, the upper arm scars can become hypertrophic and as a result, quite visible. Also, in contrast to scars on the neck, these scars are easier to hide under clothing. As previously stated, the patient should always be forewarned of the possible need of additional scars on the neck, arm, or legs [46–49].

Discussion

Although the scenarios outlined in this chapter are rare, occurring in less than 3% of cases, the techniques described here will allow microsurgeons to salvage flaps that would otherwise be lost. The author's preferred technique is to utilize the IM system. On those occasions where the IM vein is inadequate or flap found to be congested postoperatively, the author defaults to the cephalic vein for outflow due to its reliable length, diameter, and position in the surgical field. This strategy has proven successful in salvaging compromised flaps.

References

1. Fujino T, Harashina T, Enomoto K. Primary breast reconstruction after a standard radical mastectomy by a free flap transfer. Case report. Plast Reconstr Surg. 1976;58(3):371–4.
2. Hefel L, Schwabegger A, Ninković M, Wechselberger G, Moriggl B, Waldenberger P, et al. Internal mammary vessels: anatomical and clinical considerations. Br J Plast Surg. 1995;48(8):527–32.
3. Ninković M, Anderl H, Hefel L, Schwabegger A, Wechselberger G. Internal mammary vessels: a reliable recipient system for free flaps in breast reconstruction. Br J Plast Surg. 1995;48(8):533–9.
4. Taylor GI. Corlett d RJ, Boyd JB. The versatile deep inferior epigastric (inferior rectus abdominis) flap. Br J Plast Surg. 1984;37(3):330–50.
5. Allen RJ, Tucker C. Superior gluteal artery perforator free flap for breast reconstruction. Plast Reconstr Surg. 1995;95(7):1207–12.
6. Arnez ZM, Valdatta L, Tyler MP, Planinsek F. Anatomy of the internal mammary veins and their use in free TRAM flap breast reconstruction. Br J Plast Surg. 1995;48(8):540–5.
7. Dupin CL, Allen RJ, Glass CA, Bunch R. The internal mammary artery and vein as a recipient site for free-flap breast reconstruction: a report of 110 consecutive cases. Plast Reconstr Surg. 1996;98(4):682–5.
8. Feng LJ. Recipient vessels in free-flap breast reconstruction: a study of the internal mammary and thoracodorsal vessels. Plast Reconstr Surg. 1997;99(2):405–16.
9. Fortin AJ, Evans HB, Chu MW. The cardiac implications of breast reconstruction using the internal mammary artery as the recipient vessel. Can J Plast Surg. 2012;20(1):e16–8.
10. Rozen WM, Ye X, Guio-Aguilar PL, Alonso-Burgos A, Goldblatt J, Ashton MW, Whitaker IS. Autologous microsurgical breast reconstruction and coronary artery bypass grafting: an anatomical study and clinical implications. Breast Cancer Res Treat. 2012;134(1):181–98.
11. Wennstig A-K, Garmo H, Isacsson U, Gagliardi G, Rintelä N, Lagerqvist B, et al. The relationship between radiation doses to coronary arteries and location of coronary stenosis requiring intervention in breast cancer survivors. Radiat Oncol. 2019;14(1):40.
12. Clark CP, Rohrich RJ, Copit S, Pittman CE, Robinson J. An anatomic study of the internal mammary veins: clinical implications for free-tissue-transfer breast reconstruction. Plast Reconstr Surg. 1997;99(2):400–4.
13. Muto M, Satake T, Masuda Y, Kobayashi S, Tamura S, Kobayashi S, et al. Absent internal mammary recipient vein in autologous breast reconstruction. Plast Reconstr Surg Glob Open. 2020;8(2):e2660.
14. Mauch JT, Rhemtulla IA, Katzel EB, Hernandez JA, Broach RB, Serletti JM. Does size matter: evaluating the difference between right and left internal mammary veins in free flap breast reconstruction. J Reconstr Microsurg. 2019;35(9):677–81.
15. Casey WJ, Rebecca AM, Smith AA, Craft RO, Buchel EW. The cephalic and external jugular veins: important alternative recipient vessels in left-sided microvascular breast reconstruction. Microsurgery. 2007;27(5):465–9.

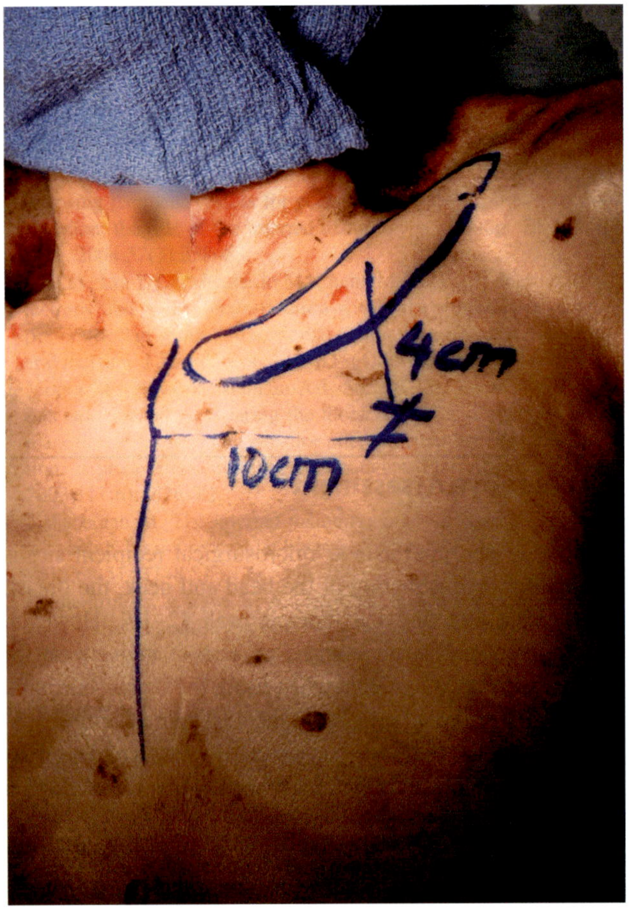

Fig. 14.1 The pectoral branch is found within 4 cm distance from the midclavicular line. Markings over the skin of the left chest for identification of the thoracoacromial vessels (indicated with X) in a cadaver

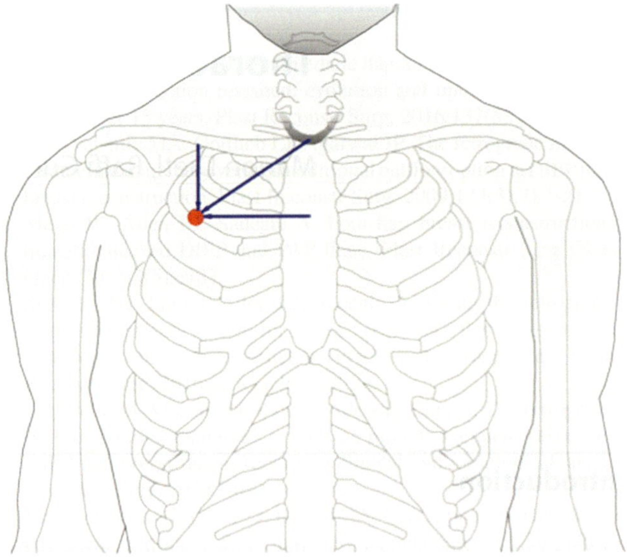

Fig. 14.2 Schematic illustration of the defined reference point indicated as red dot (10 cm distance from the manubrium (sternal notch) and midsternal line and 4.0 cm distance vertically from the clavicle) for cutaneous marking to identify pectoral branch

Table 14.1 Sonographic data for the definition of the reference point [17]

Distance in cm	Right hemithorax	Left hemithorax
Sternal notch	9.6 ± 1.0	10.1 ± 0.9
Midsternal line	9.0 ± 0.9	9.7 ± 0.8
Clavicle	3.7 ± 1.0	4.3 ± 1.2

(Fig. 14.1) [20]. Sonographic evaluation of healthy volunteers revealed that the exact location of the pectoral branch is constant with in average 10 cm distance from the manubrium (sternal notch) and midsternal line and 4.0 cm distance vertically from the clavicle [17]. These data define the reference point for cutaneous marking, as depicted in Fig. 14.2. Exact data of the sonographic measurement in healthy volunteers are documented in Table 14.1 [17]. At the level of the upper border of the third rib, the artery reaches a diameter of 1 mm, whereas the vein measures 0.9 ± 0.1 mm [17] and is therefore best suitable for microsurgical anastomosis.

Applied Anatomy

The thoracoacromial artery arises from the second part of the axillary artery, and its origin is located posterior to the pectoralis minor. The thoracoacromial artery is characterized by a short trunk which passes the medial margin of the pectoralis minor tendon. After piercing the clavipectoral fascia, the vessel classically divides into four branches, pectoral, acromial, clavicular, and deltoid, which supply the pectoralis major and minor muscle, the anterior part of the deltoid muscle, and the skin over the clavipectoral fascia [21, 22]. A schematic illustration of the thoracoacromial axis and its branches are demonstrated in Fig. 14.3.

The deltoid branch of the thoracoacromial artery parallels the cephalic vein in the deltopectoral groove [22, 23]. The acromial branch runs deep to the deltoid muscle by passing the coracoid process and subsequent anastomoses with branches of the suprascapular artery [22, 23]. The clavicular branch runs medially along the clavicular portion of the pectoralis major muscle and supplies the subclavius muscle and the sternoclavicular joint [22].

However, the pectoral branch is the only described recipient vessel of the thoracoacromial axis in microsurgical procedures. The pectoral branch is the dominant vessel and can easily be located on the posterior side of the pectoralis major muscle above the level of the third rib [17, 22]. However, along its course in the distal half of the muscle, it can no longer be well identified [22]. The pectoral branch sends small vessels to the pectoralis minor before descending on the deep surface of the pectoralis major within the epimysial sheath of the muscle and enveloped by protective perivascular fatty tissue [17, 18, 21]. Some perforators pierce the

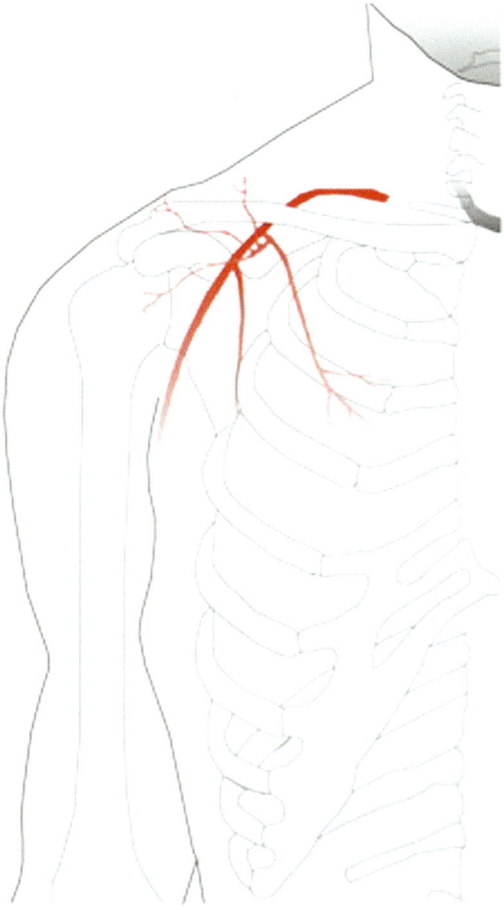

Fig. 14.3 Schematic illustration of the thoracoacromial axis and its branches

surface of the muscle and supply the overlying skin, whereas the terminal branches of the pectoral artery pass the inferolateral border of the pectoralis major to reach the skin [21]. An anatomical and sonographic study showed that the course of the vessels can differ, as some vessels pursue a caudomedial course from the acromion to the xiphoid, whereas others run primarily in a caudolateral direction reaching the lateral border of the pectoralis major muscle and afterward in a medial direction [17]. The medial and inferior branches of the pectoral artery anastomose with perforators of the internal mammary artery, whereas lateral branches may anastomose with perforators of the lateral thoracic artery [17, 19, 21, 22]. Data show that the pectoral branches on the right side descend most frequently in parallel to the median line, but descend mainly medially to the median line on the left side [24]. Nevertheless, the pectoral branch can be mainly found within 1 cm distance from the midclavicular line at both sides [20]. The pectoral branch is mainly accompanied by two adequate venae comitantes, but the lateral vein is mostly the dominant one [17]. However, the majority of vessels afterward divide into two major branches, whereas a division in three branches is possible [17]. Moreover, branches of the lateral thoracic nerve accompany the vessels underneath [1, 17]. Furthermore, a significant subcutaneous artery arises from the pectoral branch in about 25% of the cases. After its origin, this cutaneous artery pierces the deep fascia in the infraclavicular fossa and runs afterward in the subcutaneous fat in an inferior direction [21]. However, this artery is not clinically relevant when dissecting the main pectoral branch. Data reveal that at the origin of the pectoral branch from the thoracoacromial vessels, both the pectoral artery and vein measure about 3.1 mm on average [17]. However, in cadaver dissection, Geddes et al. describe an average diameter of the pectoral branch of 1.7 ± 0.6 mm [19].

Surgical Site Exposure

The preoperative assessment (including a profound clinical examination, Doppler examination, and cutaneous marking of the vascular landmarks) is essential in procedure planning. Patient's positioning for the access to the thoracoacromial vessels can vary depending on the flap harvest site and the reconstructive procedure. Preparation of the thoracoacromial axis is possible both in lateral decubitus and in supine position. Depending on the reconstructive procedure, exposure of the thoracoacromial recipient site is possible via a transmuscular or a retromuscular approach.

Transmuscular Approach

Exposure of the recipient site, as performed by the authors and described by other colleagues, is relatively straightforward through an incision 2–4 cm below the clavicle in the midclavicular line [25]. The skin incision should be about 5 cm in length. After incision through the skin und subcutis, a 10 cm to 10 cm pocket can be bluntly dissected over the muscle in a caudal direction. This pocket facilitates the access to the recipient vessel by moving the cutis to the necessary extent for subsequent microsurgical procedure. After blunt dissection and retraction of the subcutis, the pectoralis major muscle can be identified (Fig. 14.4) and fibers be split 5 cm from the clavicle in a longitudinal direction.

Both nerves and vessels enter the underside of the muscle by piercing the clavipectoral fascia. However, in this area, the vessels are surrounded by a fibrofatty layer and have yet no contact with the pectoralis major muscle. Therefore, identification of the vascular trunk and the pectoralis nerve is safely possible after retraction of the two parts of the divided pectoralis major muscle.

However, as the dissection is continued from the clavicle toward caudal, the side branches of the thoracoacromial vessel (clavicular, acromial and deltoid branch) arise. These

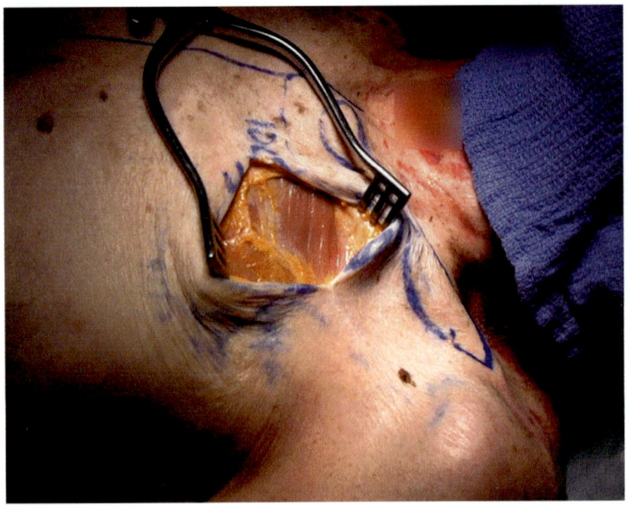

Fig. 14.4 Transmuscular approach: the pectoralis major muscle is identified after incision through the skin and subcutis in the same cadaver

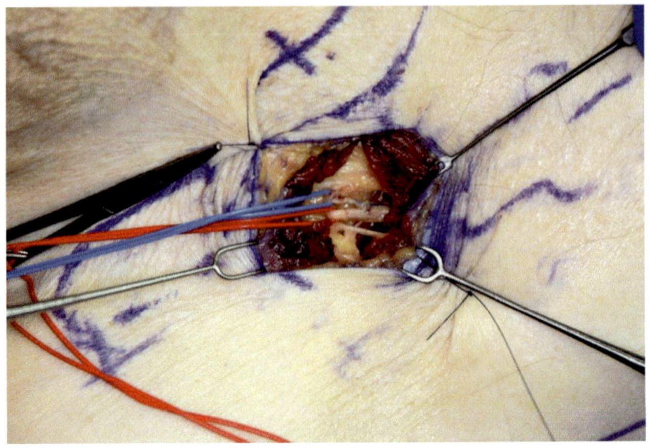

Fig. 14.5 Transmuscular approach: intraoperative exposure of the pectoral artery and vein

branches should be separated from the surrounding tissue one by one and if necessary ligated in order to extend the length and working size of the pectoral recipient vessel. Using this technique, a pedicle length of a minimum of 3 cm can be achieved (Video 14.1). Singh et al. described a similar approach to the recipient site and reported a pedicle length of 5.5 cm on the left side and 5.0 cm on the right side [25]. The pectoral branch of the thoracoacromial artery is mainly accompanied by two venae comitantes which are usually located above the artery. Therefore, the first step in vessel preparation is the dissection of the venous recipient vessels. Furthermore, lateral nerve fibers are running side by side with vessels and can generally be spared when dissecting artery and vein [17].

At the level of the third rib, the pectoral artery and vein measure 1 mm in average and are therefore best suited for microsurgical anastomosis [17] (Fig. 14.5). Authors performing a similar approach to the recipient site report an average preparation time of 10 minutes on the left side and of 13 minutes on the right side [25].

Retromuscular Approach

Access to the thoracoacromial axis is additionally possible using a retromuscular approach, when procedures on the anterior chest wall are performed. In the clinical practice of the authors, the preparation of the thoracoacromial vessels in this case is even easier and can be performed by undermining the pectoralis major muscle from caudal to cranial. The recipient pedicle is immediately visually identifiable by lifting the muscle up. The vessels emerge on the back of the pectoralis major and are running toward the clavicle.

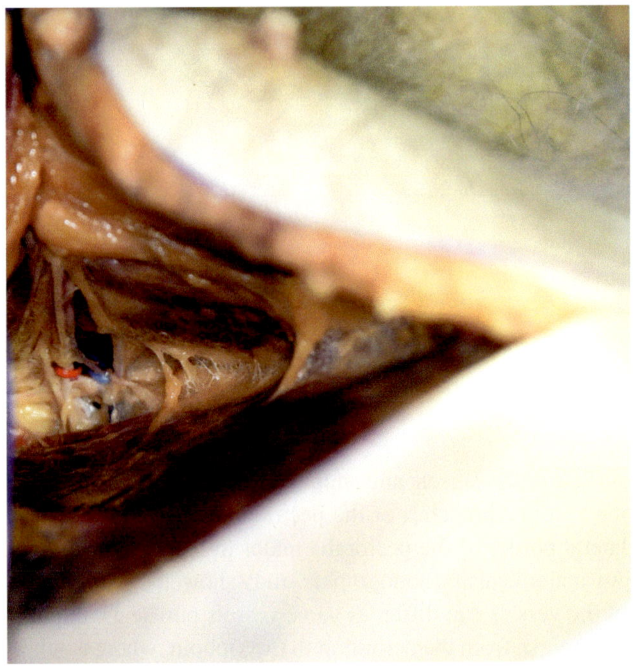

Fig. 14.6 Retromuscular approach: intraoperative exposure of the pectoral artery and vein by lifting up the pectoralis major muscle

However, in some cases, the pectoralis major muscle can already be resected and therefore recipient vessels can be accessed directly (Fig. 14.6). In both cases, anastomosis is possible without further local skin incision.

Discussion

The selection of suitable recipient vessels in microsurgery is crucial for the success of reconstructive free flap procedures. The thoracoacromial axis and its pectoral branch are mainly used as recipient vessel in the reconstructive procedures of the head and neck and ventral chest wall including the breast. However, in clinical practice, the thoracoacromial vessel is not the first choice as recipient pedicle in any of these regions. The advantages of the pectoral branch of the thoracoacromial axis are a consistent anatomy, a predictable location, and a suitable diameter of artery and vein. Both have a consistent cutoff point of 1 mm located on the upper border of the third rib [17]. The location on the ventral hemithorax enables a straightforward and therefore time-saving preparation when accessing the vessel [17, 25], in both open retromuscular and ventral transmuscular approaches. In addition, microvascular anastomoses are technically perfectly feasible due to the anatomical location and the possibility of a direct positioning of the microscope over the operative field. Furthermore, when using the pectoral branch for microsurgical anastomosis, sufficient blood supply can be still provided for the pectoralis major muscle via perforators of the internal mammary artery and the lateral thoracic artery [26]. Surgical site exposure is possible in lateral as well as supine position of the patient.

In breast reconstruction, the internal mammary artery mainly serves as recipient vessel when performing autologous free tissue transfer. However, preparation for access to these vessels is an invasive and time-consuming procedure [27]. In addition, if removal of the costal cartilage is performed, postoperative pain can increase [25] and developments of postoperative chest wall deformities are possible [27]. Hence, the thoracoacromial recipient site may be superior, as its preparation is simple and less traumatic. Furthermore, the sole use of the venous pectoral branch for additional venous drainage in autologous breast reconstruction has been recently described [11–15].

In head and neck reconstruction, including free tissue jejunal/ileal transfer [2, 8], the thoracoacromial recipient site may be superior after extensive surgical resection and/or radiation therapy in areas of preferred recipient vessels [2–8].

However, when using the pectoral branch as recipient, it has to be taken into account that the length suitable for microvascular anastomosis is limited. Thus, only flaps with a long pedicle can be used. Furthermore, in cases where the lateral thoracic artery arises from the thoracoacromial axis [28, 29], a potential reduction of the diameter of the vessel is possible and can make anastomosis increasingly difficult.

Microsurgical procedures are not uncommon in the elderly patient population. However, arteriosclerotic changes in the thoracoacromial vessels are currently not described. Therefore, the quality of vessels has to be evaluated preoperatively.

Despite few disadvantages, the thoracoacromial vessels may be used as recipient site in the microsurgical reconstruction of the head and neck, the breast, and the ventral thoracic wall.

Summary

- In the vast majority of cases, the thoracoacromial vessels are not the primary resource for revascularization of microsurgical flaps.
- In select patients, the pectoral branch of thoracoacromial vessels may be used as an alternative recipient for microsurgical reconstruction of the head and neck, breast, as well as chest wall.
- The pectoral branch has a consistent anatomy and a predictable location.
- However, preoperative imaging is recommended to confirm patency.
- Exposure of thoracoacromial vessels can be performed through trans-pectoral approach or retromuscular approach.

References

1. Ariyan S. The pectoralis major myocutaneous flap: a versatile flap for reconstruction in the head and neck. Plast Reconstr Surg. 1979;63:73–81.
2. Harashina T, Kakegawa T, Imai T, Suguro Y. Secondary reconstruction of oesophagus with free revascularized ileal transfer. Br J Plast Surg. 1981;34:17.
3. Takamatsu A, Harashina T, Inoue T. Selection of appropriate recipient vessels in difficult, microsurgical head and neck reconstruction. J Reconstr Microsurg. 1996;12:499.
4. Onoda S, Sakuraba M, Asano T, Miyamoto S, Hayashi R, Asai M, et al. Thoracoacromial vessels as recipient for head and neck reconstruction and cause of vascular complications. Microsurgery. 2011;31(8):628–31.
5. Jacobson AS, Eloy JA, Park E, Roman B, Genden EM. Vessel-depleted neck: techniques for achieving microvascular reconstruction. Head Neck. 2008;30(2):201–7.
6. Harris JP, Lueg E, Genden E, Urken ML. The thoracoacromial/cephalic vascular system for microvascular anastomoses in the vessel-depleted neck. Arch Otolatyngol Head Neck Surg. 2002;128(3):319–23.
7. Aycock JK, Stenson KM, Gottlieb LJ. The thoracoacromial trunk: alternative recipient vessels in reoperative head and neck reconstructive microsurgery. Plast Reconstr Surg. 2008;121(1):88–94.
8. Numajiri T, Fujiwara T, Nishino K, Sowa Y, Uenaka M, Shimada T, et al. The thoracoacromial artery as the recipient artery for safer free jejunal transfer in patients with irradiated, extensively scarred necks. Br J Oral Maxillofac Surg. 2009;47(1):73–4.
9. Castello JR, Taglialatela Scafati S, Sanchez O, Del Rio M. Microsurgical reconstruction of a huge mediastinal defect using thoracoacromial vessels as recipient pedicle. Plast Reconstr Surg. 2012;129(6):1021e–1023e.
10. Harashina T, Inoue T, Sasaki K, Tanaka I, Kiyoizumi T. Reconstruction of breast after super-radical mastectomy with a pedicled latissimus dorsi flap and a free TRAM flap. Br J Plast Surg. 1988;41:361.
11. Kim EJ, Lee HJ, Mun GH. Muscle-splitting approach to thoracoacromial vein for superdrainage in deep inferior epigastric artery perforator flap breast reconstruction. Microsurgery. 2019;39(3):228–33.

12. Chun JK, Harmaty M, Ting J. Thoracoacromial vessels as the recipients for supercharged muscle-sparing transverse rectus abdominis myocutaneous flaps. J Reconstr Microsurg. 2007;23(3):125–9.
13. Ayestaray B, Yonekura K, Motomura H, Ziade M. A comparative study between deep inferior epigastric artery perforator and thoracoacromial venous supercharged deep inferior epigastric artery perforator flaps. Ann Plast Surg. 2016;76(1):78–82.
14. Tarakji M, Bartow MJ, Dupin C, Tessler O. Using the venous pectoral branch from the thoracoacromial system as a lifeboat in autologous breast reconstruction. Plast Reconstr Surg Glob Open. 2017;5(6):e1367.
15. Eom JS, Sun SH, Lee TJ. Selection of the recipient veins for additional anastomosis of the superficial inferior epigastric vein in breast reconstruction with free transverse rectus abdominis musculocutaneous or deep inferior epigastric artery perforator flaps. Ann Plast Surg. 2011;67(5):505–9.
16. Chow WT, Rozen WM, Patel NG. RamakrishnanVV. Five recipient vessels for metachronous chest wall reconstruction: case report and literature review. Microsurgery. 2017;37(1):66–70.
17. Kompatscher P, Manestar M, Schuster A, Lang A, Beer GM. The Thoracoacromial vessels as recipient vessels in microsurgery and Supermicrosurgery: an anatomical and sonographic study. Plast Reconstr Surg. 2005;115:77–83.
18. Friedrich Q, Lierse W, Herberhold C. Myocutaneous vascular territory of the thoracoacromial artery. A topographical and morphometric study of the arterial vascularization of the pectoralis major myocutaneous flap. Acta Anat (Basel). 1988;131(4):284–91.
19. Geddes CR, Tang M, Yang D, Morris SF. An assessment of the anatomical basis of the thoracoacromial artery perforator flap. Can J Plast Surg. 2003;11(1):23–7.
20. Park HD, Min YS, Kwak HH, Youn KH, Lee EW, Kim HJ. Anatomical study concerning the origin and course of the pectoral branch of the thoracoacromial trunk for the pectoralis major flap. Surg Radiol Anat. 2004;26(6):428–32.
21. Cormack GC, Lamberty BGH. The arterial anatomy of skin flaps. 2nd ed. Edinburgh: Churchill Livingstone; 1986. p. 410–1.
22. McCraw J, Arnold PG. McCraw and Arnold's atlas of muscle and musculocutaneous flaps. Norfolk: Hampton Press Publishing Company; 1986. p. 97–8.
23. Hue E, Gagey O, Mestdagh H, Fontaine C, Drizenko A, Maynou C. The blood supply of the deltoid muscle. Application to the deltoid flap technique. Surg Radiol Anat. 1998;20(3):161–5.
24. Nakajima K, Ide Y, Abe S, Okada M, Kikuchi A, Ide Y. Anatomical study of the pectoral branch of thoracoacromial artery. Bull Tokyo Dent Coll. 1997;38(3):207–15.
25. Singh DP, Bluebond-Langner R, Chopra K, Gowda AU. Transverse infraclavicular approach to the thoracoacromial pedicle for microsurgical breast reconstruction. Ann Plast Surg. 2017;78(3):299–303.
26. Feeman JL, Walker EP, Shaw HJ. The vascular anatomy of the pectoralis major myocutaneous flap. Br J Plast Surg. 1981;34:3.
27. Schwabegger AH, Gschnitzer C, Ninkovic MM. Contour deformity at the internal mammary recipient site. Br J Plast Surg. 1999;52:674.
28. Loukas M, du Plessis M, Owens DG, Kinsella CR Jr, Litchfield CR, Nacar A, et al. The lateral thoracic artery revisited. Surg Radiol Anat. 2013;36:543–9.
29. Paraskevas GK. High or low incidence of the lateral thoracic artery's origin from the thoracoacromial artery? Surg Radiol Anat. 2015;37:887–9.

Deep Inferior Epigastric Vessels

15

Raffi Gurunian, Rebecca Knackstedt, Karlina Kegecik, and Richard L. Drake

Introduction

The deep inferior epigastric (DIE) vessels are typically known as donor vessels for microsurgical reconstruction using the free rectus abdominis, TRAM, or deep inferior epigastric artery perforator (DIEP) flap. Microsurgical flaps based on these vessels have been employed for a multitude of reasons in the head and neck [1, 2], breast [3–5], chest wall [6, 7], hip [8], and upper and lower extremity reconstruction [9, 10].

The DIEA and DIEV can also be isolated as recipient vessels for microsurgical reconstruction of the abdomen, chest, pelvic, and posterior trunk defects. This chapter reviews the applied anatomy and surgical exposure of the DIE vessels for use as recipient in microsurgical flap reconstruction.

Supplementary Information The online version of this chapter (https://doi.org/10.1007/978-3-030-75389-4_15) contains supplementary material, which is available to authorized users.

R. Gurunian (✉)
Department of Plastic Surgery, Cleveland Clinic, Cleveland, OH, USA

Cleveland Clinic Lerner College of Medicine, Case Western Reserve University, Cleveland, OH, USA
e-mail: gurunir@ccf.org

R. Knackstedt
Department of Plastic Surgery, Cleveland Clinic, Cleveland, OH, USA
e-mail: KNACKSR@ccf.org

K. Kegecik
Cleveland State University, Cleveland, OH, USA

R. L. Drake
Department of Anatomy, Cleveland Clinic Lerner College of Medicine, Cleveland, OH, USA
e-mail: DRAKER@ccf.org

Preoperative Assessment

The decision of which recipient vessel to utilize for microsurgical reconstruction depends on numerous patient and flap factors as well as wound characteristics. The patient's body habitus and unique anatomy influence the ease by which a vessel could be isolated. Additionally, the nature of the defect and possible zone of injury impact the availability and quality of vessels in that region. The length and caliber of the donor vessels should also be factored into decision-making process. Preoperative imaging such as Doppler ultrasound, computed tomography angiography, or magnetic resonance angiography may be warranted to assess the DIE vessels prior to surgery. This is especially pertinent for patients who have a history of complex abdominal surgeries or vascular surgeries requiring intra-abdominal procedures, or history of abdominopelvic radiation therapy as the intended DIE recipient vessels may have been injured or resected. Alternative recipient sites and/or use of arteriovenous loop grafts or vein grafts should be considered in such cases.

Applied Anatomy

The deep inferior epigastric artery (DIEA) leaves the external iliac just proximal to the inguinal ligament and curves forward in the extraperitoneal tissue in a lateral to medial direction. It then pierces the transversalis fascia and the attenuated part of the rectus sheath. It ascends between the rectus abdominis and posterior lamina of the rectus sheath [11, 12].

Cephalad to the arcuate line, the DIEA typically divides into three branching patterns [13]. The most common DIEA vascular pattern is Type 2 (57–84%), consisting of a simple bifurcation cephalad to the arcuate line [14–16], as lateral and medial branches that give rise to lateral and medial row perforators [15–20].

R. Gurunian, R. Djohan (eds.), *Recipient Vessels in Reconstructive Microsurgery*, https://doi.org/10.1007/978-3-030-75389-4_15

The lateral branch usually gives rise to multiple lateral segmental branches, accompanying the segmental nerves, which communicate with the deep intercostal arteries. The lateral branch eventually terminates as a periumbilical perforating artery. After giving off a major branch to the umbilicus, the medial branch continues cephalad, providing multiple muscle and musculocutaneous perforators. The medial branch terminates cephalad in multiple choke vessels, which communicate directly with the deep superior epigastric artery in a watershed fashion [21].

Type 1 pattern, with a single inferior vessel, is less commonly described (27–29%), followed by Type 2 pattern (14–16%), which consists of a single inferior vessel that trifurcates at the level of the arcuate line. In two studies, some patients exhibited a unilateral absent DIEA, which was identified by preoperative imaging [22, 23].

The increased use of preoperative imaging, particularly with computed tomographic angiography (CTA), has enabled visualization of the DIEA and its branches in vivo, providing a functional view of this anatomy. The branching patterns of the DIEA were found to be different in vivo compared with cadaveric studies, with a higher than previously reported incidence of Type 1 patterns and lower than reported incidence of Type 3 patterns, and that some patterns exist which were not included within the previous nomenclature (namely, Type 0 or absent DIEA and Type 4 or four-trunk DIEA) [24].

The deep inferior epigastric vein is the union of the venae comitantes of the inferior epigastric veins; it joins the external iliac vein about 1 cm proximal to the inguinal ligament. It can run laterally, medially, or centrally under the rectus muscle as it ascends cranially. According to a cadaver study by El-Mrakby and Milner [25], the DIE artery was accompanied by two veins (90%). Only in 10% of the dissections, there was only one vena comitans.

Another study conducted in 44 cadavers (88 vessel bundles, 25 males, 19 females) showed that a double emptying into major veins was present in 22.7% on the right side, in 34.1% on the left side, and in only 13.6% bilaterally; the remaining veins emptied as a stem (as a confluence of always two accompanying veins), with a variable length of 1–57 mm [26]. The literature contains a great variety of reports of accompanying veins and their emptying as a common stem into major veins [13, 27].

DIE vessels have adequate length and caliber for use as recipient. At its origin, the artery has its external diameter of 3.4 mm, and from its point of entrance into the posterior rectus sheath, its length is approximately 7.6 cm. DIEV diameters are 4 mm [21, 28].

Strauch and his associates [29] note that the average arterial length from its origin to its entrance to the rectus is 10.9 cm (range 7.1–14.7 cm). Vessel diameters at the origin and entrance are, the inferior epigastric artery measurements in diameter at the origin, respectively, 2.7 mm (range 1.6–3.5 mm) and 2.0 mm (range 1.5–2.6 mm). The artery has two venae comitantes, the diameter of which is 3.0 mm (range 1.7–3.8 mm) at the origin and 2.2 mm (range 0.8–3.1 mm) at the entrance.

Surgical Site Exposure

Isolation of the DIEA and DIEV can be accomplished from an external approach or intra-abdominally depending on the surgical defect and planned procedure (Video 15.1).

External Approach

Orientation and exact location of the skin incision is dictated by the reconstructive need. Horizontal and/or longitudinal, curvilinear incisions may be used. When a horizontal incision is made, it typically courses along a line from the anterior iliac spine and suprapubic area. Again, the width and exact location of the incision depends on the location and size of the defect. Also, the incision should be made carefully, to preserve the superficial inferior epigastric vein (SIEV), which can be utilized for additional venous drainage, if necessary. Alternatively, a longitudinal paramedian incision can be utilized over the rectus muscle. Regardless of the incision orientation, the incision is carried down to the anterior rectus sheath that must be opened to expose the lateral rectus muscle border. When the rectus lateral border is retracted medially, the DIEA and vein (DIEV) can be visualized traveling along the posterior border of the muscle. Depending on the location of reconstruction required, the vessel can be traced beneath the rectus muscle cranially. However, as the vessels are traced cranially, they will take a variable course within the substance of the muscle requiring careful dissection. Multiple branches will require clipping. The medial or lateral branch may be ligated to extend the pedicle length. In any case, an adequate length and caliber should be obtained to allow a safe and healthy microvascular anastomosis (Figs. 15.1 and 15.2).

Intra-abdominal Approach

The DIE vessels can be readily available for use as recipient in cases where abdominal cavity has been entered for various reasons such as during laparotomy for abdomino-

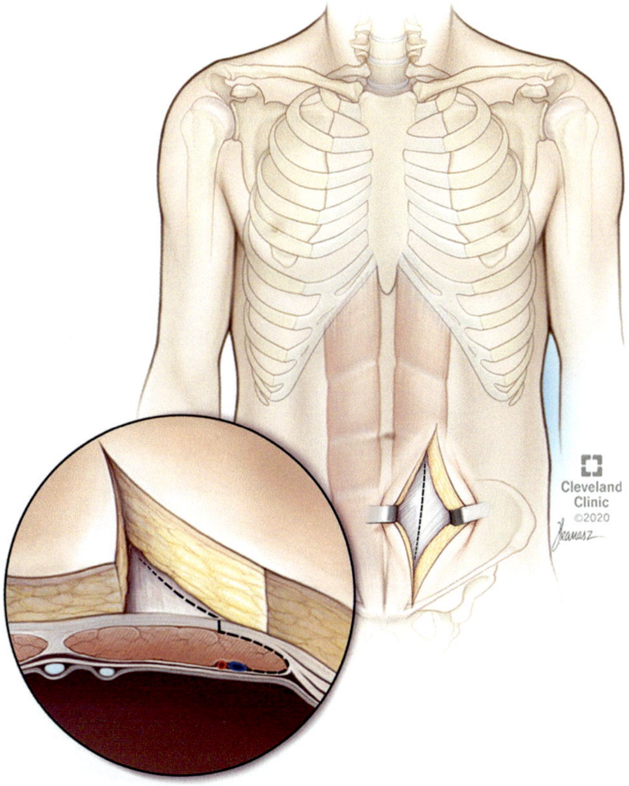

Fig. 15.1 Surgical exposure of the deep inferior epigastric vessels through external approach using a paramedian incision. Dashed line demonstrates the incision made over the lateral third of the anterior rectus sheath to expose the DIE vessels under the rectus abdominis muscle. (Reprinted with permission, Cleveland Clinic Center for Medical Art & Photography © 2020. All Rights Reserved)

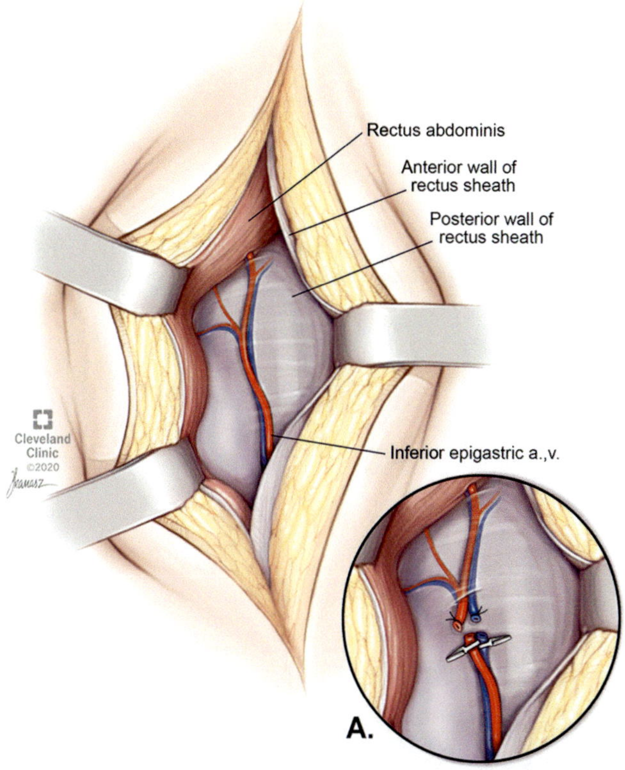

Fig. 15.2 The rectus abdominis muscle is lifted off the posterior rectus sheath and retracted medially for further dissection of DIE vessels to prepare for microvascular anastomosis. (**A**) Close-up drawing of DIEA and DIEV that are divided and prepared for microvascular anastomosis. (Reprinted with permission, Cleveland Clinic Center for Medical Art & Photography © 2020. All Rights Reserved)

perineal resections, full-thickness resections for abdominal wall tumors, or complex abdominal hernia and/or defect repairs.

When performing complex abdominal wall reconstruction using components separation techniques, in particular the transversus abdominis release (TAR) and posterior component separation, the deep inferior epigastric vessels can be approached from within the abdominal cavity [30, 31].

In the retrorectus plane, when posterior rectus sheath dissection is carried out laterally toward the semilunar line, the DIEA and DIEV can be identified and carefully prepared for microsurgical reconstruction of the abdominal wall defects [31] (Figs. 15.3 and 15.4).

A case of complex abdominal wall defect who underwent abdominal wall reconstruction using mesh construct along with posterior components separation and microsurgical anterolateral thigh flap for soft tissue coverage is presented in Figs. 15.5, 15.6, 15.7, and 15.8. Also Video 15.1 demonstrates few abdominal wall reconstruction cases that received microsurgical flap reconstruction using the DIE vessels as recipient.

Discussion

In vivo imaging and cadaver studies point out to the fact that DIE artery has a predictable anatomy but with varying branching patterns. It is recommended to obtain a preoperative imaging to confirm their patency and course.

Depending on the size and location of the defect to be reconstructed, the DIE vessels can be used within the abdomen or transposed superficially to revascularize microsurgical flaps for various reconstructive purposes. If a microsurgical flap with a short pedicle is utilized, to gain the pedicle length required of the DIEA and DIEV, tedious muscular dissection is necessary. But as dissection moves cranially, the diameter of the artery may decrease as it branches into medial and lateral rows. An intraoperative decision is made regarding the transection level of the DIE vessels to be used for anastomoses, taking the donor flap pedicle length and caliber into account for the best possible match and tension-free microvascular anastomosis. The DIE vessels can be ligated prior to entering the substance of the rectus muscle if a flap with a long pedicle is chosen. Vein grafts or arteriovenous (AV) loops should always be considered

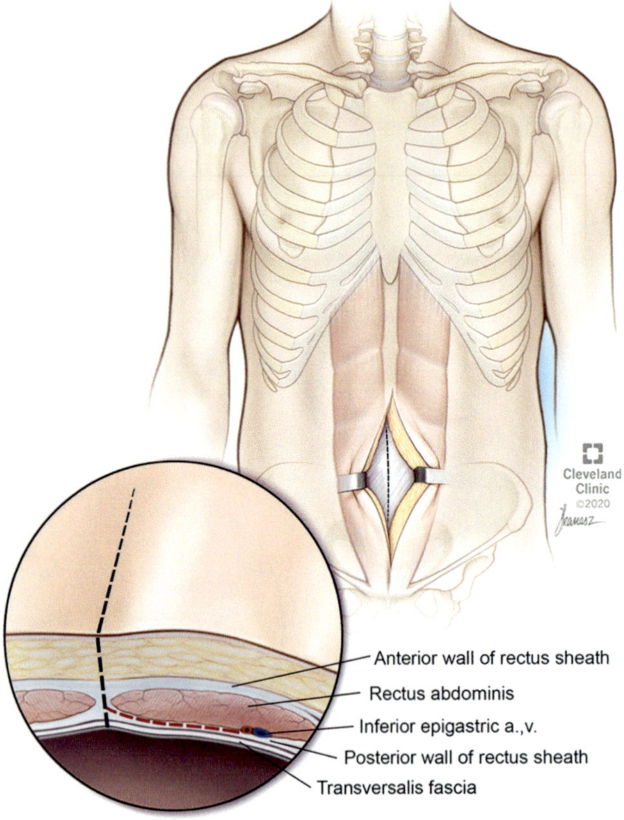

Fig. 15.3 Surgical exposure of the deep inferior epigastric vessels using intra-abdominal approach. The black dashed line indicates the laparotomy incision that is performed to enter the abdominal cavity. Please note that patients with loss of domain and large abdominal wall defect may have rectus abdominis muscle displaced laterally or even absent. Therefore, after getting into the abdomen, a careful dissection of the posterior rectus sheath and transversalis fascia underneath the rectus abdominis muscle is required to expose the DIEA and DIEV (red dashed line). (Reprinted with permission, Cleveland Clinic Center for Medical Art & Photography © 2020. All Rights Reserved)

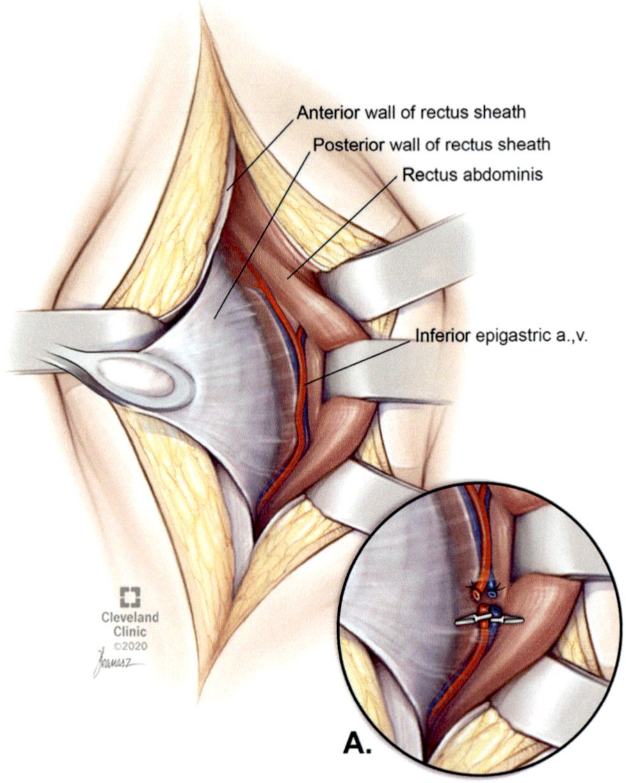

Fig. 15.4 In the retrorectus plane, when posterior rectus sheath dissection is carried out laterally toward the semilunar line, the DIEA and DIEV can be identified and prepared as recipient for microsurgical reconstruction of the abdominal wall defects. (**A**) Close-up drawing of DIEA and DIEV that are divided and prepared for microvascular anastomosis. (Reprinted with permission, Cleveland Clinic Center for Medical Art & Photography © 2020. All Rights Reserved)

preoperatively as well as intraoperatively as a backup plan in case of inadequate vessel reach [32] (Chaps. 18 and 42).

The DIEA and DIEV have been used as recipient for reconstruction using microsurgical flaps. A systematic review by the senior author on the recipient vessels for microsurgical flap reconstruction of the abdominal wall defects showed that the inferior epigastric system was the most commonly employed system for anastomosis [33].

The DIEA and DIEV have been successfully utilized for microsurgical reconstruction of the penis [34] and vagina and pelvic defects after abdominoperineal resections [35] and lumbosacral region [36].

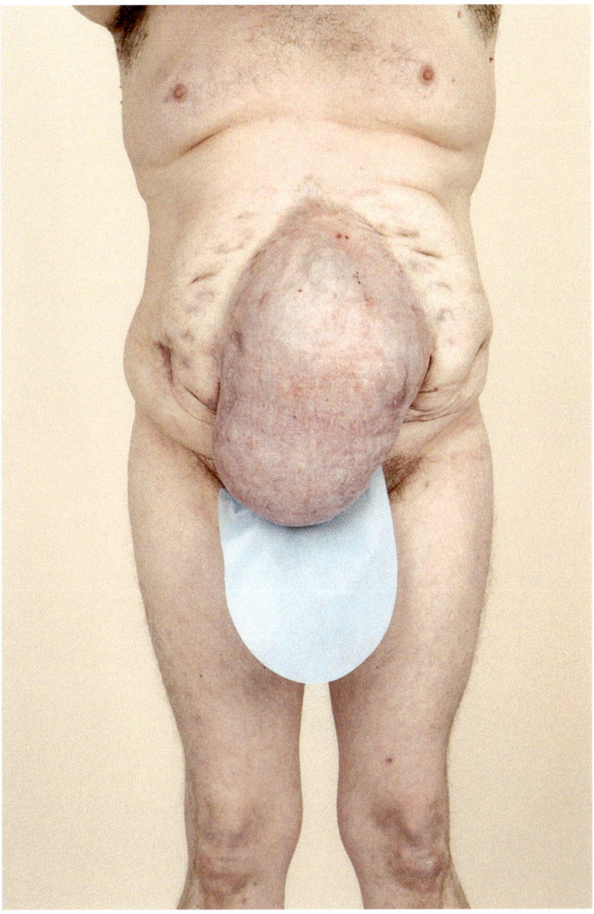

Fig. 15.5 Preoperative frontal view: Patient with complex abdominal defect with loss of domain

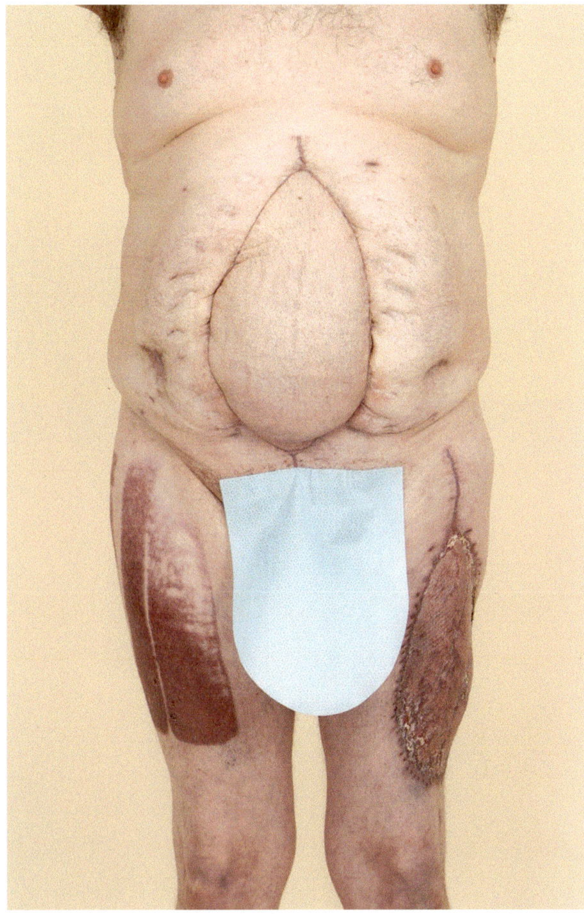

Fig. 15.6 Postoperative frontal view: Patient underwent posterior components separation and transversus abdominis release along with synthetic mesh in the retrorectus plane. Soft tissue reconstruction was performed using free anterolateral thigh flap. Right deep inferior epigastric vessels were used for recipient

Conclusion

The DIE vessels are reliable and have a predictable anatomy. Nevertheless, preoperative imaging allows for surgical planning in regard to the course of the artery and branching pattern. The DIEA and DIEV can be isolated through external approach or intra-abdominally for use as recipient in various microsurgical flaps. The approach to use depends on the reconstructive goals and specifics of each individual case.

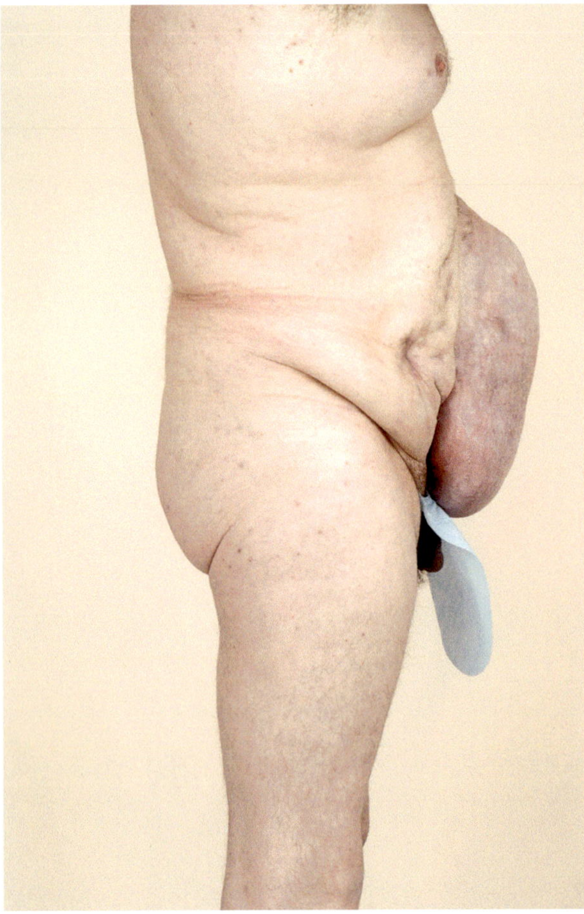

Fig. 15.7 Preoperative side view

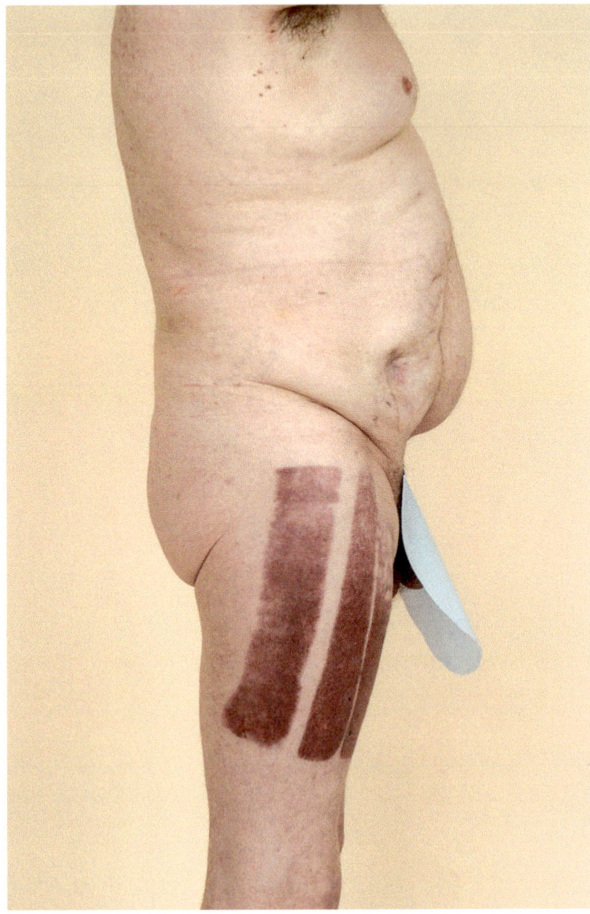

Fig. 15.8 Postoperative side view

References

1. Gurunluoglu R, Gatherwright J. Microsurgical reconstruction of complex maxillofacial gunshot wounds: outcomes analysis and algorithm. Microsurgery. 2019;39(5):384–94.
2. Leonhardt H, Mai R, Pradel W, Markwardt J, Pinzer T, Spassov A, Lauer G. Free DIEP-flap reconstruction of tumour related defects in head and neck. J Physiol Pharmacol. 2008;59(Suppl 5):59–67.
3. Nahabedian MY, et al. Breast reconstruction with the free TRAM or DIEP flap: patient selection, choice of flap, and outcome. Plast Reconstr Surg. 2002;110(2):466–75; discussion 476–7.
4. Gurunluoglu R, Shafighi M, Schwabegger A, Ninkovic M. Secondary breast reconstruction with deepithelialized free flaps from the lower abdomen for intractable capsular contracture and maintenance of breast volume. J Reconstr Microsurg. 2005;21(1):35–41.
5. Granzow JW, Levine JL, Chiu ES, Allen RJ. Breast reconstruction using perforator flaps. J Surg Oncol. 2006;94(6):441–54.
6. Tukiainen E. Chest wall reconstruction after oncological resections. Scand J Surg. 2013;102(1):9–13.
7. Gilman K, Ipaktchi K, Moore EE, Barnett C, Gurunluoglu R. Reconstruction of an emergency thoracotomy wound with free rectus abdominis flap: anatomic and radiologic basis for the surgical technique. World J Emerg Surg. 2010;5:12.
8. Gurunluoglu R. The ascending branch of the lateral circumflex femoral vessels: review of the anatomy and its utilization as recipient vessel for free-flap reconstruction of the hip region. J Reconstr Microsurg. 2010;26(6):359–66.
9. Kostakoğlu N, Keçik A. Deep inferior epigastric artery (DIEA) skin flap: clinical experience of 15 cases. Br J Plast Surg. 1998;51(1):25–31.
10. Van Landuyt K, Blondeel P, Hamdi M, Tonnard P, Verpaele A, Monstrey S. The versatile DIEP flap: its use in lower extremity reconstruction. Br J Plast Surg. 2005;58(1):2–13.
11. Williams P, Warwick R, Dyson M, Bannister LH. Gray's anatomy. In: Angiology. 37th ed. New York: Churchill Livingstone; 1989. p. 780–815.
12. Rueda M, Rueda S, Alleyne B, Drake RL, Gurunluoglu R. Chapter 4: Anatomy of the trunk. In: Bruce MA, editor. Plastic surgery: a practical guide to operative care. New York: Thieme Publishers; 2020.
13. Moon HK, Taylor GI. The vascular anatomy of rectus abdominis musculocutaneous flaps based on the deep superior epigastric system. Plast Reconstr Surg. 1988;82:815–32.
14. Itoh Y, Arai K. The deep inferior epigastric artery free skin flap: anatomic study and clinical application. Plast Reconstr Surg. 1993;91:853–63; discussion 864.
15. Rozen WM, Palmer KP, Suami H, et al. The DIEA branching pattern and its relationship to perforators: the importance of preoperative computed tomographic angiography for DIEA perforator flaps. Plast Reconstr Surg. 2008;121:367–73.
16. Ireton JE, Lakhiani C, Saint-Cyr M. Vascular anatomy of the deep inferior epigastric artery perforator flap: a systematic review. Plast Reconstr Surg. 2014;134(5):810e–21e.

17. Vandevoort M, Vranckx JJ, Fabre G. Perforator topography of the deep inferior epigastric perforator flap in 100 cases of breast reconstruction. Plast Reconstr Surg. 2002;109:1912–8.
18. Munhoz AM, Ishida LH, Sturtz GP, et al. Importance of lateral row perforator vessels in deep inferior epigastric perforator flap harvesting. Plast Reconstr Surg. 2004;113:517–24.
19. Bailey SH, Saint-Cyr M, Wong C, et al. The single dominant medial row perforator DIEP flap in breast reconstruction: three-dimensional perforasome and clinical results. Plast Reconstr Surg. 2010;126:739–51.
20. Wong C, Saint-Cyr M, Mojallal A, et al. Perforasomes of the DIEP flap: vascular anatomy of the lateral versus medial row perforators and clinical implications. Plast Reconstr Surg. 2010;125:772–82.
21. Oswald TM, Lineaweaver WC, Hui K. Recipient vessels for microsurgical flaps to the groin and pelvis: a review. J Reconstr Microsurg. 2006;22(1):5–14.
22. Xin M, Luan J, Mu L, Zhao Z, Mu D, Chen X. The efficacy of preoperative vascular mapping by MDCTA in selecting flap in abdominal flap breast reconstruction. Breast J. 2011;17:138–42.
23. Whitaker IS, Rozen WM, Smit JM, Dimopoulou A, Ashton MW, Acosta R. Peritoneo-cutaneous perforators in deep inferior epigastric perforator flaps: a cadaveric dissection and computed tomographic angiography study. Microsurgery. 2009;29:124–7.
24. Rozen WM, Ashton MW, Grinsell D. The branching pattern of the deep inferior epigastric artery revisited in-vivo: a new classification based on CT angiography. Clin Anat. 2010;23(1):87–92.
25. El-Mrakby HH, Milner RH. The vascular anatomy of the lower anterior abdominal wall: a microdissection study on the deep inferior epigastric vessels and the perforator branches. Plast Reconstr Surg. 2002;109(2):539–43; discussion 544–7.
26. Voppichler M. Untersuchung der Vasa epigastrica inferior im hinblick auf die mikrochirurgische Verwendung beim Rectus-abdominis Lappen (Thesis). Innsbruck. 1998.
27. Shafighi M, Schwabegger AH, Michelle E, Gurunluoglu R. A cadaver study: the course of the inferior epigastric vessels. Plast Reconstr Surg. 2003;112(1):341–3.
28. Serafin D. Atlas of microsurgery composite tissue transplantation. Philadelphia: WB Saunders Co; 1996. p. 210–215, 445–453, 462–464.
29. Strauch B, Yu HL, Chen ZW, Liebling R. Atlas of microvascular surgery. New York: Thieme Medical Publishers, Inc; 1993. p. 448–83.
30. Novitsky YW, Elliott HL, Orenstein SB, Rosen MJ. Transversus abdominis muscle release: a novel approach to posterior component separation during complex abdominal wall reconstruction. Am J Surg. 2012;204(5):709–16.
31. Aliotta RE, Gatherwright J, Krpata D, Rosenblatt S, Rosen M, Gurunluoglu R. Complex abdominal wall reconstruction, harnessing the power of a specialized multidisciplinary team to improve pain and quality of life. Hernia. 2019;23(2):205–15.
32. Knackstedt R, Aliotta R, Gatherwright J, Djohan R, Gastman B, Schwarz G, Hendrickson M, Gurunluoglu R. Single-stage versus two-stage arteriovenous loop microsurgical reconstruction: a meta-analysis of the literature. Microsurgery. 2018;38(6):706–17.
33. Gurunluoglu R, Rosen MJ. Recipient vessels for microsurgical flaps to the abdomen: a systematic review. Microsurgery. 2017;37(6):707–16.
34. Kropp B, Cohn JE, Wang W, Sokoya M, Ducic Y. Free tissue transfer penile reconstruction. Semin Plast Surg. 2019;33:24–9.
35. Wong A, Sbitany H. Reconstruction of intrapelvic defects using the free anterolateral thigh flap: expanding the traditional algorithm. Ann Plast Surg. 2020;84(5):554–8. https://doi.org/10.1097/SAP.0000000000002048.
36. Hung S, Chen H, Wei F. Free flaps for reconstruction of the lower back and sacral area. Microsurgery. 2000;20:72–6.

Intra-abdominal/Intraperitoneal Vessels

16

Hiroshi Matsumoto and Yoshihiro Kimata

Introduction

The gastroepiploic, jejunal, gastroduodenal, and inferior mesenteric vessels have been reported as recipient vessels for microsurgical reconstruction of the abdominal defects [1–13]. The arteries have a large caliber with a thick vascular wall, but the intraperitoneal veins have very thin walls; thus, careful surgical manipulation is required for the dissection and anastomosis of veins.

Preoperative Assessment

Preoperative assessment should include medical and surgical history. If the patient has a history of intra-abdominal surgery or irradiation, perivascular adhesion or scarring may have occurred, and planning of the selection of recipient vessels should be performed with the possibility that intraperitoneal vessels cannot be used. Three-dimensional angiography using computed tomography is very useful for preoperative evaluation (Fig. 16.1).

Applied Anatomy

Gastroepiploic Vessels

The right and left gastroepiploic arteries branch from the gastroduodenal and splenic arteries, respectively, and each artery runs the surface of the greater omentum along the greater curvature of the stomach (Fig. 16.2). The right and left gastroepiploic arteries are anastomosed at the middle of the stomach, and the length from the origin to the anastomotic point is 26.5 ± 5.15 cm and 14.1 ± 3.12 cm for the right and left gastroepiploic arteries, respectively. The vascular diameter was 2.71 ± 0.5 mm and 1.63 ± 0.6 mm in the right and left gastroepiploic arteries, respectively [14]. There are three patterns of anastomoses between the right and left gastroepiploic arteries in the middle of the stomach. The incidence of anastomoses varies from 23.5% to 70.6% in clear anastomosis and arterial arch formation, 15.3–27.8% in fine reticular anastomosis, and 5.9–50.3% in no anastomosis [15–17].

Jejunal Vessels

The number of jejunal artery branches that emerge from the superior mesenteric artery is 5–7 on average (Fig. 16.3). Each jejunal artery runs in the mesentery of the small intestine, forms an arterial arcade with the adjoining jejunal artery, and further branches, eventually becoming a numerous vasa recta and distributing to the intestine. The recipient vessel is usually selected from the second to the fourth jejunal vessel, with arteries and veins averaging 4.0 and 5.0 mm in diameter, respectively. The length of the vascular pedicle that can be dissected as a recipient vessel is 4.1 cm on average from the bifurcation of the superior mesenteric artery to the arterial arcade [13, 18].

Gastroduodenal Vessels

The gastroduodenal artery branches from the common hepatic artery, runs ventral to the pancreas, and branches into the right gastroepiploic and anterior superior pancreaticoduodenal arteries. The length of the vascular pedicle depends on the bifurcation from the common hepatic artery. The

Supplementary Information The online version of this chapter (https://doi.org/10.1007/978-3-030-75389-4_16) contains supplementary material, which is available to authorized users.

H. Matsumoto (✉) · Y. Kimata
Department of Plastic and Reconstructive Surgery, Okayama University, Graduate School of Medicine, Dentistry, and Pharmaceutical Sciences, Okayama-city, Okayama, Japan
e-mail: ojyarumatsu@ninus.ocn.ne.jp; ykimata@cc.okayama-u.ac.jp

R. Gurunian, R. Djohan (eds.), *Recipient Vessels in Reconstructive Microsurgery*, https://doi.org/10.1007/978-3-030-75389-4_16

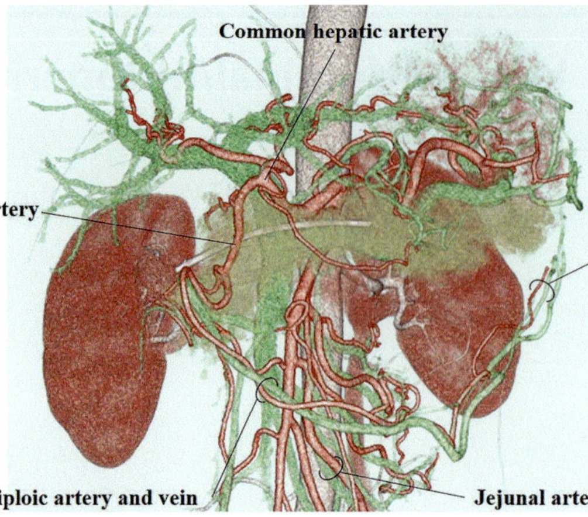

Fig. 16.1 Three-dimensional angiogram using computed tomography

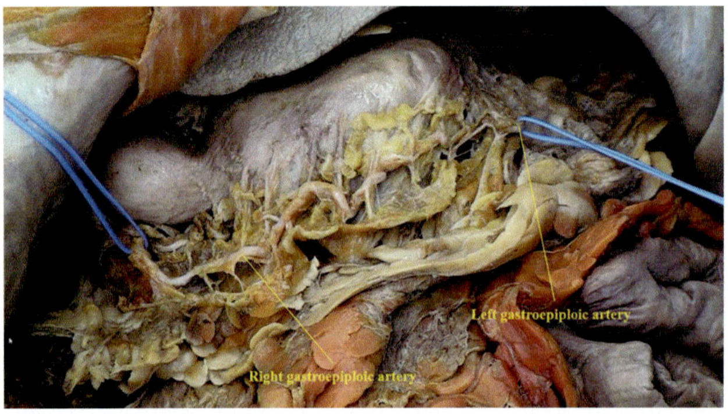

Fig. 16.2 Anatomical course of the gastroepiploic artery

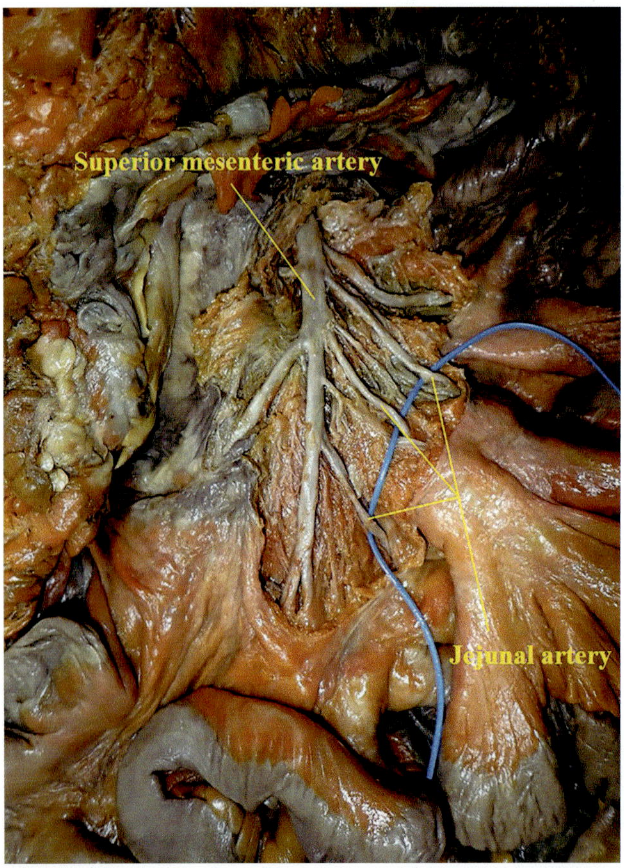

Fig. 16.3 Anatomical course of the jejunal artery

length is 3.09 ± 1.31 cm (range, 0–5.93 cm) in Howell et al. [19] and from 0.5 to 4 cm in Bradley [20]. The vascular diameter is similar to that of the common hepatic artery [20] (Fig. 16.4).

Inferior Mesenteric Vessels

The inferior mesenteric artery branches from the abdominal aorta at the level of the third lumbar vertebra, and its diameter ranges from 1.2 to 5.5 mm (mean 3.3 mm) (Fig. 16.5). The length from the inferior mesenteric artery to the left colic artery is 3–6 cm, which is used as the recipient vessel [9].

Surgical Site Exposure

When there is a full-thickness abdominal wall defect, the approach to the intra-abdominal blood vessels is relatively straight. Dissection of the artery and vein(s) is critical to the success of the microsurgical reconstruction. Intra-abdominal veins have very thin walls; therefore, venous dissection should be performed with special care and attention. Table 16.1 summarizes the potential veins that can be used for venous anastomoses.

Gastroepiploic Vessels

The right gastroepiploic artery branches from the gastroduodenal artery at the dorsal end of the pylorus and runs along the greater curvature of the stomach through the superficial layer of the greater omentum 10–20 mm caudal to the gastric attachment site of the greater omentum (Video 16.1). On the other hand, the left gastroepiploic artery branches from the splenic artery below the spleen and runs along the superficial layer of the greater omentum, similar to the right gastroepiploic artery. There are many branches from the gastroepiploic vessels that supply the anteroposterior surface of the

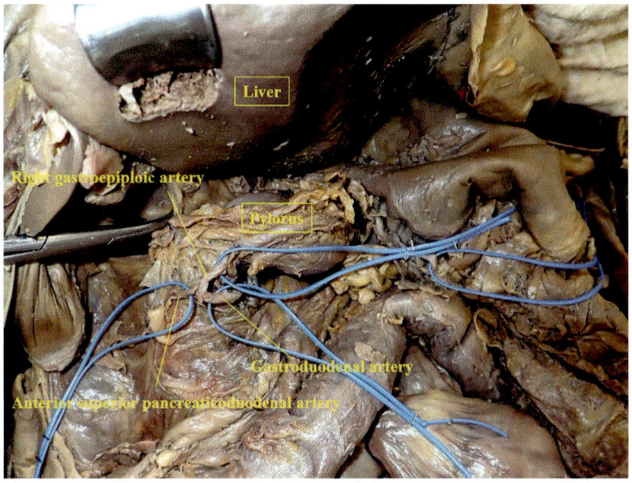

Fig. 16.4 Gastroduodenal artery and circumferential anatomy

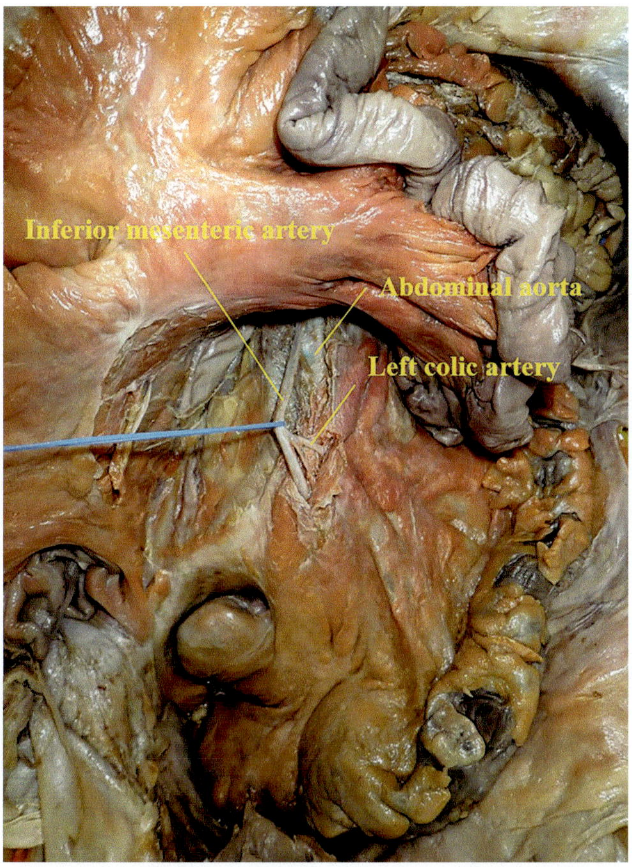

Fig. 16.5 Anatomical course of the inferior mesenteric artery

stomach and greater omentum, and these branches must be ligated when the recipient vessel is dissected. Given that the venous wall is very thin and vasospasm can easily occur, it is safer to dissect the blood vessels with the surrounding fatty tissue.

Jejunal Vessels

The second to fourth jejunal arteries are used as the recipient vessel. One of the second to fourth jejunal arteries is selected according to the length and diameter of the vascular pedicle of the donor vessel. Then, an incision is made in the mesentery of the small intestine just above the selected jejunal vessels, which are dissected until the arterial arcade. After the vascular pedicle is dissected, the arterial occlusion test should be performed to ensure that the jejunal blood flow is maintained through the arterial arcade.

Gastroduodenal Vessels

There are two approaches to the gastroduodenal artery. The first method involves approaching the superior margin of the pancreas across the omentum to identify the common hepatic artery. Next, the common hepatic artery is dissected to the distal side, the bifurcation of the gastroduodenal artery is identified, and the gastroduodenal artery is dissected from the ventral side of the head of the pancreas. Another approach involves elevating the stomach ventrally to identify the periphery of the gastroduodenal artery and dissecting it proximally. The latter approach allows easier dissection of the gastroduodenal artery. Moreover, the combination of the two approaches facilitates the dissection of the gastroduodenal artery from the head of the pancreas, particularly if a long recipient vessel is required.

Inferior Mesenteric Vessels

In the approach to the inferior mesenteric artery, first, the whole mesentery of the small intestine is mobilized to the right side, and the abdominal aorta and its bifurcation are confirmed at the midline of the abdomen. The inferior mesenteric artery is 3–4 cm cranially from the left-to-right bifur-

Table 16.1 Potential intraperitoneal recipient arteries and veins for use in microsurgical flap reconstruction of the abdominal wall defects

	Gastroepiploic vessels	Jejunal vessels	Gastroduodenal vessels	Inferior mesenteric vessels
Artery	Gastroepiploic artery	Jejunal artery	Gastroduodenal artery	Inferior mesenteric artery
Vein	Venae comitantes	Venae comitantes	Right gastroepiploic vein Middle colic vein	Inferior mesenteric vein

cation of the abdominal aorta, and it branches out slightly from the left side of the aorta. An incision is made on the surface of the mesosigmoid to expose the inferior mesenteric artery. The inferior mesenteric vein can be identified on the left side of the artery.

Discussion

Intraperitoneal vessels can be reliably used as recipient for microsurgical reconstruction of full-thickness abdominal wall defects after resection for malignancy. The gastroepiploic, jejunal, gastroduodenal, and inferior mesenteric vessels have been reported [1–13]. They are particularly useful when extraperitoneal vessels cannot be used as recipient vessels due to preexisting trauma/surgery or radiotherapy in the inguinal and pelvic regions. In addition, use of intraperitoneal vessels allows circumferential fascial closure using the vascularized fascia as part of the microsurgical flap.

Vessel selection is determined by the site of the defect and the diameter and length of the donor vessel. The authors conducted a study to select the recipient site based on the location of the abdominal wall defect. They used a cadaver with the *x*-*y* coordinate centered on the umbilicus dividing the abdomen in four quadrants. Assuming the use of an anterolateral thigh flap, the most frequently used microsurgical flap in abdominal wall reconstruction, the recipient vessel of choice at each defect was suggested as follows if the length of the donor vessel was 15 cm (Fig. 16.6): right upper quadrant, right gastroepiploic and gastroduodenal vessels; left upper quadrant, right gastroepiploic, left gastroepiploic, and jejunal vessels; right lower quadrant, right gastroepiploic, jejunal, and inferior mesenteric vessels; and left lower quadrant, jejunal and inferior mesenteric vessels.

Recipient vessel selection also depends on the following features.

Gastroepiploic Artery There are three types of anastomosis in the middle of the stomach, which are as follows: (1) the type in which the right and left arteries communicate clearly, (2) the type in which the gastroepiploic artery anastomoses have a fine reticular network, and (3) the type in which there is no anastomosis. Therefore, when the right and left gastroepiploic arteries are used as a long vascular pedicle sequentially, the left and right sides of the gastroepiploic artery must be clamped separately to ensure that the pulsation is maintained in either state. If the pulsation is absent or diminished, the right and left connections are insufficient and cannot be used sequentially (Video 16.2).

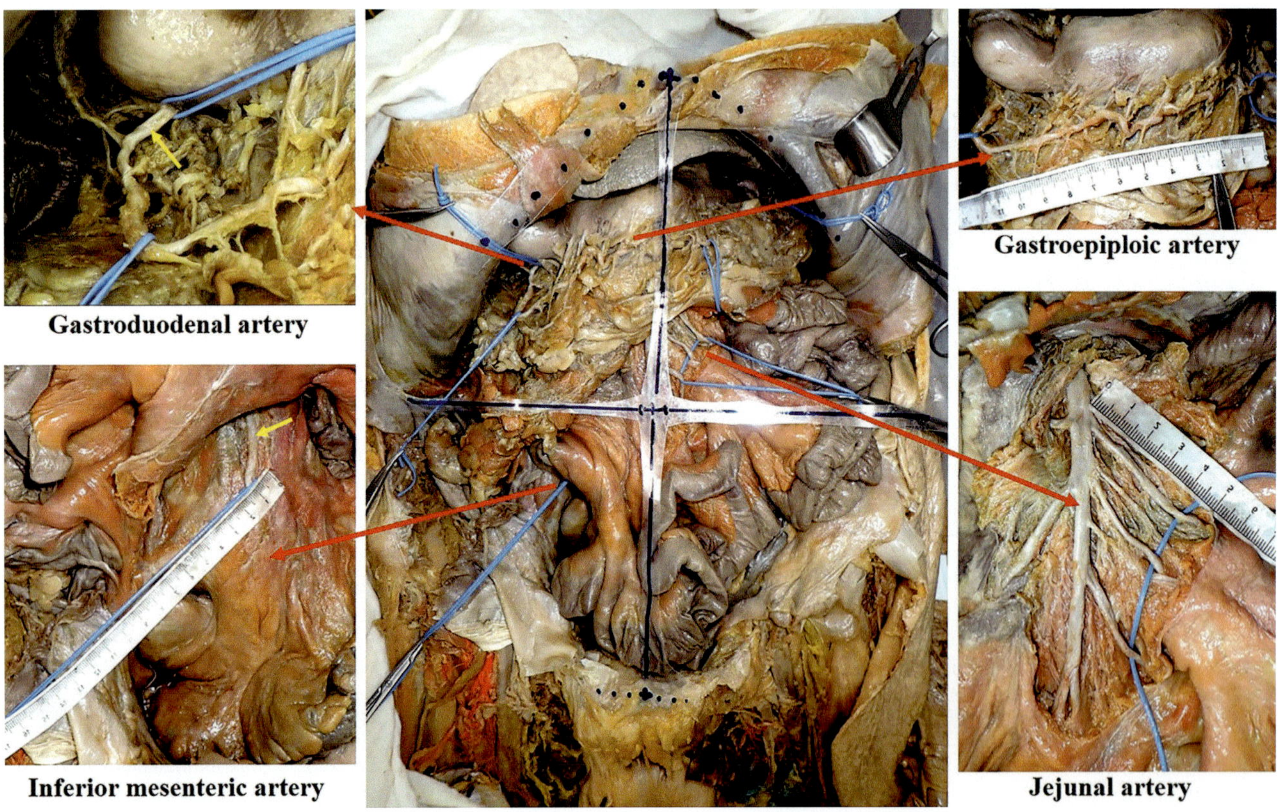

Fig. 16.6 The *x*-*y* coordinate centered on the umbilicus and the anatomical position of the recipient vessel

Jejunal Artery The first jejunal artery frequently has a common trunk with the inferior pancreatic duodenal artery. Given that the common trunk branched out from the dorsal side of the superior mesenteric artery, the first jejunal artery is located in the deep region and the length of vascular pedicle is also short. Therefore, it is difficult to use as a recipient vessel. The second to fourth jejunal arteries branch directly from the superior mesenteric artery in the 3 o'clock direction, and either of these arteries is used.

Gastroduodenal Artery Although the periphery of the gastroduodenal artery contributes to the pancreatic blood flow, it is usually safe to use it as a recipient vessel because it maintains pancreatic blood flow through the arcades from the superior mesenteric arteries. However, if the right gastroepiploic artery can be used, the gastroduodenal artery is generally not the first choice. In the meantime, if the gastroepiploic artery is being removed in the case after gastrectomy, the gastroduodenal artery becomes a candidate as a recipient vessel. However, since there is no accompanying vein in the gastroduodenal artery, the immediate surrounding veins such as the middle colic vein need to be identified and dissected.

Inferior Mesenteric Artery (IMA) IMA is not considered to be used as the first choice for recipient vessel. However, if no other usable recipient vessel can be found inside or outside the abdomen, the use of IMA should be considered. When using the IMA, the condition of the Riolan arch connecting the superior and inferior mesenteric arteries should be confirmed by preoperative contrast-enhanced computed tomography, and the degree of patency should be confirmed by the intraoperative occlusion test. If the Riolan arch is absent or poorly developed, the use of IMA should be avoided because there is a possibility of intestinal necrosis due to impaired blood flow in the inferior mesenteric artery. The IMA is located in the deep region of the pelvis, and the length of the vascular pedicle is as short as approximately 3 cm. Therefore, a flap with a long vascular pedicle (>15 cm) must be selected for reconstruction of the surface layer of the abdominal wall.

Key Points

- Intraperitoneal vessels can be used as recipient for microsurgical reconstruction of complex abdominal defects.
- When intra-abdominal adhesions are involved, the use of intraperitoneal vessels may be difficult.
- Computed tomography angiography is useful for preoperative evaluation of intraperitoneal vessels, which then needs intraoperative confirmation by occlusion test.
- The use of intraperitoneal vessels allows circumferential fascia closure.
- Vessel selection is determined by the site of the defect and the diameter and length of the donor vessel.
- When intraperitoneal vessels are used as recipient, it is assumed that the blood flow in the area nourishing each vessel is maintained by collateral circulation. Therefore, careful observation of vascular arcades with neighboring vessels is essential prior to their use.
- In addition to the gastroepiploic artery, the jejunal artery, the gastroduodenal artery, and inferior mesenteric artery, the ileocolic, middle colic, and sigmoid arteries can be potentially used as recipient vessel if there is no problem in the vascular occlusion test, because blood flow is maintained from the adjacent vessels through the arcade.
- The arteries may or may not have venae comitantes. Nevertheless, for each artery, the potential veins as listed in Table 16.1 can be selected. Also the intraperitoneal veins have very thin walls and tedious dissection is required to avoid injury. A protective fatty tissue should be preserved around the vessels.
- There are only few detailed studies of the intraperitoneal veins for use as recipient vessels in the literature; therefore, detailed anatomical studies on veins will be necessary.
- Anastomosis in the peritoneal cavity may be difficult due to respiration and site of the selected recipient vessel. In that context, vascular anastomosis can be facilitated by manually switching the ventilator and temporarily stopping ventilation.
- Postoperative complications due to use of intraperitoneal vessels include intra-abdominal adhesions, hernia, and intra-abdominal organ ischemia.

References

1. Clement RW, Young VL, Marsh JL. Use of the greater omentum as a vascular supply for free-flap transfer. Plast Reconstr Surg. 1984;74(1):131–2.
2. Chiu HW. Tensor fasciae latae free flap for full-thickness abdominal wall reconstruction utilizing the greater omentum as a vascular supply. Plast Reconstr Surg. 1985;75(4):607.
3. Penington AJ, Theile DR, MacLeod AM, Morrison WA. Free tensor fasciae latae flap reconstruction of defects of the chest and abdominal wall: selection of recipient vessels. Scand J Plast Reconstr Surg Hand Surg. 1996;30(4):299–305.
4. Sekido M, Yamamoto Y, Sugihara T, Nohira K, Shintomi Y. Microsurgical reconstruction of chest- and abdominal-wall defects associated with intraperitoneal vessels. J Reconstr Microsurg. 1996;12(7):425–30.
5. Kimata Y, Uchiyama K, Sekido M, Sakuraba M, Iida H, Nakatsuka T, et al. Anterolateral thigh flap for abdominal wall reconstruction. Plast Reconstr Surg. 1999;103(4):1191–7.
6. Koshima I, Nanba Y, Tutsui T, Takahashi Y, Itoh S, Kobayashi R. Dynamic reconstruction of large abdominal defects using a free

rectus femoris musculocutaneous flap with normal motor function. Ann Plast Surg. 2003;50(4):420–4.
7. Oswald TM, Lineaweaver WC, Hui K. Recipient vessels for microsurgical flaps to the groin and pelvis: a review. J Reconstr Microsurg. 2006;22(1):5–14.
8. Wong CH, Lin CH, Fu B, Fang JF. Reconstruction of complex abdominal wall defects with free flaps: indications and clinical outcome. Plast Reconstr Surg. 2009;124(2):500–9.
9. Petrie NC, Chan JK, Chave H, McGuiness CN. The inferior mesenteric vessels as recipients when performing free tissue transfer for pelvic defects following abdomino-perineal resection. A novel technique and review of intra-peritoneal recipient vessel options for microvascular transfer. J Plast Reconstr Aesthet Surg. 2010;63(12):2133–40.
10. Kayano S, Sakuraba M, Miyamoto S, Nagamatsu S, Taji M, Umezawa H, Kimata Y. Comparison of pedicled and free anterolateral thigh flaps for reconstruction of complex defects of the abdominal wall: review of 20 consecutive cases. J Plast Reconstr Aesthet Surg. 2012;65(11):1525–9.
11. Aliano KA, Agulnick M, Cohen B, Gonya G, Low C, Stavrides S, et al. Spinal reconstruction for osteomyelitis with free vascularized fibular grafts using intra-abdominal recipient vessels: a series of three cases. Microsurgery. 2013;33(7):560–6.
12. Hahn E Jr, Lee ES, Keith JD. A neurotized anterolateral thigh flap with a unique anastomosis to the gastroepiploic artery: a case report of a reconstruction of composite abdominal wall defect. Eplasty. 2016;16:ic29.
13. Gurunluoglu R, Rosen MJ. Recipient vessels for microsurgical flaps to the abdomen: a systematic review. Microsurgery. 2017;37(6):707–16.
14. Tomioka K, Murakami M, Saito A, Ezure H, Moriyama H, Mori R, et al. Morphometric and quantitative evaluation of the gastroepiploic artery. Okajimas Folia Anat Jpn. 2015;92(2):33–5.
15. Tomioka K, Murakami M, Saito A, Ezure H, Moriyama H, Mori R, et al. Anatomical and surgical evaluation of gastroepiploic artery. Okajimas Folia Anat Jpn. 2016;92(3–4):49–52.
16. Hannoun L, Le Breton C, Bors V, Helenon C, Bigot JM, Parc R. Radiological anatomy of the right gastroepiploic artery. Anat Clin. 1984;5(4):265–71.
17. Yamato T, Hamanaka Y, Hirata S, Sakai K. Esophagoplasty with an autogenous tubed gastric flap. Am J Surg. 1979;137(5):597–602.
18. Strauch B, Yu HL. Atlas of microvascular surgery: anatomy and operative techniques. 2nd ed. New York: Thieme; 2006. p. 543–60.
19. Howell AC, Gould DJ, Mayfield C, Samakar K, Hassani C, Patel KM. Anatomical basis of the gastroepiploic vascularized lymph node transfer: a radiographic evaluation using computed tomographic angiography. Plast Reconstr Surg. 2018;142(4):1046–52.
20. Bradley RL. Surgical anatomy of the gastroduodenal artery. Int Surg. 1973;58(6):393–6.

Common and Superficial Femoral Vessels

17

Margaret S. Roubaud and Charles E. Butler

Introduction

The common and superficial femoral arteries and veins are large caliber vessels that support numerous local flaps and may also serve as excellent recipients for distant free flaps. In particular, these vessels are invaluable for difficult microsurgical reconstructions of the lower abdomen and groin.

Preoperative Assessment

Although microsurgery generally concerns coaptation of smaller branches of the femoral vessels, the presence and patency of the common and superficial femoral vessels are paramount to successful reconstruction of the trunk region. The common femoral artery is usually directly palpable near the inguinal ligament, although assessment of the common femoral vein and superficial femoral vessels may require imaging studies. Color Doppler ultrasound imaging provides excellent information about patency and flow velocities, while studies such as computed tomography angiography (CTA) or magnetic resonance angiography (MRA) may give better detail regarding vessel location and aberrant branching. In particular, CTA and MRA imaging is warranted in the presence of previous trauma, radiation, or lymph node dissection.

M. S. Roubaud (✉)
Department of Plastic Surgery, The University of Texas MD Anderson Cancer Center, Houston, TX, USA
e-mail: MSRoubaud@mdanderson.org

C. E. Butler
Department of Plastic Surgery, Charles B. Barker Endowed Chair in Surgery, The University of Texas MD Anderson Cancer Center, Houston, TX, USA
e-mail: cbutler@mdanderson.org

Applied Anatomy

The common femoral artery and vein are direct extensions of the external iliac artery and vein. The femoral vein lies medial to the femoral artery as the vessels exit the abdominal cavity via the femoral ring. The femoral vasculature lies directly over the psoas muscle with the femoral nerve lateral to the vessels. The vessels can be easily located by palpation within the femoral triangle, which consists of the inguinal ligament superiorly, the adductor longus medially, and the sartorius laterally. The common femoral artery then branches into the superficial femoral artery and the deep femoral artery (also known as the profunda femoris). Similarly, the common femoral vein branches into the superficial femoral vein (also known as the femoral vein), the deep femoral vein, and the greater saphenous vein. The superficial vein is most commonly referred to as the femoral vein, as it is anatomically in a deep position and it is predisposed to deep vein thrombosis.

The common femoral artery gives off several important segmental branches, prior to the division into the deep and superficial vessels. In particular, the superficial circumflex artery, the superficial epigastric artery, and the superficial and deep external pudendal arteries are all segmental branches originating within the femoral triangle. The superficial femoral artery courses posterior to the sartorius muscle and anterior to the femoral vein in the adductor canal. It gives off multiple muscular branches to the anterior and medial compartments of the thigh before it terminates into the popliteal artery. One of its most important branches, the descending geniculate artery, supplies blood to the knee.

The common femoral vein also has important tributaries within the femoral triangle. The venae comitantes associated with the superficial circumflex, superficial epigastric, and pudendal all drain to the common femoral vein in parallel with their arterial counterparts. Arguably, for the microsurgeon, the greater saphenous vein is the most important branch of the common femoral vein. The greater saphenous

R. Gurunian, R. Djohan (eds.), *Recipient Vessels in Reconstructive Microsurgery*,
https://doi.org/10.1007/978-3-030-75389-4_17

vein is located in the subcutaneous tissue of the medial thigh, between the deep investing fascia of the thigh and the superficial fascia. Approximately 1–3 cm from the inguinal ligament, it pierces the deep fascia of the thigh at the saphenous hiatus to drain into the femoral vein at the saphenofemoral junction (SFJ) in the femoral triangle. Within the thigh, the saphenous vein and the femoral (superficial femoral) vein have multiple tributaries that connect the superficial and deep vein systems. The femoral vein is the main deep vein of the thigh and has numerous tributaries from all compartments.

Anatomical studies have assessed the vessel diameter and flow within the common and superficial femoral vasculature. The common femoral artery is approximately 7–9 mm in diameter, with larger diameters in males as expected [1, 2]. Mean flow volumes at rest have been estimated between 350 and 430 ml/min [1–3]. Correspondingly, the superficial femoral artery is 5–7 mm in diameter on average, with flow volumes 130–210 ml/min [2, 4–6].

In comparison, the common femoral vein is approximately 10–13 mm in diameter, with males having a slightly larger diameter as expected for height and BMI [7, 8]. The superficial femoral vein remains large distal to the saphenofemoral (SFJ) junction, with diameters between 6 and 8 mm up to 35 cm distal to the SFJ [8]. At the SFJ, the saphenous vein is usually a minimum of 3–4 mm in diameter. In vivo studies of the flow in the common femoral, superficial femoral, and greater saphenous veins have been found to be on average 360 ml/min, 147 ml/min, and 38 ml/min, respectively, although this can change significantly with dynamic dilation and constriction [9].

Surgical Site Exposure

The exposure of the common femoral and superficial femoral vasculature can be achieved through a variety of incisions that approach the femoral triangle. The pubic symphysis and anterior iliac spine should be palpated and a connecting line drawn to estimate the location of the inguinal ligament. In thin patients, the adductor longus can be palpated at the medial border of the femoral triangle. The sartorius muscle can be difficult to palpate except in very thin patients, and direct palpation of the common femoral artery can help define the lateral border. In obese or radiated groins, the midway point of the inguinal ligament can be used as a rough estimate.

In instances where there is a preexisting defect, direct exposure of the femoral triangle through existing incisions is recommended. For example, during extirpation of large abdominal or groin tumors, the inguinal ligament is frequently sacrificed and the vessels are readily exposed (Fig. 17.1a–c). If a midline laparotomy incision has been used without direct exposure of the groin, an oblique counterincision can be made 2–4 cm below the inguinal ligament to limit the dermal vasculature disruption to the abdominal wall. When the common femoral or superficial femoral vasculature is used as recipient for a free flap, and the defect is not immediately close, the surgeon can make a clinical decision whether to tunnel the flap or directly open the skin between the recipient vessels and the defect. Expected motion at the groin crease and presence of tendinous insertions are of utmost consideration when planning reconstruction. Due to large degrees of motion at the hip joint, it is exceptionally difficult to control patient hip flexion and extension in the postoperative period. Tension on microsurgical anastomoses or soft tissue inset will be poorly tolerated and prone to ischemia with postoperative edema.

Discussion

The common femoral and superficial femoral vasculatures are large caliber vessels with high flow rates. Due to extensive arborization and advanced microsurgical techniques, the microsurgeon frequently uses segmental branches of these vessels for locoregional flaps and microanastomoses. In a systematic review of recipient vessels for microsurgical flaps to the abdomen, the inferior epigastric system or intraperitoneal vessels, such as the gastroepiploic, were the most commonly utilized [10]. These vessels are favored for their proximity to the abdominal or groin defect and vessel diameter compatibility. In the same study, femoral vessels were used directly or along with a vein graft in 9.3% of patients. This may be for several reasons, including distance from the defect and technical difficulty of end-to-side anastomoses. While the reconstructive surgeon must recognize these "hurdles," there are instances when these vessels become of utmost importance, such as in cases of significant trauma, extensive tumor extirpation, or previous radiation. Management of these difficulties deserves special attention.

As stated previously, the common and superficial femoral vessels are best suited for pedicled locoregional flaps of the abdomen or groin, or as recipient vessels for this anatomic region as well. As the common femoral artery and superficial artery are the primary blood supply to the lower leg, they should not be sacrificed for reconstruction. Alternatively, the common femoral artery and superficial artery can be used as excellent recipients for end-to-side anastomoses, whether directly to a pedicle or an arteriovenous (AV) loop. The large diameter and high flow of both vessels allow a sizeable arteriotomy without the risk of steal phenomenon. Furthermore, the vessels have sufficient flow to support flaps of any size which may be significant in abdominal wall reconstruction. Of importance, the common femoral artery or superficial femoral artery can be

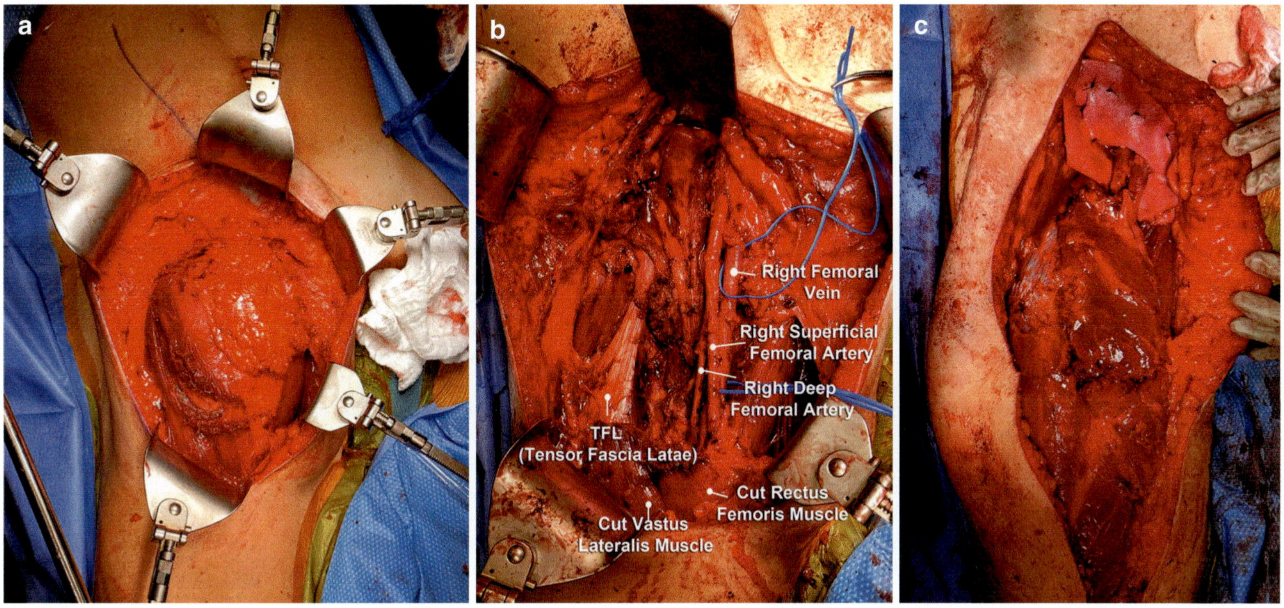

Fig. 17.1 (**a**) A recurrent liposarcoma of the right retroperitoneum and groin in a 62-year-old male that extended along the right iliopsoas muscle into the groin. The tumor abutted the external iliac, common femoral, and superficial femoral vessels. The patient was treated 6 years previously with chemoradiation and radical resection via a midline laparotomy incision. (**b**) Radical tumor resection was performed via an oblique incision over the right pelvis and groin. The common and superficial femoral vessels were skeletonized and spared, although all segmental branches were ligated with the tumor including the deep and superficial epigastric, superficial circumflex, and medial and lateral circumflex femoral systems. The greater saphenous vein, sartorius muscle, and inguinal ligament were also resected. The resultant defect created an incisional hernia with prolapse of peritoneal contents and a large dead space in the groin and upper thigh. (**c**) The abdominal wall muscle and incisional hernia were repaired with biologic mesh. To cover the mesh and exposed neurovascular structures, as well as obliterate dead space, a free vastus lateralis muscle was harvested from the ipsilateral thigh and end-to-side microsurgical anastomosis performed to the common femoral artery and vein

afflicted by significant peripheral vascular disease and calcific plaques. A successful anastomosis frequently requires stronger microsurgical suture and needle, such as an 8-0 Nylon or 6-0 Prolene, and large full-thickness bites to avoid disrupting the intima.

As discussed in Chap. 18 within this text, AV loops may be critical to bridging the distance between appropriate recipients and the reconstructive target. The saphenous vein serves as an excellent donor in this region, either as saphenous transposition or as a free anastomosis. The saphenous vein can be accessed directly at the saphenofemoral junction if it is intact, or harvested via direct incision over the medial thigh. The surgeon should plan to use an AV loop when preexisting vertical and horizontal scars on the abdomen suggest that the internal thoracic, deep inferior epigastric, or superficial circumflex systems are no longer viable [11]. Additionally, large extirpations in the retroperitoneum or groin may require ligation of multiple named branches. Additional consideration should be given to an immediate or delayed use of AV loops in microsurgical procedures. Immediate use of AV loops may eliminate the need for additional surgery and decrease the risk of thrombosis, although some authors warn that the AV loops should be given time to mature before flap anastomosis [12–17]. It is the author's practice to perform immediate AV loop anastomoses in this anatomic area due to high flow in the recipient vessels, with AV transposition (leaving the saphenofemoral junction intact) preferred to interposition.

Summary

The common and superficial femoral vessels are large caliber, high-flow vessels that arborize significantly. Locoregional flaps for the abdomen and groin are based on their segmental branches, including the superficial circumflex and superficial epigastric. When required, the common and superficial femoral systems serve as excellent recipients for free flaps given their large diameter, but require a more technically demanding end-to-side anastomosis.

References

1. Liang HL. Doppler flow measurement of lower extremity arteries adjusted by pulsatility index. Am J Roentgenol. 2020;214:10–7.
2. Holland CK, Borwn JM, Scoutt LM, et al. Lower extremity volumetric arterial blood flow in normal subjects. Ultrasound Med Biol. 1998;24:1079–86.

3. Lin YY, Shie RF, Liu KS, et al. Diameter change of common femoral arteries after percutaneous endovascular aortic repair with the use of the preclose technique. J Vasc Surg. 2014;60:50–6.
4. Lewis P, Psaila JV, Davies WT, et al. Measurement of volume flow in the human common femoral artery using a duplex ultrasound system. Ultrasound Med Biol. 1986;12:777–84.
5. Field JP, Musson AM, Zwolak RM, et al. Duplex arterial flow measurement in normal lower extremities. J Vasc Tech. 1989;13:13–9.
6. Hussain ST, Smith RE, Wood RFM, et al. Observer variability in volumetric blood flow measurements in leg arteries using duplex ultrasound. Ultrasound Med Biol. 1996;22:287–91.
7. Mednick RE, Alvi HM, Morgan CE, et al. Femoral vein blood flow during a total hip arthroplasty using a modified Heuter approach. J Arthroplast. 2015;30:786–9.
8. Keiler J, Schulze M, Claasen H, et al. Human femoral vein diameter and topography of valves and tributaries: a post mortem analysis. Clin Anat. 2018;31:1065–76.
9. Ogawa T, Lurie F, Kistner RL, et al. Reproducibility of ultrasound scan in the assessment of volume flow in the veins of the lower extremities. J Vasc Surg. 2002;35:527–31.
10. Gurunluoglu R, Rosen MJ. Recipient vessels for microsurgical flaps to the abdomen: a systematic review. Microsurgery. 2017;37:707–16.
11. Gurunluoglu R, Ghaznavi A, Krpata D, et al. Arteriovenous loop graft in abdominal wall reconstruction using free tissue transfer. J Plast Reconstr Aesthet Surg. 2016;69:1513–5.
12. Cavadas PC. Arteriovenous vascular loops in free flap reconstruction of the extremities. Plast Reconstr Surg. 2008;121:514–20.
13. Inbal A, Silva AK, Humphries LS, et al. Bridging the gap: a 20-year experience with vein grafts for free flap reconstruction. The odds for success. Plast Reconstr Surg. 2018;142:786–94.
14. Oswald TM, Stover SA, Gerzenstein J, et al. Immediate and delayed use of arteriovenous fistulae in microsurgical flap procedures: a clinical series and review of published cases. Ann Plast Surg. 2007;58:61–3.
15. Henn D, Wahmann MS, Horsch M, et al. One-stage versus two-stage arteriovenous loop reconstructions: an experience on 103 cases from a single center. Plast Reconstr Surg. 2019;143:912–24.
16. Vogt PM, Steinau HU, Spies M, et al. Outcome of simultaneous and staged microvascular free tissue transfer connected to arteriovenous loops in areas lacking recipient vessels. Plast Reconstr Surg. 2007;120:1568–75.
17. Arkudas A, Morch RE, Regus S, et al. Retrospective cohort study of combined approach for trunk reconstruction using arteriovenous loops and free flaps. J Plast Reconstr Aesthet Surg. 2018;71:394–401.

Saphenous Arteriovenous Loop

18

Erkki Tukiainen and Katariina Laurila

Introduction

Arteriovenous (AV) fistulas are abnormal connections between the arterial and the venous circulatory systems. The fistulas can be congenital or acquired. The latter can result from trauma or surgical procedures [1]. Therapeutic AV fistulas were first originally created to facilitate hemodialysis access as described by Brescia et al., who developed the radio-cephalic shunt, and this still remains in clinical use today [2]. When an autologous vein graft or comparable substitute (allograft or synthetic) interposition is used to connect a major artery and vein, it is called an arteriovenous loop.

Sometimes, there are no suitable recipient vessels in close proximity to the defect to be covered with a microvascular flap. In these cases, an AV loop can provide a solution. Threlfall et al. were the first to publish the use of an AV fistula as the recipient vessel for a free flap in the lower limb [3]. Since then, this method has been used in head and neck, trunk, and extremity reconstruction as an adjunct to free flap surgery both in single-stage or two-stage manner [4–6]. Usually, the venous loop has two anastomoses – one at both ends.

The saphenous loop is a modification of the venous loop. It avoids one anastomosis by virtue of using the natural connection of the great saphenous vein (oval fossa) as an outlet. Only the distal end of the saphenous vein needs to be anastomosed end-to-side to the femoral artery to create an AV loop.

Indications

When microvascular flap reconstructions are performed, the flap artery and vein should be connected to healthy recipient vessels to avoid thrombosis and flap loss. If the local recipient vessels are not appropriate for the free flap anastomoses, an AV loop can provide a solution.

The aim of the AV loop is to provide optimal recipient vessels for the free flap within close proximity to the defect. Vascular disease, previous radiotherapy, trauma, infection or inflammation, high-flow vascular malformation, or previous reconstructive operations may result in indications to use the AV loop. In addition in certain anatomical areas, the recipient vessels can be missing or too small for anastomoses. The autologous venous loop provides a healthy vessel with proper caliber and flow.

Furthermore, the blood pressure both in arterial and venous sides must be suitable for a microsurgical flap, i.e., both the inflow and the outflow of the loop should be close to the physiologic values after the loop has been divided in the middle and the anastomoses performed. On the arterial side, the recipient artery must have a certain blood pressure and flow. This usually means anastomosing the loop proximal to any affected, narrow segment. The right segment for arterial end-to-side anastomosis is selected by using preoperative imaging and intraoperative blood flow and pressure measurements. If necessary, preoperative angiographic imaging such as magnetic resonance angiography or digital subtraction angiography is evaluated to exclude proximal stenosis and significant atherosclerosis of the artery. According to our experience, the pressure on the main artery (suitable for loop anastomosis) should be at least 2/3 of the systemic pressure recorded in the radial artery at the same time.

Also the venous side should be carefully evaluated and any obstacles to the venous outflow should be excluded. The venous outflow requires healthy vessels and physiologic intraluminal venous pressure for the AV loop. Previous high deep venous thrombosis or high-flow vascular malformation affecting the area may result in increased venous pressure that is too high for safe free flap anastomosis. If necessary, the patency and flow of the deep vein are easily assessed by duplex ultrasonography.

E. Tukiainen (✉) · K. Laurila
Department of Plastic Surgery, Helsinki University Hospital, Helsinki, Finland
e-mail: Erkki.Tukiainen@hus.fi; Katariina.Laurila@hus.fi

R. Gurunian, R. Djohan (eds.), *Recipient Vessels in Reconstructive Microsurgery*,
https://doi.org/10.1007/978-3-030-75389-4_18

Depending on the length of the loop, even distant sites can be reached, and the loop can be turned toward the defect to be reconstructed. This allows the surgeon to reconstruct, for instance, a mangled extremity using vessels outside the zone of injury [7, 8].

In certain anatomical areas such as the chest and abdominal cavity, possible compression caused by visceral organs (ileus, expanded lungs, etc.) can cause problems. Therefore, in the reconstruction of full-thickness chest wall or abdominal cavity defects, it may be beneficial to plan the anastomoses outside the chest or abdominal cavity. A saphenous AV loop from inguinal vessels allows more freedom in choosing the location of the free flap anastomoses. The loop can be placed in a new anatomical location with the advantages of better reach for vessels and avoiding the pressure changes in the cavities that may cause compression or traction of the flap pedicle [9, 10].

The saphenous loop has several advantages. A two-team approach is often possible allowing one team to prepare the recipient vessels, i.e., the AV loop, while the other team harvests the flap. The anatomy of the great saphenous vein is rather constant and the diameter of vein usually is suitable for anastomosis. Large vessel caliber and low resistance create a high-flow AV fistula with the flow being 100–200 ml/min in our measurements by transit time flowmeter. When the saphenous loop is formed and cut distally to create the venous and the arterial side, there will be only one anastomosis on the venous side and two on the arterial side. The first anastomosis is the anastomosis of the distal end of the saphenous vein to the femoral artery. Subsequently, when the loop has been divided, the flap anastomosis can be performed relatively easily in good exposition. This is an important aspect in free flap surgery where thrombotic complications mostly occur at the site of the anastomosis. The anastomoses are performed in big vessels, the femoral artery provides excellent inflow for the flap, and the venous outflow is directed to the femoral vein (Table 18.1).

Table 18.1 Possible indications for the use of the saphenous loop

Peripheral vascular disease
High-dose radiotherapy
Trauma
Infection
Inflammation
Vascular malformation
Previous operations

Table 18.2 Defects suitable for the saphenous loop and free flap reconstruction (when local or pedicled flap options are not feasible)

Upper abdominal wall defects
Thoracoabdominal defects
Large flank defects
Large abdominal wall defects
Large lumbosacral or pelvic defects (in posterior defects both saphenous veins can be used)

Preoperative Planning

Preoperatively, the patency, location, and caliber of the greater saphenous vein should be examined with duplex ultrasound. The route of the vessel can be marked on the skin to facilitate the dissection [11]. The whole donor lower limb should be prepared for the operation. If any doubt arises regarding the condition of the vessels in the preoperative ultrasound, the other lower limb should also be prepared. In the event of atherosclerotic disease, then the preoperative angiogram (MRA or DSA) is mandatory to make sure there is no significant proximal stenosis in the iliac vessels which could reduce the flow in the femoral artery. From the imaging, the condition of and possible calcification of the femoral vessels can also be assessed.

Surgical Technique

The vein is exposed and dissected via either small longitudinal incisions placed according to the previously marked route of the vein or through a long vertical incision. To expose the proximal femoral area, a vertical 10 cm incision is performed giving access to the femoral artery and vein and proximal saphenous vein. All the side branches of the saphenous vein must be ligated and divided to allow full mobility of the vein from the oval fossa. Distally, the saphenous vein is transected at the preferred site, usually at the level of the knee joint, making sure that the loop becomes sufficiently long. The saphenous vein must be dissected more than 30 cm to give a loop reaching about 15 cm, which is usually enough even for thoracoabdominal defects or lateral flank defects. To avoid torsion, the dorsal surface of the saphenous vein can be marked with dashed line using a surgical pen (Table 18.2).

The loop is placed preliminarily toward the area of tissue defect. Any torsion or kinking should be avoided. Systemic heparin is administered prior to clamping of the femoral artery proximally and distally. The arteriotomy is performed close to the level of the oval fossa on the femoral artery with a longitudinal incision or an oval incision measuring 10 × 5 mm. The distal end of the saphenous vein is anastomosed end-to-side with a 7-0 continuous suture (Figs. 18.1 and 18.2). If the artery is atherosclerotic or previously irradiated, it must be handled with great care. The sutures should run from inside to outward of the femoral artery to avoid dissection of the vessel wall layers. Care must be taken to place the end of the loop so that the arterial flow can smoothly enter the vein without any acute angle causing turbulence. The

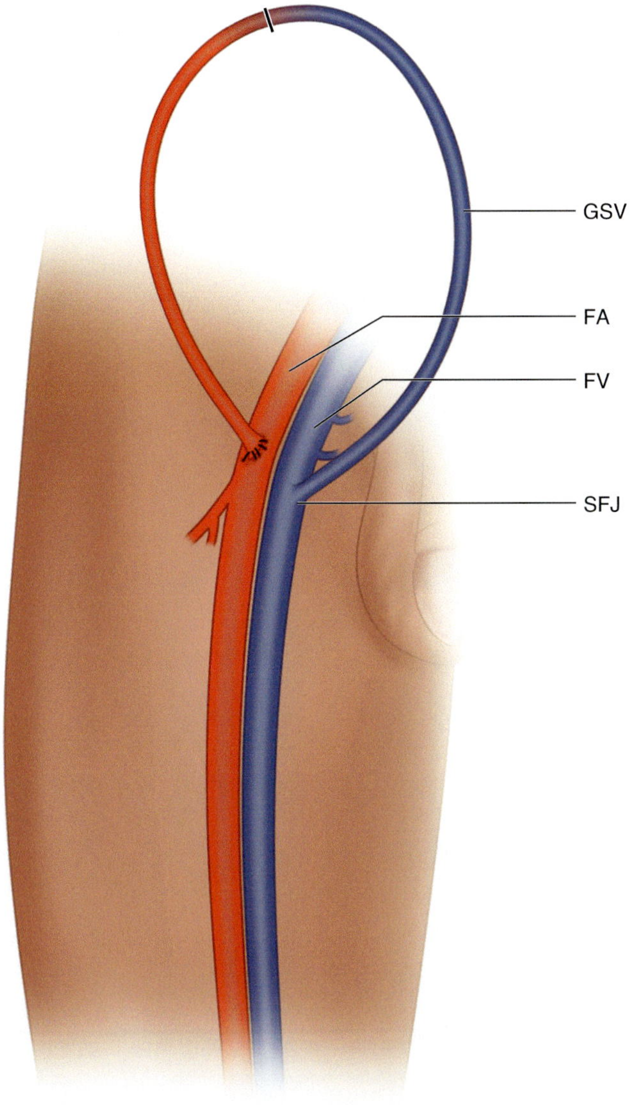

Fig. 18.1 Drawing of the anatomy of the saphenous AV loop: The arterial portion of the AV loop in red illustrating the end-to-side anastomosis of the saphenous vein to the femoral artery and the venous part of the AV loop in blue demonstrating the outflow to the femoral vein via the oval fossa. Dash line indicates the division site of the AV loop. FA, femoral artery; FV, femoral vein; SFJ, saphenofemoral junction; GSV, great saphenous vein

pulsating loop is observed carefully to detect any bleeding, stenosis, or torsion.

A subcutaneous tunnel is dissected, at least 3–4 fingers wide, and the pulsating loop is carefully delivered through the tunnel toward the defect on the upper abdomen, flank, etc. using a vascular routing instrument or a plastic bag, etc. The loop can be filled with heparin solution to avoid thrombosis and the loop is then divided in the midpoint. Any torsion can still be corrected at this stage. End-to-end anastomoses connecting the loop ends to the free flap vessels are performed as usual. It is not uncommon to have some

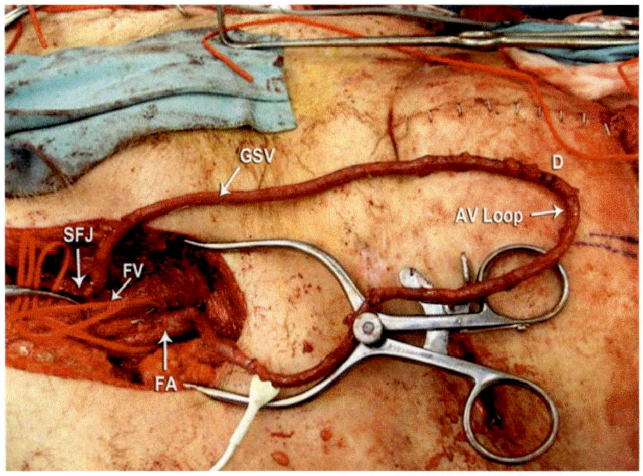

Fig. 18.2 Perioperative image of the AV loop reconstructed in the left groin: Transit time flowmeter is connected to the loop for flow measurements. Saphenous AV loop construct prior to division (D) for microsurgical flap reconstruction: The saphenous vein is anastomosed to the femoral artery (FA) in an end-to-side manner to create the AV loop. (GSV, great saphenous vein; SFJ, saphenofemoral junction; FV, femoral vein)

mismatch in the caliber of the vessels which has to be taken into account: the saphenous vein tends to be wider than the vessels of the free flap. In addition, there is a tendency toward a water hammer phenomenon, because of the high original loop flow (up to 200 ml/min). This flow is directed to the smaller artery of the free flap (flow around 20–50 ml/min, depending on the composition and size of the flap), and the flow then eventually settles to the lower level according to the flap requirements [12]. Figure 18.3a presents cases undergoing free flap reconstruction of the upper abdomen, flank, and lumbosacral regions using the saphenous AV loop.

Complications

Postoperative complications include local complications such as bleeding and wound healing problems, infection, and seroma in the groin area. Careful anatomic dissection in the groin area is mandatory to preserve the local lymphatic vessels and to avoid extensive seroma formation.

During the first two postoperative weeks, hip flexion and extension must be limited because excessive flexion (sitting on a normal or low chair) can cause compression of the vessels. In addition, uncontrolled, forceful extension of the hip in early recovery phase may result in a rupture of the anastomosis and profuse arterial bleeding.

The rationale behind the one-stage operation is to avoid the potential hemodynamic effects of a shunting AV fistula. Excessive shunting for a prolonged period of time can lead to an increased cardiac preload and potentially to heart failure. However, this is rarely encountered when the AV loop is

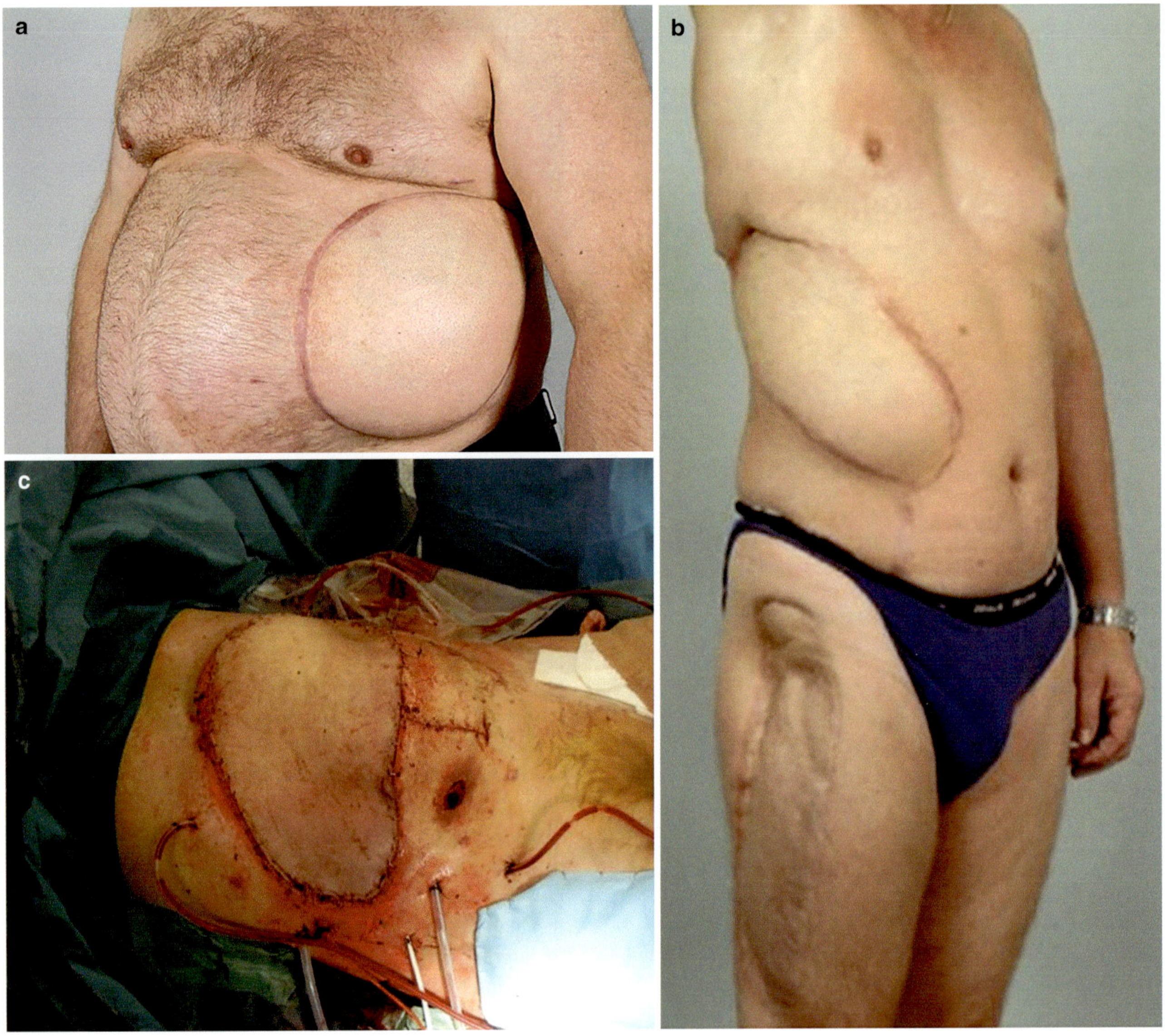

Fig. 18.3 (**a**) Postoperative image of a large TFL (tensor fascia latae) flap for the reconstruction of thoracoabdominal region using an AV loop. (**b**) Postoperative image: Microsurgical reconstruction of right flank and thoracoabdominal defect with free TFL flap using saphenous AV loop as recipient. (**c**) Intraoperative image of a TFL flap for microsurgical reconstruction of the abdomen using saphenous AV loop

reconstructed to provide recipient vessels because the flow is not as high as the flow in therapeutic AV fistulas and the flap is anastomosed without delay to the divided loop ends in one operation.

The same applies to the steal phenomenon: a stenosis on the arterial side could potentially lead to distal ischemia of the lower limb when the blood is shunted preferentially through high-flow AV fistula having a low resistance. However, after the flap has been connected, the steal effect is usually not significant because the flow is directed into the flap within the requirements of the flap. The high original flow of the fistula will be decreased to the flow required by the flap, and the flap does not function as a fistula stealing from the extremity.

Conclusion

Saphenous AV loop can be used as recipient vessels for microsurgical flaps when there is lack of workable and reliable recipient vessels in the vicinity. This technique has proved an efficient modality to overcome difficult microsurgical flap reconstructions of thoracoabdominal, lumbosacral, pelvic, and flank defects.

References

1. Rutherford RB. Arteriovenous fistulas, vascular malformations and vascular tumors. Overview. In: Rutherfor RB, editor. Vascular surgery. 6th ed. Philadelphia: Elsevier Saunders; 2005. p. 1597–601.
2. Brescia MJ, Cimino JE, Appel K, Hurwich BJ. Chronic hemodialysis using venipuncture and a surgically created arteriovenous fistula. N Engl J Med. 1966;275(20):1089–92.
3. Threlfall GN, Little JM, Cummine J. Free flap transfer-preliminary establishment of an arteriovenous fistula: a case report. Aust N Z J Surg. 1982;52(2):182–4.
4. Rand RP, Gruss JB. The saphenous arteriovenous fistula in microsurgical head and neck reconstruction. Am J Otolaryngol. 1994;15(3):215–8.
5. Karanas YL, Yim KK, Johannet P, Hui K, Lineaweaver WC. Use of 20 cm or longer interposition vein grafts in free flap reconstruction of the trunk. Plast Reconstr Surg. 1998;101(5):1262–7.
6. Hallock GG. Forearm arterial loop as an expedient source for inflow to upper extremity free flaps. Microsurgery. 1995;16(7):445–9.
7. Cavadas PC. Arteriovenous vascular loops in free flap reconstruction of the extremities. Plast Reconstr Surg. 2008;121(2):514–20.
8. Lin CH, Mardini S, Lin YT, Yeh JT, Wei FC, Chen HC. Sixty-five clinical cases of free tissue transfer using long arteriovenous fistulas or vein grafts. J Trauma. 2004;56(5):1107–17.
9. Tukiainen E, Popov P, Asko-Seljavaara S. Microvascular reconstructions of full-thickness oncological chest wall defects. Ann Surg. 2003;238(6):794–801.
10. Tukiainen E, Leppäniemi A. Reconstruction of extensive abdominal wall defects with microvascular tensor fascia latae flap. Br J Surg. 2011;98(6):880–4.
11. Albäck A, Saarinen E, Venermo M. Vein harvesting and techniques for infrainguinal bypass. J Cardiovasc Surg. 2016;57(2):292–301.
12. Lorenzetti F, Suominen S, Tukiainen E, Kuokkanen H, Suominen E, Vuola J, Asko-Seljavaara S. Evaluation of blood flow in free microvascular flaps. J Reconstr Microsurg. 2001;17(3):163–7.

Superficial Circumflex Iliac and Superficial Inferior Epigastric Vessels

19

Brendan Alleyne, Cemile Nurdan Ozturk, Lena Gurunian, and Raffi Gurunian

Introduction

Successful free tissue transfer not only relies on the raising of a viable flap but also on selection of adequate recipient vessels as a critical component of reconstructive planning. Conditions necessitating free flap coverage in the abdominal/groin area may have exhausted some of the recipient options, which are already scarce in this anatomical area. Surgeons may find themselves in challenging situations, having to resort to unusual recipients, or utilize more complex techniques including vein rerouting, vein grafting, or AV loops (also see Chaps. 18 and 42). In this regard, superficial vasculature of the lower abdominal/groin area may be considered as an alternative recipient site.

The superficial circumflex iliac artery/vein (SCIA/V) and superficial inferior epigastric artery/vein (SIEA/V) are usually only mentioned in the context of perforator free flap or pedicled flap options. Having these vessels available in the armamentarium of recipient sites is also important given their relative reliability in size and location, as well as their easy access. At times when first-line options are unavailable, due to previous surgery, radiation, or encroaching zones of injury, these superficial vessels may be prudent choices as recipient site for abdominal, pelvic, groin, and flank free flap reconstruction.

Supplementary Information The online version of this chapter (https://doi.org/10.1007/978-3-030-75389-4_19) contains supplementary material, which is available to authorized users.

B. Alleyne
Department of Plastic Surgery, Cleveland Clinic, Cleveland, OH, USA
e-mail: alleynb@ccf.org

C. N. Ozturk
Department of Head, Neck & Plastic Surgery, Roswell Park Comprehensive Cancer Center, Buffalo, NY, USA
e-mail: cemile.ozturk@roswellpark.org

L. Gurunian
Loyola Marymount University, Los Angelos, CA, USA

R. Gurunian (✉)
Department of Plastic Surgery, Cleveland Clinic, Cleveland, OH, USA

Cleveland Clinic Lerner College of Medicine, Case Western Reserve University, Cleveland, OH, USA
e-mail: gurunir@ccf.org

Preoperative Assessment

Reconstructive planning starts with a careful assessment of missing tissue components and loss of function. Choosing the correct procedure for a patient by incorporating relevant medical and surgical history, risk factors, as well as patient and family goals is essential for a successful outcome. For patients requiring free tissue transfer, availability of flap donor sites and recipient vessels are assessed, with specific attention given to location of previous scars or radiation. Zone of injury at recipient area may extend well beyond visible borders. Choice of recipient vessels is based on diameter, length, proximity to the defect to be reconstructed, and lack of trauma or radiation damage. Imaging should be obtained either via computed tomographic angiography (CTA) or magnetic resonance angiography (MRA) when vessel viability is in question [1]. Obtaining a CTA or an MRA not only helps visualize patency of vessels but also assists in identifying aberrant anatomy and alternative recipient vessel sites. These studies should be used in concert with a thorough physical exam involving Doppler ultrasound and vascular flow index studies when indicated.

Applied Anatomy

The majority of anatomical investigation involving the superficial circumflex iliac artery (SCIA) and vein (SCIV) is through its use as a perforator flap, a modification of the groin flap. The study by Suh et al. [2] corroborates other

R. Gurunian, R. Djohan (eds.), *Recipient Vessels in Reconstructive Microsurgery*, https://doi.org/10.1007/978-3-030-75389-4_19

anatomical descriptions showing that the artery typically arises directly from anterolateral aspect of the common femoral artery in majority of cases, approximately 2.5 cm below the inguinal ligament [3–5] (Fig. 19.1). It courses superficial to the fascia lata and sartorius muscle, traveling laterally and parallel to the inguinal ligament toward the anterior superior iliac spine (ASIS). A consistent description is found of a lateral deep branch as well as a more superficial medial branch [2, 4, 6, 7]. The lateral deep branch initially runs beneath the deep fascia of the sartorius muscle, penetrating this layer at the lateral border of the muscle [7, 8]. It is crossed by the lateral cutaneous nerve of the thigh [4]. The medial superficial branch immediately travels over the deep fascia (in subcutaneous fat) parallel and inferior to the inguinal ligament, toward ASIS [1, 4, 7]. According to SCIA perforator flap studies, the medial branch is absent in a small number of patients, but this may be attributed to inferolateral design of the perforator flap [1, 4, 7, 9]. SCIA common stem (proximal to superficial and deep branch takeoff) measures about 1.5 cm in length and 0.7–1.9 mm in diameter [3–5, 8] (also see Chap. 44 and Table 44.1). The bifurcation is found on average 30 mm inferior and 61 mm lateral from the midline along a line connecting the pubic tubercle to the anterior

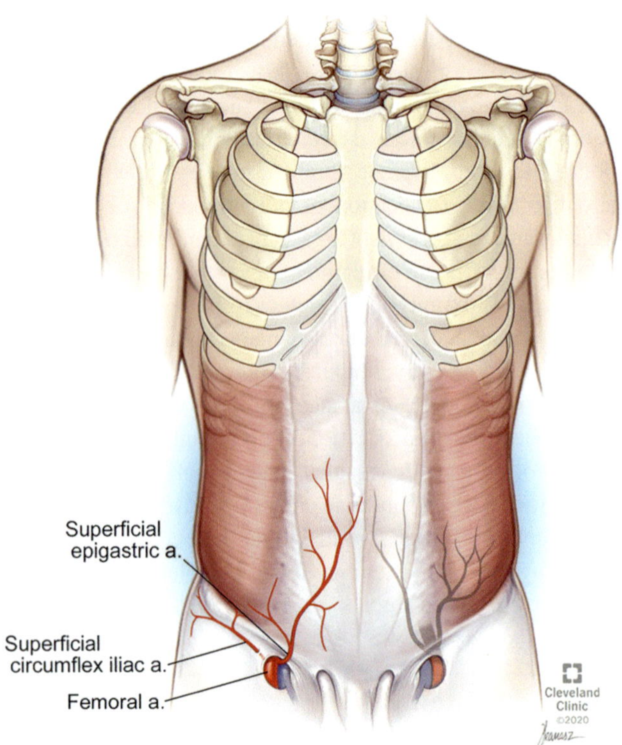

Fig. 19.1 Illustration of SCIA (superficial circumflex iliac artery) and SIEA (superficial inferior epigastric artery) branching off the femoral artery below the inguinal ligament. (Reprinted with permission, Cleveland Clinic Center for Medical Art & Photography © 2020. All Rights Reserved)

superior iliac spine [1]. The length of SCIA, as measured from origin to its disappearance into the subcutaneous tissues (as in SCIA perforator flap pedicle), ranges from 3 to 13 cm with a mean of 4.8 cm [4, 5, 8].

The superficial inferior epigastric artery (SIEA) arises from the anterior surface of the femoral artery usually within 2 cm below the inguinal ligament [10, 11] (Fig. 19.1). Initial course is superolateral before turning superiorly, traveling below Scarpa's fascia, deep and lateral to the SIEV [11, 12]. Just above the inguinal ligament, it pierces the fascia to lie in the subcutaneous tissue [11, 13]. Its position relative to the linea semilunaris was found to be highly variable, on average lying 2 cm lateral to this point [12]. Average diameter ranges 0.3–3.1 mm [3, 10–12, 14] (also see Chap. 44 and Table 44.1). Variations in origin include the common trunk of SCIA and SIEA, and independent emergence, the latter yielding smaller diameters for both vessels [14]. The length, as measured from origin to its disappearance into the subcutaneous tissues (as in SIEA flap pedicle), ranges from 3 to 7 cm with a mean of 5.2 cm [10].

The dominant venous system in the groin area is the superficial cutaneous veins that are located superficial to Scarpa's fascia [15]. SIEV, after receiving tributaries such as SCIV and venae comitantes, drains into either the superficial femoral vein, saphenous bulb, or great saphenous vein [10, 15]. The mean diameter of SIEV (or common trunk) measures about 2–2.5 mm [3, 10, 15]. There are also venae comitantes of the SCIA and SIEA that travel deep to Scarpa's fascia; however, their diameter is smaller in the range of 0.5–1 mm [7, 8]. The mean length of SIEV, as measured from subcutaneous tissues to the drainage point, is 6.4 cm [10].

Surgical Site Exposure

The ASIS (anterior superior iliac spine), pubic tubercle, and trajectory of the inguinal ligament are marked as landmarks (Video 19.1). A handheld Doppler can be useful to assist in marking the medial and lateral perforating branches of the SCIA. The lateral deep perforator transitions from deep to superficial approximately two finger widths medial to the ASIS [16]. An incision inferior and parallel to the inguinal ligament is made through the superficial fascia and down to the deep fascia from lateral to medial (Fig. 19.2). This allows for identification of the lateral SCIA perforator which can then be dissected down to the main pedicle through the deep fascia and chased medially [2, 17]. Alternatively, medial SCIA perforator branch can be located in subcutaneous tissues and dissected to the common trunk. By understanding the course of the perforating vessels, as described above, we can reliably direct our course toward the source vessel (Fig. 19.3).

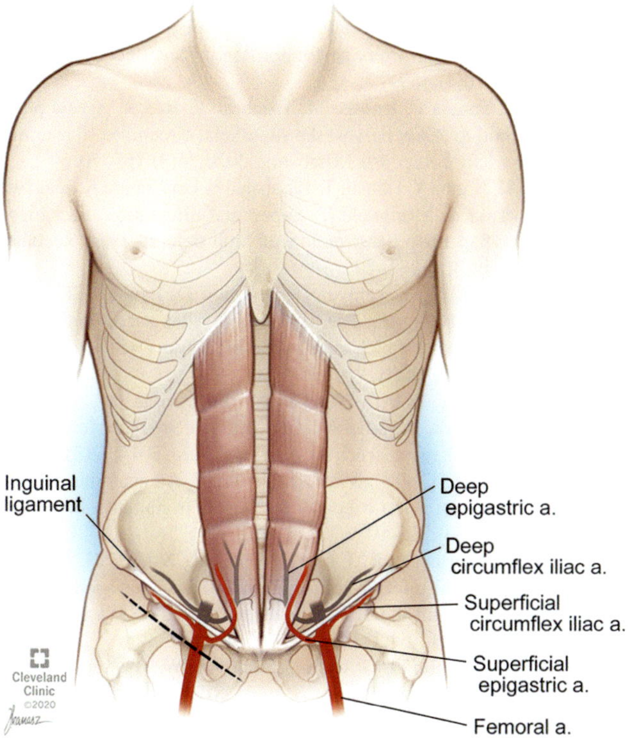

Fig. 19.2 Illustration demonstrating the incision (dashed line) on the right groin for surgical exposure of the SCIA (superficial circumflex iliac artery) and SIEA (superficial inferior epigastric artery). (Reprinted with permission, Cleveland Clinic Center for Medical Art & Photography © 2020. All Rights Reserved)

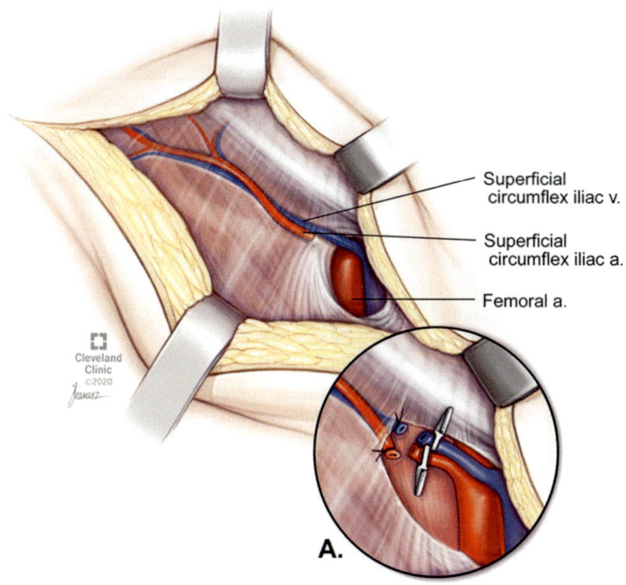

Fig. 19.3 Illustration of surgical exposure of the SCIA (superficial circumflex iliac artery). Close-up view (A): preparation of the vessels as recipient for microsurgical anastomoses. (Reprinted with permission, Cleveland Clinic Center for Medical Art & Photography © 2020. All Rights Reserved)

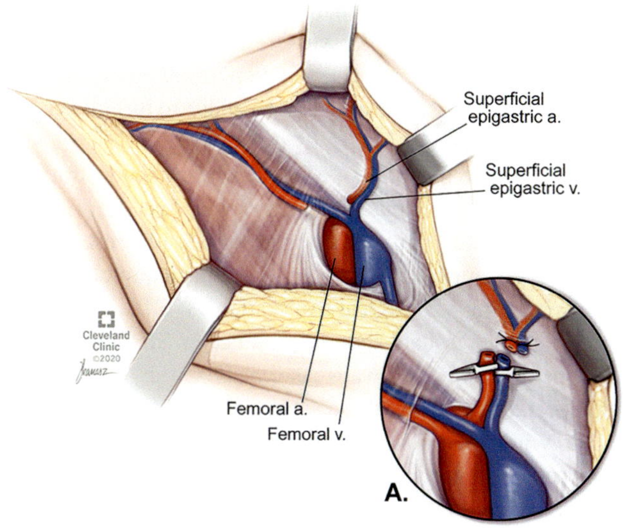

Fig. 19.4 Illustration of surgical exposure of the SIEA (superficial inferior epigastric artery). Close-up view (A): preparation of the vessels as recipient for microsurgical anastomoses. (Reprinted with permission, Cleveland Clinic Center for Medical Art & Photography © 2020. All Rights Reserved)

A similar surgical approach can be utilized to locate SIEA, utilizing an incision parallel to or overlying the inguinal ligament. The vessel can be commonly identified within 1 cm of midpoint of the inguinal ligament, but caution is advised because it can also be located laterally or medially [10]. The SIEA is then traced toward femoral vessels (Fig. 19.4). SIEV is usually located more medial and can be found in the subcutaneous tissues above the suprapubic area. Its location can be found with a handheld Doppler prior to incision.

Discussion

The SCIA/V and SIEA/V are not typically used as primary recipient vessels for reconstruction of the abdominal and inguinal area as other more dominant vessels are in close proximity. These include deep inferior epigastric system, intraperitoneal vessels, common or superficial femoral artery/vein, superior epigastrics, and deep circumflex iliac vasculature [18]. Some of the aforementioned vessels are difficult to expose, whereas others need vein grafts due to distance. SCIA/V and SIEA/V, on the other hand, are readily accessible in the lower abdominal wall as long as they have not been damaged or divided due to their superficial location. On condition that they have appropriate diameter, SCIA/V and SIEA/V have the potential to provide a quick exposure and straightforward microanastomosis without vein grafting.

They can be traced proximally for increased caliber, but it should be noted that the vessels may become tortuous, especially when there is a common trunk, making them unsuitable for anastomosis at this level due to turbulence and risk of thrombosis.

The variable anatomy of SIEA has been demonstrated in a multitude of publications since it was first described in 1975 [12, 19–22]. The variance in its rate of presence and size can be attributed to differences in methodology, i.e., cadaver studies vs. surgical exploration vs. CTA. One of the largest studies to date showed presence of SIEA in 94% of 500 hemi-abdominal walls as visualized by CTA [12]. However, only 24% of these were with a diameter >1.5 mm. SIEA/V are not the first choice for many surgeons, both as a flap pedicle and as a recipient, because of interindividual variations and the small diameter sometimes being too small for microsurgery. Similar issues exist with SCIA system, with anatomical variations accepted and regarded as one of the main challenges in raising perforator flaps in this region [5]. Presence and average size of SIEV are much more favorable, with reports showing consistent caliber suitable for microsurgery [12].

Preoperative investigation of the SIEA and SCIA with CTA provides valuable details about the existence, course, and caliber of these vessels. Color Doppler US can also be obtained for information on hemodynamics. Intraoperatively, blood flow should be clinically assessed prior to microsurgery. It is important to remember that reciprocal relations exist between adjacent vascular systems. If one of the arterial systems is hypoplastic, the others are bound to be hyperplastic. With this knowledge, surgeons should carefully observe anatomical variations and explore alternative vessels if necessary.

References

1. Yoshimatsu H, Steinbacher J, Meng S, Hamscha UM, Weninger WJ, Tinhofer IE, Harima M, Fuse Y, Yamamoto T, Tzou CHJ. Superficial circumflex iliac artery perforator flap: an anatomical study of the correlation of the superficial and the deep branches of the artery and evaluation of perfusion from the deep branch to the sartorius muscle and the iliac bone. Plast Reconstr Surg. 2019;143(2):589–602.
2. Suh HS, Jeong HH, Choi DH, Hong JP. Study of the medial superficial perforator of the superficial circumflex iliac artery perforator flap using computed tomographic angiography and surgical anatomy in 142 patients. Plast Reconstr Surg. 2017;139(3):738–48.
3. Strauch B, Yu HL, Chen ZW, Liebling R. Iliac and inferior epigastric flap. In: Atlas of microvascular surgery. New York: Thieme Medical Publishers, Inc; 1993. p. 120–8.
4. Hsu WM, Chao WN, Yang C, Fang CL, Huang KF, Lin YS, Lee TH. Evolution of the free groin flap: the superficial circumflex iliac artery perforator flap. Plast Reconstr Surg. 2007;119(5):1491–8.
5. Feng S, Xi W, Zhang Z, Tremp M, Schaefer DJ, Sadigh PL, Zhang W, Zhang YX. A reappraisal of the surgical planning of the superficial circumflex iliac artery perforator flap. J Plast Reconstr Aesthet Surg. 2017;70(4):469–77.
6. Pereira N, Parada L, Kufeke M, Troncoso E, Roa R. A new planning method to easily harvest the superficial circumflex iliac artery perforator flap. J Reconstr Microsurg. 2020;36(3):165–70.
7. Koshima I, Nanba Y, Tsutsui T, Takahashi Y, Urushibara K, Inagawa K, Hamasaki T, Moriguchi T. Superficial circumflex iliac artery perforator flap for reconstruction of limb defects. Plast Reconstr Surg. 2004;113(1):233–40.
8. Sinna R, Hajji H, Qassemyar Q, Perignon D, Benhaim T, Havet E. Anatomical background of the perforator flap based on the deep branch of the superficial circumflex iliac artery (SCIP Flap): a cadaveric study. Eplasty. 2010;10:e11.
9. Iida T, Mihara M, Yoshimatsu H, Narushima M, Koshima I. Versatility of the superficial circumflex iliac artery perforator flap in head and neck reconstruction. Ann Plast Surg. 2014;72(3):332–6.
10. Reardon CM, O'Ceallaigh S, O'Sullivan ST. An anatomical study of the superficial inferior epigastric vessels in humans. Br J Plast Surg. 2004;57(6):515–9.
11. Fukaya E, Kuwatsuru R, Iimura H, Ihara K, Sakurai H. Imaging of the superficial inferior epigastric vascular anatomy and preoperative planning for the SIEA flap using MDCTA. J Plast Reconstr Aesthet Surg. 2011;64(1):63–8.
12. Rozen WM, Chubb D, Grinsell D, Ashton MW. The variability of the superficial inferior epigastric artery (SIEA) and its angiosome: a clinical anatomical study. Microsurgery. 2010;30(5):386–91.
13. Hester TR Jr, Nahai F, Beegle PE, Bostwick J 3rd. Blood supply of the abdomen revisited, with emphasis on the superficial inferior epigastric artery. Plast Reconstr Surg. 1984;74(5):657–70.
14. Kita Y, Fukunaga Y, Arikawa M, Kagaya Y, Miyamoto S. Anatomy of the arterial and venous systems of the superficial inferior epigastric artery flap: a retrospective study based on computed tomographic angiography. J Plast Reconstr Aesthet Surg. 2020;73(5):870–5.
15. Rozen WM, Pan WR, Le Roux CM, Taylor GI, Ashton MW. The venous anatomy of the anterior abdominal wall: an anatomical and clinical study. Plast Reconstr Surg. 2009;124(3):848–53.
16. Chuang DC, Colony LH, Chen HC, Wei FC. Groin flap design and versatility. Plast Reconstr Surg. 1989;84(1):100–7.
17. Han H, Ahn M, Lee J. Penoscrotal reconstruction with superficial circumflex iliac artery perforator propeller flap. Microsurgery. 2019;39:688–95.
18. Gurunluoglu R, Rosen MJ. Recipient vessels for microsurgical flaps to the abdomen: a systematic review. Microsurgery. 2017;37(6):707–16.
19. Taylor GI, Daniel RK. The anatomy of several free flap donor sites. Plast Reconstr Surg. 1975;56(3):243–53.
20. Herrera FA, Selber JC, Buntic R, Brooks D, Buncke GM, Antony AK. How often is the superficial inferior epigastric artery adequate? An observational correlation. J Plast Reconstr Aesthet Surg. 2010;63(3):e310–1.
21. Spiegel AJ, Khan FN. An intraoperative algorithm for use of the SIEA flap for breast reconstruction. Plast Reconstr Surg. 2007;120(6):1450–9.
22. Holm C, Mayr M, Höfter E, Ninkovic M. The versatility of the SIEA flap: a clinical assessment of the vascular territory of the superficial epigastric inferior artery. J Plast Reconstr Aesthet Surg. 2007;60(8):946–51.

Superior Epigastric Vessels

20

Brandon C. Specht and Raffi Gurunian

Introduction

The superior epigastric arteries and veins are often thought of as a backup source of blood supply in the world of microsurgery. Familiarity with exposure and utilization of the superior epigastric system for free flap techniques is quite infrequent. Often, there are multiple alternative options within the abdomen and chest for vascular anastomosis that take precedence. The deep inferior epigastric vessels (discussed in Chap. 15) are a dominant recipient system for abdominal wall reconstruction, but when unavailable, the superior epigastric vessels may be considered as an alternative recipient site.

Preoperative Assessment

A thorough history, especially regarding any previous surgical history or trauma and radiation, should be obtained in each and every case. Patients with a history of coronary artery bypass graft should be questioned regarding the harvest of internal mammary arteries. The superior epigastric artery would not be reliable in this circumstance as it is one of the branches of the internal mammary artery [1].

An extensive physical exam of the soft tissues should be performed for any sign of surgical scar or trauma and radiation in the vicinity of recipient vessels intended for use for microvascular anastomosis. Often, patients requiring abdominal wall reconstruction have a history of multiple abdominal surgeries in the past, and operative notes with specific details are not always available. Furthermore, there are times when patients do not even recall having certain procedures done. In addition, with the increased use of laparoscopic surgery, the small scars can be indicative of a potential region of accidental vascular injury. Bhatti et al. [2] described a guide to safe laparoscopic port insertion to avoid injury to the superior epigastric vessels in the upper abdomen. The safe zones were within 3 cm from midline or 9 cm lateral from midline.

Therefore, when the suspicion arises regarding the patency and reliability of the selected vasculature as the recipient site, imaging should be obtained either via computed tomographic angiography (CTA) or magnetic resonance angiography (MRA) depending on surgeon preference and appropriateness for each specific patient [3]. Obtaining a CTA or MRA not only helps identify any aberrant anatomy or prior surgical trauma but also assists in surgical planning and characterization of potential recipient vessel sites including the internal thoracic, the superior epigastric, and the deep inferior epigastric vessels.

Applied Anatomy

The superior epigastric artery (SEA) and vein (SEV) are derived from the internal mammary arteries/veins (IMA/IMV) as they course the chest inferiorly toward the abdomen (Fig. 20.1). The IMA splits into its two branches at around the level of the sixth and seventh costal cartilages creating the superior epigastric artery and the musculophrenic artery. The superior epigastric artery and vein enter the abdomen from the thoracic cavity at the level of xiphoid. In the anterior abdominal wall plane, the SEA/SEV takes an inferior lateral course from the lateral sternum to between the rectus

Supplementary Information The online version of this chapter (https://doi.org/10.1007/978-3-030-75389-4_20) contains supplementary material, which is available to authorized users.

B. C. Specht
Department of Plastic Surgery, Cleveland Clinic, Cleveland, OH, USA

R. Gurunian (✉)
Department of Plastic Surgery, Cleveland Clinic, Cleveland, OH, USA

Cleveland Clinic Lerner College of Medicine, Case Western Reserve University, Cleveland, OH, USA
e-mail: gurunir@ccf.org

R. Gurunian, R. Djohan (eds.), *Recipient Vessels in Reconstructive Microsurgery*, https://doi.org/10.1007/978-3-030-75389-4_20

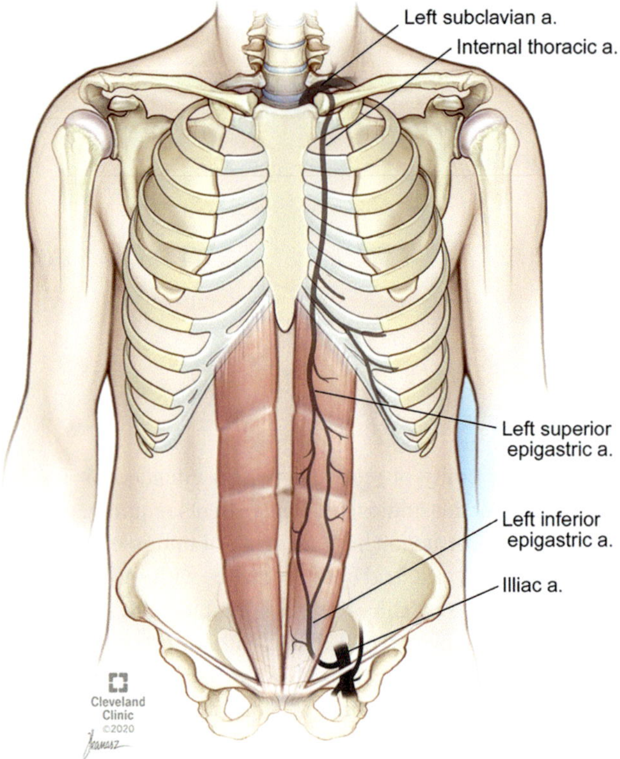

Fig. 20.1 The anatomical illustration of the rectus abdominis muscles, the superior epigastric artery, the internal thoracic artery, and the deep inferior epigastric artery: Line drawing that illustrates the anatomy of the rectus abdominis muscles, the superior epigastric artery, its relation with the internal thoracic artery, and the deep inferior epigastric artery. The superior epigastric artery originates from the internal thoracic artery at the level of the sixth and seventh rib. It then descends to enter the rectus sheath, at first behind the rectus abdominis muscle, and then anastomoses with the deep inferior epigastric branch of the external iliac. (Reprinted with permission, Cleveland Clinic Center for Medical Art & Photography © 2020. All Rights Reserved)

abdominis muscle anteriorly and the rectus sheath posteriorly [4, 5]. Typically, within the rectus abdominis muscle, the SEA will divide into at least two main branches as it courses inferiorly. The DIEA and SEA typically anastomose superiorly to the umbilicus. In cadaveric studies, the superior epigastric artery has been shown to be approximately 3–8.5 cm lateral to the midline bilaterally [2]. However, there is a great deal of variability in laterality of the vessels depending on how far superior or inferior on the abdomen. Saber et al. investigated the location of these vessels further utilizing CT imaging. They found that at the level of the xiphoid, the SEA was roughly 4.41–4.53 cm from the midline. Midway between the xiphoid and umbilicus, the vessel would course 5.36–5.50 cm from midline [6].

The caliber of the SEA and SEV can be variable and unreliable at times. As an extension of the internal mammary artery, the SEA can have a diameter of 1–2.5 mm and a pedicle length of 3–4 cm. The corresponding SEV may have a diameter of ~2.5 mm and a pedicle length similarly of 3–4 cm [7, 8]. More often than not, the ipsilateral deep inferior epigastric vessel will be of larger caliber and more reliable. However, in cadaver studies, it has been shown that some patients will have an SEA that is similar in diameter to their DIEA [9]. Likewise, Moon et al. [4] identified that there are varying anastomotic branching systems between the superior epigastric arterial system and your deep inferior arterial system. This is important because having one main vessel versus multiple branches may be a good predictor of potential caliber size and usability for microsurgery.

Surgical Site Exposure

Utilization of the superior epigastric vessels usually is performed out of necessity and not by preferred choice for many microsurgeons. With performing larger abdominal wall reconstruction, the resultant wound itself will often have some level of exposure to the axis of the superior epigastric vessels. It is imperative, with any combination surgical cases, that the other surgical teams are aware of this potential vascular pedicle to minimize iatrogenic trauma and subsequent loss of the potential recipient site. Utilization of any nearby existing skin incisions or extension of a preexisting incision is a reasonable choice for exposure of the superior epigastric vessels. This all would depend on the location, characteristics of the defect, and its proximity to the superior epigastric vessels.

With no preexisting incisions in place, the superior epigastric vessels can be accessed through a paramedian or preferably midline incision that is made in the upper third of the abdomen. A midline skin incision allows the option to potentially expose bilateral vascular pedicles if one site appears not reliable. The dissection will then carry deeply through subcutaneous tissues until the anterior rectus sheath is encountered. The skin flaps are raised off the anterior rectus sheath medially and laterally to facilitate the exposure. The dissection is carried out with total muscle relaxation. The sheath is sharply incised without energy, about 3 cm off the midline, overtop and parallel to the rectus muscle. The anterior rectus sheath fascia is carefully peeled off the rectus muscle medially and laterally. Medially, the rectus muscle is identified and the retrorectus plane is entered (Figs. 20.2 and 20.3). This plane is relatively avascular, and the dissection can be continued bluntly in a medial to lateral direction to identify the superior epigastric vessels posteriorly to the muscle. Dissection then may proceed superiorly and inferiorly to identify further length and to evaluate caliber of the vessels (Fig. 20.4). Distally, the vessels are divided and traced superiorly with delicate dissection and ligation of side branches. Final preparation of the superior epigastric artery and vein should proceed in a standard fashion. The superior epigastric vessels can be brought to the surface through the

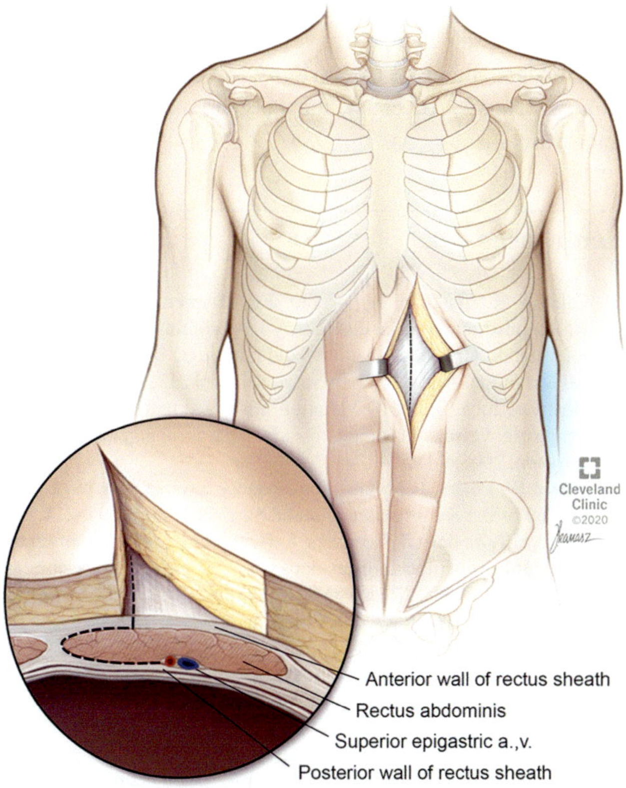

Fig. 20.2 Line drawing that illustrates the approach for exposure of the superior epigastric vessels. (Reprinted with permission, Cleveland Clinic Center for Medical Art & Photography © 2020. All Rights Reserved)

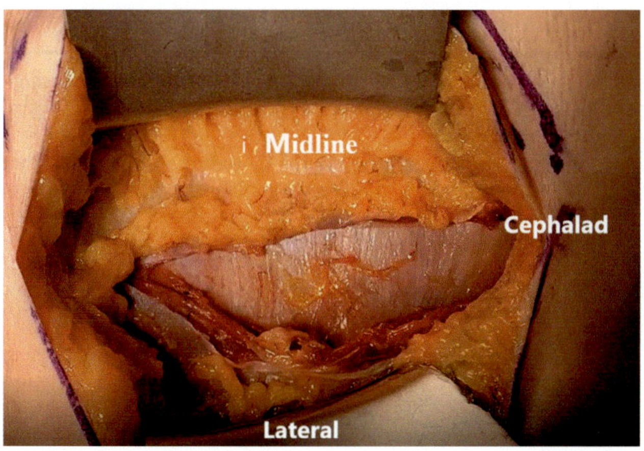

Fig. 20.3 Cadaver dissection: Note the anterior rectus sheath was incised off of midline after paramedian skin incision. The rectus muscle was retracted laterally exposing the safe plane of the posterior rectus sheath

rectus muscle or left behind the rectus muscle to allow anastomosis medial to the muscle (Figs. 20.5 and 20.6; Video 20.1). In either scenario, an adequate workable length and caliber should be obtained for microvascular anastomosis, and any potential areas of kinking, twisting, or compression should be avoided.

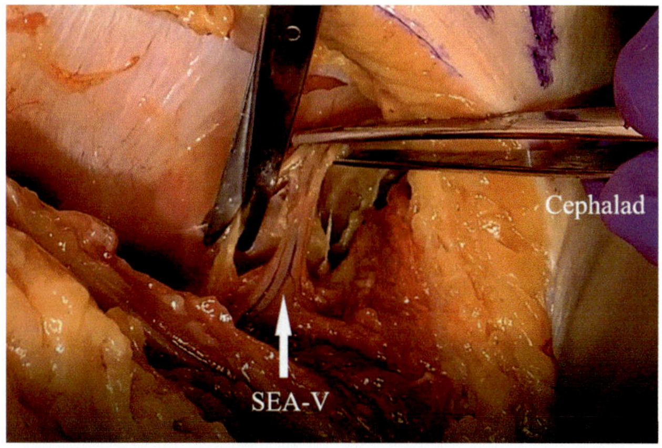

Fig. 20.4 In the same cadaver dissection, one can easily visualize the superior epigastric pedicle running along the posterior surface of the rectus muscle as it descends from the chest. The artery will enter into the muscle belly and may divide into multiple separate branches as it courses inferiorly toward the umbilicus

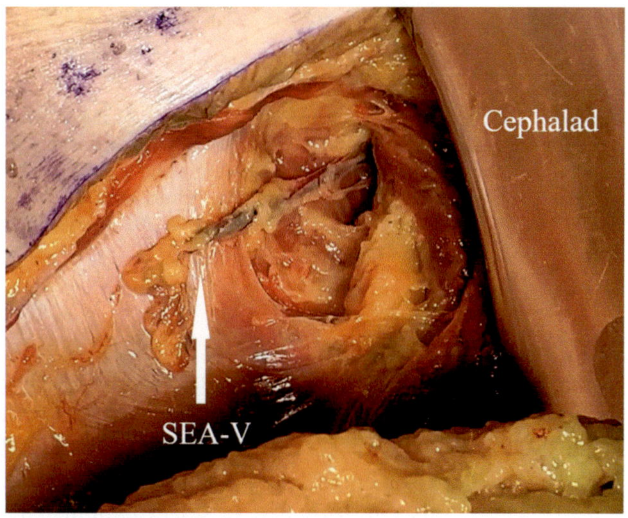

Fig. 20.5 In this image, one can see the completely isolated pedicle of the superior epigastric vessels. Note the dissection has proceeded superiorly to gain more length and mobility of the pedicle. This should be done prior to any final vessel preparation for anastomosis

Discussion

The superior epigastric vessels typically are not the first-choice recipient vessels for an abdominal or chest wall reconstruction with a free flap. In complex abdominal reconstruction using microsurgical flaps, most surgeons prefer to utilize the deep inferior epigastric pedicles for blood supply. However, those same vessels may be unavailable secondary to hernia mesh placement, trauma, and other previous surgeries. Alternative recipient vessels should then be sought out for microsurgical reconstruction. The superior epigastric vessels may be considered for reconstructions in the upper to mid-abdomen and the chest.

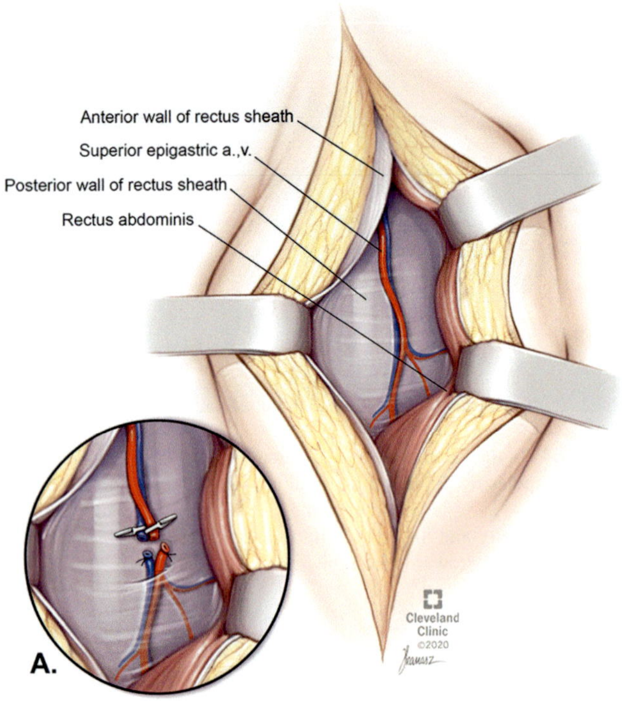

Fig. 20.6 Line drawing that illustrates the dissection of the superior epigastric vessels for use as recipient for microvascular anastomosis. A: Close-up illustration of the superior epigastric vessels prepared for microvascular anastomosis. (Reprinted with permission, Cleveland Clinic Center for Medical Art & Photography © 2020. All Rights Reserved)

In a systematic review of 38 articles performed by Gurunluoglu et al. [10], it was shown that only 1 case among 149 patients undergoing complex abdominal wall reconstruction using microsurgical free flaps involved utilizing the superior epigastric vessels as the recipient site. However, this confirms that in select patients, the superior epigastric vessels may be the only option for anastomosis [11].

Even though the indications for the use of the superior epigastric vessels as recipient vessel is very limited, having a clear understanding of the anatomy and their surgical exposure will surely diversify the surgical repertoire of any microvascular surgeon.

References

1. Gilman K, Ipaktchi K, Moore EE, Barnett C, Gurunluoglu R. Reconstruction of an emergency thoracotomy wound with free rectus abdominis flap: anatomic and radiologic basis for the surgical technique. World J Emerg Surg. 2010;5(1):12.
2. Bhatti A, Iqbal S, Lee T. Variation in surface marking of superior epigastric vessels. A guide to safe laparoscopic port insertion. Surgeon. 2008;6(1):50–2.
3. Vasile JV, Levine JL. Magnetic resonance angiography in perforator flap breast reconstruction. Gland Surg. 2016;5(2):197–211.
4. Moon HK, Taylor GI, Bostwick J. The vascular anatomy of rectus abdominis musculocutaneous flaps based on the deep superior epigastric system. Plast Reconstr Surg. 1988;82(5):830–2.
5. Kandinata N. Anatomy, abdomen and pelvis, epigastric artery [Internet]. In: StatPearls [Internet]. U.S. National Library of Medicine. Treasure Island: StatPearls Publishing; 2018. [cited 2019 Dec]. Available from: https://www.ncbi.nlm.nih.gov/books/NBK537156/.
6. Saber AA, Meslemani AM, Davis R, Pimentel R. Safety zones for anterior abdominal wall entry during laparoscopy. Ann Surg. 2004;239(2):182–5.
7. Wei F, Mardini S. Perforator-based work horse flaps. In: Flaps and reconstructive surgery. 1st ed. Philadelphia: Saunders; 2009. p. 625–38.
8. Strauch B, Yu HL, Chen ZW, Liebling R. Atlas of micro-vascular surgery. New York: Thieme Medical Publishers Inc; 1993. p. 448–83.
9. Abdul-Ameer HH, Jaffar AA, Hassan HA. Surgical anatomy of the superior epigastric artery. Iraqi J Med Sci. 2006;5(1):3–7.
10. Gurunluoglu R, Rosen MJ. Recipient vessels for microsurgical flaps to the abdomen: a systematic review. Microsurgery. 2017;37(6):707–16.
11. Ninković M, Kronberger P, Harpf C, Rumer A, Anderl H. Free innervated latissimus dorsi muscle flap for reconstruction of full-thickness abdominal wall defects. Plast Reconstr Surg. 1998;101(4):971–8.

Lumbar Vessels

21

Fatma Betul Tuncer, Isis Scomacao, Richard L. Drake, Lia Gurunian, and Raffi Gurunian

Introduction

Lumbosacral or sacral defects are usually covered with locoregional flaps when available. However, large defects or unstable wounds due to radiation or infection may require reconstruction with free flap. Recipient vessel selection in this region represents a unique challenge. Conventional recipients include superior and inferior gluteal vessels. However, these sites may not be available due to previous trauma or radiation. Even if they are available, vein grafts may be required to support the microsurgical flap. Also, interposition vein grafts or arteriovenous loops may be required from other recipient sites to circumvent the paucity of recipient vessels in the lumbosacral region [1]. However, they may increase the risk of thrombosis, number of surgeries, and free flap failure [2]. In select cases, lumbar perforators can offer a solution and be used as a local recipient vessel to avoid long AV loops and interposition vein grafts. This chapter will discuss anatomy, dissection, and surgical considerations of the lumbar artery as a recipient vessel in microsurgical flap reconstruction.

Supplementary Information The online version of this chapter (https://doi.org/10.1007/978-3-030-75389-4_21) contains supplementary material, which is available to authorized users.

F. B. Tuncer
Division of Plastic Surgery, University of Utah, Salt Lake City, UT, USA

Department of Plastic Surgery, Cleveland Clinic, Cleveland, OH, USA
e-mail: fatma.tuncer@hsc.utah.edu

I. Scomacao
Department of Plastic Surgery, Cleveland Clinic, Cleveland, OH, USA
e-mail: SCOMACI@ccf.org

Preoperative Assessment

As it will be explained later in the chapter, there is a great variability in the size and location of the lumbar artery perforators. CT angiography (CTA) is recommended for preoperative planning and for mapping the location of lumbar artery perforators based on anatomical landmarks. The size, length, and course of the lumbar arteries can be assessed on the CTA. A lumbar artery with a large caliber and septocutaneous course can be chosen as a recipient vessel. Appropriate perforator is mapped out on the skin by using measurements on the CT scan and a handheld Doppler.

Applied Anatomy

There are four pairs of lumbar arteries that arise from the posterior surface of the abdominal aorta in series with the intercostal arteries. The lumbar arteries run laterally on the bodies of the lumbar vertebra, dorsal to the sympathetic trunk, and pass between the adjacent transverse processes. They course between the psoas major muscles and sympathetic trunk anteriorly and transverse processes of the vertebrae posteriorly. Between the transverse processes of the vertebrae, each lumbar artery divides into a dorsal and an abdominal (ventral) branch. The abdominal branch pierces the aponeurosis of the transversus abdominis muscle and

R. L. Drake
Director of Anatomy, Cleveland Clinic Lerner College of Medicine, Cleveland, OH, USA
e-mail: DRAKER@ccf.org

L. Gurunian
Saddleback College, Mission Viejo, CA, USA

R. Gurunian (✉)
Department of Plastic Surgery, Cleveland Clinic, Cleveland, OH, USA

Cleveland Clinic Lerner College of Medicine, Case Western Reserve University, Cleveland, OH, USA
e-mail: gurunir@ccf.org

R. Gurunian, R. Djohan (eds.), *Recipient Vessels in Reconstructive Microsurgery*,
https://doi.org/10.1007/978-3-030-75389-4_21

runs between the transversus abdominis and internal oblique muscles until it anastomoses with the intercostal, subcostal, iliolumbar, deep circumflex, and inferior epigastric arteries. The dorsal branch supplies the skin and muscles of the back. It initially gives off a spinal branch which enters the vertebral canal through the intervertebral foramina [3]. The dorsal branch courses inside the psoas major muscle and then either passes through the quadratus lumborum (musculocutaneous perforator) or courses inside the septum between the erector spinae and quadratus lumborum (septocutaneous perforator) [4] (Fig. 21.1). The perforator pierces the thoracolumbar fascia and branches into the skin (Fig. 21.2) [4, 5]. Skin perforators are located 5–9 cm lateral to the midline (mean 7.2 cm) [6]. Kato et al. showed in their cadaver studies that one lumbar artery perforator can supply a skin territory from posterior midline to the lateral border of the rectus abdominis on the same side [7]. Each lumbar artery is accompanied by one or two veins, one of two is larger than the artery, and the other has the same or smaller diameter than the artery [4]. The mean diameter of the lumbar artery is 1.0 mm (0.8–1.3 mm) and of the lumbar vein is 1.2 (0.9–1.5 mm) [4]. The lumbar vessel length and diameters tend to increase in caliber from L1 to L4 lumbar artery [4]. L4 has the largest diameter and is usually septocutaneous [4, 7].

Surgical Site Exposure

The lumbar artery perforators can be mapped out on the skin based on the posterior midline and iliac crest on preoperative CT or MR. Dominant perforators usually originate from third and fourth lumbar vertebrae and they tend to be septo-

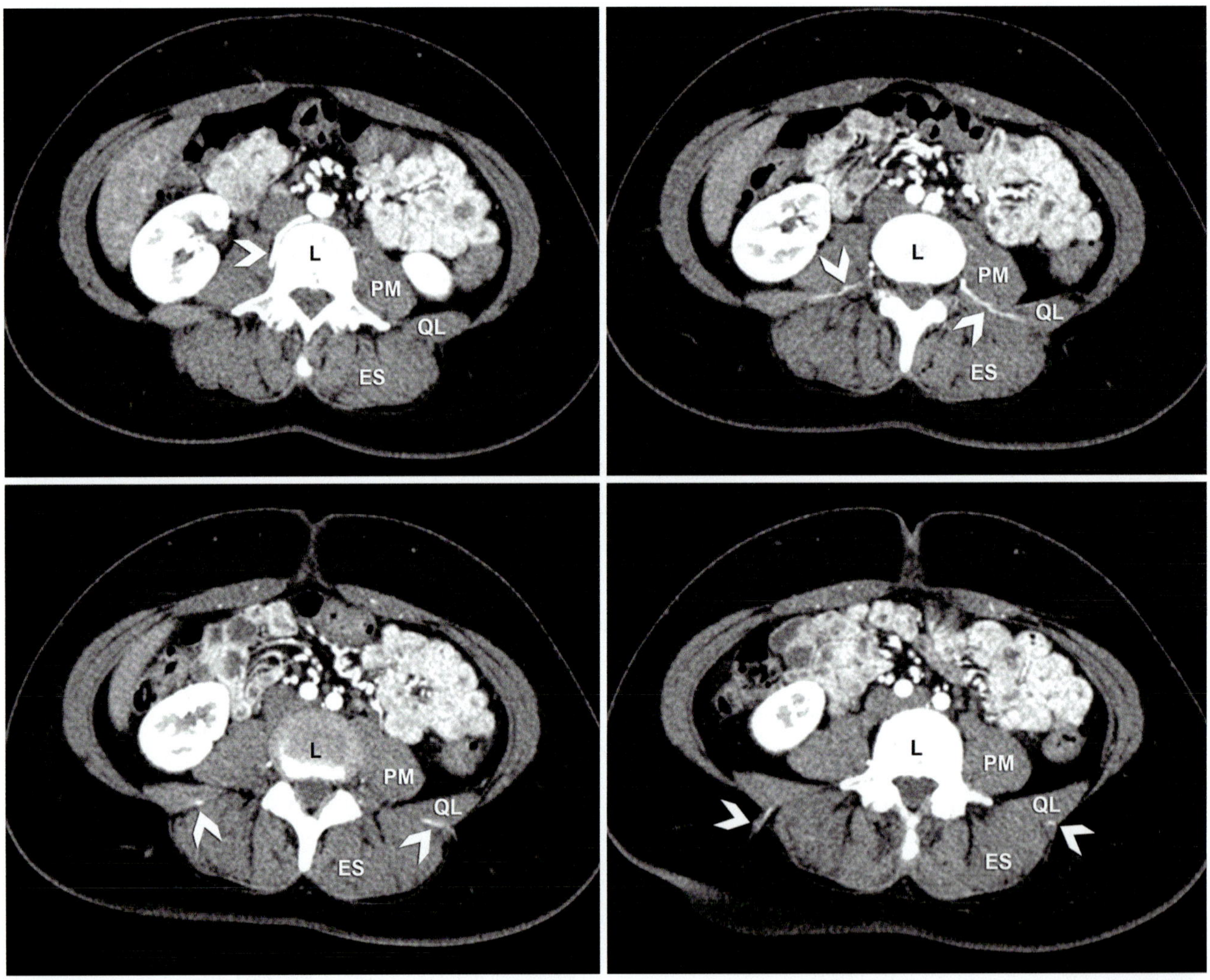

Fig. 21.1 CTA of the pelvis at the fourth lumbar vertebral level. Left upper: Arrowhead indicates the lumbar artery. Right upper: Arrowheads indicate the septocutaneous perforators on each side. These perforators initially run between psoas major and erector spine muscles. Left lower: The dorsal branch of the lumbar artery (arrowhead) has a septocutaneous course (arrowhead) between erector spinae (ES) and quadratus lumborum (QL) muscles. Right lower: Arrowheads show the terminal portions of the perforators. (L, lumbar vertebra; PM, psoas major)

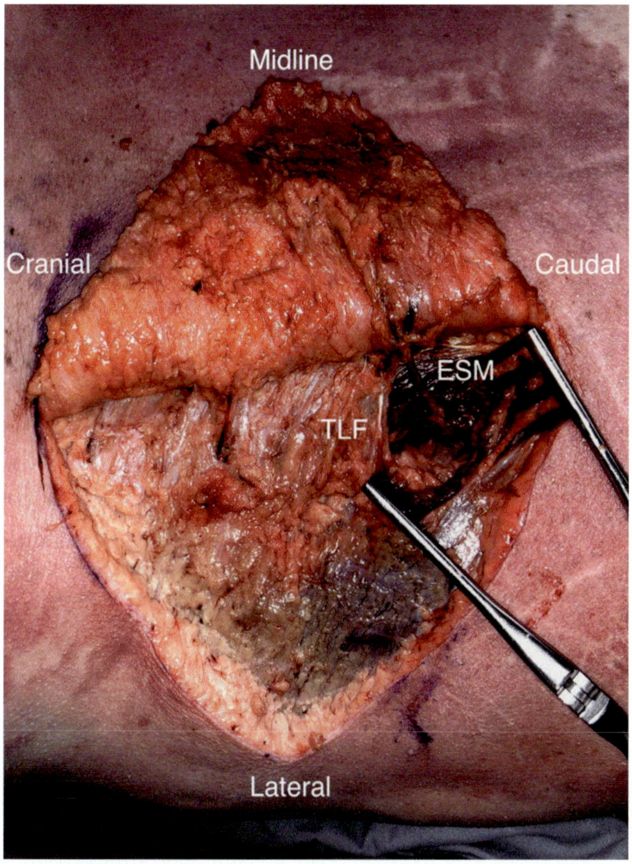

Fig. 21.2 Cadaveric dissection showing one perforator (left) piercing the thoracolumbar fascia and another perforator (right) dissected. (TLF, thoracolumbar fascia; ESM, erector spinae muscle)

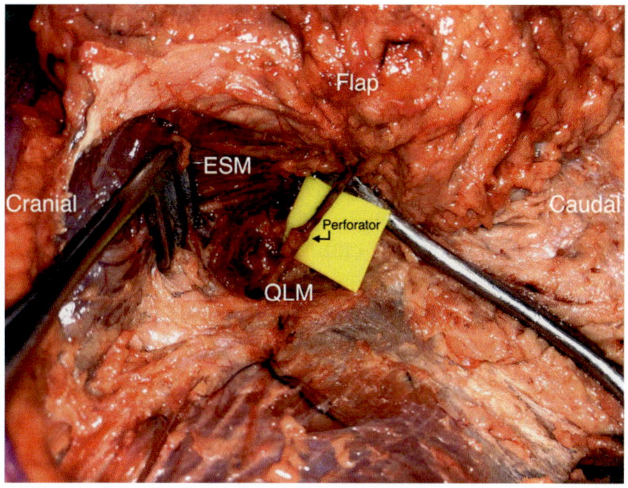

Fig. 21.3 Cadaveric dissection: complete perforator dissection. (ESM, erector spinae muscle; QLM, quadratus lumborum muscle)

cutaneous [8, 9]. Their presence can be confirmed preoperatively with a handheld Doppler or duplex Doppler ultrasound. The location of perforators is marked on the skin. Depending on the location of the defect and the recipient lumbar artery, an existing incision can be extended in the direction of the selected lumbar artery. The dissection initially starts in the suprafascial plane and switches to the subfascial plane close to the marked location of the perforator (Video 21.1). Perforators are usually found 7–10 cm lateral to the midline [8, 9]. Perforator dissection is continued until appropriate length and caliber are achieved for microsurgical anastomosis, but not deeper than transverse processes of the vertebrae. Septocutaneous perforators are easier to dissect than musculocutaneous perforators. Regardless, both types of perforators give muscular branches throughout their course. Dissection is usually stopped at or before the transverse processes of the lumbar vertebra to prevent any inadvertent damage to spinal nerves. The average length of the vessels after perforator dissection is around 4 cm, and the mean diameter is between 0.8 and 1 mm (Fig. 21.3) [10]. Because of size mismatch between the recipient and flap vessels, interposition grafts can be used to provide better caliber match and increase the length of recipient vessels. For instance, Opsomer et al. reported routine harvest of interposition grafts from the deep inferior epigastric artery and vein when they perform breast reconstruction with lumbar artery perforator flaps [10]. Perforator-to-perforator anastomosis can be done where appropriate in order to avoid interposition grafts and additional anastomoses [11].

Discussion

Locoregional flaps are usually sufficient to close most of the lumbosacral wounds. However, reconstruction with free flap may be required in patients with large defects. Free flaps have several advantages over regional flaps, such as minimal tension in the suture line and obliteration of the dead space. In addition, local flaps are sometimes affected by radiation, may violate the function of muscles, and can develop marginal tissue necrosis where coverage is the most needed.

Potential recipient vessels for lumbosacral defects are the posterior intercostal vessels, the superior gluteal vessels (also see Chap. 22), the inferior gluteal vessels (also see Chap. 23), the internal iliac vessels, double vein grafts or arteriovenous loops to the thoracodorsal, the superficial and deep femoral vessels, and the deep inferior epigastric vessels [4, 12].

The decision for which one of these recipient vessels to use depends on many factors that include vessel proximity, patency and availability, vessel length and caliber, donor vessel characteristics, type and location of the defect, as well as type and size of the flap. All of these factors should be carefully assessed for selection of the proper vessel based on the specifics of each microsurgical case.

In select cases, the lumbar artery may be used as alternative recipient, and this approach may alleviate the use of AV loops and vein grafts [13]. However, the artery may have a small caliber and shows anatomic variation. The mean diameter of the lumbar artery is 1.0 mm (0.8–1.3 mm) and of the lumbar vein is 1.2 (0.9–1.5 mm) [4, 5]. The size mismatch can be overcome by using various microsurgery techniques such as dilation, oblique cutting, evenly placed sutures, and perforator-to-perforator anastomosis. The lumbar artery that has visual pulsation, arterial spurting, strong Doppler signal, and a diameter larger than 0.8 mm is ideal for anastomosis. Preoperative CTA scan helps to choose a perforator with a large caliber and favorable anatomy. Kiil et al. showed in their cadaveric and radiologic study that diameters and locations of the perforators varied highly between specimens. They noted a trend toward increase in size when descending from L1 to L4 [4]. Septocutaneous perforators (mostly at L4 level) are preferred for an easier dissection and decreased donor site morbidity. CTA also demonstrates the course of the lumbar artery perforator and other anatomical variants such as the Adamkiewicz artery. Because of the variations in size and location of the lumbar arteries, a backup plan (e.g., AV loops, vein grafts) should be made in case the lumbar artery or vein does not meet criteria for microsurgical anastomosis.

Conclusion

The lumbar artery and vein can be used as recipient vessels in the lumbosacral region in select patients. Preoperative imaging is recommended to identify the artery with a favorable size and course.

References

1. Harris GD, Lewis VL, Nagle DJ, Edelson RJ, Kim PS. Free flap reconstruction of the lower back and posterior pelvis: indications, principles, and techniques. J Reconstr Microsurg. 1988;4(3):169–78. https://doi.org/10.1055/s-2007-1006916.
2. Khouri RK, Cooley BC, Kunselman AR, et al. A prospective study of microvascular free-flap surgery and outcome. Plast Reconstr Surg. 1998;102(3):711–21. https://doi.org/10.1097/00006534-199809030-00015.
3. Gray H. Gray's anatomy. New York: Barnes & Noble; 2010.
4. Kiil BJ, Rozen WM, Pan WR, et al. The lumbar artery perforators: a cadaveric and clinical anatomical study. Plast Reconstr Surg. 2009;123(4):1229–38. https://doi.org/10.1097/PRS.0b013e31819f299e.
5. Bissell MB, Greenspun DT, Levine J, et al. The lumbar artery perforator flap: 3-dimensional anatomical study and clinical applications. Ann Plast Surg. 2016;77(4):469–76. https://doi.org/10.1097/SAP.0000000000000646.
6. Roche NA, Van Landuyt K, Blondeel PN, Matton G, Monstrey SJ. The use of pedicled perforator flaps for reconstruction of lumbosacral defects. Ann Plast Surg. 2000;45(1):7–14. https://doi.org/10.1097/00000637-200045010-00002.
7. Kato H, Hasegawa M, Takada T, Torii S. The lumbar artery perforator based island flap: anatomical study and case reports. Br J Plast Surg. 1999;52(7):541–6. https://doi.org/10.1054/bjps.1999.3120.
8. Sommeling CE, Colebunders B, Pardon HE, Stillaert FB, Blondeel PN, van Landuyt K. Lumbar artery perforators: an anatomical study based on computed tomographic angiography imaging. Acta Chir Belg. 2017;117(4):223–6. https://doi.org/10.1080/00015458.2017.1284431.
9. Hamdi M, Craggs B, Brussaard C, Seidenstueker K, Hendrickx B, Zeltzer A. Lumbar artery perforator flap: an anatomical study using multidetector computed tomographic scan and surgical pearls for breast reconstruction. Plast Reconstr Surg. 2016;138(2):343–52. https://doi.org/10.1097/PRS.0000000000002347.
10. Opsomer D, Stillaert F, Blondeel P, Van Landuyt K. The lumbar artery perforator flap in autologous breast reconstruction: initial experience with 100 cases. Plast Reconstr Surg. 2018;142(1):1e–8e. https://doi.org/10.1097/PRS.0000000000004522.
11. Mureau MAM, Hofer SOP. Perforator-to-perforator musculocutaneous anterolateral thigh flap for reconstruction of a lumbosacral defect using the lumbar artery perforator as recipient vessel. J Reconstr Microsurg. 2008;24(4):295–9. https://doi.org/10.1055/s-2008-1080532.
12. Park S. Muscle-splitting approach to superior and inferior gluteal vessels: versatile source of recipient vessels for free-tissue transfer to sacral, gluteal, and ischial regions. Plast Reconstr Surg. 2000;106(1):81–6. https://doi.org/10.1097/00006534-200007000-00015.
13. Arkudas A, Horch RE, Regus S, et al. Retrospective cohort study of combined approach for trunk reconstruction using arteriovenous loops and free flaps. J Plast Reconstr Aesthet Surg. 2018;71(3):394–401. https://doi.org/10.1016/j.bjps.2017.08.025.

Superior Gluteal Vessels

22

DeAsia D. Jacob, David Kashan, Richard L. Drake, and Raffi Gurunian

Introduction

The vast majority of defects requiring flap coverage in the gluteal, lumbosacral, and perineal regions can be managed using locoregional flaps. However, in the occasional instance, microsurgical flap reconstruction may be required. The superior gluteal vessels can be used as recipient vessels for microsurgical reconstruction of defects in the gluteal, lumbar, sacral, and perineal regions that arise from tumors, trauma, pressure sores, or radiation injury [1]. Significant microsurgical experience is required to obtain vessels of good caliber and length that are suitable to use for microvascular anastomosis because of their deep and intramuscular location with many perforating branches.

Preoperative Assessment

Preoperative assessment should include patient medical conditions that can influence microsurgical reconstructive outcome such as hypercoagulable state, anemia, advanced age, gender, smoking, and comorbidities [2, 3]. Comorbidities associated with poorer outcomes include diabetes mellitus, peripheral vascular disease, chronic obstructive pulmonary disease (COPD), malnutrition, obesity, and high American Society of Anesthesiologists (ASA) classification [2, 3]. While flap failure cannot be attributed to the patient-related factors alone, inherent non-patient-dependent risks include length of operative time [2–5], defect location [2, 5], and type of reconstruction performed [2]. Other patient factors such as previous surgical procedures, trauma, or radiation must also be considered. While radiation does not preclude use of the superior gluteal vessels, it can make the dissection even more difficult [1]. If there is any doubt about the integrity of the vasculature, preoperative angiography should be obtained to confirm patency.

The experience and creativity of the reconstructive microsurgeon are of utmost importance in determining a solution to each and every reconstructive problem. Essentially, microsurgical flaps that can be harvested from the back are preferable as majority of patients requiring reconstruction for lumbosacral/gluteal regions will be positioned prone or lateral decubitus. Therefore, scapular, parascapular, thoracodorsal artery perforator, latissimus dorsi, and serratus flap can be viable options in solo or in various combinations depending on the wound characteristics. These flap choices would allow two teams working simultaneously for flap dissection and recipient site vessel preparation.

Intraoperative Considerations

Anesthesiologists are an integral part of the team to ensure successful completion of microsurgical procedures. Even starting from the beginning of the procedure, choice of induction and maintenance anesthetic agents can have an impact on microcirculation [2]. The surgeon must have clear communication with the anesthesia team regarding transfusion of blood products [2, 5] and intravenous fluid

Supplementary Information The online version of this chapter (https://doi.org/10.1007/978-3-030-75389-4_22) contains supplementary material, which is available to authorized users.

D. D. Jacob · D. Kashan
Department of Plastic Surgery, Cleveland Clinic, Cleveland, OH, USA
e-mail: Jacobd@ccf.org; Kashand@ccf.org

R. L. Drake
Department of Anatomy, Cleveland Clinic Lerner College of Medicine, Cleveland, OH, USA
e-mail: DRAKER@ccf.org

R. Gurunian (✉)
Department of Plastic Surgery, Cleveland Clinic, Cleveland, OH, USA

Cleveland Clinic Lerner College of Medicine, Case Western Reserve University, Cleveland, OH, USA
e-mail: gurunir@ccf.org

R. Gurunian, R. Djohan (eds.), *Recipient Vessels in Reconstructive Microsurgery*, https://doi.org/10.1007/978-3-030-75389-4_22

resuscitation as mismanagement can have deleterious effects [2, 4, 6]. While the preparation of donor and recipient vessels for microsurgical anastomosis requires extreme focus, it is important to be aware of maintaining normothermia [2, 7], even before starting the case.

As the procedure begins, even before the surgeon embarks on the daunting task of microsurgical reconstruction, the existing wound must be adequately addressed. Most patients in need of this type of surgery are in this situation because they have a soft tissue defect that cannot be sufficiently addressed with other means of reconstruction [8]. Chronicity of the wound may vary from patient to patient, but once it is decided that microvascular reconstruction is necessary, it is imperative that the wound bed be addressed. The microsurgeon must use their judgment to determine when the wound is ready for coverage and must plan for serial debridements if required. While there are many available adjuncts at the microsurgeon's discretion, surgical debridement is the gold standard for wound bed preparation [8–12].

While many of the already discussed preoperative factors also have implications intraoperatively, there are a few intraoperative measures to consider to maximize free flap success. With all of the aforementioned factors, including prolonged operative time and anesthetic agents, vasopressors may be required to maintain blood pressure. While the literature suggests that the use of vasopressors is not associated with increased flap failure, they should be used cautiously in microsurgical flap operations [13–15].

After a thorough dissection of recipient and donor vessels is performed, the microsurgeon must decide when it is time to harvest the flap. The flap must not be harvested prior to ensuring the patency of the recipient vessels. Prolonged ischemia times have been associated with poorer outcomes [16]. Technical issues can lead to flap problems such as damage to the vessel intima, poor vessel positioning resulting in kinking, and technical problems with the execution of the anastomosis [2]. It is beyond the scope of this chapter to discuss indications for intraoperative use of vasodilatory or thrombolytic agents, but it is imperative that the microsurgeon be familiar with when their use is indicated and their potential effect on flap success [4, 17, 18].

Applied Anatomy

The superior gluteal vessels arise as the largest and terminal branch of the internal iliac system, a branch of the common iliac artery, in the pelvis [19–24]. They are a part of the extrapelvic branches that supply the gluteal region. The superior gluteal artery provides the majority of the blood supply to the gluteus medius and minimus while also supplying secondary vessels to the gluteus maximus [25]. It has been shown to have many anatomical differences and the surgeon must be prepared to encounter variations [26]. Fatu et al. showed that there are variations in the internal iliac artery length and caliber between different ethnic groups and among genders. It is these variations that make it plausible that there are also variations in its terminal branch, the superior gluteal artery [21]. The Adachi classification describes the way in which the superior gluteal artery can arise from the internal iliac artery: a common ischio-gluteal trunk; a trifurcation into the superior gluteal artery, inferior gluteal artery and the internal pudendal artery; and a common pudendo-gluteal trunk [21].

The superior gluteal artery exits the pelvis through the greater sciatic foramen and passes above the piriformis muscle and inferior to the gluteus medius [1, 20, 22, 25] (Fig. 22.1). It then divides into two branches: *superficial and deep*. The more superficial branch supplies the gluteus maximus and runs along its deep surface before it anastomoses with the inferior gluteal artery (see Chap. 23) and the lateral sacral arteries [23–25]. The deeper branch supplies the gluteus medius and minimus as it runs laterally between the iliac bone and the gluteus medius [22–25]. This branch further subdivides into a superior and inferior division. The superior division continues superiorly along the gluteus

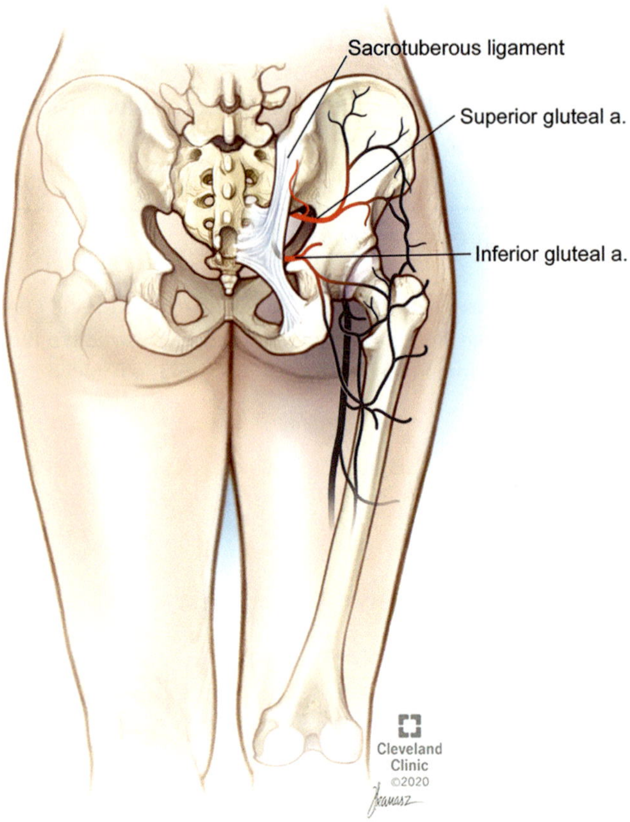

Fig. 22.1 Illustration of the arterial anatomy of the superior gluteal artery and inferior gluteal artery through the greater sciatic foramen. Note that the piriformis muscle has been removed. (Reprinted with permission, Cleveland Clinic Center for Medical Art & Photography © 2020. All Rights Reserved)

minimus toward the anterior superior iliac spine where it anastomoses with the deep iliac circumflex and with the ascending branch of the lateral femoral circumflex artery (see Chap. 31). The inferior division travels toward the greater trochanter and establishes vascular connections with the ascending branches of both medial and lateral femoral circumflex arteries and with the inferior gluteal artery [23].

The vascular anatomy of perforators from the superior gluteal artery has been well studied. Knowledge of this anatomy is useful for the microsurgeon to be able to identify the perforators and perform microvascular dissection to isolate the vascular pedicle. Ahmadzadeh et al. performed arterial injection studies in six cadavers to delineate perforator anatomy of the superior gluteal artery. They found that all perforators were musculocutaneous, with half traversing the gluteus maximus muscle and the other half the gluteus medius muscle [22]. As compared to the inferior gluteal artery perforating vessels, the superior gluteal artery perforators were more vertical as they pierced the muscle. Their group found that the average number of perforators from the superior gluteal artery was 5 ± 2 and the average vessel diameter was 0.6 ± 0.1 mm [22]. A similar cadaveric three-dimensional angiographic analysis was done by Lui et al. to determine perforator anatomy of the superior gluteal artery, and they also found that there was an average of five superior gluteal artery musculocutaneous perforators with a diameter of 0.6 mm [26].

Knowledge of the superior gluteal vessels in relation to bony and ligamentous anatomy is also important as the microsurgeon may find themselves working in close proximity to these structures in patients with acquired defects from other surgical procedures. Kieser et al. performed cadaveric dissections to help better understand this anatomy. Their group found that the sacrospinous/sacrotuberous ligament complex overlies the gluteal vessels when approached posteriorly [27]. The vessels were on average 13 mm deep to the sacrospinous/sacrotuberous ligament complex. They became deeper as they coursed away from the internal iliac [27]. In their study, the superior gluteal artery was found within 5 mm of the posterior-inferior sacroiliac joint, and it was tethered here by a constant branch just inferior to this joint before supplying the area around the sacroiliac joint [27]. In the area of the lateral sacrum, the depth of the vessels was 24 mm on average, and a perforator of the sacrospinous/sacrotuberous ligament complex tethers the vessels to this complex [27]. Similarly, a cadaveric study by Zoccali et al. investigated the relationship of the vessels to bony landmarks and its clinical implications. Their group found that the superior gluteal vessels are found in the lateral portion of L5–S1 and S1–S2 osteotomies [28]. With this information, they conclude that a high osteotomy such as S1–2 osteotomy is dangerous to the gluteal vessels, but there is only a minor bleeding risk with a S2–3 osteotomy or lower [28]. They equally caution about resection of L5 during sacrectomy as this can cause damage to the internal iliac vessels [28].

Surgical Site Exposure

Great microsurgical prowess is required for the delicate dissection of the superior gluteal vessels [29]. Because of the intramuscular course of the perforating vessels [1, 22, 26], dissection of these vessels requires some degree of sacrifice of the gluteus maximus, and caution should be used in ambulatory patients [1, 22, 26, 29]. The superior gluteal vessels can be used as recipient vessels for the reconstruction of defects in the hip, lumbosacral gluteal, and perineal regions [1, 22, 26]. Dissection in this area must proceed cautiously as damage to the gluteal vessels, especially the superior gluteal vein or its venae comitantes, can lead to bleeding into the pelvis that is difficult to control [20, 27]. While preoperative imaging is not routinely required, superior gluteal artery damage is a well-described complication of blunt pelvic trauma, and the integrity of these recipient vessels should be further investigated in the appropriate clinical scenario [23] as well as in patients with possible iatrogenic injury from hip surgery.

The procedure begins with the patient positioned in the prone or lateral decubitus position, depending on surgeon preference. Patient needs to be relaxed to facilitate the dissection. Preoperatively determined area of flap harvest may also dictate patient positioning. As lengthy operative times are often expected, it is imperative to ensure appropriate patient positioning to prevent pressure ulcers and peripheral neuropathy [30, 31]. Knowledge of the surface anatomy of the superior gluteal artery aids in identification of the vessels. The piriformis is found above a line between the superior aspect of the greater trochanter and a point halfway between the posterior superior iliac spine and the coccyx [24]. The emergence of the superior gluteal artery from the greater sciatic foramen is found at the border of the sacrum approximately one-third of the distance on a line drawn from the posterior superior iliac spine to the greater trochanter (Fig. 22.2a and b) [24, 29]. It has also been described as 6.5 cm below the posterior superior iliac spine and 4.5 cm lateral to the midline of the sacrum [20]. The perforating vessels are found adjacent to the medial two-thirds of this same described line [22, 26] (Fig. 22.3). As previously discussed, preoperative imaging is not routinely obtained, but prior to starting the procedure, a handheld Doppler is used to find perforators and they are marked on the skin [20, 29]. The superior gluteal vessels can be approached from different surgical exposures: medially, muscle-splitting, superior-lateral, and lateral approaches. Loupe magnification is required to perform the dissection. The authors strongly recommend using operating microscope to avoid injury to the superior gluteal vessels especially during deep dissection.

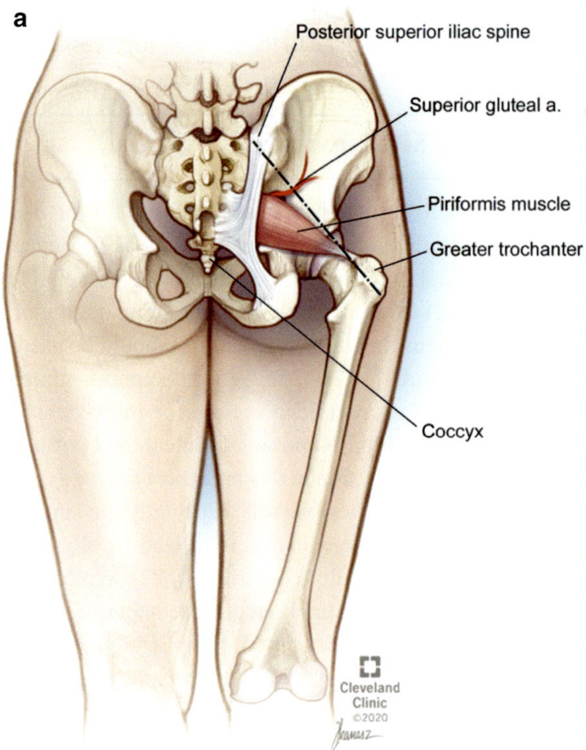

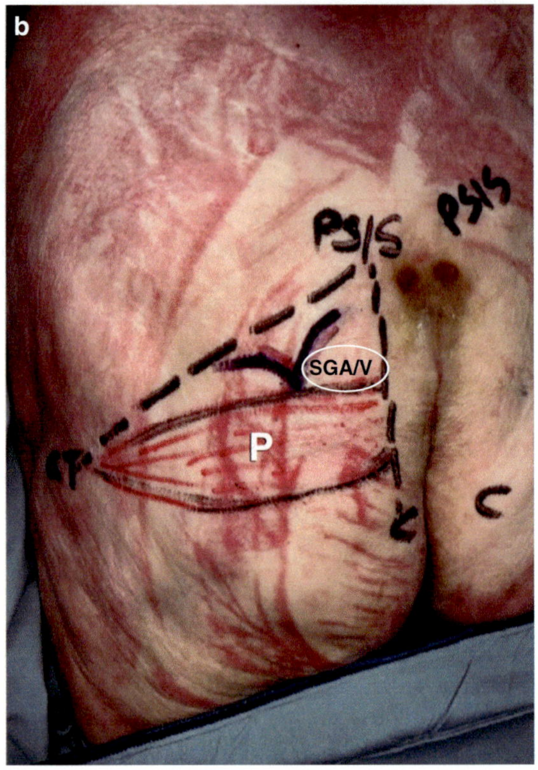

Fig. 22.2 Illustration of the surface anatomy markings for the superior gluteal artery (**a**) (Reprinted with permission, Cleveland Clinic Center for Medical Art & Photography © 2020. All Rights Reserved) and in a cadaver (**b**). The posterior superior iliac spine, PSIS, and the greater trochanter, GT, are identified. A line is drawn between these two points and then the line is divided into thirds. The superior gluteal artery (SGA) emerges from the greater sciatic foramen at the junction of the first and second thirds of this line superior to the piriformis muscle (P)

Medial Approach

The medial approach is not frequently used because of risk of damage to the superior gluteal vessels. When using this approach, the lateral sacrum is followed to visualize the vessels, which can appear rather suddenly from beneath the bone [1, 32].

Muscle-Splitting Approach

This approach has been previously described in cadaver dissection by Park and Koh [32]. The authors of the current chapter have used this approach in three patients requiring microsurgical reconstruction of lumbosacral and perineal defects. This approach is similar to superior gluteal artery perforator flap dissection [33].

The projected course of the superior gluteal vessels is marked on the skin as described in the applied anatomy section (Figs. 22.1 and 22.2). A handheld Doppler is useful for identifying their location. A lengthy skin incision is performed a few centimeters superiorly. As the dissection continues, one or two perforators are identified. Preferably, the dominant perforator is followed and all other branches are ligated. Frequent use of intraoperative handheld Doppler will help guide the dissection of the perforator(s) down to the main vessels. The identified dominant perforator(s) are ligated and divided. They can then serve as a pedicle to facilitate the dissection. Side branches are ligated and divided as needed. Dissection of these vessels then proceeds down to the gluteus maximus muscle fascia which is split. The selected vessel(s) is further tracked deeper by splitting the gluteus maximus muscle in the direction of its fibers (Figs. 22.4 and 22.5). This minimizes the damage to the muscle fibers and is especially important in ambulatory patients. Various self-retaining retractors and hooks are very useful to facilitate the dissection. Maintaining hemostasis and a bloodless field is vital in this step as bleeding can result in loss of clear vision and possibly lead to vascular damage. It is at this stage that an operating microscope may be useful for meticulous dissection. Reckless dissection may result in excess

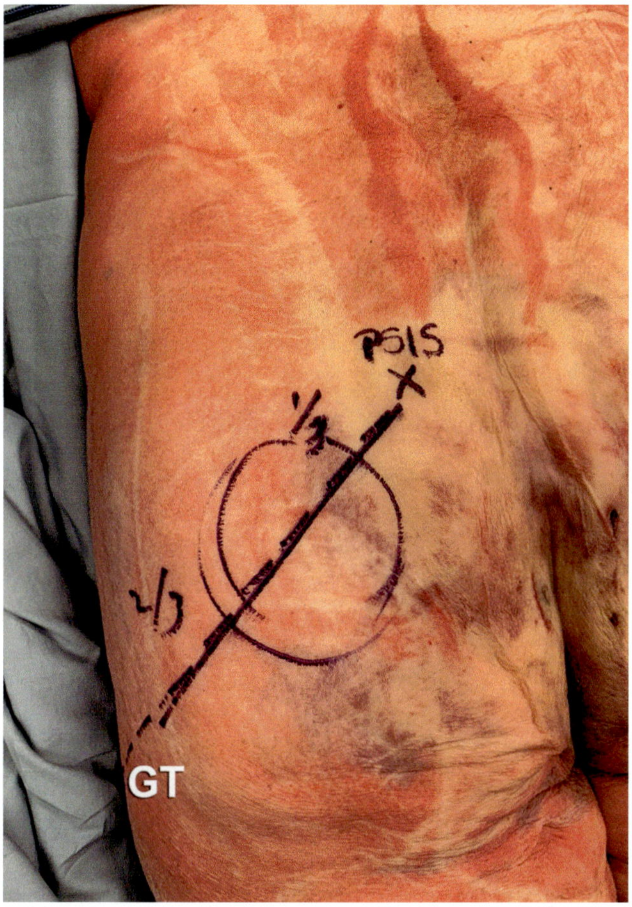

Fig. 22.3 The perforators (denoted within the circled area) are found along the medial two-thirds of a line drawn between the posterior superior iliac spine (PSIS) and the greater trochanter (GT). The superior gluteal musculocutaneous perforators are identified as they emerge through the gluteus maximus muscle and pierce the muscle fascia. The fascia and muscle fibers must be split in order to trace the perforating vessels to their origin from the superior gluteal artery

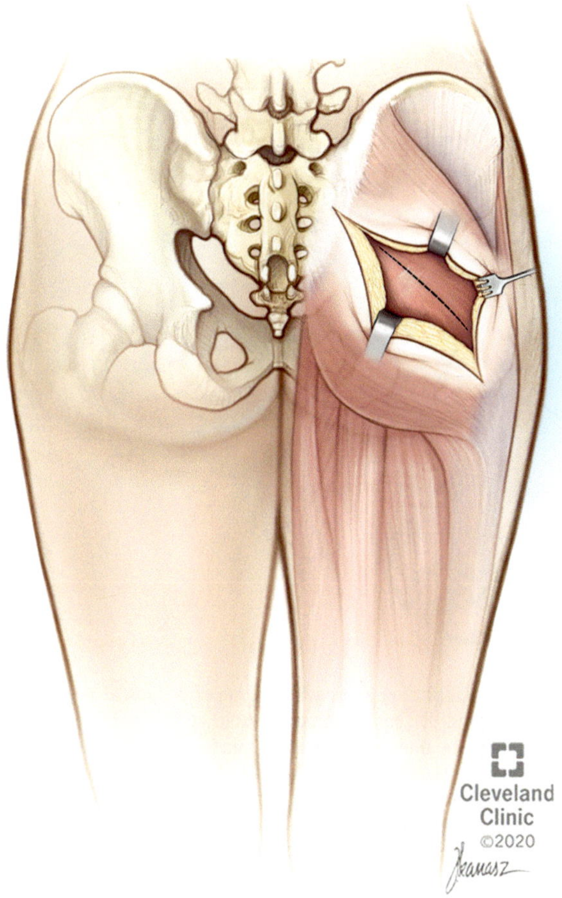

Fig. 22.4 Demonstration of skin incision down to the gluteus maximus muscle for surgical exposure of the superior gluteal vessels. (Reprinted with permission, Cleveland Clinic Center for Medical Art & Photography © 2020. All Rights Reserved)

blood loss as vessels retract into the fat or muscle. As the dissection is carried down between the piriformis and gluteus medius/minimus, branches of the superior gluteal vessels are carefully ligated and divided. When vessels with an appropriate size match to the target artery and vein are found, they are prepared for microvascular anastomosis using the operating microscope (Fig. 22.6; Video 22.1). Venous anatomy may be variable and multiple branches may require ligation to obtain the best workable vein or veins.

Superior-Lateral Approach

In this approach, the skin incision is slightly higher than the muscle-splitting approach. This would allow the identification of the gluteus maximus muscle medially and superiorly. The gluteus maximus is transected medially and superiorly at the iliac origin. The dissection then proceeds under the gluteus maximus. A search for a branch or branches is initiated. Once identified, these branches are traced deeper until the interval between the gluteus medius and piriformis muscles. Handheld Doppler is useful during dissection. Dissection is stopped when adequate size and length is obtained for microvascular anastomosis (Fig. 22.7; Video 22.2).

Lateral Approach

The main difference with this approach is a small portion of the gluteus maximus muscle is divided, elevated from the underlying gluteal medius and retracted superomedially. This allows the vessels to be identified on the undersurface of the gluteus maximus muscle. These vessels are then dissected toward the main pedicle similar to the muscle-splitting technique or the superior approach described above [1, 32].

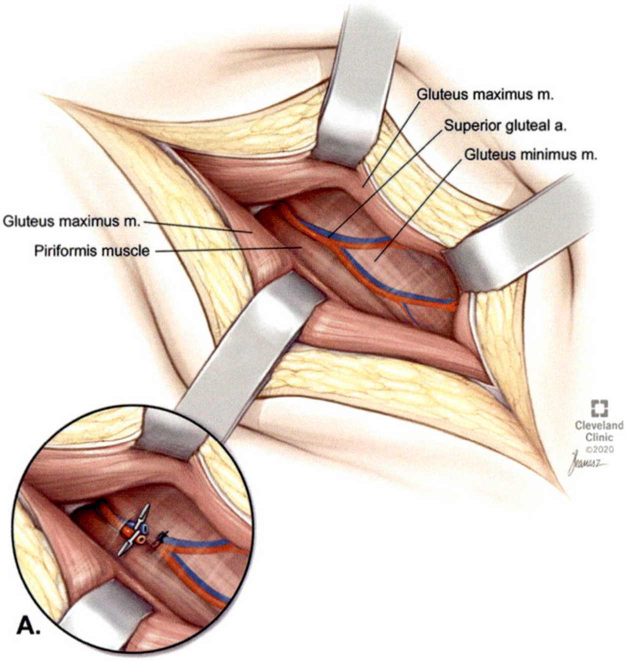

Fig. 22.5 Muscle-splitting approach: The superior gluteal vessels are dissected following gluteus maximus muscle splitting. Dissection is continued toward the interval between the piriformis and gluteus minimus until adequate size and length is obtained for microvascular anastomosis. A: Close-up of the superior gluteal vessels prepared as recipient. (Reprinted with permission, Cleveland Clinic Center for Medical Art & Photography © 2020. All Rights Reserved)

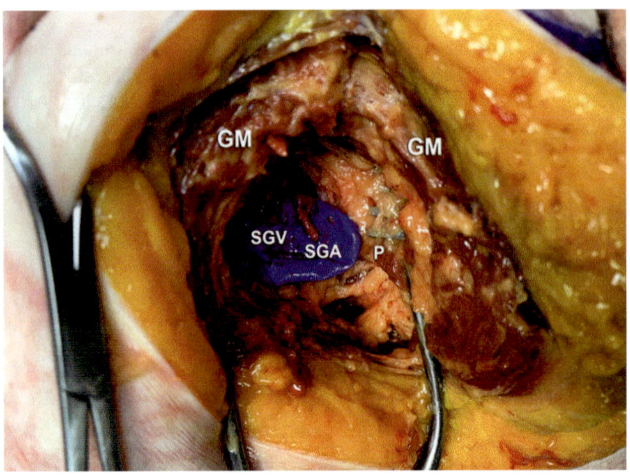

Fig. 22.6 As the perforator is traced through the substance of the gluteus maximus muscle (GM), it continues through to the interval between the gluteus minimus muscle (above) and the piriformis muscle (P). Adequate retraction is needed in this area to continue dissection down to the greater sciatic foramen to prepare the superior gluteal artery (SGA) and vein(s) (SGV)

Briefly, an oblique or curvilinear skin incision is marked superior to the axis from the posterior iliac spine to the greater trochanter. The planned incision should stay superior to expected location of the superior gluteal vessels. A hand-

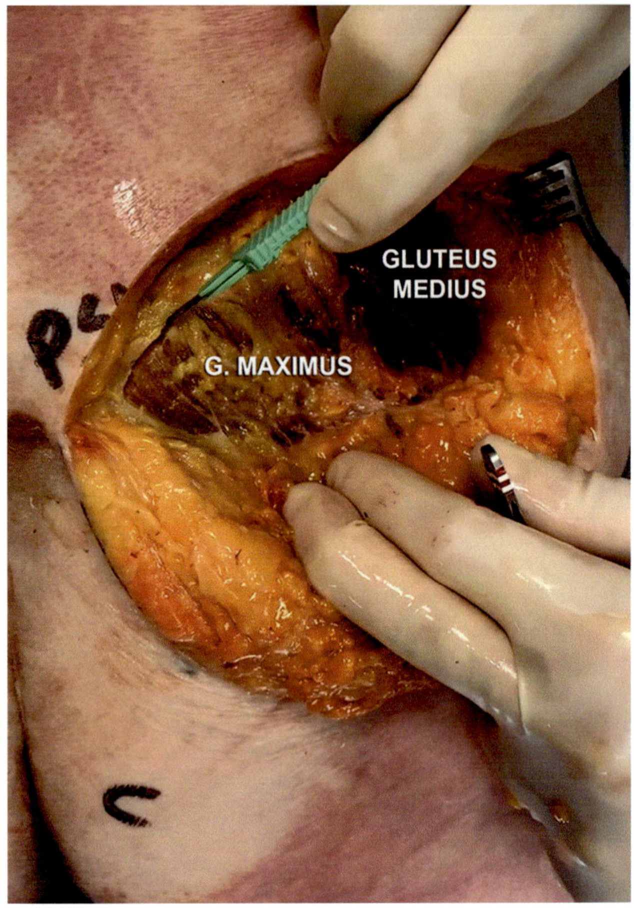

Fig. 22.7 Superior-lateral approach: After the skin and subcutaneous incisions are carried down to the gluteus maximus muscle, the interval between the gluteus medius laterally and gluteus maximus medially is identified. The insertion of the gluteus maximus muscle should be incised to raise the gluteus maximus muscle for exposure of the superior gluteal vessels

held Doppler may be useful. A wide surgical exposure is needed to help facilitate an already difficult dissection. Incision proceeds through the skin and subcutaneous tissue down to the gluteus maximus muscle. The muscle is divided and raised superomedially to allow visualization of the superficial branch of the superior gluteal vessels under the gluteus maximus muscle. The vessels are then tracked toward the suprapiriformis area. The dissection is carried out under the operating microscope. This portion of the procedure can be tedious as many small branches will be encountered that need to be ligated to ensure hemostasis.

Regardless of the approach that is used, in some cases, the dissection may continue even deeper requiring to proceed to the interval between the piriformis muscle inferiorly and the gluteus medius/minimus superiorly. Transection of the sacrospinous and/or sacrotuberous ligaments may be required to obtain satisfactory vessel length and caliber for microvascular anastomoses. In this region, there are venous plexuses that must be carefully handled to prevent bleeding [29].

As the superior gluteal vessels emerge from the pelvis, the artery averages 2.2 mm and the vein averages 3.0 mm in diameter [1, 32, 34–36]. There are usually two veins, one on either side of the artery, and they are thin-walled [32] (Fig. 22.6). Depending on the caliber of the vessels from the flap donor, the dissection can be stopped at any point when the appropriate recipient vessel caliber and pedicle length is obtained. The pedicle length is rather short at 2–3 cm [1, 32]. It is advantageous to the surgeon to safely obtain as much length as possible given the depth of the superior gluteal vessels. Just as with any other microsurgical procedure, the microsurgeon should ensure that there is sufficient exposure to safely perform an ergonomically sound microvascular anastomosis [37].

Postoperative Considerations

After successful completion of the microsurgical anastomosis and completion of the case, the surgeon has still to be cognizant of signs of impending flap compromise. Starting preoperatively and continuing into the postoperative period, free flap monitoring should be initiated [38].

Largely dependent on surgeon experience and the institutional resources, a plan must be developed for patient positioning, flap monitoring method, anticoagulation, mobilization protocol, blood pressure monitoring, and maintaining a good nutritional status to promote wound healing [39, 40]. Complications include flap compromise which requires immediate take-back and exploration, thrombectomy, TPA, and repeat vascular anastomoses for flap salvage. Vein grafts may be required for salvage, which is extremely challenging. Also, wound complications are not uncommon in the reconstruction of lumbosacral, gluteal, and perineal areas. Operative vs. nonoperative management must be determined individually [39].

Discussion

The vast majority of defects of the gluteal, lumbosacral, ischial, and perineal areas can be reconstructed using locoregional flaps. Occasionally, microsurgical flaps are needed for reconstruction. Generally, there is a paucity of recipient vessels. However, the inferior gluteal vessels (also see Chaps. 23 and 43), superior gluteal vessels (also see Chap. 43), as well as lumbar perforators (also see Chap. 21) may potentially be utilized as recipient site vessels. The decision as to whether which vessel to use depends on many factors that include vessel patency and availability, vessel length and caliber, donor vessel characteristics, type and location of the defect, as well as type and size of the flap. All of these factors should be carefully assessed for selection of the proper vessel.

The superior gluteal vessels can serve as reliable recipient vessels for microsurgical flaps, if a microsurgical flap is indicated [32, 41, 42]. Preoperative imaging is useful to confirm their patency. The regional anatomy of the bony landmarks, gluteal muscles, piriformis muscle, and ligaments in relation to the superior gluteal vessels should be well-known. Various techniques for surgical exposure of the superior gluteal vessels have been described in this chapter based on the available literature and the authors' own experience. In the muscle-splitting approach, functional preservation of the gluteus maximus muscle can be achieved in ambulatory patients by minimizing injury to the muscle fibers. Regardless of the approach, however, dissection of the superior gluteal vessels is challenging and requires significant experience. Dissection of these vessels should be carried out meticulously and tediously given their deep location until adequate size and length of the artery and vein(s) is obtained for microvascular anastomoses.

References

1. Oswald TM, Lineaweaver WC, Hui K. Recipient vessels for microsurgical flaps to the groin and pelvis: a review. J Reconstr Microsurg. 2006;22(1):5–14.
2. Stepanovs J, Ozoliņa A, Rovīte V, Mamaja B, Vanags I. Factors affecting the risk of free flap failure in microvascular surgery. Proc Latv Acad Sci B. 2016;70(6):356–64.
3. Sanati-Mehrizy P, Massenburg B, Rosa J, Taub P. Risk factors associated with free flap failure – an analysis of 2103 patients. Plast Reconstr Surg. 2015;136(4S-1):18–9.
4. Lin Y, He J, Zhang X, Wang H. Intraoperative factors associated with free flap failure in the head and neck region: a four-year retrospective study of 216 patients and review of the literature. Int J Oral Maxillofac Surg. 2019;48(4):447–51.
5. Nguyen T, Shahabi A, Vidar E, Chan L, Baker R, Schooler W, et al. 106: Risk factors associated with microvascular free flap failure: data from the ACS-National Surgical Quality Improvement Project (ACS-NSQIP). Plast Reconstr Surg. 2011;127(5):61.
6. Zhong T, Neinstein R, Massey C, McCluskey S, Lipa J, Neligan P, et al. Intravenous fluid infusion rate in microsurgical breast reconstruction. Plast Reconstr Surg. 2011;128(6):1153–60.
7. Young V, Watson M. Prevention of perioperative hypothermia in plastic surgery. Aesthet Surg J. 2006;26(5):551–71.
8. Saint-Cyr M, Wong C, Buchel E, Colohan S, Pederson W. Free tissue transfers and replantation. Plast Reconstr Surg. 2012;130(6):858e–78e.
9. Attinger C, Bulan E, Blume P. Surgical debridement. The key to successful wound healing and reconstruction. Clin Podiatr Med Surg. 2000;17(4):599–630.
10. Attinger C, Bulan E. Debridement. The key initial first step in wound healing. Foot Ankle Clin. 2001;6(4):627–60.
11. Cornell R, Meyr A, Steinberg J, Attinger C. Debridement of the noninfected wound. J Vasc Surg. 2010;52(3):31S–6S.
12. Wei C, Granick M. Surgical management of chronic wounds. Wounds. 2008;20(3):62–6.
13. Fang L, Liu J, Yu C, Hanasono M, Zheng G, Yu P. Intraoperative use of vasopressors does not increase the risk of free flap compromise and failure in cancer patients. Ann Surg. 2018;268(2):379–84.

14. Knackstedt R, Gatherwright J, Gurunluoglu R. A literature review and meta-analysis of outcomes in microsurgical reconstruction using vasopressors. Microsurgery. 2018;39(3):267–75.
15. Goh C, Ng M, Song D, Ooi A. Perioperative vasopressor use in free flap surgery: a systematic review and meta-analysis. J Reconstr Microsurg. 2019;35(7):529–40.
16. Crawley M, Sweeny L, Ravipati P, Heffelfinger R, Krein H, Luginbuhl A, et al. Factors associated with free flap failures in head and neck reconstruction. Otolaryngol Head Neck Surg. 2019;161(4):598–604.
17. Vargas C, Iorio M, Lee B. A systematic review of topical vasodilators for the treatment of intraoperative vasospasm in reconstructive microsurgery. Plast Reconstr Surg. 2015;136(2):411–22.
18. Froemel D, Fitzsimons S, Frank J, Sauerbier M, Meurer A, Barker J. A review of thrombosis and antithrombotic therapy in microvascular surgery. Eur Surg Res. 2013;50(1):32–43.
19. Rueda M, Rueda S, Alleyne B, Drake RL, Gurunluoglu R. Chapter 4: Anatomy of the trunk. In: Bruce MA, editor. Plastic surgery: a practical guide to operative care. New York: Thieme Publishers; 2020.
20. Buntic R. Superior gluteal artery perforator (SGAP) flap. In: Online atlas of microsurgery. 2020. https://www.microsurgeon.org/sgap. Accessed 13 Jan 2020.
21. Fătu C, Puişoru M, Fătu I. Morphometry of the internal iliac artery in different ethnic groups. Ann Anat. 2006;188:541–6.
22. Ahmadzadeh R, Bergeron L, Tang M, Morris S. The superior and inferior gluteal artery perforator flaps. Plast Reconstr Surg. 2007;120(6):1551–6.
23. Bosse M, Poka A, Reinert C, Brumback R, Bathon H, Burgess A. Preoperative angiographic assessment of the superior gluteal artery in acetabular fractures requiring extensile surgical exposures. J Orthop Trauma. 1988;2(4):303–7.
24. Verpaele A, Blondeel P, Van Landuyt K, Tonnard P, Decordier B, Monstrey S, et al. The superior gluteal artery perforator flap: an additional tool in the treatment of sacral pressure sores. Br J Plast Surg. 1999;52:385–91.
25. Wheeless C. Superior gluteal artery. In: Wheeless' textbook of orthopaedics. 2015. http://www.wheelessonline.com/ortho/superior_gluteal_artery. Accessed 13 Jan 2020.
26. Lui K, Hu S, Ahmad N, Tang M. Three-dimensional angiography of the superior gluteal artery and lumbar artery perforator flap. Plast Reconstr Surg. 2009;123(1):79–86.
27. Kieser D, Coudert P, Cawley D, Gaignard E, Fujishiro T, Farah K, et al. Identifying the superior and inferior gluteal arteries during a sacrectomy via a posterior approach. J Spine Surg. 2017;3(4):624–9.
28. Zoccali C, Skoch J, Patel A, Walter C, Maykowski P, Baaj A. The surgical neurovascular anatomy relating to partial and complete sacral and sacroiliac resections: a cadaveric, anatomic study. Eur Spine J. 2015;24:1109–13.
29. Boyd J, Gelfand M, Da Lio A, Shaw W, Watson J. Comparison of superior gluteal artery musculocutaneous and superior gluteal artery perforator flaps for microvascular breast reconstruction. Plast Reconstr Surg. 2009;123(6):1641–7.
30. Practice advisory for the prevention of perioperative peripheral neuropathies 2018: an updated report by the American Society of Anesthesiologists task force on prevention of perioperative peripheral neuropathies. Anesthesiology. 2018;128(1):11–26.
31. Black J, Fawcett D, Scott S. Ten top tips: preventing pressure ulcers in the surgical patient. Wounds Int. 2014;5(4):14–8.
32. Park S, Koh KS. Superior gluteal vessel as recipient for free flap reconstruction of lumbosacral defect. Plast Reconstr Surg. 1998;101(7):1842–9.
33. Gurunluoglu R, Spanio S, Rainer C, Ninkovic M. Skin expansion before breast reconstruction with the superior gluteal artery perforator flap improves aesthetic outcome. Ann Plast Surg. 2003;50(5):475–9.
34. Fujino T, Harashina T, Enomoto K. Primary breast reconstruction after a standard radical mastectomy by a free flap transfer: case report. Plast Reconstr Surg. 1976;58(3):371–4.
35. Shaw W. Breast reconstruction by superior gluteal microvascular free flaps without silicone implants. Plast Reconstr Surg. 1983;72:490–501.
36. Strauch B, Yu HL. Gluteal region. In: Strauch B, Yu HL, editors. Atlas of microvascular surgery: anatomy and operative approaches. New York: Thieme Medical; 1993. p. 102–19.
37. Lakhiani C, Fisher S, Janhofer D, Song D. Ergonomics in microsurgery. J Surg Oncol. 2018;118(5):840–4.
38. Gurunluoglu R. Free flap monitoring in the intensive care unit. In: Pieracci FM, Moore EE, editors. Handbook of surgical critical care – the practice and the evidence. Singapore: World Scientific Publishing Co. Pte. Ltd; 2015. p. 747–64.
39. Lo S, Yen Y, Lee P, Liu C, Pu C. Factors influencing postoperative complications in reconstructive microsurgery for head and neck cancer. J Oral Maxillofac Surg. 2017;75(4):867–73.
40. Sigaux N, Philouze P, Boucher F, Jacquemart M, Frobert P, Breton P. Efficacy of the postoperative management after microsurgical free tissue transfer. J Stomatol Oral Maxillofac Surg. 2017;118(3):173–7.
41. Hung SJ, Chen HC, Wei FC. Free flaps for reconstruction of the lower back and sacral area. Microsurgery. 2000;20(2):72–6.
42. Park S. Muscle-splitting approach to superior and inferior gluteal vessels: versatile source of recipient vessels for free-tissue transfer to sacral, gluteal, and ischial regions. Plast Reconstr Surg. 2000;106(1):81–6.

Inferior Gluteal Vessels

23

David Kashan, DeAsia D. Jacob, Richard L. Drake, and Raffi Gurunian

Introduction

The inferior gluteal vessels are typically known as donor vessels of locoregional flaps for the reconstruction of gluteal, ischial, and perineal buttock wounds [1–5]. Also, they serve as the pedicle for microsurgical breast reconstruction using inferior gluteal skin and/or muscle flap [6–10].

Although the gold standard for soft tissue defects of the sacral, gluteal, and perineal regions remains locoregional flaps, in certain rare cases, microsurgical flaps may be indicated for reconstruction. These include circumstances where local flaps are not safe or adequate due to previous surgery, trauma, or radiation. Another indication may be an extensive wound for which previous local flaps have failed.

While a microsurgical flap can offer a reconstructive solution to complex defects of the sacrum, gluteal, and ischial regions, there is a relative paucity of potential recipient vessels in this region. Typically, the superior or inferior gluteal vessels are considered as first-line recipient vessels (also see Chaps. 22 and 43). The decision for which one of these recipient vessels to use depends on many factors that include vessel proximity, patency and availability, vessel length and caliber, donor vessel characteristics, type and location of the defect, as well as type and size of the flap. All of these factors should be carefully assessed for selection of the proper vessel based on the specifics of each microsurgical case. This chapter reviews the relevant anatomy, preoperative assessment, and surgical site exposure of the inferior gluteal vessels.

Applied Anatomy

The inferior gluteal artery is a branch of the anterior internal iliac artery that lends its blood supply to the thigh and buttock region. The inferior gluteal and internal pudendal arteries are often a common stem from the internal iliac. It can be found exiting the greater sciatic foramen for which it travels alongside the greater sciatic nerve, internal pudendal artery and vein, and posterior femoral cutaneous nerve [11, 12].

Once under the inferior portion of the gluteus maximus, perforating vessels are seen branching out through the substance of the muscle to feed the overlying skin and fat. These perforators exit inferior to the piriformis muscle, deep to the gluteus maximus muscle.

The direction of the perforating vessels can be superior, lateral, or inferior. Perforating vessels that nourish the medial and inferior portions of the buttock have relatively short intramuscular lengths, between 5 and 7 cm, depending on the thickness of the muscle. Perforators that nourish the lateral portions of the overlying buttock skin are observed traveling through the muscle substance in an oblique manner 4–6 cm before turning upward toward the skin surface. By traveling through the muscle for relatively long distances, these vessels are longer than their medially based counterparts. The perforating vessels can be separated from the underlying gluteus maximus muscle and fascia and traced down to the parent vessel, forming the basis for the inferior gluteal artery perforator flap. Between two and four perforating vessels

Supplementary Information The online version of this chapter (https://doi.org/10.1007/978-3-030-75389-4_23) contains supplementary material, which is available to authorized users.

D. Kashan · D. D. Jacob
Department of Plastic Surgery, Cleveland Clinic, Cleveland, OH, USA
e-mail: Kashand@ccf.org; Jacobd@ccf.org

R. L. Drake
Department of Anatomy, Cleveland Clinic Lerner College of Medicine, Cleveland, OH, USA
e-mail: DRAKER@ccf.org

R. Gurunian (✉)
Department of Plastic Surgery, Cleveland Clinic, Cleveland, OH, USA

Cleveland Clinic Lerner College of Medicine, Case Western Reserve University, Cleveland, OH, USA
e-mail: gurunir@ccf.org

R. Gurunian, R. Djohan (eds.), *Recipient Vessels in Reconstructive Microsurgery*,
https://doi.org/10.1007/978-3-030-75389-4_23

originating from the inferior gluteal artery are located in the lower half of the gluteus maximus [9]. After giving off perforators in the buttocks, the inferior gluteal artery then descends into the thigh accompanied by the posterior femoral cutaneous nerve and follows a long course, eventually surfacing to supply the skin of the posterior thigh [9].

Knowledge regarding inferior gluteal vascular pedicle characteristics are largely derived from the previously published literature on the inferior gluteal artery perforator flap. The diameter of the inferior gluteal vessels is noted to be 2.5–3.5 mm for the artery, and 2.5–4.0 mm for the vein according to various authors [7, 13, 14]. Therefore, the inferior gluteal vessels have excellent caliber proximally. However, their length may vary from 2–3 cm up to 8–10 cm. Procurement of a workable pedicle length that can serve as a reliable recipient may potentially lead to the reduction of the vessel diameter. Ultimately, when the inferior gluteal vessels are going to be used as recipient, sufficient length and caliber should be obtained for safe and tension-free microvascular anastomosis.

Preoperative Assessment

As with all free flap-based surgery, smoking cessation, nutritional status, functional status, and patient expectations should be identified and reviewed prior to surgery. The authors would recommend a CTA to fully assess the underlying arterial and functional anatomy, especially in the cases of trauma and oncological resections as anatomy can often be distorted. Previous pelvic surgeries may have resulted in vascular damage to the internal iliac vessels, which would disqualify the use of the inferior gluteal vessels as recipient. The use of Doppler may assist the surgeon intraoperatively to help localize the perforators on the skin. The author will also intermittently use the Doppler throughout the surgery to ensure the dissection is safe and accurate and to avoid any accidental injury to the pedicle. This is especially helpful when the pedicle has a long intramuscular course.

Discussion with the patient regarding postoperative positioning and management is discussed in the preoperative visit as well to ensure a safe environment after discharge. It is not infrequent that these patients require acute or subacute rehabilitation after the surgery, which is discussed with both the patient and case managers prior to surgical intervention to assist with an easy transition of care.

Surgical Site Exposure

The patient should be marked in a similar fashion in which one would perform an inferior gluteal artery perforator (IGAP) flap. While in the standing position, the posterior inferior iliac spine (PSIS), coccyx, and greater trochanter are marked preoperatively. The inferior gluteal vessels exit the sciatic foramen inferior to the piriformis muscle which can be located on a line extending from the greater trochanter to halfway between the PSIS and coccyx (Fig. 23.1).

Depending on the site of flap harvest, the patient can be placed in either lateral decubitus or prone positioning. Once positioned, the surgeon should Doppler areas out where perforators are located according to the anatomic landmarks [7–9]. The perforators can usually be identified inferior to a line drawn from the greater trochanter to the midpoint of a line between the PSIS and coccyx. The gluteal fold is the most inferior border for which to check for signals. If a CTA has been performed prior to surgery, it would be prudent to use anatomical landmarks and measurements based on the imaging to help guide in the identification of the larger perforators. A skin incision is performed horizontally either inferior to the selected perforator(s) or laterally using a curvilinear incision (Fig. 23.2). It is also important to remember that inferior gluteal vessels lie in the subcutaneous tissue plane halfway between the ischial tuberosity and the greater

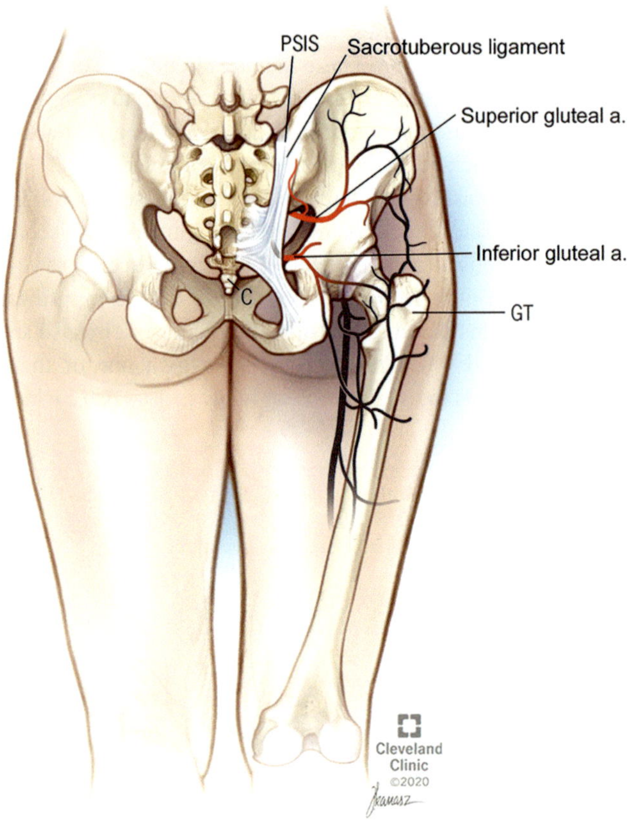

Fig. 23.1 The inferior gluteal vessels exit the sciatic foramen inferior to the piriformis muscle which can be located on a line extending from the greater trochanter (GT) to halfway between the posterior superior iliac spine (PSIS) and coccyx (C). (Reprinted with permission, Cleveland Clinic Center for Medical Art & Photography © 2020. All Rights Reserved)

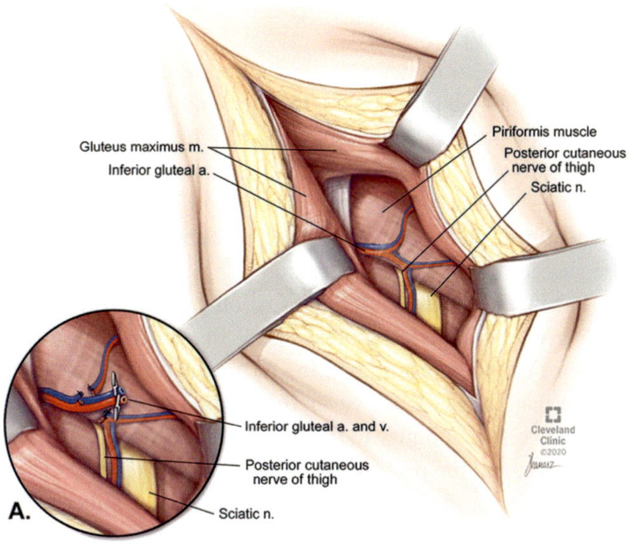

Fig. 23.2 Demonstration of skin incision down to the gluteus maximus muscle for surgical exposure of the inferior gluteal vessels. Muscle-splitting approach: The inferior gluteal vessels are dissected following gluteus maximus muscle splitting. Dissection is continued until adequate size and length is obtained for microvascular anastomosis. A: Close-up of the inferior gluteal vessels prepared as recipient. (Reprinted with permission, Cleveland Clinic Center for Medical Art & Photography © 2020. All Rights Reserved)

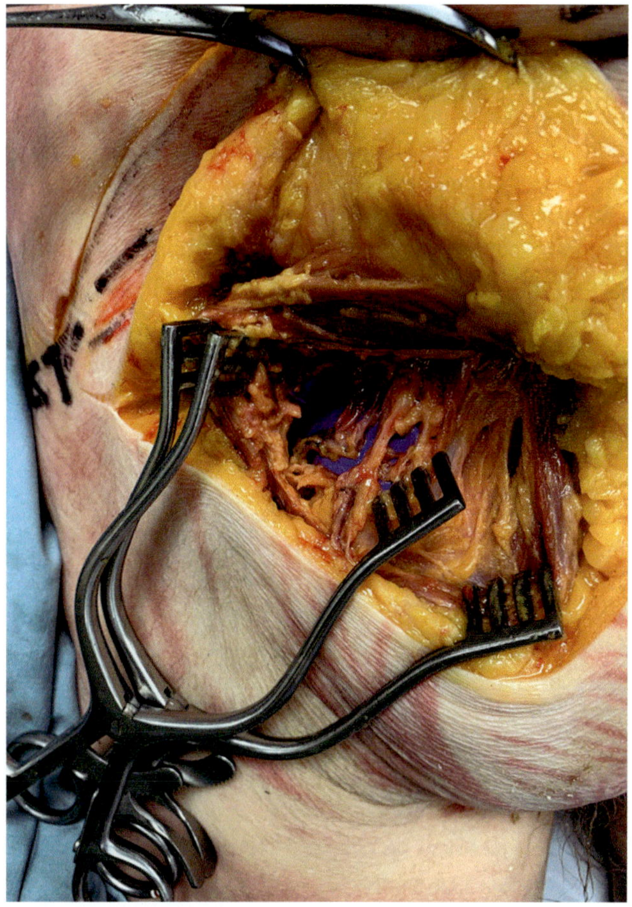

Fig. 23.3 Muscle-splitting approach in a cadaver dissection to expose the inferior gluteal vessels

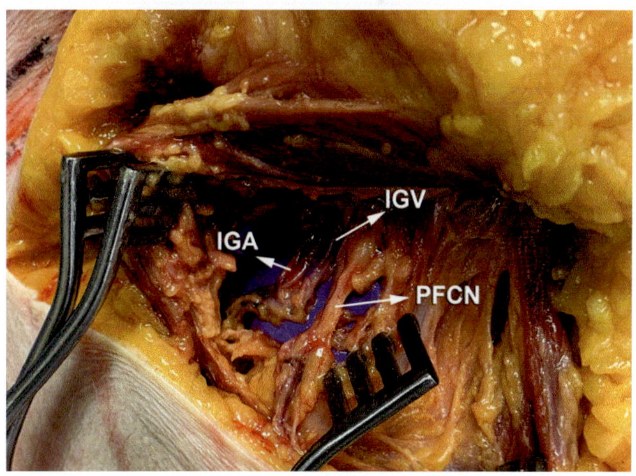

Fig. 23.4 Close-up of the inferior gluteal vessels: IGV, inferior gluteal vein; IGA, inferior gluteal artery; PFCN, posterior femoral cutaneous nerve

trochanter. Therefore, if a longitudinally oriented incision is considered, it should aim to stay lateral to this anatomic landmark.

Basically, the dissection is carried down to trace a perforator or two toward the main inferior gluteal pedicle. A hand Doppler is used frequently to trace the perforators toward the parent vessel. The perforator(s) should be dissected out in a retrograde fashion which will involve splitting of the gluteus maximus along its fibers (Fig. 23.2). Patient needs to be relaxed to facilitate the dissection through the muscle. Care must be taken when dissecting the pedicle out proximally to avoid injuring several branches of the inferior gluteal nerve. These nerves supply the remainder of attached gluteus muscle function that has not been detached. In order to maximize the length of the pedicle, all perforating branches along the length of the pedicle are clipped and transected. It is important to identify and spare the posterior femoral cutaneous nerve as it is found lateral to the IGA. The artery tends to have a long intramuscular oblique course. Care must be taken to avoid damage to the aforementioned nerves during dissection. Various self-retaining retractors and hooks are very useful to facilitate the dissection (Figs. 23.3 and 23.4). Maintaining hemostasis and a bloodless field is essential as bleeding can result in loss of clear vision. Operating microscope aids in more delicate dissection and should be utilized in the deeper parts of the dissection.

The authors ensure that the patient understands preoperatively there is the possibility of transient or permanent numbness to the posterior thigh secondary to a neuropraxia or trauma to the posterior femoral cutaneous nerve. The remainder of the dissection takes place in either the submuscular or sub-sacral fascial plane. It is important to undermine enough to allow for exposure without disrupting the insertion points of the gluteus maximus; however, if needed, the gluteus maximus can be elevated off the sacrum to facilitate dissection. The remaining blood supply to the muscle will be from the femoral circumflex vessels. When in the subfascial plane, one must be extremely careful not to damage the extensive venous plexus. When vessels with an appropriate size match to the target artery and vein are found, they are prepared for microvascular anastomosis using the operating microscope (Video 23.1).

Postoperative Management

Postoperatively, patients should be observed in ICU. The authors strongly recommend positioning the patient in the lateral decubitus or prone to avoid pressure to the flap and pedicle. The flap receives a Doppler check as well as observing for change in color, capillary refill, temperature, and turgor every hour for the first 24 hours. The authors transition to every 2 hours on postoperative day 2 and ultimately to every 4 hours until discharged [15].

Drain(s) in the reconstruction site is removed when output is less than 25 mL for two consecutive days. The Foley catheter is removed on either postoperative day 1 or 2, and the patient is encouraged to ambulate with assistance on postoperative day 1.

The authors recommend an appropriate bed based on patients' activity level as well as type of body support. Positioning is managed to ensure the patients do not develop any pressure sores during their stay at the hospital. Turning is performed every hour by the nursing staff. No pressure is allowed over the flap for about 4 weeks. Patients can usually be discharged in 1 week after surgery. They are seen either by a physician or nurse practitioner at 1, 4, 8, and 12 weeks after discharge for routine follow-up.

Discussion

The majority of patients requiring reconstruction for lumbosacral/gluteal regions will be positioned prone or lateral decubitus. Therefore, microsurgical flaps that can be harvested from the back are preferable. Scapular/parascapular flap, thoracodorsal artery perforator flap, posterior thigh perforator flap, latissimus dorsi, and serratus flap can be viable options in solo or in various combinations depending on the wound characteristics. These flap choices will allow two teams working simultaneously for flap dissection and recipient vessel site exposure.

The superior or inferior gluteal vessels can potentially be used as recipient vessels in this region. Successful microsurgical reconstructions have been reported using either of these vessels [16–19].

Vessel selection depends on the specifics of each case, length of the flap pedicle, and location and size of the defect to be reconstructed. Regardless, dissection of these vessels is technically very challenging and requires experience and expertise. The authors recommend anatomical dissections in cadaver prior to actual case, if such an opportunity exists for the surgeon in his or her institution.

The inferior gluteal artery dissection may have the advantage over the superior gluteal artery dissection for several reasons; the pedicle length of the IGA on average tends to be longer than the SGA. However, dissection of the arterial pedicle may result in injury to the inferior gluteal nerve, the sciatic nerve, and the posterior femoral cutaneous nerve.

The inferior gluteal artery has a comparable caliber to the superior gluteal artery. As the superior gluteal vessels emerge from the pelvis, the artery averages 2.2 mm and the vein averages 3.0 mm in diameter. The pedicle length is rather short at 2–3 cm (Chap. 22). Dimensions of inferior gluteal vessels are 2.5–3.5 mm the artery and 2.5–4.0 mm the vein, with a pedicle length of 2–3 cm [14].

The inferior gluteal vascular pedicle can be extended when considered for use as recipient vessel.

The course of the inferior gluteal artery perforating vessels is more oblique through the substance of the gluteus maximus muscle than the course of the superior gluteal artery perforators, which tend to travel more directly to the superficial tissue up through the muscle. This anatomic difference accounts for a longer inferior gluteal vascular pedicle that can be used as recipient, when compared to the superior gluteal vessels.

Also, a longer pedicle may be obtained by transecting the inferior gluteal vessels more distally; however, this would be at the cost of vessel diameter reduction. Therefore, inferior gluteal pedicle length and caliber should be weighed against the donor vessel characteristics to determine the best possible match and tension-free microvascular anastomosis.

If two teams are working simultaneously for flap harvest and recipient site preparation, frequent cross-checking of vessel features during dissection between the members of the team is absolutely necessary.

Conclusion

Dissection of the inferior gluteal vessels is technically challenging. Muscle-splitting approach allows functional preservation of the gluteus maximus muscle in ambulatory patients by minimizing injury to the muscle fibers. Dissection should be carried out meticulously and tediously given their deep location until adequate size and length of the artery and vein(s) is obtained for microvascular anastomoses.

References

1. Hurwitz DJ. Closure of a large defect of the pelvic cavity by an extended compound myocutaneous flap based on the inferior gluteal artery. Br J Plast Surg. 1980;33(2):256–61.
2. Hurwitz DJ, Swartz WM, Mathes SJ. The gluteal thigh flap: a reliable, sensate flap for the closure of buttock and perineal wounds. Plast Reconstr Surg. 1981;68(4):521–32.
3. Higgins JP, Orlando GS, Blondeel PN. Ischial pressure sore reconstruction using an inferior gluteal artery perforator (IGAP) flap. Br J Plast Surg. 2002;55(1):83–5.
4. Kim YS, Lew DH, Roh TS, Yoo WM, Lee WJ, Tark KC. Inferior gluteal artery perforator flap: a viable alternative for ischial pressure sores. J Plast Reconstr Aesthet Surg. 2009;62(10):1347–54.
5. Sinna R, Qassemyar Q, Benhaim T, Lauzanne P, Sabbagh C, Regimbeau JM, Mauvais F. Perforator flaps: a new option in perineal reconstruction. J Plast Reconstr Aesthet Surg. 2010;63(11):e766–74.
6. Paletta CE, Bostwick J 3rd, Nahai F. The inferior gluteal free flap in breast reconstruction. Plast Reconstr Surg. 1989;84(6):875–83; discussion 884–5.
7. Allen RJ, Levine JL, Granzow JW. The in-the-crease inferior gluteal artery perforator flap for breast reconstruction. Plast Reconstr Surg. 2006;118(2):333–9.
8. Levine JL, Miller Q, Vasile J, Khoobehi K, Craigie J, Wise MW, Allen RJ. Simultaneous bilateral breast reconstruction with in-the-crease inferior gluteal artery perforator flaps. Ann Plast Surg. 2009;63(3):249–54.
9. LoTempio MM, Allen RJ. Breast reconstruction with SGAP and IGAP flaps. Plast Reconstr Surg. 2010;126(2):393–401.
10. Weichman KE. Inferior gluteal artery perforator breast reconstruction. In: Operative techniques in plastic surgery. Philadelphia: Wolters Kluwer; 2019. p. 1452–8.
11. Rueda M, Rueda S, Alleyne B, Drake RL, Gurunluoglu R. Chapter 4: Anatomy of the trunk. In: Bruce MA, editor. Plastic surgery: a practical guide to operative care. New York: Thieme Publishers; 2020.
12. Williams P, Warwick R, Dyson M, Bannister LH. Gray's anatomy. In: William PL, Worwick R, Dyson M, Bannister LH, editors. Angiology. 37th ed. New York: Churchill Livingstone; 1989. p. 779.
13. Hamdi M, Gagnon AR. Conventional workhorse flaps. In: Wei FC, Mardini S, editors. Flaps and reconstructive surgery. 2nd ed. Philadelphia: Elsevier; 2009. p. 377–95.
14. Strauch B, Yu HL. Gluteal region. In: Strauch B, Yu HL, editors. Atlas of microvascular surgery: anatomy and operative approaches. New York: Thieme Medical; 1993. p. 102–19.
15. Gurunluoglu R. Free flap monitoring in the intensive care unit. In: Pieracci FM, Moore EE, editors. Handbook of surgical critical care – the practice and the evidence. Singapore: World Scientific Publishing Co. Pte. Ltd; 2015. p. 747–64.
16. Oswald TM, Lineaweaver WC, Hui K. Recipient vessels for microsurgical flaps to the groin and pelvis: a review. J Reconstr Microsurg. 2006;22(1):5–14.
17. Anthony J, Ritter F, Moelleken B. Utility of the inferior gluteal vessels in free flap coverage of sacral wounds. Ann Plast Surg. 1992;29:371–5.
18. Park S. Muscle-splitting approach to superior and inferior gluteal vessels: versatile source of recipient vessels for free-tissue transfer to sacral, gluteal, and ischial regions. Plast Reconstr Surg. 2000;106(1):81–6.
19. Hung SJ, Chen HC, Wei FC. Free flaps for reconstruction of the lower back and sacral area. Microsurgery. 2000;20(2):72–6.

Part IV

Upper Extremity Reconstruction

Brachial Artery and Basilic/Cephalic Veins

24

Rachel E. Aliotta, DeAsia D. Jacob, Richard L. Drake, Lia Gurunian, and Raffi Gurunian

Introduction

Large vessel disease is often managed by vascular surgeons and cardiothoracic specialists; however, disease or surgical intervention at or distal to the brachial artery often becomes the territory of both vascular surgeons and reconstructive surgeons. Therefore, knowledge of the vascular anatomy of the upper extremity is essential when considering reconstructive options for injuries or structural deficiencies requiring soft tissue and/or bone reconstruction of the upper extremity. The established workhorse vessels for microsurgical anastomoses in the upper extremity are the brachial artery and the deep brachial artery in the arm, the brachial bifurcation with its distal branches of the radial and ulnar arteries in the antecubital region [1].

Supplementary Information The online version of this chapter (https://doi.org/10.1007/978-3-030-75389-4_24) contains supplementary material, which is available to authorized users.

R. E. Aliotta · D. D. Jacob
Department of Plastic Surgery, Cleveland, OH, USA
e-mail: ALIOTTR@ccf.org; Jacobd@ccf.org

R. L. Drake
Department of Anatomy, Cleveland Clinic Lerner College of Medicine, Cleveland, OH, USA
e-mail: DRAKER@ccf.org

L. Gurunian
Saddleback College, Mission Viejo, CA, USA

R. Gurunian (✉)
Department of Plastic Surgery, Cleveland Clinic, Cleveland, OH, USA

Cleveland Clinic Lerner College of Medicine, Case Western Reserve University, Cleveland, OH, USA
e-mail: gurunir@ccf.org

Preoperative Assessment

Consideration of medical comorbidities such diabetes and rheumatologic or immunologic chronic disease, chronic vascular/thromboembolic disease, and any history of trauma or neoplastic disease should be given. Prior to considering free tissue transfer, a proper clinical and diagnostic evaluation of the patients' blood supply to the upper extremity in question is necessary. Clinical examination should include characterizing the color, temperature, and texture of the skin and soft tissues. Allen's test should be used to identify the presence or absence of dual (radial and ulnar arterial) blood supply flow to the hand.

If distal radial and ulnar pulses or proximal brachial pulses are not appreciated in the extremity, a pencil Doppler can be used to identify and characterize blood flow. If more comprehensive and definitive views are required, then advanced evaluation with upper extremity catheter angiography [2], computed tomography angiography (CTA), and/or magnetic resonance arteriography (MRA) [3, 4] can be employed. The imaging studies are recommended given the anatomical variations of the brachial artery and its branches when considering a microsurgical flap reconstruction [5–7].

Applied Anatomy

The arm is enclosed in a strong sheath of deep fascia, known as the brachial fascia. Two intermuscular septa extend from this fascia, medial and lateral intermuscular septa, which divide the arm into anterior and posterior fascial compartments. The anterior compartment also known as the flexor compartment contains the coracobrachialis muscle, biceps brachii, and brachialis muscles, which are all innervated by the musculocutaneous nerve [8].

Major nerves coming from the brachial plexus such as the ulnar and median nerve course through the proximal upper extremity in the anterior compartment adjacent to the

R. Gurunian, R. Djohan (eds.), *Recipient Vessels in Reconstructive Microsurgery*, https://doi.org/10.1007/978-3-030-75389-4_24

vasculature. The lateral cord of the brachial plexus gives rise to the musculocutaneous nerve (MCN) and distally to the lateral cutaneous nerve sensory branch of the MCN, which branches at the distal 1/4 of the arm between the biceps and brachialis muscles. The blood supply of the anterior compartment is from the brachial artery [8].

The muscles of the posterior compartment, also known as the extensor compartment, are the triceps brachii and anconeus muscle. These are innervated by radial nerve and their blood supply is from the deep brachial artery [8].

The Brachial Artery

The brachial artery is the continuation of the axillary artery, which begins at the distal border of the tendon of the teres major (Figs. 24.1 and 24.2). Proximally, it runs between the coracobrachialis and biceps brachii muscles deep and then between the biceps brachii and triceps brachii (long and medial heads) muscles in the bicipital groove. The artery is covered anteriorly only by the skin and superficial and deep fascia. The bicipital aponeurosis (lacertus fibrosus) crosses it anteriorly at the elbow. The median nerve crosses it latero-medially near the distal attachment of the coracobrachialis. The medial antebrachial cutaneous nerve and ulnar nerve are medial to the brachial artery proximally. Distally, the median nerve and basilic vein are medial to the artery. With the artery are two vena comitantes (brachial veins) connected by transverse and oblique branches [9] (Fig. 24.2).

The deep brachial artery is the largest branch of the brachial artery, which arises from the posteromedial aspect of the brachial artery, distal to the teres major (Fig. 24.2). It follows the radial nerve closely, at first back between the long and medial heads of the triceps, and then in the nerve's groove covered by the lateral head of the triceps. Here, it divides into terminal branches. In addition to the muscular branches that are distributed to the coracobrachialis, biceps and brachialis, it supplies the nutrient artery of the humerus, deltoid, middle collateral, and radial collateral arteries. The middle collateral branch, the larger terminal branch, arises behind the humerus and descends in the medial head of the triceps to the elbow. It anastomoses with the interosseous recurrent artery behind the lateral epicondyle [9]. The radial collateral, the other terminal branch, is the artery's continuation. It accompanies the radial nerve through the lateral intermuscular septum between the brachialis and lateral head of the triceps brachii, descending between the brachialis and brachioradialis anterior to the lateral epicondyle [9–11] (Fig. 24.3). The radial collateral artery anastomoses with the radial recurrent artery (branch of the radial artery) at the anterior cubital fossa (Fig. 24.4). The posterior cutaneous nerve of the forearm, arising from the radial nerve in the spiral groove, accompanies the posterior radial

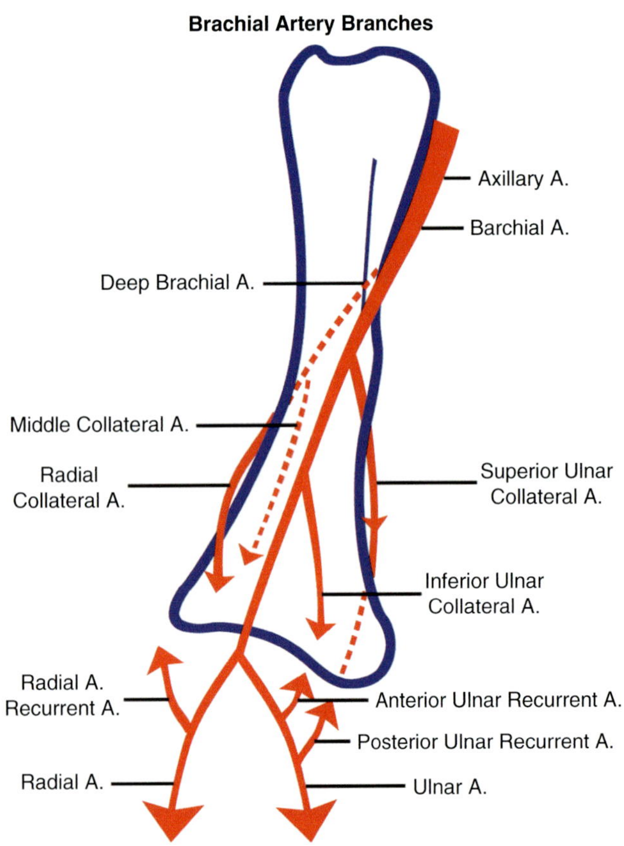

Fig. 24.1 Schematic drawing illustrating the brachial artery and its branches (in red) in relation to the humerus that is outlined with blue. Dotted red lines indicate posterior location of vessels. The arrows point out to the communication between radial collateral a. and radial recurrent a., between superior ulnar collateral a. and posterior ulnar recurrent a, between inferior ulnar collateral a. and anterior ulnar recurrent a., and finally between middle collateral a. and interosseous recurrent a. (which is not shown here)

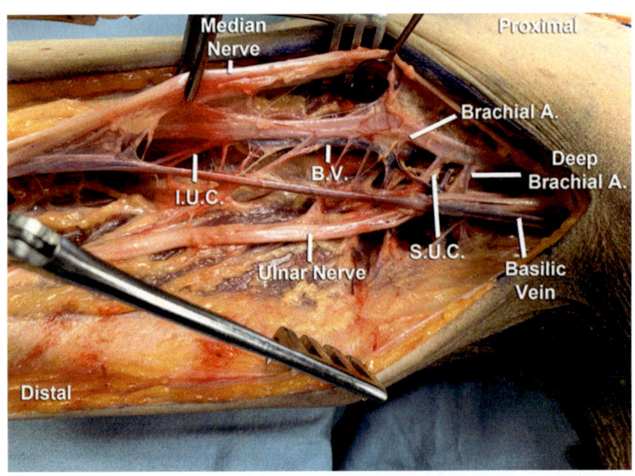

Fig. 24.2 Cadaver dissection: Surgical exposure of the brachial artery and its branches in a cadaver through a skin incision along the bicipital groove. Note that ulnar nerve travels with the superior ulnar collateral a. (SUC). IUC: inferior ulnar collateral a

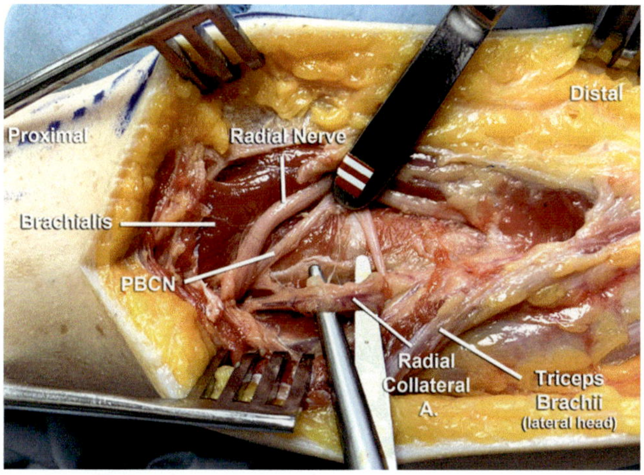

Fig. 24.3 Surgical exposure of the radial collateral artery in a cadaver dissection. Skin incision is made along a line drawn from lateral epicondyle of the humerus to the insertion of the deltoid muscle; this line delineates the lateral intermuscular septum. Dissection is then carried down to the lateral intermuscular septum between the brachialis and triceps brachii to dissect the radial collateral artery. The radial nerve and posterior antebrachial nerve should be preserved and protected during dissection

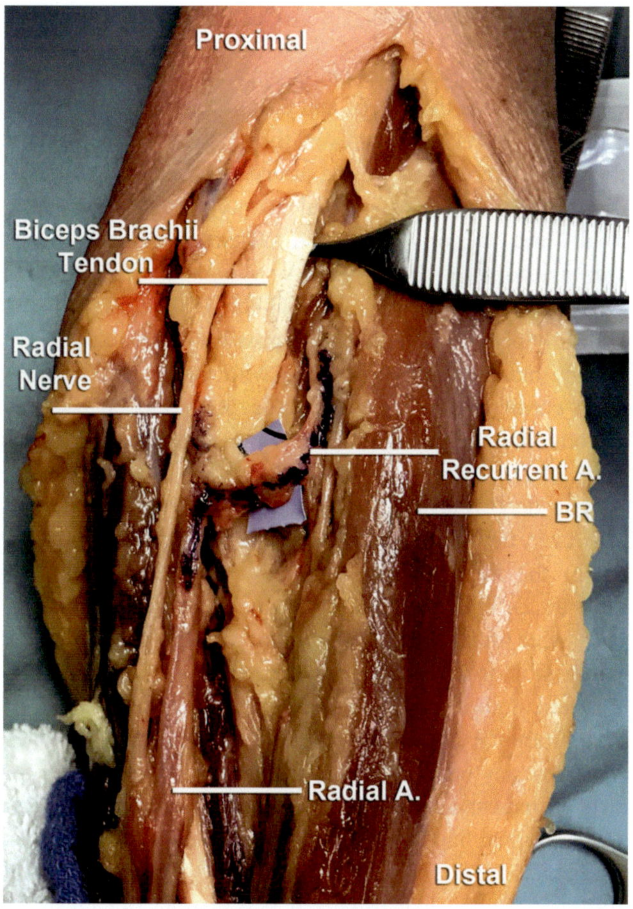

Fig. 24.4 Cadaver dissection for surgical exposure of the radial recurrent artery which is a valuable recipient artery in the microsurgical reconstruction of the upper extremity. (BR: Brachioradialis)

collateral artery and innervates the skin of the posterior forearm [9, 11].

The superior ulnar collateral artery (SUCA) is the second branch of the brachial artery that arises a little distal to the mid-upper arm (Figs. 24.1 and 24.2). Occasionally, it comes off the deep brachial artery. It accompanies the ulnar nerve, piercing the medial intermuscular septum to descend between the medial epicondyle and olecranon, ending deep to the flexor carpi ulnaris by anastomosing with the posterior ulnar recurrent and inferior collateral arteries [9, 10].

The inferior ulnar collateral artery (IUCA) begins about 5 cm proximal to the elbow. It runs medially along the brachialis muscle before piercing the medial intermuscular septum (Figs. 24.1 and 24.2). It then curls round the humerus between the triceps and bone, forming by its junction with the middle collateral branch of the deep brachial artery. It has branches descending anterior to the medial epicondyle to anastomose with the anterior ulnar recurrent artery [9].

The brachial artery dives deeply into the cubital fossa at the elbow. It divides near the neck of the radius into its terminal branches, the radial (see Chap. 25) and ulnar (see Chap. 26) arteries. The diameter of the brachial artery and its branches are outlined in Table 24.1.

The Cephalic, Basilic, and Brachial Veins

Veins of the arm and forearm can be grouped as superficial and deep, which are widely connected. Superficial veins include the cephalic, basilic, median cubital, and additional antebrachial veins and their branches.

The cephalic vein is commonly formed over the anatomical snuffbox. It curves proximally around the radial side of the forearm to its volar aspect. Distal to the elbow, a branch, the median cubital vein, joined by a branch from the deep veins, diverges proximally and medially to reach the basilic vein. The cephalic vein ascends in front of the elbow superficial to a groove between the brachioradialis and biceps. It ascends lateral to the biceps and between the pectoralis major and the deltoid (Fig. 24.5). Entering the infraclavicular fossa to pass behind the clavicular head of the pectoralis major, it pierces the clavipectoral fascia, crosses the axillary artery, and joins the axillary vein just below the clavicular level [30].

The basilic vein begins medially in the hand's dorsal venous network, ascending posteromedially in the forearm and inclining forwards to the anterior surface distal to the elbow. Joined by the median cubital vein, it ascends superficial to and between the biceps and pronator teres. It ascends medial to biceps and penetrates the deep fascia about the mid-arm (Fig. 24.6), continuing medial to the brachial artery to the lower border of the teres major muscle, there becoming the axillary vein [30, 32].

Table 24.1 Diameter of the brachial artery and its branches, and of cephalic, basilic, brachial, radial, and ulnar veins

Vessel	Diameter
Arteries	
Brachial artery	2.39–6.62 mm [12–14]
Brachial artery perforators (posterior brachial arm flap)	0.7 ± 0.4 mm [15]
Deep brachial artery	1.25–2.7 mm [13] 1.5–2.0 mm (distal end of spiral groove) [11]
Deep brachial perforators	0.7 ± 0.2 mm [16]
Middle collateral artery	0.6–2.4 mm [17, 18]
Anterior radial collateral artery	0.5–1.5 mm [17, 19]
Posterior radial collateral artery (lateral arm flap)	0.7–2.5 mm [11, 16, 17, 20–22]
Superior ulnar collateral artery (medial arm flap)	0.8–2.5 mm [16, 23–25] 0.6–3.0 mm [26]
Inferior ulnar collateral artery	0.8 ± 0.2 mm [16]
Radial artery	2.5 mm [27]
Radial artery (at anatomic snuffbox)	1.8–2.0 mm [28]
Ulnar artery	2.5 mm [27]
Veins	
Cephalic vein	2.8–10 mm [19, 29]
Basilic vein	0.7–7.3 mm [29–32]
Brachial vein	Mean diameter 4.9 mm [30]
Radial vena comitantes	At least 2.5 mm [11]
Ulnar vena comitantes	1.3 mm [27] 2.3 mm [27]

Deep veins of the forearm run with the radial and ulnar arteries draining respectively the deep and superficial palmar venous arches. They unite near the elbow as paired brachial veins. These veins flank the brachial artery, with branches similar to the arterial ones. Near the lower margin of the subscapularis, they join the axillary vein. The deep veins have numerous anastomoses with each other and with the superficial veins [30]. The diameter of veins in the arm is outlined in Table 24.1.

Surgical Site Exposure

Optimal exposure of the brachial artery is with the patient in supine position with the shoulder abducted to 90°, the elbow at full extension, and the forearm/hand supinated on a hand surgery table (Video 24.1).

Depending on the site of interest for flap coverage, the incision is planned along the longitudinal axis of the upper arm and forearm to allow for appropriate exposure as needed. The skin incision can be extended from the existing defect over the medial arm, or the medial arm can be approached directly with an incision over the bicipital groove (Fig. 24.2). After dividing the skin, the basilic vein is located in the subcutaneous tissue and runs with the medial antebrachial cutaneous nerve (Fig. 24.6). The basilic vein can be used as recipient vein. Both the nerve and the vein are retracted posteriorly, and the deep fascia is opened along the bicipital groove between the triceps and the short head of the biceps, with muscles retracted to reveal the vascular bundle with the median nerve anterior to the artery proximally and medial distally in the arm. The brachial artery can be dissected proximally and inferiorly to obtain a workable length for end-to-side anastomosis (Fig. 24.2). As variations of the arterial patterns in the upper limb are common, dissection should be carefully performed anticipating possible variations [5].

The brachial veins run along with the artery and these vena comitantes or their tributaries can also be used for venous drainage through the same dissection approach (Fig. 24.2).

The deep brachial artery can serve as recipient artery. However, its exposure requires dissection quite proximally up to the level of the distal border of the teres major (Fig. 24.2). This branch of the brachial artery may be readily accessible after carefully performed oncologic resections (if permissible from oncologic standpoint).

Meticulous dissection along the brachial artery superiorly and inferiorly may help expose brachial artery branches. SUCA or any other muscular branch of adequate length and caliber that can suitably match to the vascular pedicle of the microsurgical flap can be searched for and dissected for use as recipient artery (Fig. 24.2). The SUCA can arise from the profunda brachii, but usually it is a distinct branch of the main brachial artery. Therefore, further cranial dissection

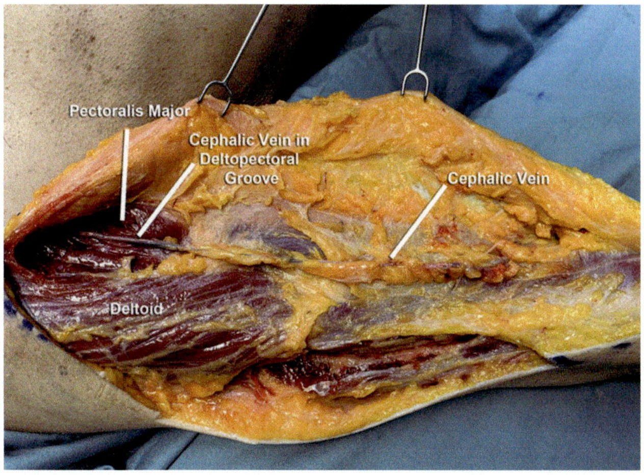

Fig. 24.5 Cadaver dissection: The cephalic vein dissected along the anterolateral surface of the forearm and arm in the subcutaneous tissue plane. It ascends lateral to the biceps in front of the elbow in the groove between the brachioradialis and biceps brachii. It courses over the arm to continue to ascend in the deltopectoral groove between the pectoralis major and the deltoid

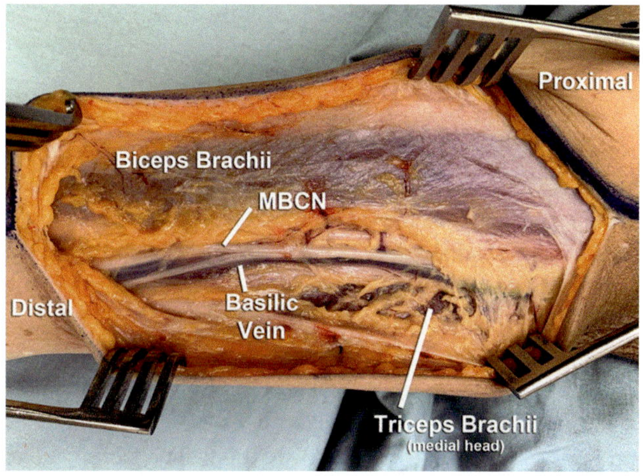

Fig. 24.6 Cadaver dissection: Medial antebrachial cutaneous nerve (MBCN) and basilic vein in the subcutaneous tissue plane; exposure through skin incision along the bicipital groove

may be required to prepare this branch. Dissection of IUCA is typically unnecessary as this branch is relatively small, making it not desirable for microvascular anastomosis. Also, in the vicinity, there are other arterial branches such as radial recurrent, radial, and ulnar arteries that can be reliably used as recipient.

Radial collateral artery, one of the terminal branches of the deep brachial artery, may be used as recipient vessel. After the deep brachial artery pierces the lateral intermuscular septum and the supinator muscle, it divides into the middle and radial collateral arteries. To expose the radial collateral artery, a line is drawn from lateral epicondyle of the humerus to the insertion of the deltoid muscle; this line delineates the lateral intermuscular septum. A skin incision is made over this line. Dissection is then carried down to the lateral intermuscular septum between the brachialis and triceps brachii. The radial nerve and posterior antebrachial nerve should be preserved and protected during dissection (Fig. 24.3).

Exposure of the brachial artery at the antecubital fossa can be performed through a skin incision that extends from the distal arm to the proximal forearm. The incision at the level of the elbow crease is made transversely to avoid skin contracture.

Subcutaneous veins, namely, the median cubital and cephalic, must be carefully preserved. The cephalic vein can be exposed over the anterolateral surface of the proximal forearm in front of the elbow in the groove between the brachioradialis and biceps brachii. These superficial veins, the radial artery and ulnar artery venae comitantes, or both can be used for venous outflow of the flap. Next, the distal bicipital aponeurosis is divided to expose the brachial artery and its flanking deep veins. These veins frequently have communicating branches anterior to the artery that must be ligated and divided for complete exposure.

The lacertus fibrosus is partially longitudinally incised and reflected. This reveals the brachial artery lying between the biceps tendon and median nerve. Approximately 2–3 cm distal to the elbow crease, entering the interval between the pronator muscle and the brachioradialis muscle, dissecting inferiorly exposes the bifurcation into the radial and ulnar arteries. Ulnar and radial vena comitantes can be used for venous outflow.

At the distal aspect of the incision, the brachioradialis is retracted radially, and the pronator teres is retracted ulnarly. The radial artery is identified by following the distal brachial artery into the interval between these two muscles. The incision can be extended distally along the line from the midpoint of the antecubital fossa to the radial styloid with the arm in supination. As one continues distally, the pronator teres dives under the radial artery to insert onto the radius. The artery courses under the medial fibers of the brachioradialis and can be found by incising the antebrachial fascia longitudinally and separating this muscle from the flexor carpi radialis (see Chap. 25).

Of interest is the radial recurrent branch coming off laterally from the radial artery. This branch lies on the supinator muscle with the nearby radial nerve visualized, and runs proximally medial to the lateral epicondyle and then within the interval between the brachioradialis and brachialis muscles (Fig. 24.4). It later naturally anastomoses with the radial collateral artery proximally above the level of the elbow.

This branch, when used either distally in the forearm or proximal in the upper arm, is robust enough in caliber to perform an end-to-end anastomosis.

At the distal aspect of the incision, the brachioradialis is retracted radially, and PT is retracted ulnarly. The ulnar artery is identified by following the distal brachial artery into the interval between these two muscles. It can be differentiated from the radial artery by its more acute takeoff from the brachial and posterior trajectory underneath the origin of the ulnar (deep) head of the pronator teres. This muscle separates it from the median nerve. Since anatomic variation is common in this area, it is important to follow the artery posteriorly to the edge of the pronator teres to ensure it has been properly identified. Exposure beyond this point either requires a separate incision or division of the pronator insertion on the ulna.

Discussion

Selection of arterial and venous recipients depends on the location of the defect, availability of healthy vessels, history of previous injury, vascular status of the upper extremity, and finally the characteristics of the microsurgical flap that is considered for reconstruction. The brachial artery and its tributaries such as the deep brachial artery and radial and ulnar arteries can reliably be used in many circumstances.

Exposure of the brachial artery, deep brachial artery, and superior ulnar collateral artery can be performed using medial arm incision. The radial collateral may be exposed through lateral arm incision and potentially be used. In certain cases such as after oncologic resections, these vessels are readily accessible in the vicinity without the extra need for further dissection.

Complicating free tissue transfer is finding a recipient vessel choice that does not threaten the distal extremity perfusion resulting in further soft tissue or functional damage for the patient. Temporary clamping of the recipient vessel to confirm persistent distal perfusion from other sources should be confirmed prior to its use and anastomosis. Also, for this reason, end-to-side anastomoses should be considered when coapting microsurgical vessels to recipients in the upper extremity, particularly when baseline flow is not ideal or adjacent limb vessel quality is otherwise diminished.

The brachial artery is of appropriate caliber along its entire course to feasibly perform end-to-side anastomoses without difficulty. For various soft tissue and/or bone reconstructions of the upper extremity, the brachial artery has been successfully used in an end-to-side fashion [33–37], (also see Chap. 27). The brachial artery has been used in an end-to-side fashion for revascularization of free fibula after oncologic resection of the humerus [36–38].

Also the deep brachial artery has been similarly used as recipient artery [37, 38]. It allows end-to-end microvascular anastomosis. Use of SUCA [39] and IUCA [40] as recipient is relatively rare.

Finally, use of terminal branches of the brachial artery, the radial artery, and the ulnar artery (including their branches) as recipient should be considered according to the size and location of the defect in conjunction with the microsurgical flap. These recipient sites are discussed in Chaps. 25 and 26 (also see Chaps. 28 and 29). Consideration should be given for end-to-side anastomosis when using ulnar and radial arteries as recipient.

The reconstructive microsurgeon should be aware of variable vascular anatomy in the upper extremity when planning to use upper arm vessels for microsurgical anastomosis [5–7]. These variations occur in up to 20% of patients [41].

Variations in the brachial artery are less common than those in the radial and ulnar arteries, but many anomalous patterns have been described. The brachial artery has been reported to be absent, as well as its profunda brachii, superior, and inferior ulnar collateral arterial branches [41]. The axillary artery served as the main collateral to the forearm.

An anomalous brachial artery has also been described that has no collateral branches, but instead it divides into two equal-sized radial and ulnar arteries in the cubital fossa [42].

In a study conducted by Rodriguez-Niedenfuhr et al. [5], variations of the arterial pattern in the upper limb were extensively investigated in 192 embalmed cadavers. The superficial brachial artery that courses in front to rather than behind the median nerve was found in about 5% of cases. The superficial brachial artery, which is important in development and normally regresses, can instead persist, and it can supply the normal territory of the main brachial artery, it runs parallel with the profunda brachii, or it can become many small cutaneous blood vessels [43].

If this superficial brachial artery persists, it remains superficial to the median nerve, instead of going deep to the median nerve. This is seen in around 5% of cases.

The accessory brachial artery is another variation. This originates above the elbow level from the upper third of the brachial artery. It can originate from the brachial or axillary artery and will then rejoin the main brachial artery in the distal arm, before its division into ulnar and radial arteries [5].

Various branching patterns of the brachial artery have also been described and one should be mindful of these during dissection. Shetty et al. [44] described a cadaver with a high bifurcation of the brachial artery in the upper arm into the radial and ulnar arteries, as opposed to the most common location in the cubital fossa. In this same report, they found that the profunda brachii had a common trunk which was the origin to the radial collateral, middle collateral, and superior ulnar collateral arteries.

The brachioradial artery is defined as a radial artery with a high origin. It was found in 53 out of 384 upper limbs (13.8%) according to the study by Rodriguez-Niedenfuhr et al. [5]. It originated from the axillary, the upper third of the brachial, and the lower third of the brachial arteries. When a brachioradial artery was present, the radial recurrent artery originated from it in 46% and from the deep brachial artery in 34% of 192 cadavers.

The superficial brachioulnar artery which is defined as an ulnar artery with a high origin courses over the superficial forearm flexor muscles. Its total incidence was 16 of 384 upper limbs (4.2%). It arose from the axillary, the upper third of the brachial, and the lower third of the brachial arteries [5].

The brachioulnar artery which is defined as an ulnar artery with a high origin and has a normal course along the forearm and hand was found 0.52% [5].

The superficial radial artery is a variation with a normal origin, but at the wrist level crossing the tendons which define the snuffbox (0.52%) [5].

The superficial brachioulnoradial artery is a superficial brachial artery branching at the elbow level into radial and ulnar arteries and coexisting with a normal brachial artery that continues as the common interosseous trunk (52%) [5].

The origin of the deep brachial artery has also been described with several anatomic variations. About 55% of the time it arises as a single trunk at the level of the teres major [6, 44].

It can originate from the axillary artery and this has been described to occur in 2–22% of cases [6, 10, 44]. Moreover, the deep brachial can originate as a common trunk with the superior ulnar collateral artery 22% of the time or as a branch of the posterior circumflex humeral artery in 7% [6, 44].

Superficial veins and/or vena comitantes can be exposed along with the arteries for microvascular anastomoses. There is a great variation in the venous anatomy in the cubital fossa, but the median cubital, basilic, cephalic, or large interconnecting branches between the deep and superficial venous systems are of adequate caliber for venous anastomosis [45].

These variations in size and length of potential veins to be used as recipient should always be remembered and anticipated. Adjustments should be made according to the specifics of each case. Selection of superficial and/or deep vein(s) for use as recipient vein depends on the exact location and characteristics of the defect to be reconstructed, length and caliber of microsurgical flap pedicle, and proximity to the arterial recipient vessel. The basilic vein can be easily dissected through medial arm incision that also gives access for brachial vein(s) exposure. Tributaries between the basilic vein and brachial veins can be used for venous drainage, if a sufficient match with the donor vein can be achieved. Similarly, the cephalic vein can be dissected through a skin incision over the anterolateral surface of the proximal forearm and distal arm between the brachioradialis and biceps. Also, the median cubital vein can easily be approached for use as recipient vein. This vein that combines the cephalic vein with the basilic vein is a great recipient resource. Deep veins accompanying the radial and ulnar arteries are always an option and can be dissected through skin incision in the proximal forearm and distal arm (also see Chaps. 25 and 26).

References

1. Bakri K. Clinical anatomy and recipient vessel selection in the upper extremity. In: Wei F-CM S, editor. Flaps and reconstructive surgery. 2nd ed. Philadelphia: Saunders/Elsevier; 2009. p. 89–114.
2. Wong VW, Katz RD, Higgins JP. Interpretation of upper extremity arteriography: vascular anatomy and pathology [corrected]. Hand Clin. 2015;31(1):121–34.
3. Ghouri MA, Gupta N, Bhat AP, et al. CT and MR imaging of the upper extremity vasculature: pearls, pitfalls, and challenges. Cardiovasc Diagn Ther. 2019;9(Suppl 1):S152–73.
4. Dave RB, Fleischmann D. Computed tomography angiography of the upper extremities. Radiol Clin N Am. 2016;54(1):101–14.
5. Rodríguez-Niedenführ M, Vázquez T, Nearn L, Ferreira B, Parkin I, Sañudo JR. Variations of the arterial pattern in the upper limb revisited: a morphological and statistical study, with a review of the literature. J Anat. 2001;199(Pt 5):547–66.
6. Celik HH, Aldur MM, Tunali S, Ozdemir MB, Aktekin M. Multiple variations of the deep artery of arm: double deep artery of arm and deep artery of arm with the superior ulnar collateral artery. A case report. Morphologie. 2004;88(283):188–90.
7. Malcic-Gürbüz J, Gürünlüoĝlu R, Ozdoĝmuş O, Yalin A. Unique case of trifurcation of the brachial artery: its clinical significance. Clin Anat. 2002;15(3):224–7.
8. Moore KL. Clinically oriented anatomy. In: The upper limb: the arm. 3rd ed. Philadelphia: Williams & Wilkins; 1992. p. 539–53.
9. Gray's anatomy. 37th ed. Angiology. William PL, Worwick R, Dyson M, Bannister LH, editors. New York: Churchill Livingstone; 1989. p. 758–60.
10. Epperson TN, Varacallo M. Anatomy, shoulder and upper limb, brachial artery. In: StatPearls. Treasure Island: StatPearls Publishing; 2020.
11. Katsaros J, Schusterman M, Beppu M, Banis JC Jr, Acland RD. The lateral upper arm flap: anatomy and clinical applications. Ann Plast Surg. 1984;12(6):489–500.
12. Maruhashi T, Soga J, Fujimura N, et al. Brachial artery diameter as a marker for cardiovascular risk assessment: FMD-J study. Atherosclerosis. 2018;268:92–8.
13. Tomiyama Y, Yoshinaga K, Fujii S, et al. Accurate quantitative measurements of brachial artery cross-sectional vascular area and vascular volume elastic modulus using automated oscillometric measurements: comparison with brachial artery ultrasound. Hypertens Res. 2015;38(7):478–84.
14. Chami HA, Keyes MJ, Vita JA, et al. Brachial artery diameter, blood flow and flow-mediated dilation in sleep-disordered breathing. Vasc Med. 2009;14(4):351–60.
15. Blondeel PN. Perforator flaps: anatomy, technique & clinical applications. 2nd ed. Quality Medical Publishing: St. Louis; 2013.
16. Blondeel PN, Morris SF, Hallock GG, Neligan PC. Perforator flaps: anatomy, technique, & clinical applications. 2nd ed. CRC Press; 2013.

17. Casoli V, Kostopoulos E, Pelissier P, Caix P, Martin D, Baudet J. The middle collateral artery: anatomic basis for the "extreme" lateral arm flap. Surg Radiol Anat. 2004;26(3):172–7.
18. Cormack GC, Lamberty BG. Fasciocutaneous vessels in the upper arm: application to the design of new fasciocutaneous flaps. Plast Reconstr Surg. 1984;74(2):244–50.
19. Wei FC, Mardini S. Flaps and reconstructive surgery. Elsevier; 2016.
20. Zenn MR, Jones G. Reconstructive surgery: anatomy, technique, and clinical application. Thieme; 2012.
21. Chung KC. Operative techniques: hand and wrist surgery E-Book. Elsevier Health Sciences; 2016.
22. Harpf C, Papp C, Ninković M, Anderl H, Hussl H. The lateral arm flap: review of 72 cases and technical refinements. J Reconstr Microsurg. 1998;14(1):39–48.
23. Breidenbach WC, Adamson W, Terzis JK. Medial arm flap revisited. Ann Plast Surg. 1987;18(2):156–63.
24. Gao XS, Mao ZR, Yang ZN, Wang BS. Medial upper arm skin flap: vascular anatomy and clinical applications. Ann Plast Surg. 1985;15(4):348–51.
25. Hou C, Chang S, Lin J, Song D. Surgical atlas of perforator flaps: a microsurgical dissection technique. Springer Netherlands; 2015.
26. Karamürsel S, Bağdatli D, Demir Z, Tüccar E, Celebioğlu S. Use of medial arm skin as a free flap. Plast Reconstr Surg. 2005;115(7):2025–31.
27. Strauch B, Yu HL, Chen ZW, Liebling R. Atlas of microvascular surgery. New York: Thieme Medical Publishers, Inc.; 1993. p. 47.
28. Strauch B, Yu HL, Chen ZW, Liebling R. Atlas of microvascular surgery. New York: Thieme Medical Publishers, Inc.; 1993. p. 85.
29. Irfan H, Ooi GS, Kyin MM, Ho P. Revealing maximal diameter of upper limb superficial vein with an elevated environmental temperature. Int J Chronic Dis. 2016;2016:8096473.
30. Sharp R, Cummings M, Childs J, et al. Measurement of vein diameter for Peripherally Inserted Central Catheter (PICC) insertion: an observational study. J Infus Nurs. 2015;38(5):351–7.
31. Baptista-Silva JCC, Dias AL, Criventi SV, Burihan E. Anatomy of the basilic vein in the arm and its importance for surgery. Braz J Morphol Sci. 2003;20:171–5.
32. Gray's Anatomy. 37th ed. Angiology. William PL, Worwick R, Dyson M, Bannister LH, editors. New York: Churchill Livingstone; 1989. p. 806–7.
33. Koteswara Rao Rayidi V, Prakash P, Srikanth R, Sreenivas J, Swathi K. Anterolateral thigh flap-the optimal flap in coverage of severe elbow injuries. Indian J Plast Surg. 2019;52(3):314–21.
34. Horch RE, Stark GB. The rectus abdominis free flap as an emergency procedure in extensive upper extremity soft-tissue defects. Plast Reconstr Surg. 1999;103(5):1421–7.
35. Shin AY, Bishop AT, Moran SL, Sim FH. Vascularized free fibula transfer for oncologic reconstruction of the humerus. Clin Orthop Relat Res. 2005;438:80–4.
36. Bilgin SS. Reconstruction of proximal humeral defects with shoulder arthrodesis using free vascularized fibular graft. J Bone Joint Surg Am. 2012;94(13):e94.
37. Adani R, Delcroix L, Innocenti M, Tarallo L, Baccarani A. Free fibula flap for humerus segmental reconstruction: report on 13 cases. Chir Organi Mov. 2008;91(1):21–6.
38. Onoda S, Sakuraba M, Asano T, et al. Use of vascularized free fibular head grafts for upper limb oncologic reconstruction. Plast Reconstr Surg. 2011;127(3):1244–53.
39. Kurlander DE, Shue S, Schwarz GS, Ghaznavi AM. Vascularized fibula epiphysis transfer for pediatric extremity reconstruction: a systematic review and meta-analysis. Ann Plast Surg. 2019;82(3):344–51.
40. Pappalardo M, Patel K, Cheng MH. Vascularized lymph node transfer for treatment of extremity lymphedema: an overview of current controversies regarding donor sites, recipient sites and outcomes. J Surg Oncol. 2018;117(7):1420–31.
41. Ciervo A, Kahn M, Pangilinan AJ, Dardik H. Absence of the brachial artery: report of a rare human variation and review of upper extremity arterial anomalies. J Vasc Surg. 2001;33(1):191–4.
42. Jurjus A, Sfeir R, Bezirdjian R. Unusual variation of the arterial pattern of the human upper limb. Anat Rec. 1986;215(1):82–3.
43. Yang HJ, Gil YC, Jung WS, Lee HY. Variations of the superficial brachial artery in Korean cadavers. J Korean Med Sci. 2008;23(5):884–7.
44. Shetty SD, Nayak BS, Madhav NV, Sirasanagandla SR, Abhinitha P. The abnormal origin, course and the distribution of the arteries of the upper limb: a case report. J Clin Diagn Res. 2012;6(8):1414–6.
45. Imanishi N, Nakajima H, Aiso S. Anatomic study of the venous drainage architecture of the forearm skin and subcutaneous tissue. Plast Reconstr Surg [Internet]. 2000 Nov [cited 2020 Mar 18];106(6):1287–94. Available from.: http://www.ncbi.nlm.nih.gov/pubmed/11083557.

Radial Artery

25

Andrew R. Bauder, Zvi Steinberger, Oded Ben Amotz,
L. Scott Levin, and Ines C. Lin

Introduction

The radial artery serves as a common recipient vessel for microsurgical reconstruction of the upper extremity. Its safe exposure relies on knowledge of its relationship with surrounding structures of critical functional importance. Fortunately, this anatomy is superficial in most of the forearm and consistent, making for expedient recipient vessel exposure. The radial artery can also be easily accessed in the dorsal hand at the snuffbox for more distal reconstructions.

Applied Anatomy

The radial artery (Fig. 25.1) is one of two continuations of the brachial artery, the other being the ulnar artery (also see Chaps. 24, 26, 28, and 29). At origin, it measures 3.0–3.5 mm in diameter [1] (Table 25.1). The brachial artery bifurcates roughly at the level of the radial tuberosity, or approximately 2.2 cm distal to the transverse elbow crease [6]. The ulnar artery comes off at nearly a right angle, while the relatively smaller radial artery continues as a more direct extension of the brachial artery. The radial artery continues to supply the superficial volar compartment of the forearm and the mobile wad [7].

In the proximal forearm, the belly of the brachioradialis muscle lies lateral to the radial artery. The muscle also overlaps the radial artery anteriorly. The pronator teres is medial to the artery. Distally, the tendon of the flexor carpi radialis is medial and that of the brachioradialis lateral to the radial artery. The superficial branch of the radial nerve is lateral in the vessel's middle third, which lies just volar to the pronator teres. Posterior are successively as follows: the tendon of biceps, supinator, the distal attachment of pronator teres, radial head of flexor digitorum superficialis, flexor pollicis longus, pronator quadratus, and the lower end of the radius.

Just proximal to the wrist crease, the radial artery can be easily palpable immediately radial to the flexor carpi radialis tendon, lying only 2 mm below the skin and measuring the mean diameter of the radial artery to be 2.2 ± 0.4 mm, ranging from 1.0 to 3.4 mm [4] (Table 25.1).

Along its course in the middle and distal thirds of the forearm, it is accompanied by two venae comitantes. There are interconnections between the venae and the superficial system along the length of the radial artery. In the cubital fossa, the two venae coalesce into a single large vein for 1–2 cm, which then connects to the cephalic vein via the profundus cubitalis vein [8–10]. This is the largest interconnection between the superficial and deep venous systems and is used by some to supply dual venous drainage of the free radial forearm flap through one venous anastomosis [11].

At the volar carpal ligament, the radial artery sends off a superficial branch before continuing deep to the ligament to anastomose with the volar branches of the ulnar artery in the

Supplementary Information The online version of this chapter (https://doi.org/10.1007/978-3-030-75389-4_25) contains supplementary material, which is available to authorized users.

A. R. Bauder
Division of Plastic Surgery, Department of Surgery, University of Pennsylvania, Philadelphia, PA, USA
e-mail: Andrew.bauder@pennmedicine.upenn.edu

Z. Steinberger
Department of Orthopaedic Surgery, University of Pennsylvania, Philadelphia, PA, USA

Department of Hand and Microsurgery, Sheba Medical Center, Tel Hashomer, Israel

O. B. Amotz
Department of Orthopaedic Surgery, University of Pennsylvania, Philadelphia, PA, USA

L. S. Levin · I. C. Lin (✉)
Division of Plastic Surgery, Department of Surgery, University of Pennsylvania, Philadelphia, PA, USA

Department of Orthopaedic Surgery, University of Pennsylvania, Philadelphia, PA, USA
e-mail: Scott.Levin@pennmedicine.upenn.edu; ines.lin@pennmedicine.upenn.edu

R. Gurunian, R. Djohan (eds.), *Recipient Vessels in Reconstructive Microsurgery*,
https://doi.org/10.1007/978-3-030-75389-4_25

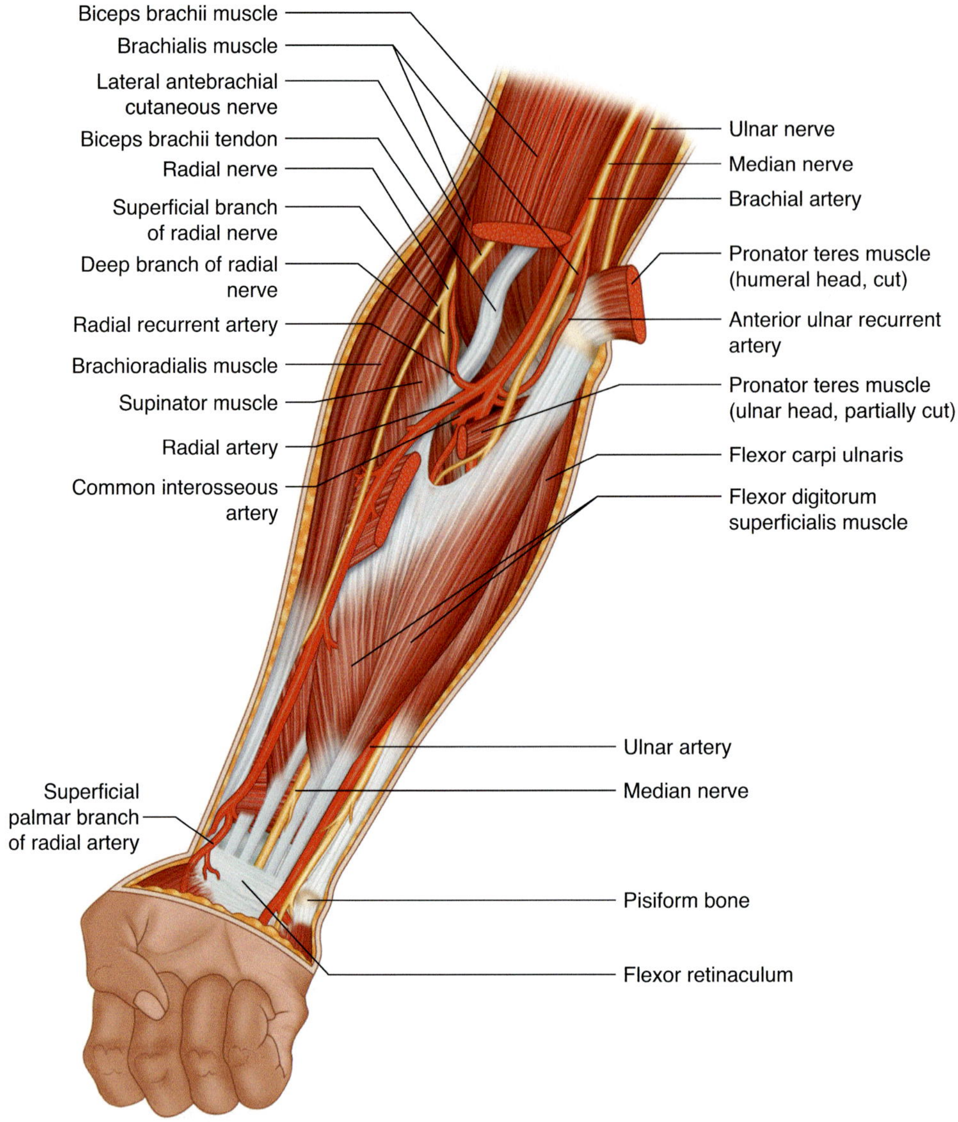

Fig. 25.1 Course of the radial artery with its branches in the forearm

Table 25.1 External diameter of the radial artery and its branches including deep and superficial palmar arches

Radial artery 2.5 mm [2]	3.0–3.5 mm (at origin) [1]
	3.14 ± 0.64 mm (range: 2.0 to 4.0 mm) [3]
Radial recurrent artery from bifurcation [3]	1.84 ± 0.59 mm (range: 1.0 mm to 2.9 mm) at the 20 mm point from bifurcation [3]
Radial artery (at wrist)	1.0–3.4 mm (mean 2.2 ± 0.4 mm) [4]
Radial artery (at snuffbox)	1.8–2.0 mm [2]
Deep palmar arch	1.4 mm [2]
	1.5 mm [5]
Princeps pollicis	1.3 mm [2]
Superficial palmar arch	1.8 mm [2, 5]

The numbers in square bracket at the end indicate the references

hand to form the deep palmar arch. The superficial branch contributes to the ulnar dominant superficial palmar arch about 45% of the time; in 45%, the superficial arch is formed by the ulnar artery alone and in the remaining 10%, the arch is incomplete [5, 12, 13]. After this, the main radial artery, which bends dorsally, gives rise to the princeps pollicis and first dorsal metacarpal arteries before diving between the heads of the first dorsal interosseous and wrapping volarly around the base of the second metacarpal [14–16]. Here, it consistently provides inflow to the deep palmar arch, which lies just volar to the metacarpals [13]. In turn, the deep arch gives rise to the three palmar metacarpal arteries.

Anatomic Variants

While the radial artery commonly begins as a bifurcation in the antecubital fossa at the level of the radial neck and continues distally deep to the antebrachial fascia of the anterior forearm, numerous anatomic variants exist. These notably include a high origin of the artery, and rarely a superficial radial artery or even congenital absence [17–20]. Rodríguez-Niedenführ reviewed the plethora of live and cadaveric descriptions of the variants of the brachial artery and its distal continuations [18]. Although it has been referenced by many different names, the most common anatomic irregularity is a high origin of the radial artery, which may occur in up to 14% of patients [17, 18]. This high origin, also named "brachioradial artery," most commonly arises from the medial aspect of the upper third of the brachial artery. However, it may also originate from the axillary artery or the lower two-thirds of the brachial artery [17]. As it traverses the cubital fossa, it can pass either anterior or posterior to the bicipital aponeurosis, and may reconnect with the brachial artery in the cubital fossa via a large cubital crossover vessel. The recurrent radial artery can then come off either the brachial artery or the brachioradial artery, when it is present.

Regardless of upper arm and cubital fossa variations, once the artery enters the distal two-thirds of the forearm, its anatomy is consistent. The rare exception is a superficial radial artery. In this case, the artery can lie superficial to the tendons of the snuffbox, and may become superficial higher in the forearm [18]. Finally, while congenital absence is exceedingly rare, it has been reported [20]. When absent, the radial artery vascular territory is replaced by the anterior interosseous or median arteries.

Radial Artery Branches

The branches of the radial artery are best organized based on anatomical location in the forearm, wrist, and hand. They are listed below based on their order of origination traveling from proximal to distal along the upper extremity.

Forearm

Radial Recurrent Artery (RRA)

The RRA is the first major branch of the radial artery, 1.5 mm to 2 mm in size at its origin [3] (Table 25.1). In three-quarters of patients, this branch originates from the radial artery either at or, more commonly, just distal to its bifurcation from the brachial artery. However, it may also come directly off the brachial or even the ulnointerosseous trunk [3, 21]. In a third of patients, it is joined by another branch, the accessory radial recurrent artery, which is clinically relevant in that it can form a vascular loop around the biceps tendon [21].

The RRA travels proximally to join the radial nerve at the proximal edge of the supinator muscle just prior to the nerve's bifurcation into the radial sensory nerve (RSN) and the posterior interosseous nerve (PIN) (Fig. 25.1). It then passes anterior to the lateral epicondyle to anastomose with the radial collateral artery, a branch of the profunda brachii. Its exposure in this area relies on careful preservation of the lateral antebrachial cutaneous nerve (LABCN) which lies superficial to the radial recurrent artery at the elbow. The LABCN is the distal continuation of the musculocutaneous nerve and exits the upper arm just lateral to the biceps tendon in the cubital fossa to become superficial and provide cutaneous innervation to the radial aspect of the forearm. This anastomosis between the RRA and radial collateral arteries is found at the lateral intermuscular septum just proximal to the elbow and continues distally. Importantly, these vessels form the basis of the lateral and reversed lateral arm flaps, which can also be based posterior to the lateral epicondyle on the anastomosis between the interosseous recurrent and posterior radial collateral arteries [22].

Muscular Branches

As the radial artery travels distally, it provides multiple perforators to muscles on the volar/radial aspect of the forearm. This includes the superficial volar compartment and, to a lesser extent, the mobile wad. The RRA most often supplies the brachioradialis, extensor carpi radialis/brevis, and supinator muscles, but these may all be supplied directly from the radial artery [3].

Septocutaneous Branches

Septocutaneous branches arise along the entire course of the radial artery within the intermuscular septum located in the proximal two-thirds of the forearm between the muscle bellies of the brachioradialis and flexor carpi radialis. The largest septocutaneous branch is the inferior cubital artery arising 3.5 centimeters distal to the elbow crease [23]. This usually originates from the lateral aspect of the radial artery, but can also come off the radial recurrent in a third of patients [23]. It then pierces the deep fascia just medial to the LABCN and brachioradialis and goes on to supply a 20 to 30 centimeter skin paddle just distal to the antecubital fossa [23].

The septocutaneous branches otherwise parallel the course of the cephalic vein in the forearm and average only 0.6 millimeters in diameter [24]. They are particularly dense in the cubital fossa and distal third of the forearm and sparse in between [7, 25]. There is a reliable cluster of septocutaneous branches 2 to 4 centimeters proximal to the radial styloid [26, 27], which is an important consideration when designing and harvesting the radial forearm, reversed radial forearm, or radial forearm perforator flaps.

Periosteal Branches

In addition to supplying the periosteal network at the metaphyseal-epiphyseal junction, the radial artery also sends off periosteal branches to the radius along its entire length. These come in the form of musculocutaneous branches, which are most dense at the origins of the flexor pollicis longus and pronator quadratus, as well as fascioperiosteal branches, which take a more direct course to the radius [28, 29]. Like septocutaneous branches, these fascioperiosteal branches are most dense in the distal third of the forearm at the lateral radius near the insertion of the brachioradialis [28, 30]. Clinically, these periosteal branches are used to harvest a segment of the distal radius with the long vascular leash of the radial artery to be used either as pedicled flaps for osseous defects of the upper extremity or as free flaps for composite microvascular reconstruction.

Wrist

Superficial Palmar Branch (SPB)

The SPB originates from the medial aspect of the radial artery 1 centimeter proximal to the radial styloid [31]. At its source, it is 1 to 1.5 millimeters in diameter, delivering a good size match for digital arteries [32]. The SPB usually travels superficial to the abductor pollicis brevis but may rarely travel between the abductor and opponens muscles [33]. In the thenar eminence, it provides branches to the thenar musculature and cutaneous branches to the overlying skin. Here it is consistently accompanied by the radial division of the palmar cutaneous branch of the median nerve. As it travels further distal, the SPB may anastomose with the terminal branches of the ulnar artery to form the superficial palmar arch. The superficial palmar arch gives rise to three common palmar digital arteries and a proper palmar ulnar digital artery [2].

Just distal to this arcade, it bifurcates into the first palmar metacarpal artery and the radialis indicis [14]. The first palmar metacarpal artery is a short artery, and its entire length lies anterior to the thenar muscles. In a cadaver study by Ramirez and Gonzalez, in every case, it branched off from the superficial palmar arch and followed an entirely different course than the princeps pollicis artery. This artery has also been given other names, including the first commissural artery and the intermetacarpal artery [14].

Palmar (Volar) Carpal Branches

At the distal edge of the pronator quadratus, the radial artery or its superficial palmar branch sends off a vessel to form the radial half of the palmar carpal arch [34, 35]. This vessel connects with both its ulnar counterpart and the anterior division of the anterior interosseous artery. Similarly, over the distal carpal row, another arch is formed named the palmar intercarpal arch. Although they are utilized less frequently than their dorsal analogues, the palmar carpal and intercarpal arches can be used to provide vascularized bone graft from the volar distal radius to reconstruct carpal defects and nonunions [34, 36, 37].

Dorsal Carpal Branches

The radial artery gives off the 1, 2 intercompartmental supraretinacular arteries, which originate from the radial artery distal to the radial styloid after the takeoff of the superficial palmar branch. These arteries travel superficial to the extensor retinaculum in a retrograde fashion between the first and second and second and third extensor compartments [35]. These branches are common sources for vascularized distal radius bone grafts for bony reconstruction of the scaphoid [35, 38].

The carpal branches of the radial and ulnar arteries form the dorsal carpal arch, which receive contributions from both the dorsal and palmar interosseous arteries. In contrast to the first dorsal metacarpal artery, which is a direct branch of the radial artery, the remaining dorsal metacarpal arteries (DMAs) arise from the dorsal carpal arch. As they run forward, they are supplemented or occasionally replaced by perforators from the deep palmar arch or palmar metacarpal arteries, which pass through the interosseous spaces proximal to the metacarpal heads. Additional perforators link the palmar and dorsal systems in the web spaces [39].

From the dorsal carpal arch, three dorsal metacarpal arteries descend on the second to fourth dorsal interosseous muscles and bifurcate into the dorsal digital branches for the adjacent sides of all four fingers. They anastomose with the palmar digital branches from the superficial palmar arch; near their origins, they also anastomose with the deep palmar arch by the proximal perforating arteries and, near their bifurcation, with the palmar digital rami of the superficial palmar arch by distal perforating arteries [40].

The second dorsal metacarpal artery is the most reliable and largest caliber, permitting the formation of the distally based dorsal hand flap and small pedicled vascularized bone grafts of the second and third metacarpals [39, 41]. The third and fourth dorsal metacarpal arteries are smaller and less reliable [42].

Hand

Princeps Pollicis Artery (PPA)

As the radial artery continues distally along the floor of the anatomic snuffbox underneath the tendons of the first and third extensor compartments, it becomes superficial and easily palpable at the bony crotch of the first webspace. Here, it gives rise to both the princeps pollicis and first dorsal metacarpal arteries and transitions into the deep palmar arch (Fig. 25.2) [14]. While there is substantial anatomic variation in the arterial supply to the thumb, the princeps pollicis is regarded as the dominant supply [14, 15]. On the ulnar side of the thumb, it forms the majority of the supply to the dorsal-ulnar thumb vessel. The PPA also contributes considerably to the volar-ulnar supply along with the first palmar metacarpal artery off the superficial branch of the radial artery. It has a less important role on the radial side of the thumb, which has a more variable pattern of blood supply. The PPA also has an overlapping angiosome with the superficial branch of the radial artery. As previously reviewed, the superficial branch of the radial artery supplies cutaneous perforators to the thenar eminence. However, the PPA also dependably sends off cutaneous perforators to the thenar eminence over the distal half of the first metacarpal [43].

First Dorsal Metacarpal Artery (FDMA)

The FDMA arises just before the radial artery dives palmarly between the heads of the first dorsal interosseous muscle. It sends branches into the first dorsal interosseous and reliably has three to four cutaneous branches [44]. The radial branch supplies the skin overlying the ulnar side of the thumb metacarpophalangeal joint and may continue as the dorso-ulnar vessel to the tip of the thumb. The intermediate branch goes on to supply the dorsal skin at the apex of the first webspace. The ulnar branch is often the most substantial and travels distally to supply the territory overlying the dorso-radial aspect of the index finger proximal phalanx. All of these branches travel along the fascia of the first dorsal interosseous muscle and can be used to create local flaps for reconstruction of the hand. In particular, the ulnar branch is by a division of the sensory branch of the radial nerve along the dorsum of the hand. This allows for creation of a sensate pedicled FDMA flap that can reach the tip of the thumb [45].

Radialis Indicis Artery

The radialis indicis branches off the radial artery, mostly off the princeps pollicis prior to transitioning to the deep palmar

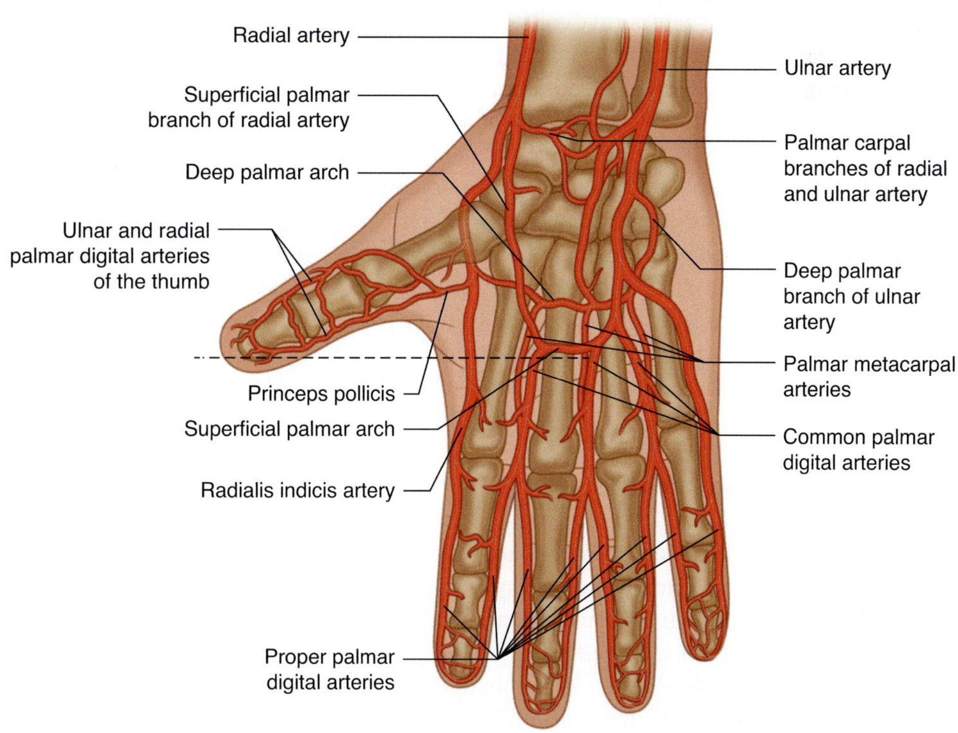

Fig. 25.2 The radial artery and its branches in the wrist and hand including the deep and superficial palmar arches

arch [2]. A cadaver study by Ramirez and Gonzalez also indicates that the radialis indicis is one of the two terminal branches of the SPB of the radial artery [14]. It can also originate directly from the superficial palmar arch [5, 13, 33]. In instances of a hypoplastic SPB or an incomplete arch, the radialis indicis artery would represent the radial-most continuation of the ulnar artery as it traverses from ulnar to radial creating the superficial arch [13].

Deep Palmar Arch

There is less variability in the deep palmar arch than in the superficial palmar arch. As the radial artery turns palmarly around the base of the second metacarpal, it forms the deep arch, which continues ulnarly to meet one or both of the deep palmar branches of the ulnar artery [10]. In most cases, the deep arch has a smaller average diameter of 1.5 mm compared to the superficial arch (1.8 mm) [5] (Table 25.1). The deep arch gives off three palmar metacarpal arteries.

Preoperative Assessment

While the ulnar artery is commonly referred to as the dominant vessel to the hand, its caliber is similar to the radial artery at the wrist [12]. Moreover, its flow margin is less than 10% greater than the radial artery. As such, while it may initially seem as if the radial artery can be sacrificed with relative impunity due to ulnar dominant flow, the arterial system may be more balanced than was originally thought [12].

Despite this, in a hand with normal collateral flow between the radial and ulnar arteries, occlusion of the radial artery appears to be relatively inconsequential because there is a compensatory increase in flow through the ulnar and anterior/posterior interosseous arteries [46]. Hand perfusion, strength, function, and cold tolerance are all preserved in the short term, and reports of long-term sequelae are rare [47–49]. However, in a hand with abnormal or incomplete connections between the two arteries, sacrifice of the radial artery can result in ulceration, ischemia, and paresthesias of the radial digits. As such, preoperative assessment remains critical to avoid these severe sequelae.

Allen Test/Modified Allen Test

The Allen test, first described by Edgar Van Nuys Allen in 1929, was developed to determine the adequacy of the collateral flow between the radial and ulnar arteries to the hand. An alternative method, the modified Allen test, proposed by Irving Wright, is considered superior and more often used. The patient is asked to keep the arm mildly flexed at the wrist. The elbow is gently extended, but overextension may lead to a false positive. The examiner compresses the radial and ulnar arteries simultaneously, stopping blood flow to the hand. Meanwhile, the patient is asked to repeatedly open and close their hand to exsanguinate the hand. The fist is then gently unclenched, and the fingers are allowed to relax in a resting posture. The hand should remain white or blanched. At this point, compression is released from the ulnar artery, and the examiner observes the hand color. Hand color should return within 10 seconds. The test is repeated, with compression released from the radial artery rather than the ulnar artery. Again, reperfusion within 10 seconds is considered normal.

The reliability of the modified Allen test for preoperative assessment has been hotly debated in the cardiac surgery literature pertaining to harvest of the radial artery for coronary bypass. Opponents argue that it is too subjective, with poor inter-relater reliability [50–52]. Despite these concerns, it has held up in multiple studies as quite specific (>95%) [53, 54], meaning if the Allen test is negative (normal collateral perfusion from the ulnar), it is safe to harvest the radial artery. This is particularly true if flow to the thumb is normal after occlusion of the radial artery [54]. The Allen test has not been shown to be nearly as sensitive as it is specific. Thus, if it is positive (abnormal collateral perfusion from the ulnar), it has been suggested that another confirmatory test be performed, such as complete radial and ulnar artery duplex ultrasound.

Additional imaging must also be considered in patients with select comorbidities. Due to the common nature of coronary artery disease, it is worth noting that patients can present with upper extremity arterial calcifications visible on plain films very early in the disease course; this may warrant additional workup with duplex ultrasonography or CT angiography [55]. While significant peripheral arterial disease (PAD) of the upper extremity is rare, and even rarer below the elbow [56], an on-table angiogram or CT angiogram should be considered with symptomatic upper extremity PAD. Patients with flow-limiting vasculitis should be handled similarly.

When considering reconstructive options, we favor preserving flow through both arteries to the hand when at all possible. This can be achieved through an end-to-side anastomosis into the radial artery or an end-to-end anastomosis using a side branch of reasonable diameter. An abnormal Allen test is a relative, but not absolute, contraindication for end-to-side anastomosis to the dominant artery during reconstruction, and end-to-end anastomosis with a side branch may be considered. The Allen test can be simulated intraoperatively after the radial artery exposure before an arteriotomy is performed, particularly if the radial artery is to be ligated. The radial artery can be temporarily occluded distally with a vascular clamp after standard methods of exsanguination of the extremity (e.g., with an Esmarch bandage, or with limb elevation and brachial artery occlusion). With the radial artery clamped and the tourniquet deflated or removed, distal hand perfusion through the ulnar artery should be confirmed, which can also be assessed using a surface Doppler signal at the thumb. Finally, direct perfusion to the hand should be closely followed intraoperatively when there is still opportunity to reconstruct the artery or revise the inflow.

Surgical Site Exposure

Exposure of the radial artery follows from knowledge of the applied anatomy and branching pattern above. Exposure in the distal two-thirds of the forearm is relatively straightforward owing to the superficial location of the artery and its straight-line course. However, exposure in the cubital fossa can be challenging owing to rotation of the forearm and the deep location of the artery and proximity to other structures. Similarly, radial artery exposure in the snuffbox deserves special consideration given its intricate association with nerves and extrinsic tendons.

Cubital Fossa and Proximal Third of the Forearm

A transverse or s-shaped antecubital incision is used to expose the distal brachial artery at its bifurcation and the proximal radial and ulnar arteries (Fig. 25.3, Video 25.1). Subcutaneous veins, namely, the median cubital and cephalic, must be carefully preserved. These superficial veins, the deep radial artery venae comitantes, or both can be used for venous outflow of the flap. Next, the distal bicipital aponeurosis is divided to expose the brachial artery and its flanking

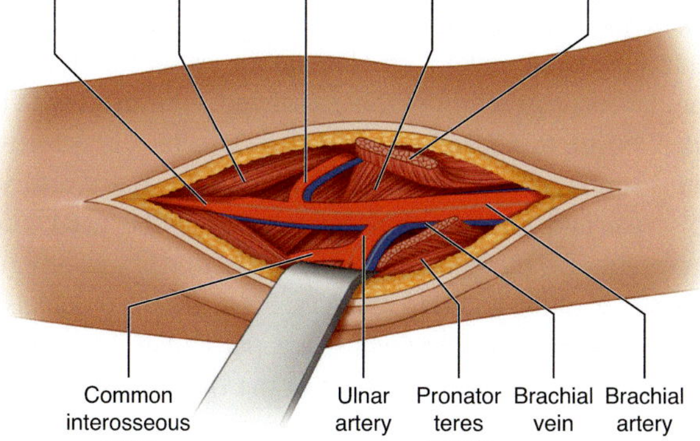

Fig. 25.3 Exposure of the radial artery in the cubital fossa

deep veins. These veins frequently have communicating branches anterior to the artery that must be ligated and divided for complete exposure.

At the distal aspect of the incision, the brachioradialis is retracted radially, and the pronator teres is retracted ulnarly. The radial artery is identified by following the distal brachial artery into the interval between these two muscles. The incision can be extended distally along the line from the midpoint of the antecubital fossa to the radial styloid with the arm in supination. As one continues distally, the pronator teres dives under the radial artery to insert onto the radius. The artery courses under the medial fibers of the brachioradialis and can be found by incising the antebrachial fascia longitudinally and separating this muscle from the flexor carpi radialis.

Microsurgical Indications

The relatively deeper location of the radial artery in the proximal forearm and cubital fossa compared to the more distal forearm makes anastomoses more challenging and thus may be a less desirable location for microsurgical anastomosis. There is also essentially no size benefit proximally because the artery is a similar caliber along its entire length from the brachial bifurcation to the wrist. However, radial artery exposure in the cubital fossa remains useful for microsurgical reconstruction of elbow defects for which the lateral arm or reversed lateral arm flap is inadequate or unavailable. Larger free flaps can also be employed for extensive forearm resurfacing and/or functional reconstruction.

The proximity of the radial artery, RRA, and the bifurcation of the radial nerve into the RSN and PIN is beneficial for free functional muscle transfers. The PIN provides two motor branches to the supinator muscle (one radial, one ulnar). Either one or both can be used for motor innervation of a free functional muscle flap for wrist and/or finger extension [57].

The anterior interosseous nerve (AIN) can also serve as a donor nerve. Its exposure through the cubital fossa incision requires finding the median nerve proximally, which is located deep and radial to the radial artery at the elbow level. Once the median nerve is located, it can be traced distally as it passes between the two heads of the pronator teres. This exposure is facilitated by releasing the bicipital aponeurosis, or lacertus fibrosus. There will be numerous small crossing vessels over the nerve that need to be divided. The anterior interosseous nerve will come off radially from the median nerve as it crosses between the two heads of the pronator teres. The AIN then hugs the anterior aspect of the interosseous membrane before innervating the pronator quadratus. It can be exposed along this entire course for additional donor nerve length if needed, but dissection involves working around the flexor muscles if they have not been debrided.

Middle and Distal Thirds of the Forearm

At the middle and distal forearm, a linear or curvilinear incision follows the axis drawn from the bicipital tendon at the antecubital fossa to the radial styloid and is made directly over the radial artery at the radial volar forearm with minimal morbidity so long as the radial sensory and distal branches of the lateral antebrachial cutaneous nerves are protected (Videos 25.1 and 25.2). The artery is ulnar to the RSN and continues to lie between the brachioradialis and flexor carpi radialis. The RSN arises from under the brachioradialis and radial wrist extensors and becomes superficial about 8 to 9 centimeters proximal to the radial styloid; thus for exposures in the wrist and distal third of the forearm, it is expected to lie superficial to the antebrachial fascia. It is important to protect the venae comitantes flanking the radial artery during its exposure at this level. Either the venae or the more dorsally located superficial venous system such as the cephalic vein can be utilized for venous egress.

Microsurgical Indications

In the middle and distal thirds of the forearm, the radial artery is utilized for microvascular reconstruction of soft tissue defects in the surrounding region of the hand and forearm when pedicled options are not available. For dorsal defects, an end-to-end anastomosis to the posterior interosseous artery can also be considered.

For defects with a large osseous component, vascularized free fibula transfer is an established reconstructive option [58], although other flaps – such as the lateral arm and iliac crest – have also been successfully used [59, 60]. The radial shaft and distal radius can be accessed through either volar Henry approach or the dorsal Thompson approach. A volar approach to the radius, between the interval of the radial artery and FCR, is in close proximity to the radial artery. Alternatively, a dorsal approach allows easy manipulation of the bone flap with low risk of injury to the artery. Furthermore, a dorsal approach can be extended distally to access the carpus and proximally to reach the radial head. This additional visualization is helpful when using the fibular head to reconstruct the radiocarpal joint in adults and restore epiphyseal growth in children [61, 62]. If the surgeon uses a dorsal approach to the radius, the volar exposure of the radial artery is still applicable, and a wide subcutaneous tunnel is created to pass the vascular pedicle toward the radial artery. Finally, the same combination of dorsal and volar incisions can be used for reconstruction of the carpal bones, such as with medial femoral condyle transfer for scaphoid nonunion of the proximal pole or Kienböck's disease, or a volar-only approach can be done for scaphoid waist nonunion with avascular necrosis and humpback deformity [63, 64].

Snuffbox

A 3 cm longitudinal (linear or curvilinear) skin incision is made in the snuffbox, between the radial styloid and the base of the first metacarpal and between the first (extensor pollicis brevis, abductor pollicis longus) and third (extensor pollicis longus) extensor compartments (Video 25.3). The cephalic vein is identified in the subcutaneous tissue and retracted. The incision is made longitudinally to minimize the possibility of inadvertent injury to the terminal branches of the radial sensory nerve. The course of the artery is obliquely oriented below this incision as it passes dorsally. There is usually one branch of the nerve that travels just radial to the first extensor compartment and is closely associated with the radial artery at the radial styloid proximally. The main continuation of the nerve trifurcates distally in the area where the artery crosses underneath the extensor pollicis longus [65].

These nerve branches are carefully exposed and retracted, as is the cephalic vein, which usually has a nerve branch running just underneath it. There are frequent connections between the superficial and deep venous systems at this level. The cephalic vein is the preferred source of venous outflow for microvascular reconstruction because of its position in the dissection field, and it is usually more sizeable than the venae comitantes in this location.

The extensor pollicis longus is then retracted ulnarly, and the extensor pollicis brevis retracted radially. The deep fascia is divided, after which the artery is easily visible and can be followed distally. The dorsal carpal branches and muscular branches to the first dorsal interosseous can be divided to free the artery proximally and distally for improved exposure in preparation for anastomosis. Vessel loops can be used to help position the artery more superficially in the snuffbox for end-to-side anastomosis.

Microsurgical Indications

The radial artery is an advantageous recipient vessel in the distal forearm and snuffbox compared to proximally. Its superficial location, large caliber, and ease of exposure around the wrist make it an ideal donor vessel for all microvascular reconstruction of the dorsal and volar hand with the exception of exclusively ulnar-sided defects. The snuffbox shares similar microsurgical indications to the radial artery at the wrist, and one location can sometimes be used interchangeably for the other. Given its more dorsal location, the snuffbox is more suited to reconstruction of dorsal defects of the hand, thumb, and first webspace, particularly if the flap's vascular pedicle is shorter, such as the lateral arm flap. The snuffbox approach to the radial artery can also access inflow for thumb replantation with a vein graft.

Princeps Pollicis Artery and the Origin of the Deep Palmar Arch

Volar Approach

A curved incision is made from the ulnar side of the base of the thumb at the first web space, along the thenar crease to the wrist between the thenar and hypothenar eminences. The palmar fascia and flexor retinaculum are divided, and the recurrent branch of median nerve, sensory branches of the thumb, and index of the median nerve are identified and carefully protected. The thenar muscles with the motor and sensory branches of the thumb are retracted radially, while the flexor pollicis longus and oblique head of the adductor pollicis are retracted ulnarly. The PPA is identified on the palmar aspect of the first metacarpal bone, under the oblique head of the adductor pollicis. If a wider exposure is required, the lateral insertion of the oblique head of the adductor pollicis can be divided. In this way, the radial indicis artery as well as origin of the palmar arch can be exposed [2].

Dorsal Approach

An incision is made from the ulnar side of the metacarpophalangeal joint of the thumb to the anatomic snuffbox. Tracing the radial artery distally, the first dorsal interosseous muscle is divided. In this way, the origins of the PPA and radialis indicis arteries, as well as the origin of the deep palmar arch, are identified and exposed [2].

Microsurgical Indications

While these vessels can be exposed via the volar and dorsal approaches as described above, use of PPA and deep palmar arch as recipient vessel for microsurgical flap reconstruction is typically not necessary, but may occasionally be used for revascularization of free tissue.

References

1. Haerle M, Häfner H-M, Dietz K, Schaller H-E, Brunelli F. Vascular dominance in the forearm. Plast Reconstr Surg. 2003;111(6):1891–8.
2. Strauch B, Yu HL, Chen ZW, Liebling R. Atlas of microvascular surgery. New York: Thieme Medical Publishers, Inc. 1993; pp. 84–100.
3. Hamahata A, Nakazawa H, Takeuchi M, Sakurai H. Usefulness of radial recurrent artery in transplant of radial forearm flap: an anatomical and clinical study. J Reconstr Microsurg. 2012;28(3):195–8.
4. Lee D, Kim JY, Kim HS, Lee KC, Lee SJ, Kwak HJ. Ultrasound evaluation of the radial artery for arterial catheterization in healthy anesthetized patients. J Clin Monit Comput. 2016;30(2):215–9.
5. Gellman H, Botte MJ, Shankwiler J, Gelberman RH. Arterial patterns of the deep and superficial palmar arches. In: Clinical orthopaedics and related research. Lippincott Williams and Wilkins; 2001. p. 41–46.
6. Serafin D. Atlas of microsurgical composite tissue transplantation. Philadelphia: Saunders; 1996. 813 p.
7. Inoue Y, Taylor GI. The angiosomes of the forearm: anatomic study and clinical implications. Plast Reconstr Surg. 1996;98(2):195–210.
8. Gottlieb LJ, Tachmes L, Pielet RW. Improved venous drainage of the radial artery forearm free flap: use of the profundus cubitalis vein. J Reconstr Microsurg. 1993;9(4):281–6.
9. Timmons MJ. The vascular basis of the radial forearm flap. Plast Reconstr Surg. 1986;77(1):80–92.
10. Shima H, Ohno K, Michi KI, Egawa K, Takiguchi R. An anatomical study on the forearm vascular system. J Cranio-Maxillo-Facial Surg. 1996;24(5):293–9.
11. Selber JC, Sanders E, Lin H, Yu P. Venous drainage of the radial forearm flap: comparison of the deep and superficial systems. Ann Plast Surg. 2011;66(4):347–50.
12. Doscher W, Viswanathan B, Stein T, Margolis IB. Hemodynamic assessment of the circulation in 200 normal hands. Ann Surg. 1983;198(6):776–9.
13. Singh S, Lazarus L, De Gama BZ, Satyapal KS. An anatomical investigation of the superficial and deep palmar arches. Folia Morphol (Warsz). 2017;76(2):219–25.
14. Ramírez AR, Gonzalez SM. Arteries of the thumb: description of anatomical variations and review of the literature. Plast Reconstr Surg. 2012;129(3): 468e–76e.
15. Miletin J, Sukop A, Baca V, Kachlik D. Arterial supply of the thumb: Systemic review. Clinical anatomy. vol. 30. Wiley; 2017. p. 963–73.
16. Webster N, Saint-Cyr M. Flaps based on the dorsal metacarpal artery. Hand clinics. vol. 36. W.B. Saunders; 2020. p. 75–83.
17. Haładaj R, Wysiadecki G, Dudkiewicz Z, Polguj M, Topol M. The high origin of the radial artery (brachioradial artery): its anatomical variations, clinical significance, and contribution to the blood supply of the hand. Biomed Res Int [Internet]. 2018 [cited 2019 Dec 29];2018:1520929. Available from.: http://www.ncbi.nlm.nih.gov/pubmed/29992133.
18. Rodríguez-Niedenführ M, Vázquez T, Nearn L, Ferreira B, Parkin I, Sañudo JR. Variations of the arterial pattern in the upper limb revisited: a morphological and statistical study, with a review of the literature. J Anat. 2001;199(5):547–66.
19. Rodríguez-Baeza A, Nebot J, Ferreira B, Reina F, Pérez J, Sañudo JR, et al. An anatomical study and ontogenetic explanation of 23 cases with variations in the main pattern of the human brachio-antebrachial arteries. J Anat [Internet]. 1995 Oct [cited 2019 Dec 29];187(Pt 2):473–9. Available from.: http://www.ncbi.nlm.nih.gov/pubmed/7592009.
20. Zheng Y, Shao L, Mao J. Bilaterally symmetrical congenital absence of radial artery: a case report. BMC Surg [Internet]. 2014 [cited 2019 Dec 29];14:15. Available from: http://www.ncbi.nlm.nih.gov/pubmed/24650137.
21. Vazquez T, Sañudo JR, Carretero J, Parkin I, Rodríguez-Niedenführ M. Variations of the radial recurrent artery of clinical interest. Surg Radiol Anat. 2013;35(8):689–94.
22. Lai CS, Lin SD, Chou CK, Tsai CC. The reverse lateral arm flap, based on the interosseous recurrent artery, for cubital fossa burns. Br J Plast Surg [Internet]. 1994 [cited 2020 Feb 12];47(5):341–5. Available from.: http://www.ncbi.nlm.nih.gov/pubmed/8087373.
23. Camuzard O, Foissac R, Clerico C, Fernandez J, Balaguer T, Ihrai T, et al. Inferior cubital artery perforator flap for soft-tissue coverage of the elbow anatomical study and clinical application. J Bone Jt Surg Am Vol. 2016;98(6):457–65.
24. Chen SH, Xu DC, Tang ML, Ding HM, Sheng WC, Peng TH. Measurement and analysis of the perforator arteries in upper extremity for the flap design. Surg Radiol Anat. 2009;31(9):687–93.
25. Sham E, Masia JA, Reddy TJ. Vascular analysis of radial artery perforator flaps. Ann Maxillofac Surg. 2018;8(1):66–72.

26. Ho AM, Chang J. Radial artery perforator flap. J Hand Surg Am. 2010;35(2):308–11.
27. Chang S-M, Hou C-L, Zhang F, Lineaweaver WC, Chen Z-W, Gu Y-D. Distally based radial forearm flap with preservation of the radial artery: anatomic, experimental, and clinical studies. Microsurgery [Internet]. 2003 [cited 2019 Dec 30];23(4):328–37. Available from.: http://www.ncbi.nlm.nih.gov/pubmed/12942523.
28. De Taddéo A, Collin B, Hardy H, Guichard B, Trouilloud P, Trost O. Can one harvest a long bone stick in the radial forearm flap? Original radioanatomical and NanoSPECT-CT Bioscan microvascular study. Ann Chir Plast Esthet. 2014;59(3):170–6.
29. Cormack GC, Duncan MJ, Lamberty G. The blood supply of the bone component of the compound osteo-cutaneous radial artery forearm flap-an anatomical study. Br J Plast Surg. 1986;39(2):173–5.
30. Zaidenberg EE, Martinez E, Zaidenberg CR. Vascularized distal radius bone graft for treatment of ulnar nonunion. J Hand Surg. W.B. Saunders. 2018;43:685.e1–e5.
31. Yang J-W, Kim J-S, Lee D-C, Ki S-H, Roh S-Y, Abdullah S, et al. The radial artery superficial palmar branch flap: a modified free thenar flap with constant innervation. J Reconstr Microsurg [Internet]. 2010 [cited 2019 Dec 30];26(8):529–38. Available from.: http://www.ncbi.nlm.nih.gov/pubmed/20648418.
32. Radunovic M, Vukcevic B, Radojevic N, Vukcevic N, Vuksanovic-Bozaric A. Superficial palmar branch of the radial artery: a study of occurrence and diameter. Ann Anat. 2018;220:55–9.
33. Ilić M, Milisavljević M, Maliković A, Laketić D, Erić D, Boljanović J, et al. The superficial palmar branch of the radial artery: a corrosion cast study. Folia Morphol (Warsz). 2018;77(4):649–55.
34. Tang P, Fischer CR. A new volar vascularization technique using the superficial palmar branch of the radial artery for the collapsed scaphoid nonunion. Tech Hand Up Extrem Surg. 2010;14(3):160–72.
35. Shin AY, Bishop AT. Vascular anatomy of the distal radius: implications for vascularized bone grafts. In: Clinical orthopaedics and related research. Lippincott Williams and Wilkins; 2001. p. 60–73.
36. Elzinga K, Chung KC. Volar radius vascularized bone flaps for the treatment of scaphoid nonunion. Hand clinics. vol. 35. W.B. Saunders; 2019. p. 353–363.
37. Gras M, Mathoulin C. Vascularized bone graft pedicled on the volar carpal artery from the volar distal radius as primary procedure for scaphoid non-union. Orthop Traumatol Surg Res [Internet]. 2011 [cited 2020 Feb 15];97(8):800–6. Available from.: http://www.ncbi.nlm.nih.gov/pubmed/22116058.
38. Kakar S, Shin AY. Vascularized bone grafting from the dorsal distal radius for Kienböck's disease: technique, indications and review of the literature. Chir Main. 2010;29(Suppl 1):S104–11.
39. Quaba AA, Davison PM. The distally-based dorsal hand flap. Br J Plast Surg. 1990;43(1):28–39.
40. Gray's anatomy. 37th ed. Angiology. William PL, Worwick R, Dyson M, Bannister LH, editors. New York: Churchill Livingstone; 1989. p. 760–2.
41. Dauphin N, Casoli V. The dorsal metacarpal arteries: anatomical study. Feasibility of pedicled metacarpal bone flaps. J Hand Surg Eur Vol. 2011;36(9):787–94.
42. de Rezende MR, Mattar Júnior R, Cho AB, Hasegawa OH, Ribak S. Anatomic study of the dorsal arterial system of the hand. Rev Hosp Clin Fac Med Sao Paulo. 2004;59(2):71–6.
43. Al-Dhamin A, Cox J, Bissell MB, Marciel-Miranda A, Morris SF. Anatomical study of the princeps pollicis artery perforator flap. Ann Plast Surg. 2016;76(5):564–8.
44. Sherif MM. First dorsal metacarpal artery flap in hand reconstruction. I. Anatomical study. J Hand Surg Am. 1994;19(1):26–31.
45. Zhang X, Shao X, Shen Q, Yu Y, Li Y, Fan A. Use of the first dorsal metacarpal artery-based fascial flap for reconstruction of small defects on the dorsum of the hands. J Hand Surg Am. 2019;44(12):1096.e1–e6.
46. Manabe S, Tabuchi N, Tanaka H, Arai H, Sunamori M. Hand circulation after radial artery harvest for coronary artery bypass grafting. J Med Dent Sci. 2005;52:101–7.
47. Dumanian GA, Segalman K, Mispireta LA, Walsh JA, Hendrickson MF, Wilgis EF. Radial artery use in bypass grafting does not change digital blood flow or hand function. Ann Thorac Surg [Internet]. 1998 [cited 2020 Jan 1];65(5):1284–7. Available from.: http://www.ncbi.nlm.nih.gov/pubmed/9594852.
48. Chim H, Bakri K, Moran SL. Complications related to radial artery occlusion, radial artery harvest, and arterial lines. Hand Clin. W.B. Saunders. 2015;31:93–100.
49. Holman WL, Davies JE, Lin JY, Wang Y, Goldman S, Bakaeen FG, et al. Consequences of radial artery harvest: results of a prospective, randomized, multicenter trial. JAMA Surg. 2013;148(11):1020–3.
50. Jarvis MA, Jarvis CL, Jones PR, Spyt TJ. Reliability of Allen's test in selection of patients for radial artery harvest. Ann Thorac Surg [Internet]. 2000 [cited 2020 Jan 1];70(4):1362–5. Available from.: http://www.ncbi.nlm.nih.gov/pubmed/11081899.
51. Bertrand OF, Carey PC, Gilchrist IC. Allen or no Allen: That is the question!. J Am Coll Cardiol. Elsevier USA. 2014; 63:1842–1844.
52. Jongsma H, Bekken JA, Akkersdijk GP, Hoeks SE, Verhagen HJ, Fioole B. Angiosome-directed revascularization in patients with critical limb ischemia. J Vasc Surg. Mosby Inc. 2017;65:1208–19. e1.
53. Kohonen M, Teerenhovi O, Terho T, Laurikka J, Tarkka M. Is the Allen test reliable enough? Eur J Cardio-Thoracic Surg [Internet]. 2007 [cited 2020 Jan 1];32(6):902–5. Available from: https://academic.oup.com/ejcts/article-lookup/doi/10.1016/j.ejcts.2007.08.017
54. Ruengsakulrach P, Brooks M, Hare DL, Gordon I, Buxton BF. Preoperative assessment of hand circulation by means of doppler ultrasonography and the modified Allen test. J Thorac Cardiovasc Surg. 2001;121(3):526–31.
55. Taylor EM, Wu WW, Ruan Q, Hall EC, Giladi AM, Iorio ML. Coronary Artery Disease Association With Arterial Calcifications on Routine Hand Radiographs. J Hand Surg Am [Internet]. 2019 [cited 2020 Jan 1];44(12):1060–5. Available from.: http://www.ncbi.nlm.nih.gov/pubmed/31677909.
56. Cheun TJ, Jayakumar L, Sheehan MK, Sideman MJ, Pounds LL, Davies MG, et al. From the Vascular Endovascular Surgery Society Outcomes of upper extremity interventions for chronic critical ischemia. [cited 2020 Jan 24]; Available from: https://doi.org/10.1016/j.jvs.2018.04.056.
57. Soldado F, Bertelli J. Free Gracilis Transfer Reinnervated by the nerve to the supinator for the reconstruction of finger and thumb extension in longstanding C7-T1 brachial plexus root avulsion. 2013 [cited 2020 Jan 24.]; Available from: https://doi.org/10.1016/j.jhsa.2013.02.009.
58. Jupiter JB, Gerhard HJ, Guerrero J, Nunley JA, Levin LS. Treatment of segmental defects of the radius with use of the vascularized osteoseptocutaneous fibular autogenous graft. J Bone Jt Surg - Ser A. 1997;79(4):542–50.
59. Windhofer C, Michlits W, Karlbauer A, Papp C. Treatment of segmental bone and soft-tissue defects of the forearm with the free osteocutaneous lateral arm flap. J Trauma Inj Infect Crit Care [Internet]. 2011 [cited 2020 Mar 17];70(5):1286–90. Available from: http://www.ncbi.nlm.nih.gov/pubmed/21610442.
60. Pic Gomis L, Gomis R. Crête iliaque vascularisée et reconstruction du radius distal. Chir Main. 2010;29(Suppl. 1):S49–58.
61. Muramatsu K, Ihara K, Azuma E, Orui R, Goto Y, Shigetomi M, et al. Free vascularized fibula grafting for reconstruction of the wrist following wide tumor excision. Microsurgery [Internet]. 2005 [cited 2020 Mar 17];25(2):101–6. Available from.: http://www.ncbi.nlm.nih.gov/pubmed/15704229.

62. Aldekhayel S, Govshievich A, Neel OF, Luc M. Vascularized proximal fibula epiphyseal transfer for distal radius reconstruction in children: a systematic review [Internet]. Microsurgery. John Wiley and Sons Inc.; 2016 [cited 2020 Mar 17]; 36:705–11. Available from: http://doi.wiley.com/10.1002/micr.22521.
63. Higgins JP, Bürger HK. Medial femoral trochlea osteochondral flap: applications for scaphoid and lunate reconstruction [Internet]. Clin Plast Surg. W.B. Saunders; 2017 [cited 2020 Mar 31];44:257–65. Available from: http://www.ncbi.nlm.nih.gov/pubmed/28340661.
64. Kazmers NH, Thibaudeau S, Levin LS. A Scapholunate Ligament–Sparing technique utilizing the medial femoral condyle corticocancellous free flap to reconstruct scaphoid nonunions with proximal pole avascular necrosis [Internet]. J Hand Surg. W.B. Saunders. 2016 [cited 2020 Mar 31]41:e309–15. Available from: http://www.ncbi.nlm.nih.gov/pubmed/27436566.
65. Robson AJ, See MS, Ellis H. Applied anatomy of the superficial branch of the radial nerve. Clin Anat. 2008;21(1):38–45.

Ulnar Artery

26

Andrew R. Bauder, Zvi Steinberger, L. Scott Levin, and Ines C. Lin

Introduction

The ulnar artery serves as a recipient vessel for microsurgical reconstruction of the upper extremity less frequently than the radial artery owing to its deep location in the proximal two thirds of the forearm. Many surgeons also believe that the ulnar artery is the dominant inflow to the hand, making its use as a recipient vessel potentially more perilous. Furthermore, its close proximity to the ulnar nerve may be a point of concern. Its safe exposure relies on knowledge of its relationship with surrounding structures of critical functional importance.

Applied Anatomy

The ulnar artery is one of two continuations of the brachial artery, the other being the radial artery (also see Chaps. 24 and 25). The brachial artery bifurcates roughly at the level of the radial tuberosity [1]. The smaller radial artery continues on as a more direct extension of the brachial artery, while the ulnar artery comes off at nearly a right angle (Fig. 26.1). The ulnar artery and its branches go on to supply nearly the entire musculature of the forearm aside from the mobile wad.

In the proximal third of the forearm, the ulnar artery dives underneath the deep head of the pronator teres (PT) and takes an oblique course between the flexor digitorum superficialis and profundus muscles to reach the ulnar border of the forearm (Fig. 26.1). From here, its course follows a line drawn between the medial epicondyle and the pisiform, and the vessel lies between the flexor carpi ulnaris (FCU) medially and flexor digitorum superficialis (FDS) laterally. In the distal third of the forearm just proximal to the wrist joint, the 2–3 mm ulnar artery can be palpable immediately radial to the FCU tendon. It is usually accompanied by two venae comitantes; these venae have superficial connections with the overlying medial antebrachial vein volarly and the basilic vein dorsally [2].

At the distal aspect of Guyon's canal, the ulnar artery sends off a deep palmar branch before continuing on to anastomose with the superficial palmar branch of the radial artery to form the superficial arch (Figs. 25.2 and 26.2). The deep palmar branch contributes to the radial dominant deep palmar arch in nearly every patient [3]. After this, the main ulnar artery gives off the ulnar palmar digital artery to the small finger as well as the common digital artery to the fourth webspace [4]. It then continues on as the superficial palmar arch, which interconnects with the superficial palmar branch to form a complete arch in the majority of patients [3]. The superficial arch provides the remaining common digital arteries.

Anatomic Variants

While the ulnar artery usually originates as a bifurcation from the brachial artery in the antecubital fossa about 5 cm distal to the elbow crease, it can originate higher on the brachial or axillary artery. The prevalence of a high origin of the

Supplementary Information The online version of this chapter (https://doi.org/10.1007/978-3-030-75389-4_26) contains supplementary material, which is available to authorized users.

A. R. Bauder
Division of Plastic Surgery, Department of Surgery, University of Pennsylvania, Philadelphia, PA, USA
e-mail: Andrew.bauder@pennmedicine.upenn.edu

Z. Steinberger
Department of Orthopaedic Surgery, University of Pennsylvania, Philadelphia, PA, USA

Department of Hand and Microsurgery, Sheba Medical Center, Tel Hashomer, Israel

L. S. Levin · I. C. Lin (✉)
Division of Plastic Surgery, Department of Surgery, University of Pennsylvania, Philadelphia, PA, USA

Department of Orthopaedic Surgery, University of Pennsylvania, Philadelphia, PA, USA
e-mail: Scott.Levin@pennmedicine.upenn.edu; ines.lin@uphs.upenn.edu

R. Gurunian, R. Djohan (eds.), *Recipient Vessels in Reconstructive Microsurgery*,
https://doi.org/10.1007/978-3-030-75389-4_26

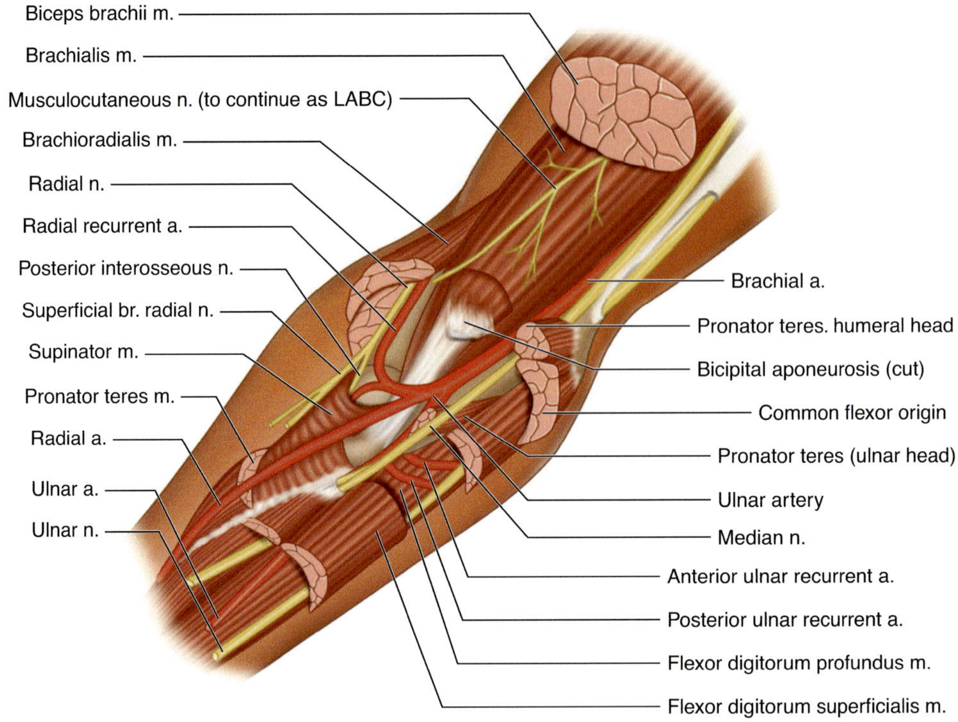

Fig. 26.1 Course of the ulnar and radial arteries with forearm musculature included. The ulnar artery takes an oblique course in the proximal third of the forearm to meet the ulnar nerve

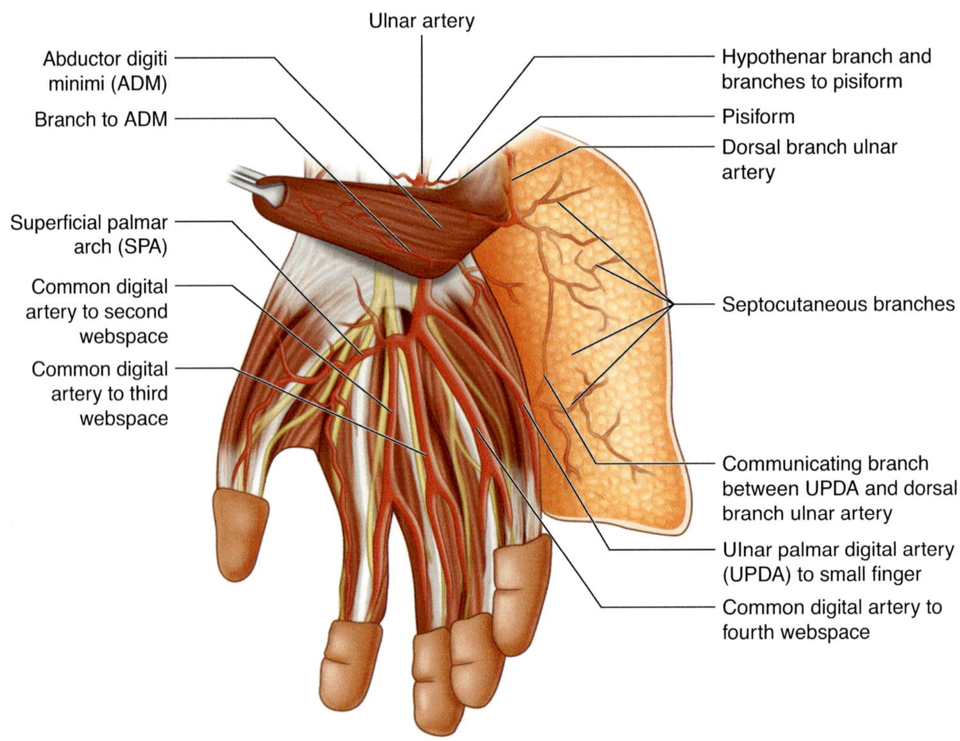

Fig. 26.2 Vascular anatomy of the hypothenar eminence and the superficial palmar arch

ulnar artery is estimated between 1% and 9%, and may vary somewhat based on ethnicity [5–7]. This variant is most common in the Indian population (9%), is least common in Asian populations (1%), and occurs in about 4% of the Caucasian population in Europe [5]. When present, it is usually found in males in the right upper extremity [5].

In cases of a high origin of the ulnar artery, it is almost always superficial and is named the superficial ulnar artery (SUA) for this reason. It passes deep to the antebrachial fascia but superficial to all of the flexor muscles of the forearm except the palmaris longus [6, 7]. It is also located slightly more radial than the normal ulnar artery and can be found just radial to the line between the intermuscular septum of the upper arm and the radial aspect of the pisiform. Very rarely, the ulnar artery may take this superficial course even though it has a normal origin from the brachial artery distal to the elbow crease [8].

This relatively prevalent anatomic variation is important to keep in mind for inadvertent cannulation of the artery during attempted intravenous line placement as well as iatrogenic surgical injury. It also provides the opportunity for easily harvested fasciocutaneous flaps based on the SUA with no septal or intramuscular dissection.

Branches

The branches of the ulnar artery are best organized based on their anatomical location in the forearm, wrist, and hand. They are listed below based on their order of origination traveling distally along the upper extremity.

Forearm

Ulnar Recurrent Arteries

Before giving off the common interosseous artery, the ulnar artery has two branches that travel medially and proximally, named the anterior and posterior ulnar recurrent arteries (Fig. 26.1). Their names reflect their relationship with the medial epicondyle, and the vessels contribute to the vascular network around the medial elbow. The posterior ulnar recurrent artery is the bigger of the two and can be nearly 2 mm in diameter.

These two arteries can originate either as a common trunk or as independent branches from the ulnar artery [9]. The anterior ulnar recurrent artery traverses proximally between the brachialis and PT to anastomose with the inferior ulnar collateral artery. The posterior ulnar recurrent artery comes off the ulnar artery distal to the anterior ulnar recurrent artery and ascends proximally between the flexor digitorum profundus (FDP) and superficialis (FDS) muscles to anastomose with the superior ulnar collateral artery.

Together, the anterior and posterior ulnar recurrent arteries form the basis of the reverse medial arm flap, which is analogous to the reverse lateral arm flap on the radial side. The posterior ulnar recurrent artery usually has a more robust contribution to the flap as it is of larger caliber, has a more discrete anastomosis with the ulnar collateral system, and sends off multiple perforators to the overlying medial arm skin along its course [9, 10]. It also forms the primary vascular pedicle to the ulnar nerve around the elbow [11].

Common Interosseous Artery

The common interosseous artery exists as a short trunk off the ulnar artery just after its divergence from the brachial artery. It is usually less than 2 cm long before branching into the anterior and posterior interosseous arteries, which are named for their relationship with the interosseous membrane between the radius and ulna.

Posterior Interosseous Artery (PIA)

After bifurcating from the common interosseous artery, the posterior interosseous artery penetrates the interosseous membrane and enters the deep posterior compartment of the arm underneath the supinator, 8–10 cm distal to the interepicondylar line of the humerus [12–14]. It travels along the line between the lateral epicondyle and the distal radioulnar joint with the arm in pronation and gives off branches to the deep and superficial posterior (dorsal) compartment musculature as well as the radius and ulna. The PIA is most intimately associated with the posterior interosseous nerve in the proximal third of the forearm, and less so in the distal third of the forearm.

Along this course, the PIA provides numerous septocutaneous perforators along the intermuscular septum between the fifth and sixth extensor compartment muscles (EDM and ECU); these are largest proximally and distally, but relatively diminutive in the middle third of the forearm [13]. Approximately 5 cm proximal to the ulnar styloid, the PIA forms an anastomosis with the recurrent branch of the anterior interosseous artery (AIA) [12, 13, 15]. The reverse PIA flap is based on this recurrent branch of the AIA and captures the vascular territory of the PIA through choke anastomoses in the middle third of the dorsal forearm [13]. This flap is often used to resurface the dorsal hand up to the metacarpophalangeal joint, although some have extended its indications to more distal dorsal finger defects [14, 16].

Interosseous Recurrent Artery (IRA)

The interosseous recurrent artery variably originates from the posterior interosseous artery, from the common interosseous artery, or at the bifurcation of the common interosseous artery into the anterior and posterior interosseous arteries [9]. The IRA ascends proximally underneath the anconeus between the lateral epicondyle and the olecranon to anastomose with the middle collateral artery, also called the posterior collateral artery. It supplies muscular branches to the anconeus and overlying skin along its course. Unlike the true anastomoses between the ulnar recurrent arteries and their associated collateral arteries around the elbow, the anastomosis between the IRA and the middle collateral artery is more often only through choke vessels [9].

Anterior Interosseous Artery (AIA)

The anterior interosseous artery bifurcates from the common interosseous artery and hugs the anterior aspect of the interosseous membrane along its course, supplying the muscles of the deep anterior (volar) compartment of the forearm and the periosteum of the radius [17]. Five centimeters proximal to the ulnar styloid, it branches into an anterior and posterior division. The posterior division immediately penetrates the interosseous membrane and then gives off the dorsal inter- and extra-compartmental arteries as well as the previously mentioned recurrent branch that forms the basis of the reverse PIA flap [18, 19]. The anterior division remains on the volar aspect of the interosseous membrane and, like the posterior division, forms a vascular arcade around the distal radius and ulna to provide the anterograde vascular basis for pedicled bone grafts of the distal radius and ulna.

Muscular Branches

The ulnar artery directly supplies branches to the proximal muscle bellies of the superficial anterior compartment of the forearm, including the PT, FCU, and FDS. All of these muscles except the FCU have a dual supply and are also nourished distally by branches from the radial artery. The deep anterior compartment is mostly supplied by branches from the anterior interosseous artery with occasional contributions from the radial and ulnar arteries. The superficial posterior compartment muscles receive branches from the posterior interosseous artery, while the mobile wad is supplied by the radial and radial recurrent arteries. Finally, the muscles of the deep posterior compartment receive dual supply from the PIA and the dorsal (posterior) branch of the AIA except the supinator, which is also supplied by the radial recurrent artery [20]. In sum, the ulnar artery and its branches (ulnar recurrent and anterior and posterior interosseous arteries) provide some muscular branches to all the compartments of the forearm except the mobile wad.

Septocutaneous Branches

Like the radial artery, the ulnar artery septocutaneous perforators are densest in the proximal and distal thirds of the forearm. These perforators lie in the interval between the FDS and FCU along the line between the medial epicondyle and the pisiform. In the proximal forearm, a reliable perforator is located about 7 cm distal to the medial epicondyle [12]. In the distal forearm, three clinically significant septocutaneous perforators of greater than 0.5 mm diameter are found approximately 5, 10, and 15 cm proximal to the pisiform [21]. The distal two perforators of this group in the distal forearm are almost always septocutaneous, while the proximal perforator sometimes takes a musculocutaneous course through the FCU [21]. A rich subdermal vascular plexus in the middle third of the forearm links the perforators in the distal forearm to those in the proximal forearm [12]. The middle third of the forearm typically lacks cutaneous perforators of clinically significant size.

The distal trio of ulnar septocutaneous perforators (Fig. 26.3) allows for an ulnar forearm flap that is analogous to the radial forearm flap [22]. The ulnar forearm flap carries less hair bearing skin than the radial forearm flap and benefits from a less conspicuous donor site that is more often able to be closed primarily [21, 23]; however, it suffers from a shorter pedicle length. Although the venae comitantes are usually used for venous egress, the superficial system can be utilized by including the basilic vein (dorsal) or the median antebrachial vein (volar).

The distal-most septocutaneous perforator can be used for propeller flap reconstruction of large ulnar-sided wrist defects [24] or as a small neurocutaneous free flap with the inclusion of the cutaneous branches of the medial antebrachial cutaneous nerve or the ulnar sensory nerve [25]. When used for sensate reconstruction of fingertip pulp defects, this ulnar artery neurocutaneous flap has demonstrated better long-term sensibility than the reversed homodigital island flap [26].

Periosteal Branches

While the ulnar artery supplies the main intramedullary nutrient vessel of the ulna about 7 cm distal to the olecranon, the ulnar artery provides no extraosseous vessels until 3 cm proximal to the ulnar styloid. Instead, the entire diaphysis of the ulna is supplied by segmental periosteal branches from the anterior and posterior interosseous arteries [27]. Finally, the rich vascular network of the ulnar carpal branches and the terminal dorsal and volar branches of the AIA supplies the metaphyseal and epiphyseal ulna.

Wrist

Dorsal Branch

The dorsal branch of the ulnar artery accompanies the dorsal branch of the ulnar nerve as it branches from the ulnar nerve about 5–6 cm proximal to the ulnar styloid. It travels on the medial aspect of the ulna with the nerve until it moves dorsally at the level of the pisiform [28]. Here, the ulnar nerve bifurcates, and the ulnar artery gives off branches to the pisiform bone that form the basis of the pisiform vascularized bone flap that has been described for treatment of scaphoid nonunion [28, 29].

Palmar (Volar) Carpal Branches

At the distal edge of the pronator quadratus, the ulnar artery sends off a vessel to form the ulnar half of the palmar carpal arch [18, 30]. This vessel connects with both its radial artery counterpart and indirectly to the anterior division of the anterior interosseous artery. Similarly, over the distal carpal row,

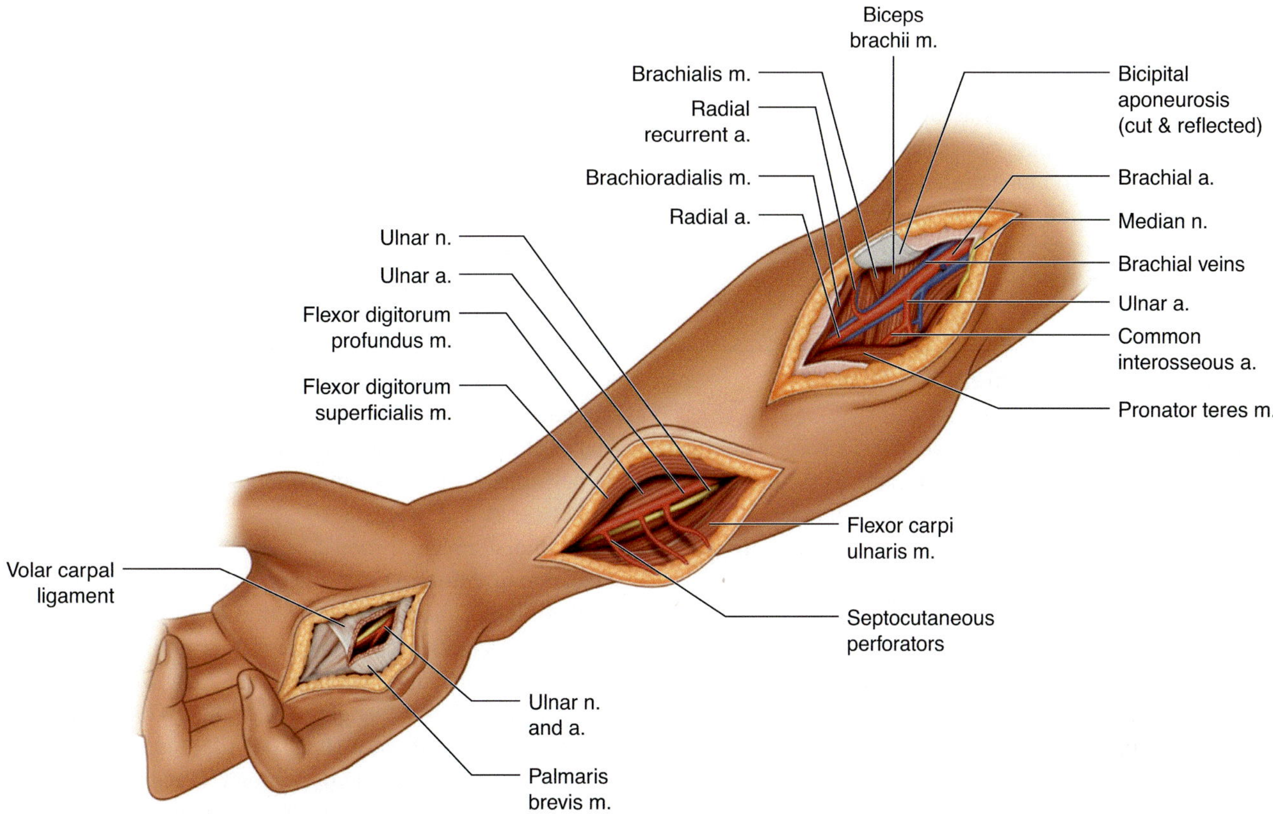

Fig. 26.3 Exposure of the ulnar artery in the forearm: proximally in the cubital fossa, between the FCU and FDS in the middle and distal thirds of the forearm, and distally in Guyon's canal

another arch, the palmar intercarpal arch, is formed. Although they are utilized less frequently than their dorsal analogues, the palmar carpal and intercarpal arches can be used to provide vascularized bone graft from the volar distal radius to reconstruct carpal defects and nonunions [29–31].

Dorsal Carpal Branches

The ulnar artery also contributes to the ulnar half of the dorsal carpal and intercarpal arches, although it has a less robust relationship with the inter- and extra-compartmental vessels than the radial artery. These vessels mostly take an oblique course toward the radial artery after branching from the posterior division of the anterior interosseous artery [18]. The ulnar artery is most intimately associated with the fifth extra-compartmental artery with which it usually has one direct connection proximally and one distally at the intercarpal arch.

Hand

The ulnar artery sends off a number of clinically relevant branches in Guyon's canal (Fig. 26.2). The first is a small hypothenar cutaneous branch immediately radial and distal to the pisiform that supplies the small free hypothenar flap with glabrous skin for fingertip pulp reconstruction [32]. The second is a branch to abductor digiti minimi (ADM) [4]. The third is the ulnar palmar digital artery (UPDA) to the small finger. Five or six septocutaneous perforators originate from the UPDA to the small finger between ADM and the fifth metacarpal [33]. This axially oriented network of perforators forms either a true (70%) or choke (30%) anastomosis with branches from the dorsal branch of the ulnar artery or the previously mentioned intercarpal arch (Fig. 26.2) [34]. The most robust of these perforators is located at the level of the small finger A1 pulley and is reliably greater than 1 mm [33, 34]. It forms the pedicle for the reverse hypothenar flap that can be used for sensate reconstruction of small finger cutaneous defects through inclusion of a division of the dorsal branch of the ulnar nerve. Finally, the ulnar artery sends off one or two volar branches to join the deep palmar arch before continuing on to form the superficial palmar arch [3, 35].

Superficial Palmar Arch

The ulnar artery is the principal supply to the superficial palmar arch, which lies just underneath the palmar aponeurosis (Figs. 25.2 and 26.2). The superficial arch averages 1.8 mm in diameter and reliably provides the common digital arteries to the second, third, and fourth webspaces [3]. It less reliably provides branches to the radial aspect of the index finger, first webspace, and thumb. The common digital branches are nearly the same diameter as the superficial palmar arch. After being joined by the volar metacarpal arteries from the deep palmar arch, these common digital arteries bifurcate into the proper palmar digital arteries. These are the distal-most extent of the ulnar artery and can be found at the mid-axial line of each finger.

Preoperative Assessment

While the ulnar artery is commonly considered the dominant vessel to the hand, its caliber is the same as the radial artery at the wrist [36]. Moreover, its flow margin is less than 10% greater than the radial artery. As such, the arterial system may be more balanced than was originally thought.

In a hand with normal collateral flow between the radial and ulnar arteries, sacrifice of the ulnar artery is relatively inconsequential because of a compensatory increase in flow through the radial artery [37]. Hand perfusion, grip strength, and cold tolerance are all preserved [23, 37]. However, in a hand with abnormal or incomplete connections between the two arteries, sacrifice of the ulnar artery can result in ulceration, ischemia, and paresthesias of the ulnar two digits, similar to some clinical presentations of hypothenar hammer syndrome. As such, preoperative assessment remains critical to avoid these severe sequelae.

Allen Test/Modified Allen Test

The Allen test, first described by Edgar Van Nuys Allen in 1929, was developed to determine the adequacy of the collateral flow between the radial and ulnar arteries to the hand. Irving Wright described the modified Allen test, which is considered superior and is more often used. The wrist is gently flexed, and the elbow is extended, avoiding overextension as it may lead to a false positive. The examiner's fingers externally compress the radial and ulnar arteries simultaneously at the volar wrist of the same extremity, stopping inflow to the hand. Meanwhile, the patient is asked to repeatedly open and close the hand, finishing in a full fist to exsanguinate the hand. The fist is then gently unclenched, and the fingers are allowed to relax in a resting posture in near full extension. The hand should remain white or blanched. At this point, compression is released from the radial artery, and the examiner observes the hand color. Hand color should return within 10 seconds to reflect adequate distal perfusion through the radial artery. The test is repeated again, with compression released from the ulnar rather than the radial artery. Again, reperfusion within 10 seconds is considered normal. It is important that distal hand perfusion through the radial artery is confirmed for safer utilization of the ulnar artery as a recipient vessel, especially if an end-to-end anastomosis is considered.

The reliability of the modified Allen test has come into question in recent years. Opponents argue that it is too subjective, with poor inter-relater reliability [38–40]. Despite these concerns, it has held up in multiple studies as quite specific (>95%), [41, 42], meaning if the Allen test is negative with normal collateral perfusion from the radial artery, it is safe to sacrifice the ulnar artery. The Allen test has not been shown to be nearly as sensitive as it is specific. Thus, if it is positive (abnormal collateral perfusion from the radial artery), it has been suggested that another confirmatory test be performed, such as complete radial and ulnar artery duplex ultrasound [41].

Additional imaging should be considered in patients with select comorbidities. Due to the common nature of coronary artery disease, patients may have intimal disorders and radiographically apparent upper extremity arterial calcifications very early in the disease course and may warrant duplex ultrasonography or CT angiography [43]. While significant peripheral arterial disease (PAD) of the upper extremity is rare [44], a diagnostic angiogram or CT angiogram should be considered for patients with symptomatic upper extremity PAD. Patients with flow limiting vasculitis should be managed similarly. These studies may aid the surgeon with surgical planning or anticipating inflow problems.

When considering reconstructive options, we favor preserving flow through both arteries to the hand when at all possible. An abnormal Allen test is a relative, but not absolute, contraindication for end-to-side anastomosis to the dominant artery during reconstruction. If sacrifice of the ulnar artery is necessary for microvascular anastomosis, perfusion to the hand should always be closely observed intraoperatively when there is still opportunity to revise the anastomosis or reconstruct the artery. In addition, the Allen test can be simulated intraoperatively after the ulnar artery exposure before an arteriotomy is performed. The ulnar artery can be temporarily occluded distally with a vascular clamp after standard methods of exsanguination of the extremity (e.g., with an Esmarch bandage or limb elevation and brachial artery occlusion). With the ulnar artery clamped, distal hand perfusion through the radial artery should be confirmed after the tourniquet has been deflated or removed, and this can also be assessed using a surface Doppler probe at the small finger.

Surgical Site Exposure

Exposure of the ulnar artery derives from knowledge of the applied anatomy and branching pattern above. It is most easily accessed in the distal third of the forearm, while exposure in the cubital fossa can be more challenging due to the deep location and posterior trajectory of the artery.

Cubital Fossa and Proximal Third of the Forearm

A transverse or curvilinear antecubital incision is used to expose the distal brachial artery at its bifurcation into the radial and ulnar arteries (Fig. 26.3, Video 26.1). Once the incision is made, subcutaneous veins must be carefully preserved, as these will likely be candidate recipient veins for microvascular reconstruction. There is a great variation in the venous anatomy in the cubital fossa, but the median cubital, basilic, cephalic, or large interconnecting branches between the deep and superficial venous systems are of adequate caliber for venous anastomosis [2]. At the distal aspect of the incision, the brachioradialis is retracted radially, and PT is retracted ulnarly. The ulnar artery is identified by following the distal brachial artery into the interval between these two muscles. It can be differentiated from the radial artery by its more acute takeoff from the brachial and posterior trajectory underneath the origin of the ulnar (deep) head of the pronator teres (Figs. 26.1 and 26.3, Video 26.1). This muscle separates it from the median nerve. Since anatomic variation is common in this area, it is important to follow the artery posteriorly to the edge of the pronator teres to ensure it has been properly identified. Exposure beyond this point either requires a separate incision or division of the pronator insertion on the ulna.

Microsurgical Indications

While it is technically feasible to access the ulnar artery in the cubital fossa and proximal forearm, there are limited indications because the radial and brachial arteries are easier to expose and prepare as recipient vessels through the same incision. Nevertheless, accessing the ulnar artery at this level could be considered for microvascular inflow of forearm or elbow flap coverage if the ulnar artery is already injured distally and is not providing distal perfusion but is patent proximally.

Middle and Distal Thirds of the Forearm

At the middle and distal forearm, a linear or gently curved incision follows the axis drawn from the medial epicondyle to the pisiform. Distally, the incision should lie just radial to the easily palpable flexor carpi ulnaris tendon. The ulnar artery can be identified by developing the plane between the FCU and FDS muscles (Fig. 26.3, Video 26.1). The FCU is retracted ulnarly, while FDS is retracted radially. The artery joins the ulnar nerve at roughly the midpoint of the forearm and lies lateral to the nerve along its course to the wrist. It is usually accompanied by two venae comitantes, one of which is similar caliber to the artery. The nearest cutaneous venous candidate for outflow is the median antebrachial vein or larger basilic vein.

All nerve branches must be carefully protected during exposure. Twelve to fourteen centimeters proximal to the ulnar styloid, the ulnar nerve gives off a palmar cutaneous branch that innervates the skin overlying the hypothenar eminence [45]. This nerve remains subfascial until just prior to the wrist. In more distal exposures, the dorsal ulnar sensory nerve will also be visualized, branching off the ulnar nerve approximately 5 cm proximal to the ulnar styloid [46, 47].

Microsurgical Indications

The ulnar artery is most commonly accessed for microsurgical reconstruction of the distal third of the forearm and hand. It is used less frequently than the radial artery partially due to the greater distance between the ulnar artery and nearby large caliber cutaneous veins for outflow and partially due to its perception as the dominant vascular inflow to the hand. It is best suited as a donor vessel for reconstruction of defects of the ulnar forearm and hypothenar eminence.

For ulnar defects that require free vascularized bone transfer, bony exposure of the ulna and the ulnar vasculature can be achieved through the same incision between the FCU and FDS. However, in the arm with multiple prior operations, the ulna itself may be accessed directly in the interval between FCU and ECU per standard orthopedic approach, and the pedicle can be tunneled volarly for microvascular anastomosis. For large segment defects, the free fibula remains the mainstay of treatment and can be converted to a double-barrel configuration for treatment of bony loss of both the radius and ulna [48, 49] (also see Chap. 28). Smaller nonunion defects have been effectively treated with the lateral arm [50] or medial femoral condyle flaps [51], while the ulnar head can be replaced with transfer of the second metatarsal head [52].

Guyon's Canal

The volar incision used to access the ulnar artery can be extended across the wrist flexion crease using a Brunner type incision. This incision is extended obliquely onto the hypothenar eminence over the radial aspect of the pisiform. The subcutaneous fat is retracted to reveal palmaris brevis and volar (palmar) carpal ligament, which form the roof of Guyon's canal [53]. These structures are transected to reveal the ulnar neurovascular bundle, with the ulnar artery radial to the ulnar nerve (Fig. 26.3).

Microsurgical Indications

Anastomosis to the ulnar artery in Guyon's canal is well suited to reconstruction of the ulnar fingers and ulnar hand, including the hypothenar eminence. Given the more difficult exposure due to its proximity to the ulnar nerve and the multiple branches from both structures, this approach is usually reserved for flaps with limited pedicle length that will not reach the ulnar artery proximal to the ulnocarpal joint or the radial artery. In addition, this incision is used for vascular sympathectomy and ulnar artery reconstruction for hypothenar hammer syndrome.

References

1. Serafin D. Atlas of microsurgical composite tissue transplantation. Philadelphia: Saunders; 1996. 813 p.
2. Imanishi N, Nakajima H, Aiso S. Anatomic study of the venous drainage architecture of the forearm skin and subcutaneous tissue. Plast Reconstr Surg [Internet]. 2000 Nov [cited 2020 Mar 18];106(6):1287–94. Available from: http://www.ncbi.nlm.nih.gov/pubmed/11083557.
3. Gellman H, Botte MJ, Shankwiler J, Gelberman RH. Arterial patterns of the deep and superficial palmar arches. In: Clinical orthopaedics and related research. Lippincott Williams and Wilkins; 2001. p. 41–46.
4. Murata K, Tamai M, Gupta A. Anatomic study of arborization patterns of the ulnar artery in Guyon's canal. J Hand Surg Am. 2006;31(2):258–63.
5. Dartnell J, Sekaran P, Ellis H. The superficial ulnar artery: incidence and Calibre in 95 cadaveric specimens. Clin Anat. 2007;20(8):929–32.
6. Devansh. Superficial ulnar artery flap. Plast Reconstr Surg. 1996;97(2):420–6.
7. Rodríguez-Niedenführ M, Vázquez T, Nearn L, Ferreira B, Parkin I, Sañudo JR. Variations of the arterial pattern in the upper limb revisited: a morphological and statistical study, with a review of the literature. J Anat. 2001;199(5):547–66.
8. Sirasanagandla SR, Pamidi N, Nayak SB, Jetti R, Thangarajan R. Superficial ulnar artery associated with anomalous origin of the common interosseous and ulnar recurrent arteries. J Clin Diagnostic Res. 2016;10(5):AD01–2.
9. Hayashi A, Maruyama Y. Anatomical study of the recurrent flaps of the upper arm. Br J Plast Surg [Internet]. 1990 [cited 2020 Feb 11];43(3):300–6. Available from: http://www.ncbi.nlm.nih.gov/pubmed/2350635.
10. Maruyama Y, Onishi K, Iwahira Y. The ulnar recurrent fasciocutaneous island flap: Reverse medial arm flap. Plast Reconstr Surg [Internet]. 1987 [cited 2020 Feb 11];79(3):381–7. Available from: http://www.ncbi.nlm.nih.gov/pubmed/3823214.
11. Li M, He Q, Hu Z, Chen S, Lv Y, Liu Z, et al. Applied anatomical study of the vascularized ulnar nerve and its blood supply for cubital tunnel syndrome at the elbow region. Neural Regen Res [Internet]. 2015 1 [cited 2020 Feb 12];10(1):141. Available from: http://www.nrronline.org/text.asp?2015/10/1/141/150723.
12. Sun C, Hou ZD, Wang B, Ding ZH. An anatomical study on the characteristics of cutaneous branches-chain perforator flap with ulnar artery pedicle. Plast Reconstr Surg. 2013;131(2):329–36.
13. Hubmer MG, Fasching T, Haas F, Koch H, Schwarzl F, Weiglein A, et al. The posterior interosseous artery in the distal part of the forearm. Is the term "recurrent branch of the anterior interosseous artery" justified? Br J Plast Surg. 2004;57(7):638–44.
14. Costa H, Pinto A, Zenha H. The posterior interosseous flap – a prime technique in hand reconstruction. The experience of 100 anatomical dissections and 102 clinical cases. J Plast Reconstr Aesthet Surg [Internet]. 2007 [cited 2020 Feb 15];60(7):740–7. Available from: http://www.ncbi.nlm.nih.gov/pubmed/17507303.
15. Hamada R, Shinaoka A, Sugiyama N, Watanabe T, Miura Y, Kimata Y. Recurrent branch of anterior interosseous artery perforator-based propeller flap for distal forearm injuries: report of 2 cases. Microsurgery [Internet]. 2018 [cited 2020 Feb 11];38(8):917–23. Available from: http://www.ncbi.nlm.nih.gov/pubmed/30380173.
16. Brunelli F, Valenti P, Dumontier C, Panciera P, Gilbert A. The posterior interosseous reverse flap: experience with 113 flaps. Ann Plast Surg [Internet]. 2001 [cited 2020 Feb 11];47(1):25–30. Available from: http://www.ncbi.nlm.nih.gov/pubmed/11756799.
17. Hu W, Martin D, Foucher G, Baudet J. [Anterior interosseous flap]. Ann Chir Plast Esthet [Internet]. 1994 [cited 2020 Feb 15];39(3):290–300. Available from: http://www.ncbi.nlm.nih.gov/pubmed/7717663.
18. Shin AY, Bishop AT. Vascular anatomy of the distal radius: implications for vascularized bone grafts. In: Clinical orthopaedics and related research. Lippincott Williams and Wilkins; 2001. p. 60–73.
19. Hasegawa H, Shimizu T, Omokawa S, Kawamura K, Sananpanich K, Mahakkanukrauh P, et al. Vascularized pedicled bone graft from the distal radius supplied by the anterior interosseous artery for treatment of ulnar shaft nonunion: an anatomical study of cadavers and a case report. Microsurgery [Internet]. 2020 [cited 2020 Feb 15];micr.30566. Available from: http://www.ncbi.nlm.nih.gov/pubmed/32048745.
20. Inoue Y, Taylor GI. The angiosomes of the forearm: anatomic study and clinical implications. Plast Reconstr Surg. 1996;98(2):195–210.
21. Yu P, Chang EI, Selber JC, Hanasono MM. Perforator patterns of the ulnar artery perforator flap. Plast Reconstr Surg. 2012;129(1):213–20.
22. Hekner DD, Roeling TAP, Van Cann EM. Perforator anatomy of the radial forearm free flap versus the ulnar forearm free flap for head and neck reconstruction. Int J Oral Maxillofac Surg [Internet]. 2016 [cited 2020 Feb 12];45(8):955–9. Available from: http://www.ncbi.nlm.nih.gov/pubmed/27012603.
23. Chang EI, Liu J. Prospective comparison of donor site morbidity following radial forearm and ulnar artery perforator flap harvest. Plast Reconstr Surg [Internet]. 2020 [cited 2020 Feb 12];1. Available from: http://journals.lww.com/10.1097/PRS.0000000000006790.
24. Jang HS, Lee YH, Kim MB, Chung JY, Seok HS, Baek GH. Fasciocutaneous propeller flap based on perforating branch of ulnar artery for soft tissue reconstruction of the hand and wrist. CiOS Clin Orthop Surg. 2018;10(1):74–9.
25. Jihui JU, Liu Y, Hou R. Ulnar artery distal cutaneous descending branch as free flap in hand reconstruction. Injury. 2009;40(12):1320–6.
26. Tu Q, Liu S, Chen T, Li S, Yan H, Li Z. A comparative study of finger pulp reconstruction using free distal ulnar artery perforator flaps and reverse dorsal Homodigital Island flaps. Ann Plast Surg. 2019;83(6):650–4.
27. Wright TW, Glowczewskie F. Vascular anatomy of the ulna. J Hand Surg Am. 1998;23(5):800–4.
28. Cavusoglu T, Ozden H, Comert A, Yazici I, Acar HI, Tellioglu AT, et al. Topographical anatomy of the dorsal branch of the ulnar nerve and artery: a cadaver study. Surg Radiol Anat. 2011;33(3):229–33.
29. Elzinga K, Chung KC. Volar radius vascularized bone flaps for the treatment of scaphoid nonunion. Hand Clin. W.B. Saunders; 2019;35:353–363.
30. Tang P, Fischer CR. A new volar vascularization technique using the superficial palmar branch of the radial artery for the collapsed scaphoid nonunion. Tech Hand Up Extrem Surg. 2010;14(3):160–72.
31. Gras M, Mathoulin C. Vascularized bone graft pedicled on the volar carpal artery from the volar distal radius as primary procedure for

scaphoid non-union. Orthop Traumatol Surg Res [Internet]. 2011 [cited 2020 Feb 15];97(8):800–6. Available from: http://www.ncbi.nlm.nih.gov/pubmed/22116058.
32. Hwang K, Han JY, Chung IH. Hypothenar flap based on a cutaneous perforator branch of the ulnar artery: an anatomic study. J Reconstr Microsurg [Internet]. 2005 [cited 2020 Feb 9];21(05):297–301. Available from: http://www.thieme-connect.de/DOI/DOI?10.1055/s-2005-871770.
33. Toia F, Marchese M, Boniforti B, Tos P, Delcroix L. The little finger ulnar palmar digital artery perforator flap: anatomical basis. Surg Radiol Anat [Internet]. 2013 [cited 2020 Feb 15];35(8):737–40. Available from: http://www.ncbi.nlm.nih.gov/pubmed/23443276.
34. Hao PD, Zhuang YH, Zheng HP, Yang XD, Lin J, Zhang CL, et al. The ulnar palmar perforator flap: anatomical study and clinical application. J Plast Reconstr Aesthetic Surg. 2014;67(5):600–6.
35. Singh S, Lazarus L, De Gama BZ, Satyapal KS. An anatomical investigation of the superficial and deep palmar arches. Folia Morphol (Warsz). 2017;76(2):219–25.
36. Doscher W, Viswanathan B, Stein T, Margolis IB. Hemodynamic assessment of the circulation in 200 normal hands. Ann Surg. 1983;198(6):776–9.
37. Rodriguez ED, Mithani SK, Bluebond-Langner R, Manson PN. Hand evaluation following ulnar forearm perforator flap harvest: a prospective study. Plast Reconstr Surg [Internet]. 2007 [cited 2020 Feb 12];120(6):1598–601. Available from: http://www.ncbi.nlm.nih.gov/pubmed/18040194.
38. Jarvis MA, Jarvis CL, Jones PR, Spyt TJ. Reliability of Allen's test in selection of patients for radial artery harvest. Ann Thorac Surg [Internet]. 2000 [cited 2020 Jan 1];70(4):1362–5. Available from: http://www.ncbi.nlm.nih.gov/pubmed/11081899.
39. Bertrand OF, Carey PC, Gilchrist IC. Allen or no Allen: that is the question! J Am Coll Cardiol. Elsevier USA; 2014;63:1842–1844.
40. Jongsma H, Bekken JA, Akkersdijk GP, Hoeks SE, Verhagen HJ, Fioole B. Angiosome-directed revascularization in patients with critical limb ischemia. J Vasc Surg. Mosby Inc.; 2017;65:1208–19.e1.
41. Kohonen M, Teerenhovi O, Terho T, Laurikka J, Tarkka M. Is the Allen test reliable enough? Eur J Cardio-Thoracic Surg [Internet]. 2007 [cited 2020 Jan 1];32(6):902–5. Available from: https://academic.oup.com/ejcts/article-lookup/doi/10.1016/j.ejcts.2007.08.017.
42. Ruengsakulrach P, Brooks M, Hare DL, Gordon I, Buxton BF. Preoperative assessment of hand circulation by means of doppler ultrasonography and the modified Allen test. J Thorac Cardiovasc Surg. 2001;121(3):526–31.
43. Taylor EM, Wu WW, Ruan Q, Hall EC, Giladi AM, Iorio ML. Coronary artery disease association with arterial calcifications on routine hand radiographs. J Hand Surg Am [Internet]. 2019 [cited 2020 Jan 1];44(12):1060–5. Available from: http://www.ncbi.nlm.nih.gov/pubmed/31677909.
44. Cheun TJ, Jayakumar L, Sheehan MK, Sideman MJ, Pounds LL, Davies MG, et al. From the Vascular Endovascular Surgery Society Outcomes of upper extremity interventions for chronic critical ischemia. [cited 2020 Jan 24]; Available from: https://doi.org/10.1016/j.jvs.2018.04.056.
45. Tubbs RS, Rogers JM, Loukas M, Cömert A, Shoja MM, Cohen-Gadol AA. Anatomy of the palmar branch of the ulnar nerve: Application to ulnar and median nerve decompressive surgery – Laboratory investigation. J Neurosurg [Internet]. 2011 [cited 2020 Feb 14];114(1):263–7. Available from: http://www.ncbi.nlm.nih.gov/pubmed/20367079.
46. Le Corroller T, Bauones S, Acid S, Champsaur P. Anatomical study of the dorsal cutaneous branch of the ulnar nerve using ultrasound. Eur Radiol. 2013;23(8):2246–51.
47. Puna R, Poon P. The anatomy of the dorsal cutaneous branch of the ulnar nerve. J Hand Surg Eur Vol [Internet]. 2010 [cited 2020 Feb 14];35(7):583–5. Available from: http://www.ncbi.nlm.nih.gov/pubmed/20498153.
48. Saint-Cyr M, Farkas J, Gupta A. Double-barrel free fibula flap for treatment of infected nonunion of both forearm bones. J Reconstr Microsurg [Internet]. 2008 [cited 2020 Apr 6];24(8):583–7. Available from: http://www.ncbi.nlm.nih.gov/pubmed/18925545.
49. Safoury Y. Free vascularized fibula for the treatment of traumatic bone defects and nonunion of the forearm bones. J Hand Surg Am. 2005;30(1):67–72.
50. Windhofer C, Michlits W, Karlbauer A, Papp C. Treatment of segmental bone and soft-tissue defects of the forearm with the free osteocutaneous lateral arm flap. J Trauma Inj Infect Crit Care [Internet]. 2011 [cited 2020 Mar 17];70(5):1286–90. Available from: http://www.ncbi.nlm.nih.gov/pubmed/21610442.
51. Fei W, Danmou X, Dong R, Wei F, Eberlin KR, Yan C, et al. Free vascularized medial femoral condyle corticocancellous flap for treatment of challenging upper extremity nonunions. J Reconstr Microsurg [Internet]. 2015 [cited 2020 Apr 6];31(2):124–31. Available from: http://www.ncbi.nlm.nih.gov/pubmed/25265070.
52. Cavadas PC, Thione A. Ulnar head reconstruction with microvascular second metatarsal. Plast Reconstr Surg Glob Open [Internet]. 2017 [cited 2020 Apr 6];5(4):e1284. Available from: http://www.ncbi.nlm.nih.gov/pubmed/28507853.
53. Cobb TK, Carmichael SW, Cooney WP. Guyon's canal revisited: an anatomic study of the carpal ulnar neurovascular space. J Hand Surg Am [Internet]. 1996 [cited 2020 Mar 18];21(5):861–9. Available from: http://www.ncbi.nlm.nih.gov/pubmed/8891986.

Recipient Vessels: Humerus Reconstruction

27

Margaret S. Roubaud and Edward I. Chang

Introduction

Bony reconstruction of the extremity has undergone tremendous advancements over time, and the free fibula flap has emerged as the workhorse flap for reconstruction of upper and lower extremity bone defects resulting from trauma and osteomyelitis and following oncologic resection [1–4]. While there are alternate vascularized osseous and osteocutaneous flaps such as the scapula and iliac crest or non-vascularized bone grafts, this chapter will focus on the use of the fibula for bony reconstruction of humeral defects.

The fibula has become the bone flap of choice as the fibula has distinct advantages compared to other options. Given the reliable anatomy and ability to harvest a long straight segment of bone with sufficient cortical bone, the fibula is well-suited for reconstruction of long bone defects. Further, the pedicle to the fibula is consistent, providing vessels of suitable length and caliber for microsurgical anastomoses. While there are inherent benefits to the fibula itself, achieving high success of bony union and limb salvage is also clearly dependent on perfusion via reliable recipient vessels [5].

Preoperative Assessment

As with any patient undergoing a microvascular free tissue transfer, a thorough history and physical are warranted. In particular, prior medical history and comorbidities that may suggest peripheral vascular disease and associated habits such as smoking should be documented. With patients undergoing oncologic resection, documentation of adjuvant therapies is also critical as prior radiation and chemotherapy can have an impact not only on bony union but also on adequate healing of the overlying soft tissue. Previous surgeries should be documented in the upper extremity as well as the donor site.

Regarding the donor site, a thorough vascular exam is also warranted. If the dorsalis pedis and posterior tibial pulse are not both strongly palpable, the authors recommend obtaining an angiogram to document adequate perfusion and runoff to the lower extremity. While a normal peripheral vascular exam does confirm adequate perfusion of the leg, it does not rule out the possibility of the anatomic variation peronea magnum where the peroneal vessels are the primary blood supply to the lower leg. In general, the authors do not obtain routine imaging of the lower extremity unless warranted by an abnormal clinical exam [6]. As the peroneal vessels are the primary blood supply to the fibula, sacrifice of the peroneal vessels during harvest of the fibula can have devastating consequences. However, in the setting that the anterior tibial vessels are utilized to perfuse the fibular head and epiphysis for a vascularized growth plate transfer, it is also critical to confirm patency of the anterior tibial vessels via a palpable dorsalis pedis pulse and also to ensure there is adequate perfusion if the anterior tibial vessels are ligated. Again, in the setting of prior trauma, an abnormal peripheral vascular exam, or numerous prior surgeries in the lower extremity, an angiogram is recommended.

Regarding the upper extremity, previous operations should be confirmed in particular whether patients have undergone prior resections for malignancy or perhaps prior interventions in the setting of trauma. The patient's hand dominance should also be noted, and the physical exam should include a thorough neurovascular exam with documentation of distal radial and ulnar pulses and an Allen's test to confirm dominance. The physical exam should also document range of motion, strength, and any sensory deficits. The overlying skin should also be examined for prior scars, any sequelae of radiation, and the pliability of the overlying soft tissue. In the setting or prior radiation, consider should be given to the possibility of needed additional soft tissue coverage of the construct. Particularly, as hardware will be necessary in nearly all cases, it is imperative

M. S. Roubaud · E. I. Chang (✉)
Department of Plastic Surgery, The University of Texas MD Anderson Cancer Center, Houston, TX, USA
e-mail: MSRoubaud@mdanderson.org; eichang@mdanderson.org

R. Gurunian, R. Djohan (eds.), *Recipient Vessels in Reconstructive Microsurgery*,
https://doi.org/10.1007/978-3-030-75389-4_27

to provide stable, durable coverage to minimize risks of extrusion and infection of the hardware.

Imaging studies should be reviewed of the upper extremity to determine the extent and location of the anticipated defect. Defects of the diaphysis are ideal for reconstruction using a segment of the fibula which is straight and will hypertrophy with time. For short segmental defects of the diaphysis, some have reported performing a double-barrel technique where two fibula segments are utilized to bridge the bony defect. In the setting of a more proximal defect or resection, consideration should be given toward reconstruction of the humeral head and also the growth plate in pediatric patients. In this setting, the fibular head can be harvested with the flap in order to reconstruct the glenohumeral joint and also for transfer of the epiphysis in patients who have not yet reached skeletal maturity. Discussion with the resecting surgeon or the orthopedic surgeon to determine the best modality of reconstruction is imperative to help design and plan the harvest of the fibula flap.

Imaging of the vasculature should be considered in the setting of an abnormal pulse exam, or in the setting of prior trauma or surgeries. In particular, with crush, penetrating, blast, or other traumatic injuries, it is critical that appropriate recipient vessels are identified and also a secondary option if the primary recipients are not available. In the upper arm, there is a relative paucity of available recipients as the brachial artery represents the primary vascular supply in the upper arm. In patients who perhaps have had a long-term catheter or port in the affected side for either long-term antibiotics or chemotherapy, consideration should also be given to a venous duplex to confirm patent venous outflow in the upper extremity. However, in the absence of clinical findings, the likelihood of a venous thrombosis is likely low.

Recipient Vessels

In the upper arm, there are a limited number of available recipient vessels; however, some options can be considered depending on the extent of the resection. For diaphyseal defects and midshaft defects, the brachial artery is the primary inflow vessel, and an end-to-side anastomosis is always a consideration. The brachial artery is the continuation of the subclavian artery which becomes the axillary artery, and then the brachial artery beyond the teres major muscle [7–9] (also see Chap. 24). However, there are potentially some branches off the brachial artery than can be considered if they are available. The profunda brachii represents a reasonable recipient as one of the larger caliber branches of the brachial artery and will be the source of the radial collateral artery which can also serve as a recipient artery. The superior ulnar collateral artery also arises from the main brachial artery and can be used as a potential recipient artery. The radial and ulnar collateral arteries form anastomoses with the radial and ulnar recurrent arteries respectively more distally toward the antecubital fossa, and can also serve as recipient vessels for more distal defects. For more proximal defects, the circumflex humeral artery can be used, but this would be in the setting of a very proximal defect where reconstruction would aim to reconstruct the glenohumeral joint. In this setting, potentially the distal continuation of branches from the axillary artery can be used such as the thoracodorsal or the lateral thoracic arteries.

The outflow of the arm can progress through the deep system or the superficial system. The venae comitantes of the brachial artery are typically of reasonable size to serve as the recipient veins. Other possible outflow vessels include the cephalic vein or the basilic vein, both of which can be divided distally for more distal defects, but the vessels can also be rotated to fibula pedicle more proximally with relative ease as well. While the arterial anastomosis can be performed in an end-to-side orientation to the brachial artery or perhaps end-to-end to a branch of the brachial artery, the venous anastomosis should always be performed in an end-to-end fashion if possible.

As with any microvascular anastomosis, the use of a vein graft or creating an arteriovenous (AV) loop is always an option. Depending on the length that is needed, a number of different options for vein graft are available. The most commonly used donor site is the saphenous vein that can provide a long length of vein of reasonable caliber, particularly if the vein is harvested more proximally in the thigh. A cautionary note on the use of the saphenous vein is that the vein has a very thick wall and does not dilate readily and perhaps is better suited for an arterial graft rather than for a venous anastomosis. However, when a long length is needed, the saphenous vein still represents the most accessible donor site. Alternatively, the cephalic vein is also a readily usable donor vein, but clearly, one would not use the cephalic vein in the ipsilateral arm if a venous outflow vessel is needed. Another consideration which can be used and would not incur any additional donor site or burn the bridge in the ipsilateral arm would be the second venae comitantes (VC) of the peroneal vessels. In general, the authors perform a single venous anastomosis, leaving the second VC as a potential donor vein if needed.

Humerus Reconstruction with Vascularized Fibula

The use of the fibula for humerus reconstruction has been well-described in the literature with high success rates for achieving bony union and for limb preservation. A number of different approaches have been described, but no definitive large-volume studies exist comparing the different approaches. However, there is no question that vascularized bony reconstruction is superior to non-vascularized bone grafts [10]. The fibula can be used to bridge the diaphyseal defect and fixated in place with an intercalary component in the remaining proximal and distal ends of the remaining humerus as a single segment, or for shorter defects, an osteotomy can be performed in the fibula creating two segments to bridge the defect in a double-barrel orientation [11–14]. In the setting that an allograft is used to span the humeral defect, a vascularized fibula flap can also be used both as an onlay and as an intercalary strut to further buttress the reconstruction. Studies have demonstrated improved outcomes with this approach compared to allograft alone as the vascularized fibula aids in faster revascularization and remodeling of the bony construct [15–17].

Despite the variety of approaches to humerus reconstruction using the free fibula flap, the overwhelming consensus demonstrates overall excellent long-term results with high restoration of function in the majority of studies [18–20]. Aside from providing adequate bone stock for reconstruction of the diaphysis, the fibula flap can also be harvested as an osteocutaneous flap or as a chimeric flap including the soleus or flexor hallucis longus muscle if additional soft tissue is needed for skin coverage or additional bulk over the hardware. Further, the fibula flap also adds the versatility of an epiphyseal growth plate transfer in pediatric patients [21–23]. In order to maximize the perfusion of the proximal fibula including the epiphysis, the flap elevation is modified compared to the traditional harvest for the diaphysis of the fibula which is perfused by the peroneal vessels. The proximal fibula including the growth plate is supplied by branches of the anterior tibial artery, and therefore, the dissection much proceed more proximally paying careful attention not to interrupt the nutrient vessels or the periosteal blood supply to the fibular head [24, 25]. In addition, with the proximal dissection, the common peroneal nerve should also be identified and carefully preserved during the fibula harvest.

Reconstruction of the proximal humerus in children providing vascularized growth plate transfer is similar to fibular head transfer for reconstruction of the glenohumeral joint in adult patients. Studies have demonstrated high success rates with proximal humerus reconstruction achieving acceptable range of motion and mobility, also maintaining function of the upper extremity in these patients [26–28]. Given the proximal nature of the dissection and the use of the anterior tibial vessels, the pedicle length is considerably shorter than the peroneal vessels used for midshaft reconstruction. In this setting, more proximal recipient vessels will be necessary, and branches arising from the axillary artery and associated veins should be used. Branches arising from the subscapular axis such as the thoracodorsal vessels can serve as recipient vessels which are preferred compared to proceeding with an end-to-side anastomosis to the axillary vessels.

Dissection of the thoracodorsal vessels is generally familiar territory for most plastic reconstructive surgeons and microsurgeons as the pedicle for the latissimus dorsi flap. Most reconstructive microsurgeons are facile at the dissection and anatomy given the use of the free latissimus dorsi muscle for reconstruction of extremity or scalp defects or the pedicle latissimus dorsi myocutaneous flap for breast reconstruction. While the thoracodorsal artery will likely be a reasonable size match for the peroneal or anterior tibial arteries, the VC of the peroneal artery may be larger than the more distal thoracodorsal vein. In this setting, as previously noted, the cephalic or basilic vein can be ligated distally with still sufficient caliber and transposed more proximally to serve as an outflow vessel for the venous anastomosis.

In certain instances, particularly in compound fractures and polytrauma, or following oncologic resection where the extremity has undergone adjuvant radiation therapy, there may be a need for additional soft tissue coverage along with the bony reconstruction. The peroneal vascular pedicle also provides branches to the surrounding musculature which can be included in the flap in a chimeric fashion. Alternatively, studies have demonstrated very reliable anatomy of perforators arising from the peroneal vessels that supply the overlying skin allowing harvest of the skin that can be used not only to help achieve closure of the incision with healthy vascularized, non-irradiated tissue but also to help serve as a monitoring segment to confirm robust perfusion of the bone construct [29].

Complications

As with any microvascular operation, the most dreaded complication is a microvascular thrombosis resulting in compromised perfusion of the free flap. Whether one opts to proceed with emergent exploration and attempt flap salvage and revascularization is surgeon dependent, and the decision to proceed with prolonged surgery to attempt salvaging the fibula flap versus leaving the fibula as a bone graft is multifactorial and dependent on discussion with the multidisciplinary team. This may increase the risks of other complications such as nonunion or infection in the setting of prior radiation, hardware placement, and non-vascularized tissue. Other long-term complications include hardware failure or fracture of the fibula flap which would mandate further surgery. Restrictions in range of motion may occur particularly in the setting of arthrodesis and resection of the humeral head and glenohumeral joint. Potential complications that are case specific may be osteomyelitis in the trauma cases or potentially recurrence following oncologic resection [30].

Regarding the donor site, harvest of the fibula is generally well tolerated with low risks. Occasionally, patients may notice difficulty with mobility of the great toe as the flexor hallucis longus muscle must be disinserted in order to harvest the fibula. However, despite these issues, most patients are able to return to their baseline level of activity without restrictions and limitations in their ability to ambulate following harvest of the fibula [31].

Summary

The free fibula flap represents the workhorse flap for long bone reconstruction including the humerus. With reliable vascular anatomy, adequate bone stock, potential for including soft tissue, and limited donor site morbidity, the free fibula is one, if not the ideal, option for humeral reconstruction. Modifications including the ability to double barrel the bone or transfer the growth plate in pediatric patients and reconstruction of the joint are attractive options demonstrating the versatility of the free fibula flap.

Case Example

A 12-year-old boy diagnosed with an osteosarcoma of the right humerus who completed induction chemotherapy and radiation was anticipated to undergo a segmental resection of the humerus with preservation of the growth plate. A free fibula osteocutaneous flap was harvested to reconstruct the bony defect and for skin closure (Fig. 27.1). The bony defect was reconstructed with internal fixation (Fig. 27.2). The arterial anastomosis was completed in an end-to-side fashion to the brachial artery with the use of a vein graft, while the venous anastomosis was completed in an end-to-end fashion

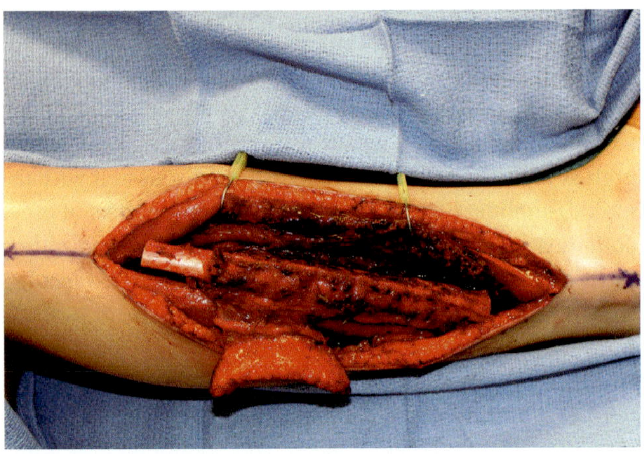

Fig. 27.1 Free fibula osteocutaneous flap harvested from the ipsilateral right leg for reconstruction of the humeral defect. A skin paddle was harvested to assist with skin closure given the prior radiation and also for postoperative monitoring

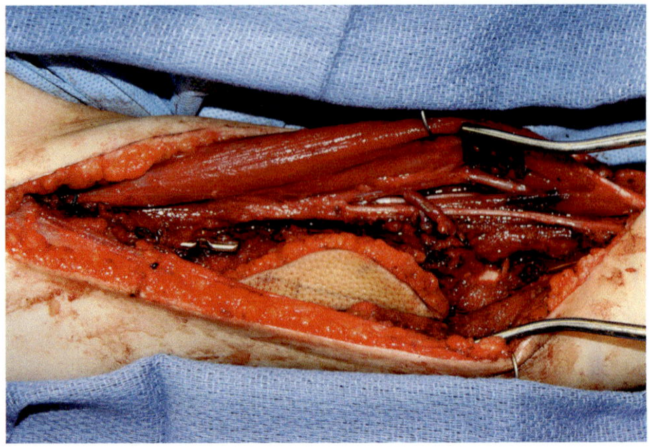

Fig. 27.2 Free fibula flap fixated in place with hardware. Note the arterial anastomosis was completed with the use of a vein graft, while the venous anastomosis was completed in an end-to-end fashion to the recipient vein

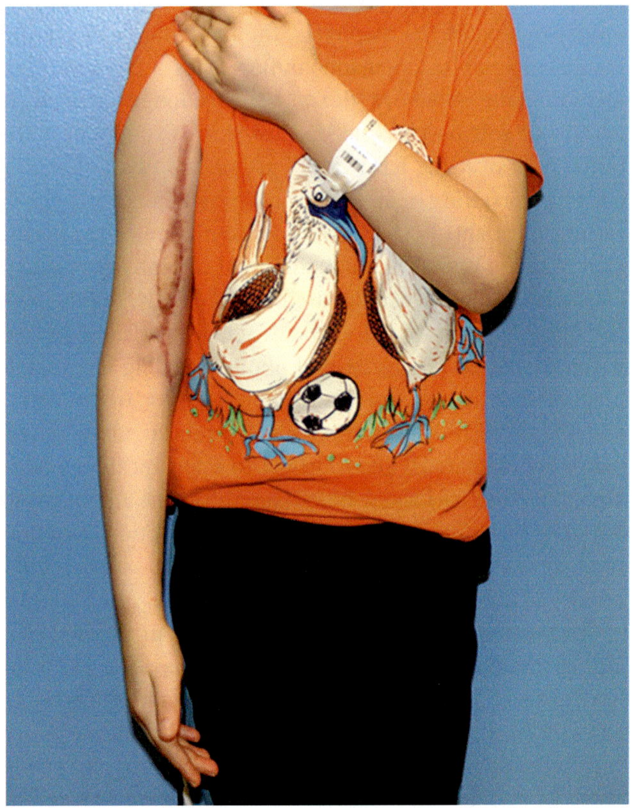

Fig. 27.3 Postoperative photo demonstrating healed skin paddle without evidence of infection, hardware extrusion, or failed fibula flap

to one of the venae comitantes of the brachial artery using a venous coupler (Synovis Micro Companies Alliance, Inc., Birmingham AL). The patient healed with an uneventful hospital course and has achieved bony union with normal function of his dominant right arm (Figs. 27.3 and 27.4).

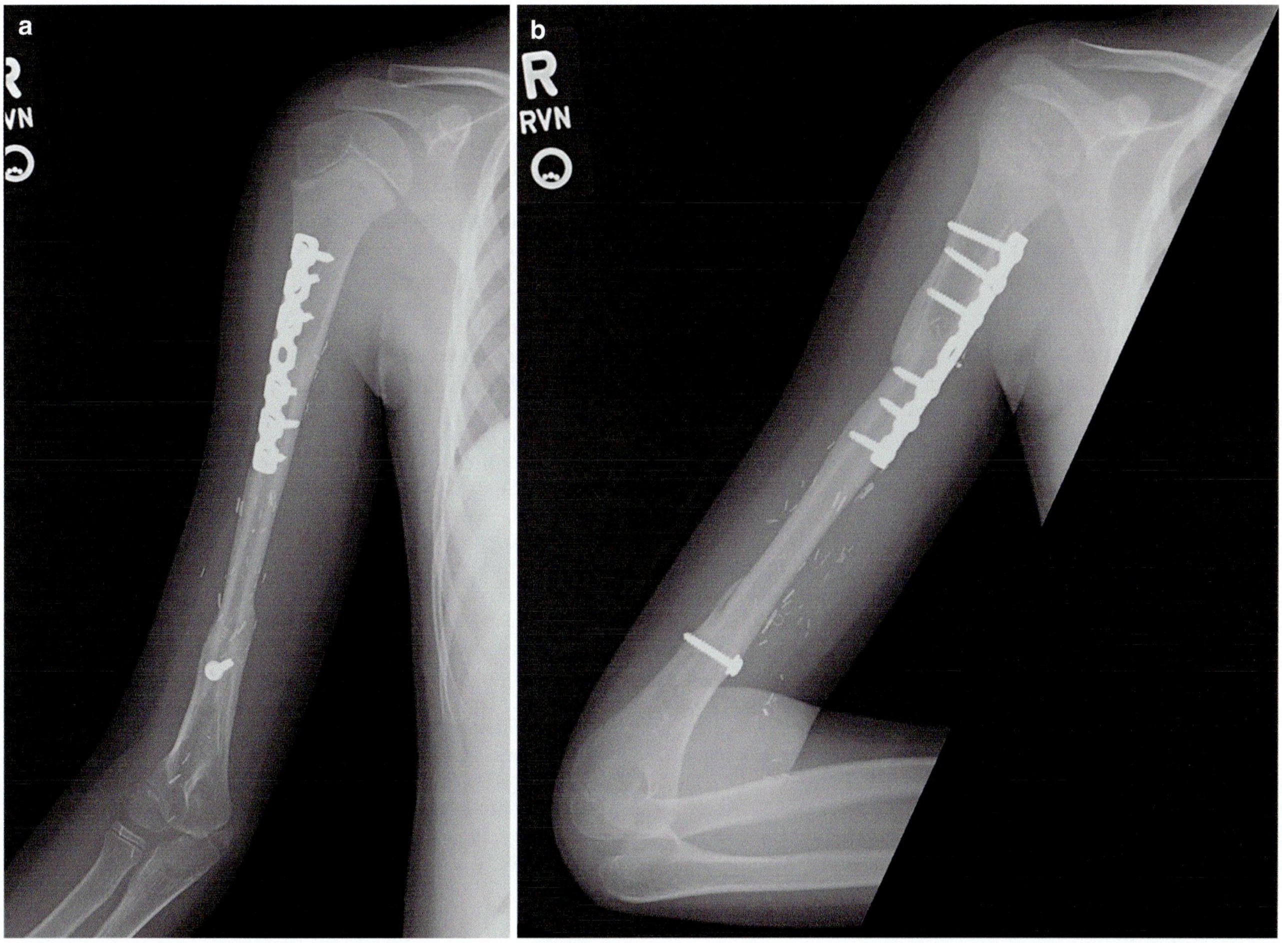

Fig. 27.4 Radiographic imaging of the arm demonstrating appropriate alignment and bony union of free fibula flap to the remaining humerus with hypertrophy of the transferred fibula ((**a**) anterior and (**b**) lateral views)

References

1. Taylor GI, Corlett RJ, Ashton MW. The evolution of free vascularized bone transfer: a 40-year experience. Plast Reconstr Surg. 2016;137(4):1292–305.
2. Houdek MT, Wagner ER, Wyles CC, Nanos GP 3rd, Moran SL. New options for vascularized bone reconstruction in the upper extremity. Semin Plast Surg. 2015;29(1):20–9.
3. Rose PS, Shin AY, Bishop AT, Moran SL, Sim FH. Vascularized free fibula transfer for oncologic reconstruction of the humerus. Clin Orthop Relat Res. 2005;438:80–4.
4. Claxton MR, Houdek MT, Tibbo ME, Wagner ER, Bakri K, Moran SL. Utility of free vascularized fibular flaps to treat radiation-associated nonunions in the upper extremity. J Plast Reconstr Aesthet Surg. 2020;73(4):633–7.
5. Landau MJ, Badash I, Yin C, Alluri RK, Patel KM. Free vascularized fibula grafting in the operative treatment of malignant bone tumors of the upper extremity: a systematic review of outcomes and complications. J Surg Oncol. 2018;117(7):1432–9.
6. Alolabi N, Dickson L, Coroneos CJ, Farrokhyar F, Levis C. Preoperative angiography for free fibula flap harvest: a meta-analysis. J Reconstr Microsurg. 2019;35(5):362–71.
7. Breeland G, Alshuqayfi HA. Anatomy, shoulder and upper limb, Profunda Brachii Artery StatPearls [Internet]. Treasure Island (FL): StatPearls Publishing; 2020 Jan-2019 May 30.
8. Epperson TN, Varacallo M. Anatomy, Shoulder and Upper Limb, Brachial Artery StatPearls [Internet] Treasure Island (FL): StatPearls Publishing; 2020 Jan-2019 Jan 4.
9. Shenoy S. Surgical anatomy of upper arm: what is needed for AVF planning. J Vasc Access. 2009;10(4):223–32.
10. Estrella EP, Wang EH. A comparison of vascularized free fibular flaps and nonvascularized fibular grafts for reconstruction of long bone defects after tumor resection. J Reconstr Microsurg. 2017;33(3):194–205.
11. Wright TW, Miller GJ, Vander Griend RA, Wheeler D, Dell PC. Reconstruction of the humerus with an intramedullary fibular graft. A clinical and biomechanical study. J Bone Joint Surg Br. 1993;75(5):804–7.
12. Chang DW, Weber KL. Use of a vascularized fibula bone flap and intercalary allograft for diaphyseal reconstruction after resection of primary extremity bone sarcomas. Plast Reconstr Surg. 2005;116(7):1918–25.
13. Tang CH. Reconstruction of the bones and joints of the upper extremity by vascularized free fibular graft: report of 46 cases. J Reconstr Microsurg. 1992;8(4):285–92.

14. Wada T, Usui M, Isu K, Yamawakii S, Ishii S. Reconstruction and limb salvage after resection for malignant bone tumour of the proximal humerus. A sling procedure using a free vascularised fibular graft. J Bone Joint Surg Br. 1999;81(5):808–13.
15. Li J, Wang Z, Pei GX, Guo Z. Biological reconstruction using massive bone allograft with intramedullary vascularized fibular flap after intercalary resection of humeral malignancy. J Surg Oncol. 2011;104(3):244–9.
16. Li J, Chen G, Lu Y, Zhu H, Ji C, Wang Z. Factors influencing osseous union following surgical treatment of bone tumors with use of the Capanna technique. J Bone Joint Surg Am. 2019;101(22):2036–43.
17. Zaretski A, Amir A, Meller I, Leshem D, Kollender Y, Barnea Y, Bickels J, Shpitzer T, Ad-El D, Gur E. Free fibula long bone reconstruction in orthopedic oncology: a surgical algorithm for reconstructive options. Plast Reconstr Surg. 2004;113(7):1989–2000.
18. del Piñal F, Innocenti M. Evolving concepts in the management of the bone gap in the upper limb. Long and small defects. J Plast Reconstr Aesthet Surg. 2007;60(7):776–92.
19. Friedrich JB, Moran SL, Bishop AT, Shin AY. Free vascularized fibula grafts for salvage of failed oncologic long bone reconstruction and pathologic fractures. Microsurgery. 2009;29(5):385–92.
20. Saleh R, Yurianto H, Pasallo P, Guatama A, Subagio ES. Good functional outcome evaluation of free vascularized fibular head graft (FVFHG) as treatment after resection of giant cell tumor (GCT) campanacci 3 at proximal humerus: a case report. Int J Surg Case Rep. 2019;61:254–8.
21. Pho RW, Patterson MH, Kour AK, Kumar VP. Free vascularised epiphyseal transplantation in upper extremity reconstruction. J Hand Surg Br. 1988;13(4):440–7.
22. Innocenti M, Ceruso M, Manfrini M, Angeloni R, Lauri G, Capanna R, Bufalini C. Free vascularized growth-plate transfer after bone tumor resection in children. J Reconstr Microsurg. 1998;14(2):137–43.
23. Erdmann D, Garcia RM, Blueschke G, Brigman BE, Levin LS. Vascularized fibula-based physis transfer for pediatric proximal humerus reconstruction. Plast Reconstr Surg. 2013;132(2):281e–7e.
24. Innocenti M, Delcroix L, Romano GF. Epiphyseal transplant: harvesting technique of the proximal fibula based on the anterior tibial artery. Microsurgery. 2005;25(4):284–92.
25. Stevenson JD, Doxey R, Abudu A, Parry M, Evans S, Peart F, Jeys L. Vascularized fibular epiphyseal transfer for proximal humeral reconstruction in children with a primary sarcoma of bone. Bone Joint J. 2018;100-B(4):535–41.
26. Shuck J, Wood BC, Zarella C, Oh AK, Henshaw RM, Rogers GF. Near-complete Humerus reconstruction in the pediatric patient with vascularized free fibula transfer. Plast Reconstr Surg Glob Open. 2016;4(12):e1143.
27. Scaglioni MF, Chang EI, Gur E, Barnea Y, Meller I, Kollander Y, Bickels J, Dadia S, Zaretski A. The role of the fibula head flap for joint reconstruction after osteoarticular resections. J Plast Reconstr Aesthet Surg. 2014;67(5):617–23.
28. Onoda S, Sakuraba M, Asano T, Miyamoto S, Beppu Y, Chuman H, Kawai A, Nakatani F, Kimata Y. Use of vascularized free fibular head grafts for upper limb oncologic reconstruction. Plast Reconstr Surg. 2011;127(3):1244–53.
29. Yu P, Chang EI, Hanasono MM. Design of a reliable skin paddle for the fibula osteocutaneous flap: perforator anatomy revisited. Plast Reconstr Surg. 2011;128(2):440–6.
30. Arai K, Toh S, Tsubo K, Nishikawa S, Narita S, Miura H. Complications of vascularized fibula graft for reconstruction of long bones. Plast Reconstr Surg. 2002;109(7):2301–6.
31. Momoh AO, Yu P, Skoracki RJ, Liu S, Feng L, Hanasono MM. A prospective cohort study of fibula free flap donor-site morbidity in 157 consecutive patients. Plast Reconstr Surg. 2011;128(3):714–20.

Recipient Vessels: Ulna Reconstruction

28

Gokhan Sert and Hung-Chi Chen

Introduction

The most important contribution of the forearm to the hand and upper extremity function is its rotational movement: supination and pronation. This motion requires coordinated movement of the proximal radioulnar joint (PRUJ), distal radioulnar joint (DRUJ), and intact interosseous membrane with stable radius and ulna. Disruption of any of these components would potentially deteriorate forearm functions. The ulnar head serves as an anatomical point of origin and insertion for important wrist stabilizer ligaments of DRUJ. Besides, distal ulna carries 20% of the load transferred from the carpus to forearm [1]. Thus, distal ulnar resections lead to wrist instability which results in pain, restricted movement, and weakness. Shortening of the ulna causes loss of grip and torsional strength of the forearm which is known as anteroposterior instability of the wrist. Impingement of the proximal stump of the ulna towards the radius may cause progressive pain. Ulnar coronoid has an important role in elbow stabilization, and ulnohumeral articulation is one of the primary static constraints for stability of the elbow joint which creates flexion and extension of the forearm. Therefore, anatomical and functional integrity of the ulna is mandatory for functioning upper extremity.

Small and noncomplex defects of the ulna can be successfully treated with conventional nonvascularized bone grafting. This method necessitates a well vascularized wound bed without infection and long immobilization time to allow graft incorporation by the process called creeping substitution. With the advances in microsurgery, transfer of a vascularized bone segment became possible. Since its first introduction by Taylor et al. in 1975, free vascularized fibula transfer has gained wide popularity for treating a variety of bone defects [2]. The advantages of vascularized bone transfers over conventional bone grafts are well known [3]. Vascularized bone can survive in poorly vascularized or potentially infected beds. Bony healing is superior because healing process does not include necrosis and regeneration sequences (creeping substitution) as in bone grafts. Structural integrity and strength of the transferred bone are preserved through the healing process. For this reason, nonunion or malunion rates are lower, and vascularized bone can allow early active mobilization of the extremity. Moreover, epiphyseal transfers have become possible with improved anatomical knowledge of vascularized bone transfers. The most popular option for ulna reconstruction is fibula osseous or osseocutaneous free flap. Additionally, various donor sites for vascularized bone transfer have been reported in the literature [4, 5]. Other flaps such as scapular flap, iliac flap, osseocutaneous radial forearm flap, osseocutaneous lateral arm flap, and second metatarsal flap can also be used in certain indications of ulnar defects. Major arteries of the forearm can provide robust and reliable inflow for transferred fibula. However, presence of an anatomical variation and complete transection of a dominant artery for end-to-end anastomosis may cause devastating complications. In order to avoid ischemic complications of the hand, circulation pattern and vascular anatomy must be evaluated preoperatively. For the same reason, end-to-side anastomosis to ulnar and radial arteries or end-to-end anastomosis to interosseous arteries may be preferable. Vascularized fibula transfer is a valuable option with good functional results for reconstruction of proximal ulna/elbow joint, ulnar shaft, and distal ulna/DRUJ. This chapter focuses on selection of recipient vessels in treatment of ulnar defects with fibula flap.

G. Sert · H.-C. Chen (✉)
Department of Plastic Surgery, International Medical Center of China Medical University Hospital, China Medical University, Taichung City, Taiwan
e-mail: D19722@mail.cmuh.org.tw

R. Gurunian, R. Djohan (eds.), *Recipient Vessels in Reconstructive Microsurgery*,
https://doi.org/10.1007/978-3-030-75389-4_28

Recipient Vessels: Radius Reconstruction

29

Dicle Aksoyler and Hung-Chi Chen

Introduction

Traumatic injuries, tumors (Ewing sarcoma, osteosarcoma, giant cell tumor), and congenital abnormalities (radial club hand, radial aplasia, phocomelia, premature plate closure) can cause bone deficiency and impair the growth of the radius. This results in discrepancy between the ulna and radius, development of ulnocarpal impingement, and progressive radial deviation of the hand. The coherent relationship between the radius and the ulna both proximally and distally allows the rotation of the forearm, i.e., the radial bone rotation around the ulnar bone. Especially in growing child, neither nonvascularized grafts nor alloplastic implants can restore the joint function or physiologic growth of the wrist [1–3]. On the other hand, vascularized bone grafts possess several advantages when compared to nonvascularized grafts. These include transplantation of living matrix and osteocytes, superior cell survival rates, increased local blood flow in the adjacent scarred soft tissue, improvement of the longitudinal growth of the growth plate, and less risk of stress fractures or osteomyelitis in the long term [3, 4].

The use of vascularized autogenous bone graft was first described by [5–8]. Owing to these studies, fibular flap has gained wide popularity for reconstruction of long bone defects. Vascularized bone grafts are typically indicated for bone defects more than 6 cm resulting from tumor resections, congenital abnormalities, trauma, osteomyelitis, and nonunions [3, 9].

The advantages of fibula flap are several-fold. It has a tubular shape and size similar to the diaphysis of the radius and ulna and can provide up to 25 cm bone length. A skin paddle over the fibula can provide additional soft tissue for reconstruction. Flexor hallucis longus and/or soleus muscles can be included for filling up dead space or restore muscle function in the forearm. Including sural nerve into the flap can provide sensation. Possibility of flowthrough anastomosis not only improves the blood supply to the flap but also acts as a vascular runoff for a second free flap. The flow-through approach can maintain the extremity perfusion especially in the presence of absent or hypoplastic vascular structures [9].

Preoperative Assessment

Preoperative planning should be made both in recipient site and donor site. The length and location of defect are assessed with plain radiographs. The vascular anatomy of the recipient site should be checked with Allen test initially. In addition, MR angiography or CT angiography should be considered especially in traumatic cases and congenital abnormalities to further evaluate the vascular structures. Patients who are candidates for radius reconstruction due to congenital bone defect should undergo systemic evaluation to determine the renal, cardiac function, or hematologic abnormalities. All devitalized tissues should be debrided in traumatic cases prior to flap reconstruction. Clinical examination of the lower extremities and assessment of pedal pulses with Doppler provide valuable information on the status of the vasculature. Also preoperative angiography of the lower extremity may be helpful to rule out the case of peronea magna and to further assess the vasculature in high-risk patients with peripheral arterial disease.

D. Aksoyler · H.-C. Chen (✉)
Department of Plastic Surgery, International Medical Center of China Medical University Hospital, China Medical University, Taichung, Taiwan
e-mail: d19722@mail.cmuh.org.tw

R. Gurunian, R. Djohan (eds.), *Recipient Vessels in Reconstructive Microsurgery*,
https://doi.org/10.1007/978-3-030-75389-4_29

Overview of Vascular Anatomy of the Forearm

At the distal margin of the teres major, the axillary artery becomes brachial artery, and it continues approximately 1 cm distal to the elbow, where it bifurcates into the ulnar and the radial artery. In the proximal arm, the brachial artery lies posterior to the median nerve, whereas distally, the median nerve lies medial to the brachial artery (also see Chap. 24). The median nerve first lies lateral and anterior to the brachial artery in the proximal arm, and then it crosses the artery to lie medial to it distally. The ulnar nerve lies on the medial side of the brachial artery along the arm. Usually two venae comitantes accompany the brachial artery. The basilic vein is located medial aspect of the brachial artery. The brachial artery gives off four branches in the arm: the profunda brachii, the nutrient artery to the humerus, superior ulnar collateral artery, and inferior ulnar collateral artery (also see Chap. 24, Video 24.1). The profunda brachii, the first and the largest branch, arises posteromedially, just distal to the teres major muscle and continues laterally between the medial and lateral heads of the triceps brachii muscle with the radial nerve in the spiral groove of the humerus before piercing the lateral intermuscular septum. The profunda brachii then divides into two terminal branches: the radial collateral artery and middle collateral artery. The middle collateral artery arrives in the medial head of the triceps and ends in the olecranon plexus of the posterior elbow. The radial collateral artery follows the course of the radial nerve before dividing into anterior and posterior divisions. It descends to the region of the lateral epicondyle with its anterior division (ARCA = anterior radial collateral artery) where it anastomoses with the radial recurrent artery (Fig. 24.4). The posterior division of the radial collateral artery (PRCA) lies in the posterior compartment and reaches the lateral intermuscular septum, where it is located between the triceps muscle posteriorly and the brachialis muscle anteriorly. It gives various septocutaneous perforators (1–15 cm proximal to the lateral epicondyle) that supply the overlying skin, forming the vascular territory of the lateral arm flap.

The ulnar artery emerges from the brachial artery 1–2 cm distal to the elbow (also see Chap. 26). It courses toward the wrist with ulnar nerve, which is located ulnar to the artery. The ulnar artery has two venae comitantes. In the proximal forearm, the artery is located deep to the flexor carpi radialis, pronator teres, palmaris longus, and flexor digitorum superficialis. In the distal half of the forearm, it lies over the flexor digitorum profundus between the flexor carpi ulnaris and flexor digitorum superficialis. Around the wrist both the artery and the vein course superficially to the flexor retinaculum. The deep palmar branch of the ulnar artery enters the Guyon's canal and contributes to the deep palmar arch (Fig. 25.2). The ulnar artery is the principal artery contributing to the superficial palmar arch. The ulnar artery gives off three branches in the forearm: anterior and posterior ulnar recurrent arteries (medially from the ulnar artery), and the common interosseous artery (laterally from the ulnar artery), which divides into the anterior and posterior interosseous arteries in the antecubital fossa. The anterior interosseous artery courses between the flexor digitorum profundus (medially) and flexor pollicis longus (radially) muscles. The anterior interosseous artery supplies these muscles and passes posterior to the pronator quadratus muscle in the distal forearm. The anterior ulnar recurrent artery communicates with the inferior ulnar collateral artery, and the posterior ulnar recurrent artery communicates with the superior ulnar collateral artery (also see Chap. 24).

The posterior interosseous artery is the other terminal branch of the common interosseous artery. It arises from the common interosseous artery at the distal border of the supinator muscle. In the proximal forearm, it pierces the upper aspect of the interosseous membrane and enters the posterior compartment of the forearm. Here, it gives off the interosseous recurrent artery, which anastomoses proximally with the middle collateral artery (also see Chap. 24).

The posterior interosseous artery descends on the posterior aspect of the interosseous membrane with the posterior interosseous nerve between the supinator (superficially) and abductor pollicis longus (deeply) muscles, supplying both. In the distal forearm it terminates by anastomosing with a branch of the anterior interosseous artery.

The radial artery is the direct continuation of the brachial artery at the level of radius neck. It travels between the brachioradialis and flexor carpi radialis muscles. It gives off its major branch at the level of antecubital fossa, the radial recurrent artery (also see Chap. 25, Video 25.1). This branch courses deep to the brachioradialis muscle and anastomoses with the radial collateral artery at the level of elbow (Fig. 24.4). Table 29.1 provides diameter of the ulnar and radial artery and their branches.

Surgical Exposure of Proximal Radius and the Recipient Vasculature

The patient is placed in supine position, with arm in extension and forearm in supination. The brachial artery can be easily palpated and located superficially at the level of medial arm. The skin incision can be extended from the existing defect over the medial arm, or the medial arm can be approached directly with an incision over the bicipital groove. A longitudinal incision can be performed 5–6 cm proximal to the flexion crease along the medial edge of the biceps muscle, which continues obliquely across the elbow flexion crease to the lateral and flexor side of the forearm,

Table 29.1 Diameters of vessels and flaps related to these vessels

Artery	Related flap	Region	Diameter/length	Diameter/length of related veins
Peroneal artery [10]	Fibula flap	Lower leg	Diameter: 1.5–2.5 mm Length: 2–6 cm	Venae comitantes: Length: 2–6 cm Diameter: 2–4 mm Superficial vein lesser saphenous; length: 2–6 cm or longer Diameter: 2–4 mm
Anterior tibial artery [11]	Fibula flap with physis	Lower leg	Diameter: 2.0–3.0 mm Length: 2.5–5 cm	Venae comitantes: Diameter:2.3 mm Small saphenous vein diameter: 3 mm
Posterior radial collateral artery [12]	Lateral arm flap	Proximal forearm	Diameter: 1.5–2 mm Pedicle length: 3.4–7 cm	Cephalic vein: 2.5–4 mm [13, 14] Venae comitantes: 2.5 mm
Posterior interosseous artery [15]	Posterior interosseous artery perforator flap	Middle-distal forearm	Diameter: 1.2–2.6 mm	Basilic vein: 3.0–3.7 mm [14]
Anterior interosseous artery [15]	Anterior interosseous artery perforator flap	Middle-distal forearm	Diameter: 2 mm	Basilic vein: 3.0–3.7 mm [13, 14]
Radial recurrent artery [16]	Reverse lateral arm flap	Proximal forearm	Diameter: 0.5–1.5 mm Length: 1.9–5.5 cm	Venae comitantes of the radial collateral artery and its posterior branch Length: 6 cm (range 4–8 cm) Diameter: 2.5 mm (range 1.5–3 mm)
Ulnar recurrent artery [17]	Ulnar recurrent artery flap (reverse medial forearm flap)	Proximal forearm	Diameter: 0.6–1 mm Length: 2.3–4.7 cm	Diameter: 0.6–1 mm
Ulnar artery [15]	Ulnar forearm flap	Proximal or distal forearm	Diameter: 2.5–2.8 mm (wrist level) Diameter: 4.1–4.6 mm (elbow level)	Venae comitantes of ulnar artery: 1.0–1.5 mm
Radial artery [16]	Radial forearm flap	Proximal or distal forearm	Diameter: 3.0–3.5 mm (elbow level) 2.5–3.1 mm (wrist level) length: 15–22 cm	Venae comitantes of radial artery: 1.0–2 mm

where it turns distally along the inner forearm (also see Chaps. 25 and 26, Videos 25.1 and 26.1).

First, the basilic vein and the medial antecubital cutaneous nerve are identified medial to the brachial artery in the subcutaneous plane of the inner upper arm (also see Chap. 24 and Video 24.1). These structures must be preserved. The deep fascia is opened along the bicipital groove between the triceps and the short head of the biceps, with muscles retracted to reveal the vascular bundle with the median nerve anterior to the artery proximally and medial to it distally in the arm. The brachial artery can be dissected proximally and inferiorly to obtain a workable length for an end-to-side anastomosis.

More distally, the deep fascia of anterior compartment is incised to enter triangular antecubital fossa. The important anatomical landmarks are the biceps tendon and the lacertus fibrosus centrally, the brachioradialis muscle laterally, and the pronator teres and flexor muscles medially. Lacertus fibrosis is incised along the edge of pronator teres, and the biceps tendon is identified centrally. The median nerve, brachial artery, and two venae comitantes are identified. Again, the brachial artery can be dissected and prepared for an end-to-side anastomosis at this location. For venous outflow, the basilic vein or brachial veins can be used in an end-to-end fashion. Also, depending on the distance from the reconstruction site, vein grafts may be considered.

Approximately 1–2 cm distal to the elbow crease, the brachial artery gives off its two major branches: the radial and ulnar arteries. The ulnar artery is usually deeper than the radial artery. Tracing the ulnar artery, the common interosseous artery that branches off the ulnar artery as a short segment proximally can be dissected. Also the anterior interosseous artery can be identified by tracing the common interosseous artery (Video 26.1). The ulnar artery continues distally its course beneath the deep head of pronator teres and subsequently enters the interval between flexor digitorum superficialis and flexor digitorum profundus muscles (Video 26.1).

The common or anterior interosseous artery, median antecubital vein, and/or any other superficial or deep vein in the vicinity can be used in an end-to-end manner. Or alternatively, the ulnar artery and its venae comitantes can be prepared for microvascular anastomoses either for an end-to-end or end-to-side fashion (Fig. 29.1).

In contrast to the ulnar artery, the radial artery is located more superficially, which is easily identified in the interval between the brachioradialis muscle and flexor carpi radialis muscle anterior to the pronator teres muscle (Video 25.1). Multiple branches arise from the radial artery at the cubital fossa; however, the largest one is the radial recurrent artery, which runs proximally and joins the anterior branch of the profunda brachii artery in the region of lateral epicondyle

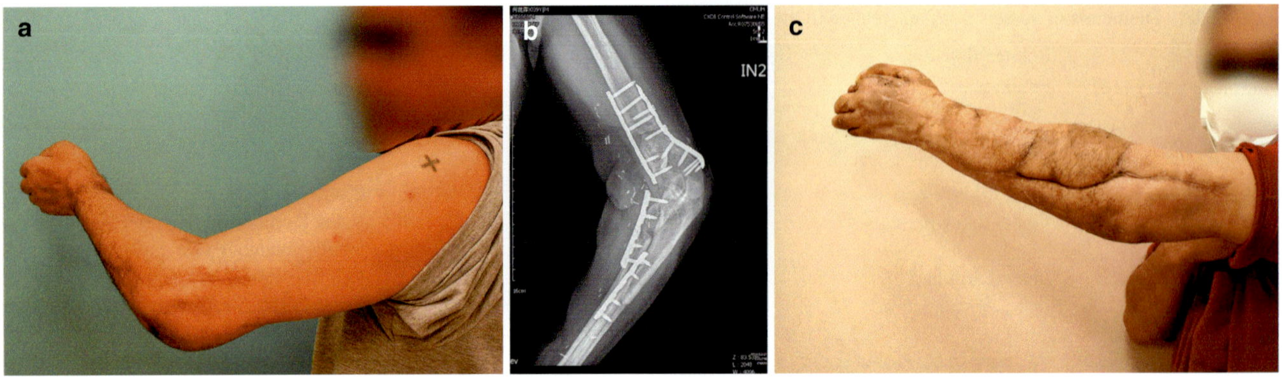

Fig. 29.1 (**a**) The 46-year-old male patient had crush injury to the left forearm, elbow, and distal humerus while working in the factory. The initial operation was done at a community hospital. Then he was referred to our hospital. He presented with significant limitation in extension of elbow extension. (**b**) Multiple plates had been done for the distal humerus, radius, and ulna. However, there was malunion at the proximal radius. Soft tissue contracture at the elbow was released. A fibular osteocutaneous flap was harvested from the left leg for reconstruction. It was used for two purposes: (a) for soft tissue coverage of the forearm after release of elbow contracture and (b) for reconstruction of proximal radius. The recipient artery was the ulnar artery which was anastomosed to the peroneal artery in end-to-side fashion; and the recipient vein was cephalic vein which was anastomosed to the peroneal vein in end-to-end fashion. (**c**) Five months after surgery, the extension of elbow was improved, leaving only 15 degrees of extension lag. Also, the radius had good union

(Fig. 24.4). The radial recurrent artery and cephalic vein can be used in an end-to-end manner. Alternatively, at this level, the radial artery and its venae comitantes can be used either end-to-end or end-to-side manner for microvascular anastomoses.

Between the pronator teres and brachioradialis muscle, the dissection continues deeply to the supinator muscle, and the insertional edge of this muscle is detached with scalpel or periosteal elevator to expose radius bone. Additional exposure of distal aspect of radius can be done by detaching the insertion of brachioradialis muscle from the bone. Radial nerve enters the forearm deep to brachioradialis muscle and continues distally, after giving its posterior interosseous nerve branch at the upper edge of the supinator muscle. This branch must be preserved during dissection of the surgical site.

Surgical Exposure of Distal Radius and Recipient Vasculature

The radius bone can be dissected through Henry's (volar), Thompson's (dorsal), or extensile-anterior flexor carpi radialis approaches which enable exposure alongside the whole radial length (RL) [18, 19].

Recent studies advocate that flexor carpi radialis approach is more convenient for the exposure of distal radius compared to other approaches [19–21]. Our preferred approach is flexor carpi radialis approach; patient with the arm in extension and forearm in supination, a longitudinal incision is made proximal to the wrist crease along the flexor carpi radialis radially to avoid injury to the palmar cutaneous branch of median nerve. The Parona space is encountered between the fascia of the pronator quadratus and the flexor digitorum profundus tendon sheath. Radially, the radial artery and, ulnarly, the ulnar artery are identified (Videos 25.2 and 26.1). Pronator quadratus insertion is reflected to expose the distal radius. The radial or ulnar artery and their venae comitantes and/or the cephalic vein can be used for revascularization of microsurgical flap (Fig. 29.2).

Operative Technique

Free Fibula Osteocutaneous or Musculoseptocutaneous Flap

If osteocutaneous flap is planned, skin island should be outlined around the septocutaneous perforators that are mostly located in the middle and distal third of the bone along the posterior intermuscular septum [22]. These perforators can be identified using a handheld Doppler as well as CTA. The lateral approach is used for dissection of the flap using a pneumonic tourniquet. First, the anterior skin border of the flap is incised, and dissection continues subfascially until the peroneus longus tendon is encountered. Then, dissection continues between the peroneus longus and soleus muscles along the posterior intermuscular septum. The septocutaneous perforators that have been identified at the posterior border of the fibula are visualized. Peroneus longus muscle is dissected off the bone leaving about 2 mm muscle cuff over the periosteum to preserve periosteal blood supply. Subsequently, the anterior intermuscular septum is incised longitudinally along the fibula to enter the anterior (extensor) leg compartment. Similarly, the extensor hallucis longus and the extensor digitorum longus are dissected off the periosteum with 2 mm muscle cuff. Extreme caution is required to

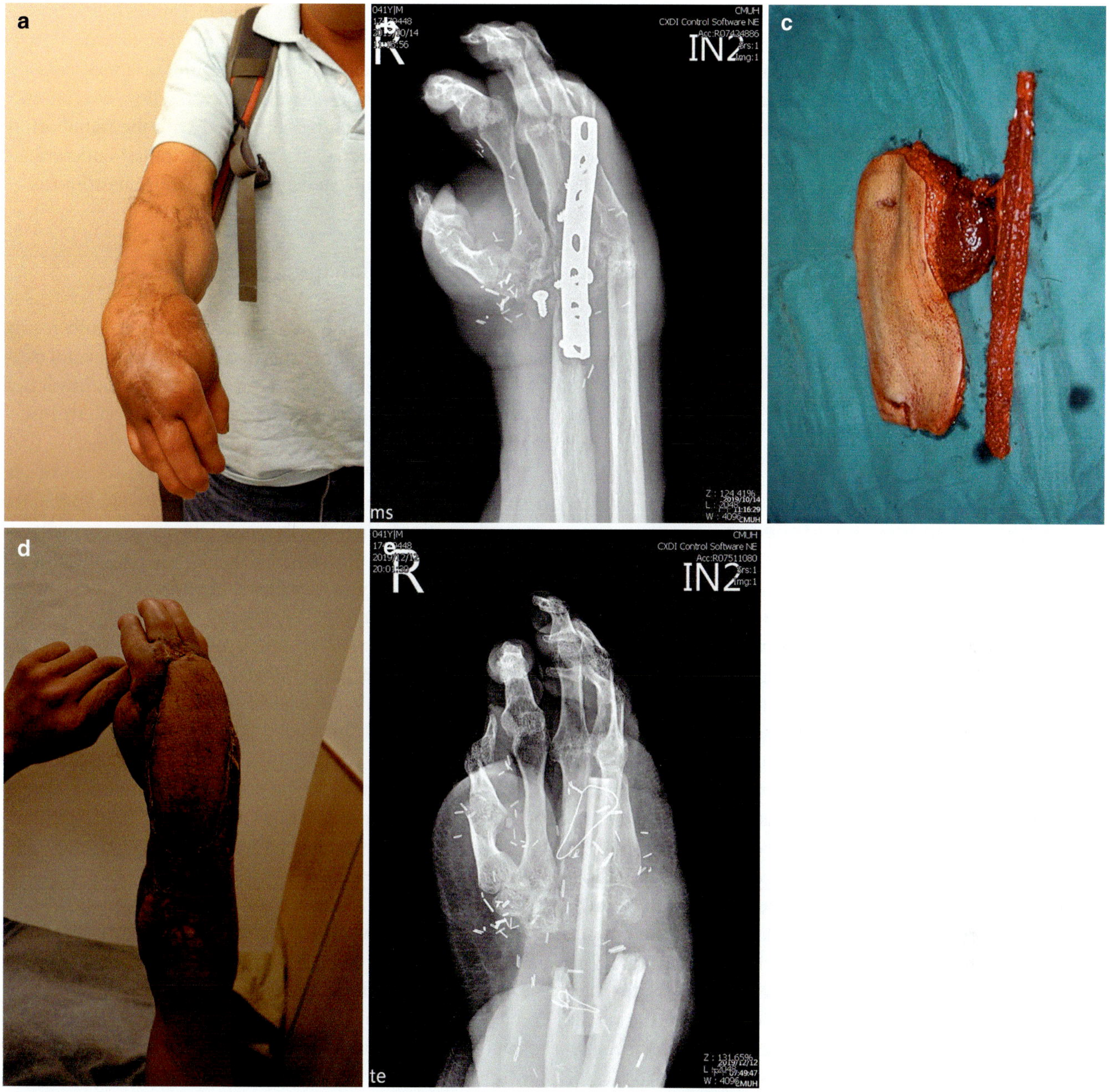

Fig. 29.2 (**a**) The 42-year-old male patient had crush injury to the right wrist and forearm due to accidental injury while working at a factory. He underwent surgery in a local hospital prior to his referral to our hospital. (**b**) There were no carpal bones in the wrist. In the previous operation, metal plate had been used for fusion between third metacarpal bone and radius. However, there was no bony union due to lack of healthy bone at the wrist. The plate was loose and separated from third metacarpal bone as shown in the X-ray. (**c**) A fibular osteocutaneous flap was used for reconstruction. The skin island was used for two purposes: (a) for replacement of the indurated skin at the dorsum of right hand and (b) to bridge the bone defect between the third metacarpal bone and the radius. The recipient artery was the radial artery which was anastomosed to the peroneal artery in end-to-side fashion, and the recipient vein was cephalic vein in end-to-end fashion. (**d**) The early postoperative photo showing good healing and healthy flap. (**e**) At 6 months after surgery, there was good bony union between the third metacarpal bone and the radius

avoid injuring the anterior tibial neurovascular bundle. Next, the anterior interosseous membrane between the tibia and fibula is exposed and incised alongside the fibula. Required osteotomies are performed proximally and distally to facilitate the dissection of the peroneal pedicle. After the dissection of pedicle, the tibialis posterior muscle is separated from the flap, and pedicle dissection continues proximally toward the tibioperoneal trunk. Distally the peroneal vessels are identified and ligated. Posterior incision of the skin island is made. If required, posterior compartment muscles, flexor halucis longus or soleus muscle, can be included in the flap. Also, sometimes, perforators may be traveling through the soleus muscle as musculocutaneous perforators which require tedious dissection. The pedicle dissection continues in the posterior compartment between the soleus and flexor hallucis longus muscles. The pedicle is carefully dissected between the tibialis posterior and flexor hallucis longus. The whole unit is elevated based on the peroneal vessels proximally. The tourniquet is released. The flap is harvested after letting perfusion into the flap for about 15 min. If both radius and ulna reconstruction are needed in the forearm, the fibula can be split at its midpoint and fixed with double barrel modification. Table 29.1 provides peroneal pedicle length and diameter.

Operative Technique

Free Fibula Osteomusculocutaneous Flap Elevating with Physis

In this method, the distal radius defect is reconstructed with proximal part of the fibula including the physis and epiphysis, which is based on the vascular pedicle of the anterior tibial artery [1]. Using anterolateral approach, an incision is performed through the intermuscular septum between the tibialis anterior and the extensor digitorum longus muscles, which extends until the biceps femoris tendon is inserted proximally. The elevation of flap starts distally. The tibialis anterior neurovascular bundle and periosteal branches supplying the diaphysis must be preserved. Proximally, 3–4 cm cuff of peroneal longus muscle and extensor digitorum longus muscle is left attached to the fibular head since it includes the recurrent epiphyseal branch of the anterior tibial artery, which arises 2 cm distal from the anterior tibial artery origin (Table 29.1). The common peroneal nerve and motor branches of the peroneal nerve must be preserved during the fibular head and neck dissection and separated from the anterior tibial vascular pedicle. After the isolation of pedicle, the proximal tibiofibular joint is opened, and a strip of biceps femoris muscle is incorporated to the flap in order to reinforce soft tissue reconstruction at the recipient site with preservation of lateral collateral ligaments of the knee as much as possible. The bony component of the flap should not exceed proximal two thirds of the fibula because of inadequate blood supply of anterior tibial artery to the periosteum more distally. The lateral collateral ligaments and residual biceps femoris tendon are reattached to the lateral aspect of tibia for knee joint stabilization [1, 23]. At the recipient site, proximal head of the fibula and distal part of the radius are fixated with plate and screws. The wrist joint is temporarily stabilized with 1.2 mm Kirschner wire, and strip of biceps femoris is anchored to the remaining distal radiocarpal capsule and ligaments and radial collateral ligaments. Due to short pedicle length of the anterior tibial artery, temporary arteriovenous fistula or vein grafts can be used. The recipient vessels that can be used include branches of the deep brachial artery and concomitant vein, posterior circumflex artery, and the concomitant vein. Alternatively, a reverse flow arterial end-to-end anastomosis can be performed with the radial artery or common interosseous artery, and the radial concomitant vein or cephalic vein can be used for venous anastomosis.

Postoperative Management

The fibula osteocutaneous flap used for upper limb reconstruction does not require extensive shaping and several osteotomies unlike the flap used for mandible reconstruction [24]. The fibula osteocutaneous flap is more prone to vascular thrombosis after more than 5 h of ischemia time.

The arterial flow velocity of the flap peaks at 3 days postoperatively, and the venous velocity begins to increase on the second to third day. Furthermore, increased velocity is accompanied by a decreased risk of vascular thrombosis. Therefore, typically, a vascular compromise occurs in the first 2 days after surgery [25–28].

Even if only osseous component of the flap is necessary for most cases, we believe that fibula flap should be harvested with a small skin paddle to enable flap monitoring. The assessment of flap viability is performed with color, temperature, and a capillary refill of the skin paddle, and a Doppler device is used on the perforators of the skin paddle to assess an adequate blood supply.

Although rare, vascular compromise to fibula flap may occur. Venous thrombosis is primarily caused by technical error and/or mechanical obstruction due to compression, such as kinking, twisting, or hematoma. Prompt correction of the mechanical cause has been shown to have a higher salvage rate than arterial-caused failures [26, 27]. We usually prefer to place a small piece of fat around the pedicle as a cushion to secure it and prevent kinking or twisting of the vessels [29]. Arterial thrombosis may be associated with technical errors and vascular disease, such as atherosclerosis and calcified plaques. Difficulty in dissecting the recipient vessels in previously operated scarred tissues may predispose to inadvertent vessel injury. Vessel mismatch may be another significant cause for failure. Each and every attempt of removing a clot and of repeating anastomosis can lead to a prolonged ischemia time with a potential risk of no-reflow phenomenon [26].

Since the loss of fibula flap has devastating consequences, every attempt should be made for its success. We developed an algorithm to minimize flap failure. If there is any doubt regarding vascular comprise, reexploration of the flap is done immediately.

First, the pedicle is explored. If present, hematoma around the pedicle and anastomotic site is washed out and removed. If the anastomoses are patent, then the pedicle is checked for potential kinking or mechanical compression. The pedicle is re-inset making sure there is no kinking or twisting.

Secondly, if only the artery is clotted, the arterial anastomosis is repeated. If this does not work, the distal side of the peroneal artery is used for anastomosis to provide arterial inflow to the flap.

Thirdly, if only the vein is thrombosed, a thrombectomy is performed, or the segment of the thrombosed vein is excised. Subsequently the venous anastomosis is repeated. If necessary, the cephalic vein or a concomitant vein is used as a new recipient vessel. If the venous congestion of the flap cannot be improved by redo venous anastomosis, it may indicate more widespread clotting inside the flap. In this case, performing anastomosis for both distal ends of peroneal artery and vein should be considered to supply the flap in retrograde manner. In this way, the arterial inflow of the flap is uninterrupted on both sides of the peroneal artery, and the retrograde venous drainage can be provided with the distal side of the peroneal vein.

Fourth, if both the arterial and venous anastomosis are occluded, arterial and venous anastomosis are performed at both sides of the flap to provide dual blood supply. If this approach is unsuccessful for vein anastomosis but there is uninterrupted arterial inflow, we remove the fixation plate and screws to provide one-sided venous leakage from the bone marrow of the fibula. We prepare for extra blood products. The skin paddle sutures are loosely approximated at few places or not at all. Patients return to the operation room 3 weeks after surgery to re-inset the skin paddle and for fixation of the bone with plates and screws. We believe that these methods will lead to a high success rate for salvaged fibular osteocutaneous flaps.

Previously used temporary Kirschner wire for wrist stabilization is removed between 3 and 6 weeks postoperatively. After 2 months postoperatively, active physiotherapy is initiated with loading and strengthening of the upper limb according to the patient's tolerance. Then, follow-up continues every 3 months after the surgery.

Nonvascular Complications of Vascularized Fibula Flap

Complications in the donor and recipient site may occur. To prevent the occurrence of compartment syndrome in the recipient site, the senior author (H.C.C.) always advocates using split thickness skin graft for closure instead of primary closure.

The temporary peroneal nerve palsy may occur during the fibular flap harvest. It usually returns in 6 months postoperatively. Inappropriate repair of flexor hallucis longus muscle may result in toe flexion contraction. Stress fracture at the ipsilateral tibia may occur especially with physis reconstruction. With the delayed union of the bone, stress fractures can occur in the long term at the graft site. To prevent this complication, vascular compromise to the flap and long-term immobilization of the graft should be avoided.

Discussion

In embryologic life, between the fourth and eighth weeks the signalization of apical ectodermal ridge (AER) provides proximal to distal limb development, the zone of polarizing activity (ZPA) maintains radioulnar limb formation, and the wingless-type signaling (Wnt) provides ventral and dorsal limb axis, and these interdependent signalization mechanisms contribute to the proper development of humerus, radius, ulna, brachial plexus, upper limb vessels, carpal bones, finger rays, phalanges, flexor-extensor abductor, and adductor muscles and tendons [30, 31]. Most congenital abnormalities occur in this fragile development period either spontaneously or genetically inherited especially accompanied with cardiac abnormalities [31, 32]. Radius bone longitudinal deficiency might be associated with VACTERL (additional spinal, renal, gastrointestinal, cardiac abnormalities), Holt-Oram (additional cardiac septal defects), TAR (thrombocytopenia, anemia), Fanconi aplastic anemia, trisomy 13 and trisomy 18, and Nager syndrome (additional craniofacial abnormalities). Some of longitudinal deficiencies cannot be treated properly by centralization of wrist, carpal bone resection, splinting, or lengthening of radius with distraction osteogenesis [33–35]. To overcome the wrist radial deviation, to improve soft tissue deficiency, and to improve the power of wrist extensors, free fibula osteocutaneous flap including with epiphyseal transfer also with soleus muscle should be considered as a main treatment.

Particularly in the advanced stage patients with the absence of physis and distal radius [36], the transplanted physis demonstrates reliable healing with continued growth at a rate similar to the contralateral side and ipsilateral ulna. Likewise, radiographs of the transplanted physis showed remodeling of the articular surface, providing a stable, functional wrist, with 70% of wrist motion compared with the contralateral side [37–39]. Even if some authors advocate that the intercommunicating musculoperiosteal and perichondrial branches enable to harvest fibular head free flap based on peroneal vessels or bipedicled flap also including the inferior lateral genicular artery, long-term results show radial or ulnar wrist deviation and diminished longitudinal growth. The advantage of anterior tibial artery is its large caliber. However, as this vessel cannot be used in flow-through manner, reverse flow should be maintained, and if necessary the vein grafts should be considered [23, 40–43]. The vascularized fibular head transfer shows an average growth rate of 0.58 cm/year. Based on peroneal artery pedicle and anterior tibial artery pedicle, average growth rate has been demonstrated to be 0.36 cm/year and 0.83 cm/year, respectively [40].

The timing of surgery for radial club hand is between the age of 2 years and school age. However, patients should obtain cleats and brackets to reduce wrist deviation before the surgery [44]. Moreover, radial artery and radial nerve are usually absent or hypoplastic in varying degrees. Even if the artery exists, it may have weak pulse. The ulnar artery is usually normal and may also deviate to the radial side [45–47].

In these instances, recipient vessels might be the branches of deep brachial artery and concomitant vein, posterior circumflex artery, and concomitant vein either with or without a vein graft. Also, a reverse flow arterial end-to-end anastomosis can be done with ulnar or common interosseous artery, concomitant veins, or cephalic vein.

The fibular epiphysis has similar shape and size with distal radius and allowing gradual remodeling of articular surface with proximal carpal row with increased wrist range of motion and stability. On the other hand, the nonvascularized transfer of fibular head results in arrest of growth and diminished epiphyseal growth. Therefore, the efficacy of reconstruction improves when it is transferred as a free flap with less risk of stress fractures or avascular necrosis in the future [40]. Although stress fracture following free bone transfer is seen in up to 17% of patients, reconstruction using free fibula has achieved excellent results by most reports, with 85–89% of patients attaining union of the graft [9].

The fibula flap anatomically provides a reliable option for forearm reconstruction; however, functional recovery is controversial due to complicated articulation of the forearm, wrist, and hand [48]. Also, skeletally immature patients with large bone defects represent a challenging problem secondary to the need to match their healthy bone growth in the upper extremity. The most reliable option involves the transfer of the proximal fibular epiphysis enabling both bony reconstruction and growth potential especially for the radius reconstruction.

Compliance with Ethical Standards

Funding: No, the authors did not take any funding in either the case or the submission process.

Conflict of Interest: All authors declare that they have no conflict of interest.

Ethical approval: All procedures performed in this study involving human participant were in accordance with the 1964 Helsinki Declaration and its later amendments or comparable ethical standards.

References

1. Innocenti M, Delcroix L, Manfrini M, Ceruso M, Capanna R. Vascularized proximal fibular epiphyseal transfer for distal radial reconstruction. J Bone Joint Surg Am. 2004;86(7):1504–11.
2. Onoda S, Sakuraba M, Asano T, Miyamoto S, Beppu Y, Chuman H, et al. Use of vascularized free fibular head grafts for upper limb oncologic reconstruction. Plast Reconstr Surg. 2011;127(3):1244–53.
3. Wood MB, Bishop AT. Massive bone defects of the upper limb: reconstruction by vascularized bone transfer. Hand Clin. 2007;23(1):49–56.
4. Yuceturk A, Tuncay C, Isiklar U, Tandogan R. Vascularised bone graft applications in upper extremity problems. Microsurgery. 1998;18(3):160–2.
5. Mckee DM. Microvascular bone transplantation. Clin Plast Surg. 1978;5(2):283–92.
6. Ueba Y, Fujikawa S. Nine years follow-up of a free vascularized fibula graft in neurofibromatosis-A case report and literature. J Orthop Trauma Surg. 1983;26:595.
7. Taylor GI, Miller GD, Ham FJ. The free vascularized bone graft. A clinical extension of microvascular techniques. Platic Reconstr Surg. 1975;55(5):533–44.
8. Zaretski A, Amir A, Meller I, Leshem D, Kollender Y, Barnea Y, et al. Free fibula long bone reconstruction in orthopedic oncology: a surgical algorithm for reconstructive options. Plast Reconstr Surg. 2004;113(7):1989–2000.
9. Houdek MT, Wagner ER, Wyles CC, Nanos GP 3rd, Moran SL. New options for vascularized bone reconstruction in the upper extremity. Semin Plast Surg. 2015;29(1):20–9.
10. Salgado C, Chim H, Moran S, Wei FC, Mardini S. Fibula flap. In: Flaps and reconstructive surgery by eds. Wei FC, Mardini S., 2nd ed. Elsevier, 2016: pp. 596–612.,
11. Xu Z, Chenglin L, Zhiwen N, Sumin W, Ruxia Y, Xu M. Use of flap based on anterior tibial artery for free transfer. J Reconstr Microsurg. 2008;24(2):103–10.
12. Katsaros J, Schusterman M, Beppu M, Banis JC Jr, Acland RD. The lateral upper arm flap: anatomy and clinical applications. Ann Plast Surg. 1984;12(6):489–500.
13. Spivack DE, Kelly P, Gaughan JP, van Bemmelen PS. Mapping of superficial extremity veins: normal diameters and trends in a vascular patient-population. Ultrasound Med Biol. 2012;38(2):190–4.
14. Sharp R, Cummings M, Childs J, Fielder A, Mikocka-Walus A, Grech C, et al. Measurement of vein diameter for Peripherally Inserted Central Catheter (PICC) insertion: an observational study. J Infus Nurs. 2015;38(5):351–7.
15. Haerle M, Hafner HM, Dietz K, Schaller HE, Brunelli F. Vascular dominance in the forearm. Plast Reconstr Surg. 2003;111(6):1891–8.
16. Trager S, Pignataro M, Anderson J, Kleinert JM. Color flow Doppler: imaging the upper extremity. J Hand Surg Am. 1993;18(4):621–5.
17. Thomas BP, Geddes CR, Tang M, Morris SF. Vascular supply of the integument of the upper extremity. In Perforator flaps: anatomy, technique, & clinical applications, 2nd ed by Blondeel PN, Morris SF, Hallock GG, Neligan PC. CRC Press, 2013:pp 299–329.
18. Holweg P, Hohenberger GM, Schwarz AM, Staresinic M, Krassnig R, Grechenig S. Comparison of volar and dorsal plate osteosynthesis for radial shaft fractures: an anatomical pilot study. Injury. 2017;48(Suppl 5):S38–40.
19. Jockel CR, Zlotolow DA, Butler RB, Becker EH. Extensile surgical exposures of the radius: a comparative anatomic study. J Hand Surg Am. 2013;38(4):745–52.
20. Lattmann T, Dietrich M, Meier C, Kilgus M, Platz A. Comparison of 2 surgical approaches for volar locking plate osteosynthesis of the distal radius. J Hand Surg Am. 2008;33(7):1135–43.
21. Wijffels MM, Orbay JL, Indriago I, Ring D. The extended flexor carpi radialis approach for partially healed malaligned fractures of the distal radius. Injury. 2012;43(7):1204–8.
22. Wei FC, Chen HC, Chuang CC, Noordhoff MS. Fibular osteoseptocutaneous flap: anatomic study and clinical application. Plast Reconstr Surg. 1986;78(2):191–200.

23. Taylor GI, Wilson KR, Rees MD, Corlett RJ, Cole WG. The anterior tibial vessels and their role in epiphyseal and diaphyseal transfer of the fibula: experimental study and clinical applications. Br J Plast Surg. 1988;41(5):451–69.
24. Chang SY, Huang JJ, Tsao CK, Nguyen A, Mittakanti K, Lin CY, et al. Does ischemia time affect the outcome of free fibula flaps for head and neck reconstruction? A review of 116 cases. Plast Reconstr Surg. 2010;126(6):1988–95.
25. Chang EI, Zhang H, Liu J, Yu P, Skoracki RJ, Hanasono MM. Analysis of risk factors for flap loss and salvage in free flap head and neck reconstruction. Head Neck. 2016;38(Suppl 1):E771–5.
26. Yu P, Chang DW, Miller MJ, Reece G, Robb GL. Analysis of 49 cases of flap compromise in 1310 free flaps for head and neck reconstruction. Head Neck. 2009;31(1):45–51.
27. Chang EI. Impact of venous outflow tract on survival of osteocutaneous free fibula flaps for mandibular reconstruction: a 14-year review. Head Neck. 2017;39(7):1454–8.
28. Hanasono MM, Barnea Y, Skoracki RJ. Microvascular surgery in the previously operated and irradiated neck. Microsurgery. 2009;29(1):1–7.
29. Mousavi SA, Chen SH, Yildirim MEC, Chen HC. Using fat graft as safe and effective pillow to prevent compression and torsion anastomosis for microvascular anastomosis. Surg Innov. 2019;26:636–7. 1553350619861559.
30. Daluiski A, Yi SE, Lyons KM. The molecular control of upper extremity development: implications for congenital hand anomalies. J Hand Surg Am. 2001;26(1):8–22.
31. Bamshad M, Watkins WS, Dixon ME, Le T, Roeder AD, Kramer BE, et al. Reconstructing the history of human limb development: lessons from birth defects. Pediatr Res. 1999;45(3):291–9.
32. Temtamy SA, McKusick VA. The genetics of hand malformations. Birth Defects Orig Artic Ser. 1978;14(3):i–xviii, 1–619.
33. Goldfarb CA, Wall L, Manske PR. Radial longitudinal deficiency: the incidence of associated medical and musculoskeletal conditions. J Hand Surg Am. 2006;31(7):1176–82.
34. Matsuno T, Ishida O, Sunagawa T, Suzuki O, Ikuta Y, Ochi M. Radius lengthening for the treatment of Bayne and Klug type II and type III radial longitudinal deficiency. J Hand Surg Am. 2006;31(5):822–9.
35. Taghinia AH, Al-Sheikh AA, Upton J. Preoperative soft-tissue distraction for radial longitudinal deficiency: an analysis of indications and outcomes. Plast Reconstr Surg. 2007;120(5):1305–12. discussion 13–4.
36. Vilkki SK. Distraction and microvascular epiphysis transfer for radial club hand. J Hand Surg Br. 1998;23(4):445–52.
37. Innocenti M, Delcroix L, Manfrini M, Ceruso M, Capanna R. Vascularized proximal fibular epiphyseal transfer for distal radial reconstruction. J Bone Joint Surg Am. 2005;87(Suppl 1 Pt 2):237–46.
38. Akinbo O, Strauch R. Physeal transfers for skeletal reconstruction. J Hand Surg Am. 2008;33(4):584–90.
39. Medrykowski F, Barbary S, Gibert N, Lascombes P, Dautel G. Vascularized proximal fibular epiphyseal transfer: two cases. Orthop Traumatol Surg Res. Elsevier, Saunders, Philadelphia, USA. 2012;98(6):728–32.
40. Aldekhayel S, Govshievich A, Neel OF, Luc M. Vascularized proximal fibula epiphyseal transfer for distal radius reconstruction in children: a systematic review. Microsurgery. 2016;36(8):705–11.
41. Pho RW, Patterson MH, Kour AK, Kumar VP. Free vascularised epiphyseal transplantation in upper extremity reconstruction. J Hand Surg Br. Elsevier, Saunders: Philadelphia, USA; 1988;13(4):440–7.
42. Sawaizumi M, Maruyama Y, Okajima K, Motegi M. Free vascularised epiphyseal transfer designed on the reverse anterior tibial artery. Br J Plast Surg. 1991;44(1):57–9.
43. Yang YF, Wang JW, Huang P, Xu ZH. Distal radius reconstruction with vascularized proximal fibular autograft after en-bloc resection of recurrent giant cell tumor. BMC Musculoskelet Disord. 2016;17(1):346.
44. Netscher DT, Scheker LR. Timing and decision-making in the treatment of congenital upper extremity deformities. Clin Plast Surg. 1990;17(1):113–31.
45. James MA, McCarroll HR Jr, Manske PR. The spectrum of radial longitudinal deficiency: a modified classification. J Hand Surg Am. 1999;24(6):1145–55.
46. VanHeest A, Grierson Y. Dorsal rotation flap for centralization in radial longitudinal deficiency. J Hand Surg Am. CRC Press, Boca Raton, FL, USA. 2007;32(6):871–5.
47. Van Allen MI, Hoyme HE, Jones KL. Vascular pathogenesis of limb defects. I. Radial artery anatomy in radial aplasia. J Pediatr. 1982;101(5):832–8.
48. Hollenbeck ST, Komatsu I, Woo S, Schoeman M, Yang J, Erdmann D, et al. The current role of the vascularized-fibular osteocutaneous graft in the treatment of segmental defects of the upper extremity. Microsurgery. CRC Press: Boca Raton, FL, USA; 2011;31(3):183–9.

Part V

Lower Extremity Reconstruction

Descending Branch of the Lateral Circumflex Femoral Vessels

30

Nathan F. Miller, Geoffrey G. Hallock, and Yee Cheng Low

Introduction

Although originally the anterolateral thigh flap introduced by Song et al. [1] as with perforator flaps in general was slow to be adopted, in most parts of the world today it has become the ideal soft tissue flap as both a local flap and a microsurgical free tissue transfer [2]. Therefore, it would be safe to say that even the occasional reconstructive surgeon is quite familiar with the course of the usual source pedicle of this flap, the descending branch of the lateral circumflex femoral vessels [LCFDB]. Even this basic knowledge of the anatomy has been found to have additional and versatile indications. Zenn et al. [3] have shown that as an autograft, the LCFDB can be a superior alternative to an arteriovenous loop that might be necessary to reach a recipient site far from a defect where there is a paucity of other local options. For that matter, the LCFDB can itself serve as that recipient site. Such has been shown possible for the proximal [4] and distal thigh [5], particularly when the more conventional major femoral vessels have been compromised or are far from a lateral defect or convenient for ectopic implantations allowing temporary insetting prior to eventual lower limb replantation [6, 7]. In addition, if none of the many local recipient site options for knee coverage are available [8], the proximal LCFDB instead has been used directly [9] or extended by vein grafts for orthograde flow to allow reach [10] or via retrograde perfusion using the distal-based LCFDB [11–13].

Supplementary Information The online version of this chapter (https://doi.org/10.1007/978-3-030-75389-4_30) contains supplementary material, which is available to authorized users.

N. F. Miller
University of Maryland/R Adams Cowley Shock Trauma Center, Baltimore, MD, USA

G. G. Hallock (✉)
Division of Plastic Surgery, St. Luke's Hospital, Sacred Heart Campus, Allentown, PA, USA

Y. C. Low
Division of Plastic and Reconstructive Surgery, Department of Surgery, Lehigh Valley Health Network, Allentown, PA, USA
e-mail: YeeCheng.Low@lvhn.org

Applied Anatomy

The descending branch of the lateral circumflex femoral system [LCFDB] typically arises from the lateral circumflex femoral vessels beneath the proximal rectus femoris [RF] muscle (Fig. 30.1) [14, 15]. At this point, the mean arterial diameter may be 3.4 mm and vein 3.9 mm [3]. Sometimes the usually paired venae comitantes at this level join together, but more often one is much larger than the other [14]. The LCFDB then passes distally in the septum between the RF and vastus lateralis [VL] muscles for a mean distance of 20.5 cm [3, 16]. Ultimately, the LCFDB typically enters the vastus lateralis muscle proper at about 6–10 cm above the center of the patella [12]. At this point Kim et al. [12] found that the artery ranged in size from 1.0 to 2.0 mm and vein 0.8 to 2.0, while more proximally at 15 cm above the patella they were 1.0–3.0 mm for both the artery and vein. Eventually, the LCFDB will encounter choke vessels of the superior lateral genicular or profunda femoris, which would be the means for any retrograde perfusion [17].

The lateral circumflex femoral vessels usually arise from the profunda femoris but rarely may instead be from the external iliac [15]. From this arises usually a single descending branch, but sometimes a bifurcation occurs with both medial and lateral descending branches [15]. Although well known that perforators have a variable pattern of origin from this source pedicle [16], if dual branches are present, they will always be from the lateral branch [15]. Most pertinent here is the finding by Valdatta et al. [15] in a cadaver study where in a single example the LCFDB ran its entire course in the intermuscular septum between the RF and vastus intermedius muscles instead of the VL.

R. Gurunian, R. Djohan (eds.), *Recipient Vessels in Reconstructive Microsurgery*,
https://doi.org/10.1007/978-3-030-75389-4_30

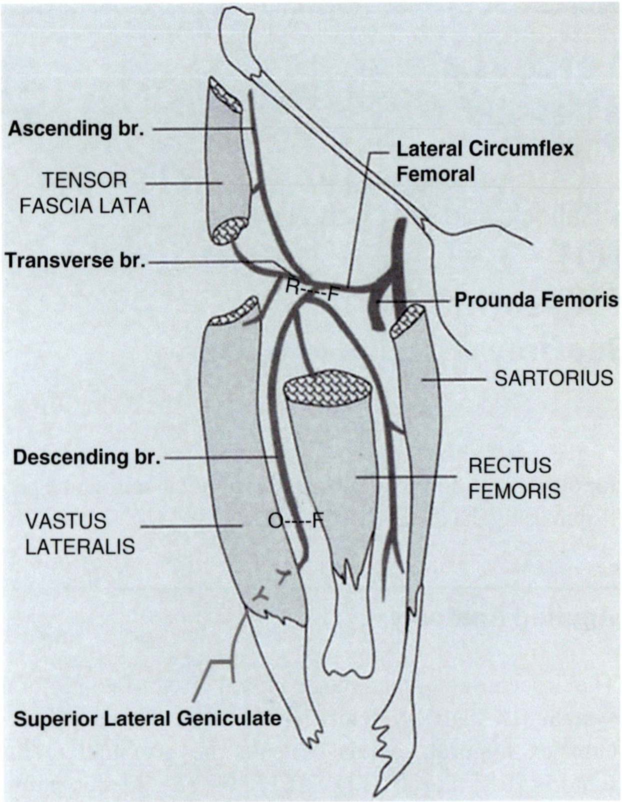

Fig. 30.1 The descending branch [DB] usually arises from the lateral circumflex femoral [LCF] vessels underneath the rectus femoris [RF] muscle and then courses distally in the septum between RF and vastus lateralis [VL] until entering the latter. When used as a reversed flow recipient site, for maximum pedicle length the LCFDB should be divided at its origin [marked "R---F"], whereas if orthograde flow is desirable, LCFDB can be divided [marked "O---F"] where length and caliber are appropriate anywhere along the septum and usually proximal to where it enters VL

Recipient Site Preparation

Whether an orthograde or reverse flow LCFDB recipient site is needed, the initial approach will be identical (Video 30.1). Just as when designing an anterolateral thigh flap, a line is drawn from the anterosuperior iliac spine to the superior lateral border of the patella. This roughly corresponds to the intermuscular septum found between the rectus femoris [RF] and vastus lateralis [VL] muscles. The center of this line is marked, and a short incision starting there is made down through the fascia lata to expose the linear vertical fat pad that characteristically distinguishes the separation of the RF from the VL muscle. With medial retraction of the RF, and if a perforator is found, that can be followed down until seen to arise from the LCFDB. Further dissection of that source pedicle will depend on the specific circumstances of the location of the defect and chosen flap, but in all cases care must be observed to protect the femoral motor nerve during this dissection to ensure function preservation.

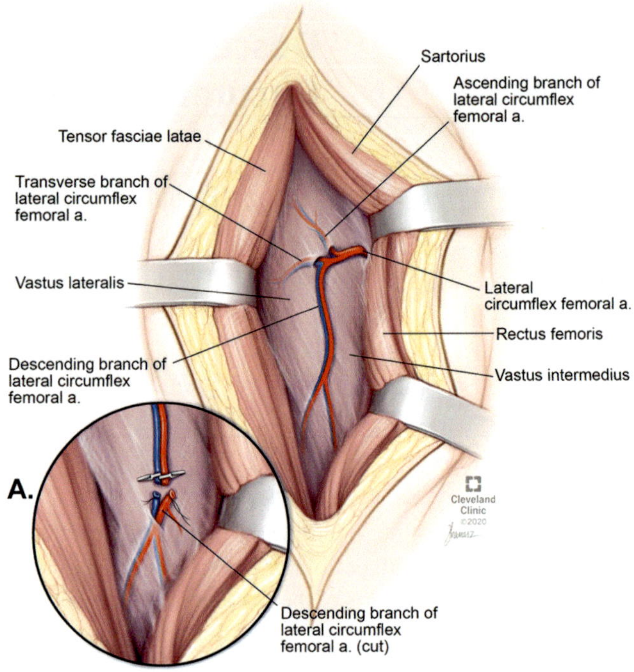

Fig. 30.2 Illustration of the LCFDB for use as recipient vessel at the mid-third of the thigh. (**A**) Close-up drawing of the LCFDB that is divided and prepared for microvascular anastomosis. (Reprinted with permission, Cleveland Clinic Center for Medical Art & Photography © 2020. All Rights Reserved)

Proximal-Based Recipient Site

If this option is selected, orthograde inflow and outflow to any flap will be ensured. The amount of recipient pedicle dissection depends on the length needed to reach where the flap will be inset, as well as the selection of a symmetrical vessel caliber or to permit elevation to a superficial site to simplify any end-to-end microanastomoses (Video 30.1, Fig. 30.2). As when taken as an arteriovenous autograft, this recipient pedicle length can reliably extend from the LCF vessels themselves proximally to where the descending branch enters the vastus lateralis muscles distally, although vessel caliber will be inversely proportional to pedicle length (Fig. 30.3). If vein grafts are chosen to extend reach [10], the caliber of the vein grafts will probably determine the site to best divide the LCFDB with then their interposition (Fig. 30.4). As an alternative, a loop of the greater saphenous vein can be the source of the arterial side vein graft while simultaneously being the source of outflow to thereby avoid a venous side vein graft.

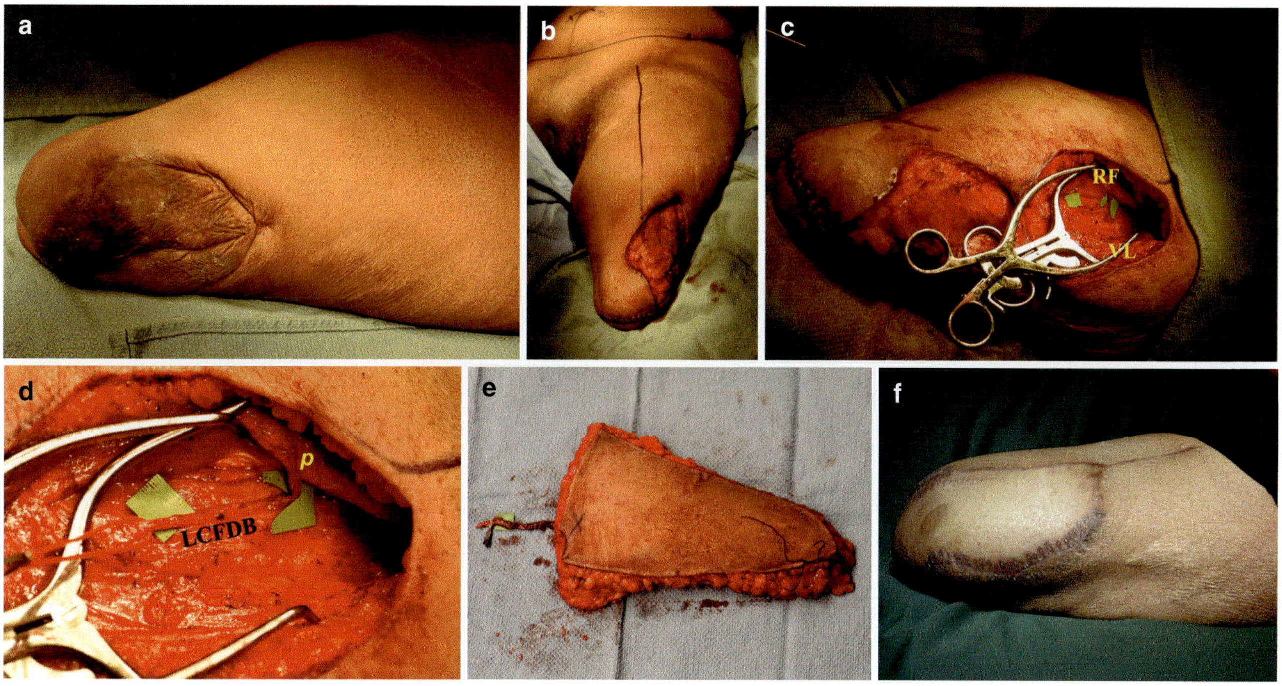

Fig. 30.3 Direct orthograde flow recipient site: (**a**) Above-knee [AK] amputation stump that was initially directly skin grafted on the lateral femur 25 years previously, with recent breakdown; (**b**) defect following removal of entire skin graft and release of adhesions to the femur, with a line drawn extending to the anterior superior iliac spine along the septum identified distally between the vastus lateralis [VL] and rectus femoris [RF] muscles; (**c**) separation of VL and RF from distal to proximal along the septum; (**d**) close-up revealed a septocutaneous perforator [p] that was followed down to readily expose the descending branch of the lateral femoral circumflex [LCFDB] vessels, which in turn was freed up enough to allow it to be brought to a superficial position to simplify all microanastomoses at the level of the vessel loop; (**e**) left hemiabdomen deep inferior epigastric artery perforator [DIEP] free flap based on medial row perforator with eccentric design to provide long reach of the flap itself in addition to keeping proximally a 10 cm vascular pedicle; (**f**) final result with DIEP free flap providing shear-stress free stable soft tissue padding over lateral AK stump

Distal-Based Recipient Site

This variation, which provides an alternative recipient site if coverage is needed for the knee or upper leg [11], may not always have reliable perfusion as inflow and outflow will be in a reverse or retrograde fashion [12]. For this reason, Gao et al. [13] in their series always used the reversed LCFDB artery only, but never the accompanying veins. Instead, the venae comitantes of any flap were anastomosed to either the available greater or lesser saphenous vein for orthograde outflow to avoid the risk of venous congestion.

If proceeding with this choice, the LCFDB recipient pedicle can be dissected all the way proximally to its origin from the LCF, where once divided allows maximal pedicle length. More distal pedicle lengthening by division of any side branches back best to no more than 15 cm above the center of the patella will preserve hopefully enough distal arterial branches for flow augmentation as arterial collaterals in addition to the theoretical presence of the superior lateral genicular system [12]. Gao et al. [13] have extended this pedicle even more by taking up to a 2-cm-wide muscle cuff around the LCFDB to create a more distal pivot point.

Discussion

Use of the descending branch of the lateral circumflex femoral vessels [LCFDB] as a recipient site with a proximal-based origin will best insure orthograde perfusion. Such an approach has been used for thigh [4, 5] and knee coverage [9, 10] with free flaps, especially for lateral defects or if the major femoral vessels or their branches have in some way been compromised, but there is no reason to not similarly allow reach to the abdomen, pubis, perineum, or even hip if the need arose and an alternative local flap was not possible. The LCFDB as a distal-based recipient site might be considered if other choices about the knee were unavailable [8]. This may be satisfactory for arterial inflow at least on the basis of reasonable retrograde pressure recordings [18], but just as for the distal-based ALT flap where venous congestion is a high risk factor, the use of a nearby subcutaneous vein would be preferable to provide orthograde outflow, as is routinely done for this ped-

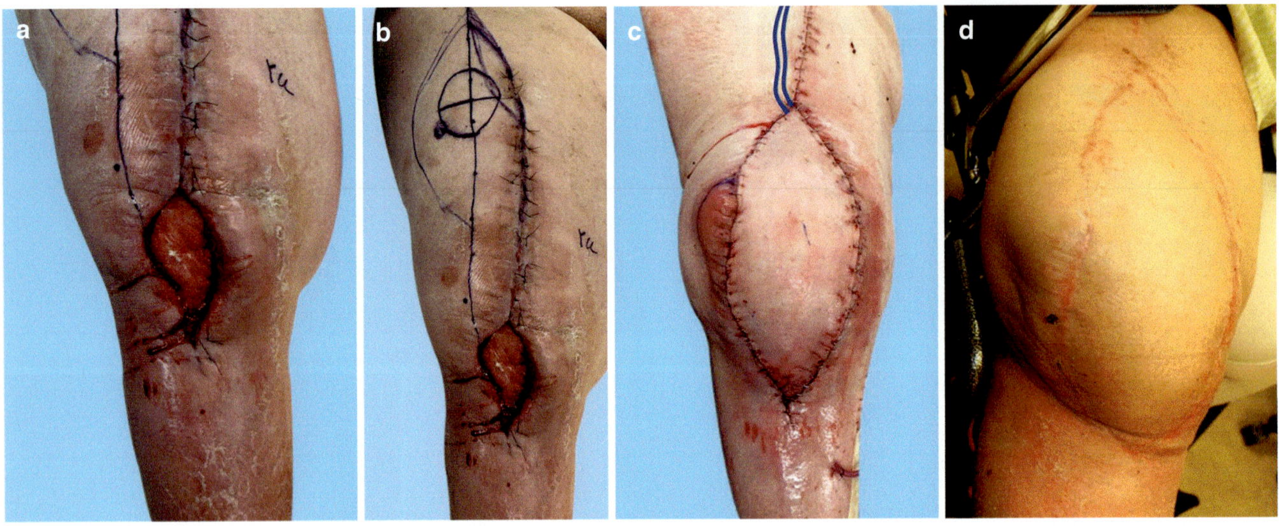

Fig. 30.4 Vein graft extended orthograde flow recipient site: (**a**) Following total knee arthroplasty complicated by periprosthetic joint infection and conversion to a knee arthrodesis, a parapatellar wound could not be closed, (**b**) an ipsilateral anterolateral thigh free flap incorporating the prior orthopedic incision was designed for coverage, (**c**) then advanced and inset into the defect by extending both the proximal descending branch artery and vein with 10-cm-long vein grafts as depicted in the overlying schematic, (**d**) allowing excellent wound healing with patient seen in wheelchair

icled ALT version by the Chung Gung group [19]. Of course, any supermicrosurgeon could just use one of the perforators arising from the LCFDB at any level and avoid source pedicle dissection altogether and any worries over direction of perfusion, if that were to be a feasible solution!

References

1. Song YG, Chen GZ, Song YL. The free thigh flap: a new free flap concept based on the Septocutaneous artery. Br J Plast Surg. 1984;37:149–59.
2. Wei FC, Jain V, Celik N, Chen HC, Chuang DCC, Lin CH. Have we found an ideal soft-tissue flap? An experience with 672 anterolateral thigh flaps. Plast Reconstr Surg. 2002;109:2219–26.
3. Zenn MR, Pribaz J, Walsh M. Use of the descending lateral femoral circumflex artery and vein for vascular grafting: a better alternative to an arteriovenous loop. Plast Reconstr Surg. 2010;126:140–2.
4. Hallock GG. Restoration of quadriceps Femoris function with a dynamic microsurgical free latissimus Dorsi muscle transfer. Ann Plast Surg. 2004;52:89–92.
5. Hallock GG. The vascular pedicle of the anterolateral thigh flap as an alternative recipient site for thigh free flaps. J Reconstr Microsurg. 2008;24:131–6.
6. Qing L, Tang J. Using temporary ectopic implantation by the distal runoff vessel of the lateral circumflex femoral system and combining with free modified Laissimus Dorsi Myocutaneous flap for salvaging an amputated leg in children. Ann Plast Surg. 2019;82:708–10.
7. Wang KC, Hung KS, Chang TY, Wu PT, Lee YC. Temporary ectopic implantation of an amputated leg using the distal runoff vessels of the anterolateral thigh flap followed by subsequent prefabricated chimeric replantation. Ann Plast Surg. 2019;82:71–5.
8. Fang T, Zhang EW, Lineaweaver WC, Zhang F. Recipient vessels in the free flap reconstruction around the knee. Ann Plast Surg. 2013;71:429–33.
9. Yuen JC, Zhou AT. Free flap coverage for knee salvage. Ann Plast Surg. 1996;37:158–66.
10. Yagi Y, Ueda K, Shirakabe M, Oba S, Omiya Y. Reconstruction of knee ligaments with a free tensor fascia Lata Myocutaneous flap transfer. Br J Plast Surg. 2002;55:155–7.
11. Chien WH, Chen IC, Tan TS, Tang YW. Salvage of knee joint tumor prosthesis using turnover reverse-flow descending branch of lateral circumflex femoral artery as recipient vessel for the free ALT flap: a case report. J Reconstr Microsurg. 2007;23:505–9.
12. Kim JS, Lee HS, Jang PY, Choi TH, Lee KS, Kim NG. Use of the descending branch of lateral circumflex femoral artery as a recipient pedicle for coverage of a knee defect with free flap: anatomical and clinical study. Microsurgery. 2010;30:32–6.
13. Gao SH, Feng SM, Chen C, Jiao C, Sun LQ, Zhang WL. A new recipient artery for reconstruction of soft-tissue defects in the lower limb with a free anterolateral thigh flap: the reversed descending branch of the lateral femoral circumflex artery. Plast Reconstr Surg. 2012;130:1059–65.
14. Shieh SJ, Chiu HY, Yu JC, Pan SC, Tsai ST, Shen CL. Free anterolateral thigh flap for reconstruction of head and neck defects following cancer ablation. Plast Reconstr Surg. 2000;105:2349–57.
15. Valdatta L, Tuinder S, Buoro M, Thione A, Faga A, Putz R. Lateral circumflex femoral arterial system and perforators of the anterolateral thigh flap: an anatomic study. Ann Plast Surg. 2002;49:145–50.
16. Kimata Y, Uchiyama K, Ebihara S, Nakatsuka. Anatomic variations and technical problems of the anterolateral thigh flap: a report of 74 cases. Plast Reconstr Surg. 1998;102:1517–23.
17. Park S, Eom JS. Selection of the recipient vessel in the free flap around the knee: the superior medial genicular vessels and the descending genicular vessels. Plast Reconstr Surg. 2001;105:1177–82.
18. Pan SC, Yu JC, Shieh SJ, Lee JW, Huang BM, Chiu HY. Distally based anterolateral thigh flap: an anatomic and clinical study. Plast Reconstr Surg. 2004;114:1768–75.
19. Lin CH, Zelken J, Hsu CC, Lin CH, Wei FC. The Distally based, venous supercharged anterolateral thigh flap. Microsurg. 2016;36:20–8.

Ascending and Transverse Branches of the Lateral Circumflex Femoral Vessels

31

Raffi Gurunian

Introduction

The lateral circumflex femoral vessels and their branches support various locoregional or microsurgical flaps in the armamentarium of reconstructive surgery. In addition, these vessels may serve as recipient for microsurgical reconstruction of soft tissue and/or bone in the hip, the thigh, the knee, and in some cases the lower abdomen.

Preoperative Assessment

Considerable amount of critical thinking and careful planning is required in each and every microsurgical flap case. When microsurgical reconstruction is indicated in the hip area, the lateral circumflex femoral artery (LCFA) and its tributaries are available for use as recipient vessels, in the majority of cases. However, imaging studies like color Doppler ultrasound, computed tomography angiography, or magnetic resonance angiography may be warranted in the presence of previous radiation and trauma. Typically, the decision that branches of the LCF vessels can be used as recipient site vessel is made intraoperatively.

Applied Anatomy

The lateral circumflex femoral artery commonly originates from the lateral side of the profunda femoris artery, passes laterally between the divisions of the femoral nerve behind the sartorius and rectus femoris muscles, and divides into ascending, transverse, and descending branches [1] (Fig. 31.1). Initially, the ascending and transverse branches are generally a common conduit and subsequently divide. In

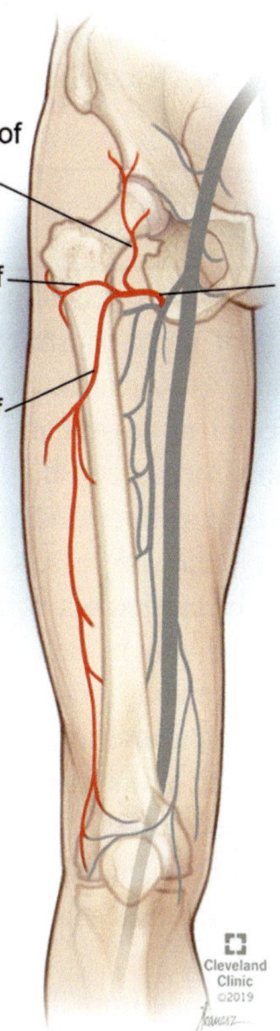

Fig. 31.1 Illustration of the ascending, the transverse, and the descending branches of the lateral circumflex femoral artery. (Printed with permission, Cleveland Clinic, Center for Medical Art & Photography © 2019. All Rights Reserved)

Supplementary Information The online version of this chapter (https://doi.org/10.1007/978-3-030-75389-4_31) contains supplementary material, which is available to authorized users.

R. Gurunian (✉)
Department of Plastic Surgery, Cleveland Clinic, Cleveland, OH, USA

Cleveland Clinic Lerner College of Medicine, Case Western Reserve University, Cleveland, OH, USA
e-mail: gurunir@ccf.org

R. Gurunian, R. Djohan (eds.), *Recipient Vessels in Reconstructive Microsurgery*, https://doi.org/10.1007/978-3-030-75389-4_31

a cadaver dissection study, Hubmer et al. demonstrated that the ascending branch emerged from the lateral circumflex femoral artery in 44 cases of 45 specimens. In one case, the ascending branch and the descending branch of the lateral circumflex femoral artery originated separately from the deep femoral artery [2]. The authors also demonstrated that the transverse branch was available in all 45 specimens studied. In 33 specimens, the transverse branch emerged from the ascending branch. In six cases, it emerged together with the descending branch from the lateral circumflex femoral artery, and in five cases, it emerged from the descending branch. In one case, the transverse branch was the first vessel to emerge from the lateral circumflex femoral artery [2].

The ascending branch is predictably located at a range of 7.5–11.0 cm distal to the anterior superior iliac spine (ASIS) on the line drawn from the ASIS to the lateral border of the patella [3, 4].

In cadaver dissections, Saadeh and his associates found that the external diameter of the ascending branch is 2.90 mm with a mean length of 3.79 cm. The artery is closely associated by two venae comitantes measuring 1.8 to 2.5 mm in diameter [5]. A three-dimensional vascular anatomy study of the tensor fascia latae by Kalander and Morris demonstrated the mean external diameter of the LCFA-ascending artery to be 2.7 mm ± 0.4 and the mean length 3.6 cm ± 0.6. The distance from the anterior superior iliac spine to point where the vascular pedicle reaches the muscle ranged from 6.7 to 10.2 cm [6].

Surgical Site Exposure

Position of the patient varies according to the flap harvest site as well as goals of the reconstruction. If possible, the positioning should allow two teams working simultaneously, one preparing the recipient vessels and the other raising the flap. These two teams should constantly be in communication regarding the length, caliber, and quality of the flap pedicle as well as the recipient site vessels.

Dissection should be carried out with the patient relaxed. An ipsilateral hip bump may be helpful. The key landmark for exposure of the ascending branch as well as the transverse branch is the anterior superior iliac spine (ASIS). When a line is drawn from this point to the lateral border of the patella edge, it coincides with the anterior edge of the tensor fascia latae muscle (TFL) and the vastus lateralis muscle. This line also roughly delineates lateral border of the rectus femoris muscle.

A skin incision extending from the margin of the defect is made over the line described earlier in the proximal anterolateral thigh. While retracting the skin and subcutaneous tissue above the TFL muscle through this incision, the suprafascial plane is dissected bluntly to identify the interval between the TFL and the rectus femoris muscle. The rectus femoris and sartorius muscles are retracted medially to facilitate exposure and dissection. The thick fascia overlying the TFL and the rectus femoris muscles is incised to enter the interval between these two muscles. Self-retaining retractors and hooks are very useful and can be used in a step-wise manner as the dissection deepens. Oftentimes the additional fascial webs/bands need to be transected in the interval to access the ascending branch. Once visualized on the deep surface of the tensor fascia latae muscle, the ascending branch is tracked medially toward the origin from the lateral circumflex femoral artery. In general, the ascending branch can be estimated to be at a point 7 to 12 cm distal to the ASIS. The vessel is transected when sufficient workable size and length is obtained for microvascular anastomosis [7]. The ascending artery usually is accompanied by two venae comitantes (Figs. 31.2 and 31.3, Video 31.1). However, this is a vein-rich area, and other suitable veins in the vicinity can

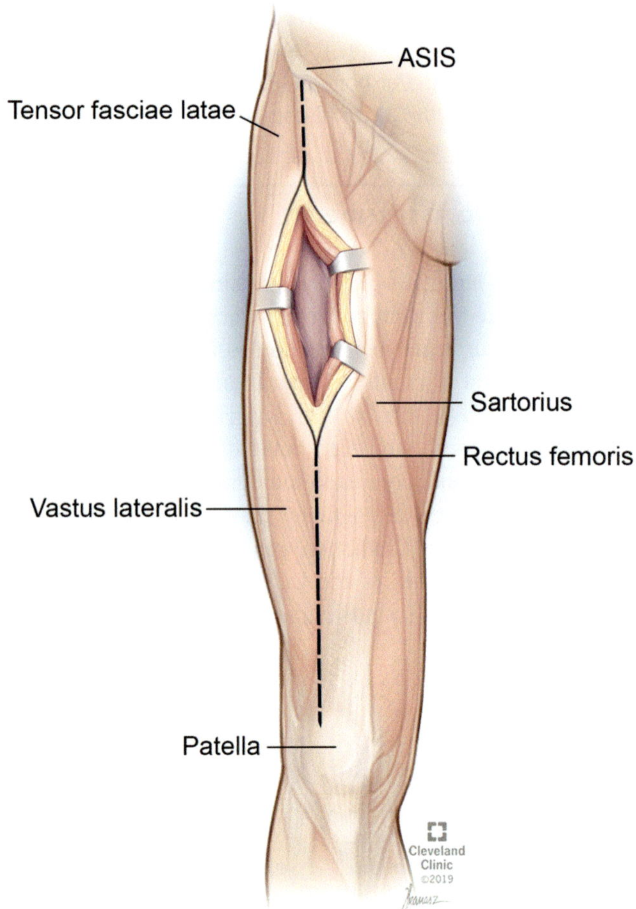

Fig. 31.2 Anatomical location of the ascending branch: A line is drawn from the anterior superior iliac spine (ASIS) to the lateral border of the patella. This line coincides with the medial and anterior border of the tensor fascia latae muscle and the vastus lateralis muscle. In general, the ascending branch of the lateral circumflex femoral artery is located at a point 7 to 12 cm distal to the anterior superior iliac spine, in the interval between the tensor fascia latae and the rectus femoris muscles. (Printed with permission, Cleveland Clinic, Center for Medical Art & Photography © 2019. All Rights Reserved)

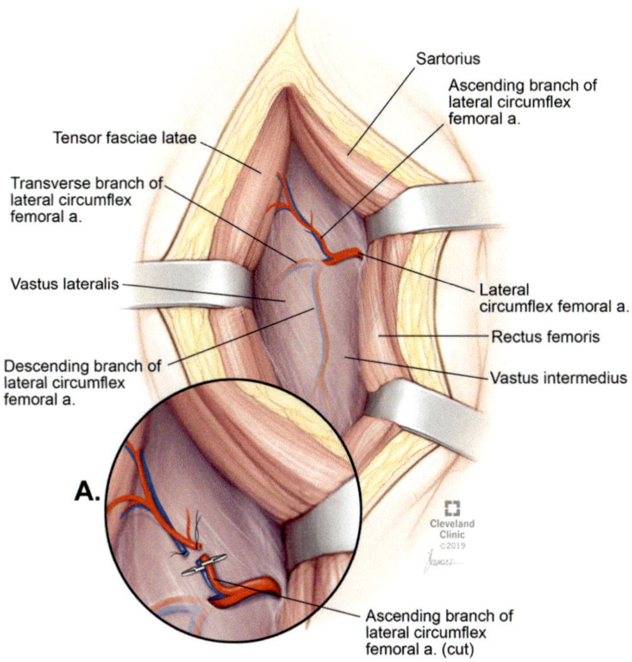

Fig. 31.3 The interval between the tensor fascia latae and the rectus femoris muscles. The ascending branch follows an oblique course behind the rectus femoris muscle to reach the tensor fascia latae muscle, laterally and superiorly in the hip. The close-up view demonstrating the ascending branch prepared as recipient vessel for microvascular anastomosis. Alternatively, the transverse branch may be used for the same purpose. It can be located more distally between the rectus femoris and the vastus lateralis muscles. The caliber and length of this vessel should be assessed to determine its suitability for recipient vessel. (**A**) Close-up drawing of the ascending branch that is divided and prepared for microvascular anastomosis. (Printed with permission, Cleveland Clinic, Center for Medical Art & Photography © 2019. All Rights Reserved)

easily be dissected and prepared. Also, the transverse branch of the lateral circumflex femoral artery can be exposed using the same approach and potentially used as recipient. However, the dissection needs to be extended more distally between the rectus femoris and vastus lateralis muscles. The transverse branch can be found about 5 cm distal to the ascending branch (Video 31.1). Its potential use as an alternative recipient needs to be assessed for length and caliber as the transverse branch is the smallest of all the branches of the lateral circumflex femoral vessels [8]. Thus, various recipient vessel options are available in this area. The choice would be at the discretion of the reconstructive microsurgeon.

Discussion

The ascending branch has some advantages when used as recipient. The clinical and anatomical evidence has demonstrated a consistent anatomy, predictable location, and sufficient length and caliber. The surgical site exposure is relatively easy and straightforward. Lateral location close to the hip makes the ascending branch more suitable for use in the lateral hip and proximal lateral thigh defects. Also, the location of the ascending branch of the lateral circumflex femoral artery is suitable for vascularization of the free fibula in the management of avascular necrosis of femoral head [9].

Use of ascending branch also bears some drawbacks. First, microvascular anastomoses can be technically challenging as it lies deep in the proximal thigh especially in patients with thick subcutaneous tissue. Second, the pedicle for the tensor fascia latae muscle flap is sacrificed, thus eliminating the potential use of this muscle flap. Third, the ascending branch rarely can be of inadequate diameter. In such cases, further dissection may be required medially toward the LCF vessels, which may reduce the workable distance of the vessel. Alternatively, the transverse branch can be exposed and examined for its suitability for microanastomosis. Also, the descending branch may potentially be used as recipient. However, it would be necessary to extend the dissection further inferiorly to obtain an effective vessel length [10]. Also, larger diameter LCFA/V can be reached by ligating the descending branch, which at their origin is 1.5–2.5 mm and 2.5–4.0 mm, respectively [11]. Final selection of the proper artery and vein is made considering the caliber and length of these vessels as well as the pedicle of the microsurgical flap.

References

1. Rueda M, Rueda S, Alleyne B, Drake RL, Gurunluoglu R. Chap. 3. Anatomy of the lower extremity. In: Bruce MA, editor. Plastic surgery: a practical guide to patient care. New York: Thieme Publishers. 2020.
2. Hubmer MG, Schwaiger N, Windisch G, Feigl G, Koch H, Haas FM, Justich I, Scharnagl E. The vascular anatomy of the tensor fasciae latae perforator flap. Plast Reconstr Surg. 2009;124(1):181–9.
3. Nahai F. The tensor fascia lata flap. Clin Plast Surg. 1980;7:51–6.
4. Cormack GC, Lamberty BGH. The arterial anatomy of skin flaps. 2nd ed. New York: Churchill Livingstone; 1994. p. 236–7.
5. Saadeh FA, Haikal FA, Abdel-Hamid FA. Blood supply of the tensor fasciae latae muscle. Clin Anat. 1998;11:236–8.
6. Kalandar A, Morris SF. Three-dimensional vascular anatomical study of the tensor fasciae Latae muscle and perforators. J Reconstr Microsurg. 2019; https://doi.org/10.1055/s-0038-1677010.
7. Gurunluoglu R. The ascending branch of the lateral circumflex femoral vessels: review of the anatomy and its utilization as recipient vessel for free-flap reconstruction of the hip region. J Reconstr Microsurg. 2010;26(6):359–66.
8. Williams PL, Warwick R, Dyson M, Bannsiter LH. Arteries of the lower limbs. In: Williams PL, Warwick R, Dyson M, Bannsiter LH, editors. Gray's Anatomy. New York: Churchill Livingstone; 1989. p. 781–91.
9. Tu Y, Chen Z, Lineaweaver WC, Zhang F. Different recipient vessels for free microsurgical fibula flaps in the treatment of avascular necrosis of the femoral head: a systematic review and meta-analysis. Ann Plast Surg. 2017;79(6):583–9.
10. Hallock GG. The vascular pedicle of the anterolateral thigh flap as an alternative recipient site for thigh free flaps. J Reconstr Microsurg. 2008;24:131–6.
11. Strauch B, Yu HL, Chen ZW, Liebling R. Tensor fascia lata flap. In: Strauch B, Yu HL, Chen ZW, Liebling R, editors. Atlas of microvascular surgery. New York: Thieme Medical Publishers; 1993. p. 174–6.

Superficial Femoral Vessels and Branches

32

DeAsia D. Jacob and Raffi Gurunian

Introduction

The superficial femoral vessels and its branches can be used as recipient vessels in microsurgical reconstruction of defects of the perineum, thigh, and the knee and also in gender confirmation surgery during phalloplasty. When considering using the superficial femoral artery as a recipient vessel, it is important to recall its role in supplying blood to the lower limb, and disruptions in blood flow to this vessel can result in critical lower limb ischemia [1]. Because of the superficial femoral artery's main role in the lower limb, anastomoses to this vessel need to be performed in an end-to-side fashion to preserve perfusion to the lower limb. There are many locations along the length of the superficial femoral vessels where microsurgical anastomoses can be performed, depending on the location of the defect. It is critical to have an understanding of the regional anatomy of the desired location of exposure to protect other critical neurovascular structures that travel with the superficial femoral vessels. This chapter will explore this anatomy and provide case examples of the superficial femoral vessels' use in microsurgical reconstruction.

Supplementary Information The online version of this chapter (https://doi.org/10.1007/978-3-030-75389-4_32) contains supplementary material, which is available to authorized users.

D. D. Jacob
Department of Plastic Surgery, Cleveland Clinic, Cleveland, OH, USA
e-mail: Jacobd@ccf.org

R. Gurunian (✉)
Department of Plastic Surgery, Cleveland Clinic, Cleveland, OH, USA

Cleveland Clinic Lerner College of Medicine, Case Western Reserve University, Cleveland, OH, USA
e-mail: gurunir@ccf.org

Preoperative Assessment

The superficial femoral artery must be used with caution in people with a history of peripheral arterial disease. Because of the superficial femoral artery's long course in the thigh with few side branches, it is subject to forces such as compression, flexion, and torsion that can change the flow through the vessels and predispose it to peripheral arterial disease [2, 3]. A careful history and physical must be obtained. Patients with a history of risk factors for peripheral arterial disease such as coronary artery disease, diabetes mellitus, hypertension, older age, gender, and smoking [4] should alert the reconstructive surgeon to perform a careful physical exam or obtain ancillary studies, such as computed tomography angiography (CTA) [5], to evaluate the patency of the desired recipient vessels. Patients with lower extremity peripheral arterial disease may present with claudication, rest pain, ischemic ulceration or gangrene, temperature or color changes of the leg, or absent pulses [4]. Caution should be used in selecting the superficial femoral vessels as recipients in these high-risk patients.

Applied Anatomy

Embryologically, the femoral artery is present at the 14 mm stage and enters the leg as a distinct artery that communicates with the axial and sciatic arteries. Around 22 mm the sciatic artery regresses, and the femoral artery becomes the sole arterial supply to the lower limb [6]. Anatomical variations of the superficial femoral artery have been described such as duplication [7, 8], hypoplasia [9, 10] and persistent sciatic arteries that supply the lower limb [11, 12]. The microvascular surgeon must be aware of these anatomical variations because they have higher rates of aneurysm formation and thromboembolic complications [13, 14]. These patients may also suffer from intermittent claudication [15]. These variants may be

R. Gurunian, R. Djohan (eds.), *Recipient Vessels in Reconstructive Microsurgery*,
https://doi.org/10.1007/978-3-030-75389-4_32

unusable and may require the use of alternative recipient vessels.

After the external iliac artery passes under the inguinal ligament, it becomes the common femoral artery (lies anterior to the femoral head), which runs for about 4 cm until the profunda femoris branches off posterolaterally, and the continuation is known as the superficial femoral artery [6, 16]. The superficial femoral artery continues down the length of the thigh and gives off the descending genicular branch before it enters the adductor hiatus which is the aperture in the aponeurotic insertion of the adductor magnus that transmits the femoral artery and vein from the adductor canal to the popliteal space [6, 17, 18]. As it exits the adductor hiatus, the superficial femoral artery becomes the popliteal artery [6, 16]. The superficial femoral artery can be exposed in the femoral triangle or in the adductor/Hunter's canal. The anatomy of each area is described below.

Femoral Triangle

The femoral triangle is located in the upper third of the thigh below the inguinal ligament. Its borders are inguinal ligament (superior), adductor longus (medial), and sartorius (lateral) [16, 19, 20]. The floor is formed by the iliopsoas, pectineus, and adductor longus. The roof is composed of the layers of skin, subcutaneous tissue, and superficial and deep fascia. The contents of the femoral triangle, from lateral to medial, are the femoral nerve, femoral artery, femoral vein, and lymphatics [19, 20] (Video 32.1). With the exception of the femoral nerve, all of the structures within the femoral triangle are encased within the femoral sheath, which is a continuation of the transversalis fascia in the abdomen and the iliac fascia. The femoral nerve is found between the iliacus and psoas major muscles but is not within the femoral sheath. Within the sheath, each neurovascular structure has its own subsheath [19, 20] (also see Chap. 17).

Adductor Canal (Hunter's Canal)

The adductor canal is a musculoaponeurotic tunnel that passes through the middle to lower third of the thigh, averaging 8.5–11.5 cm in length [21, 22]. Several of the same structures that pass through the femoral triangle also pass through the adductor canal. Its borders are vastus medialis (anterolateral), adductor longus (proximal-posterior), adductor magnus (distal-posterior), and vasoadductor membrane located deep to sartorius (medial) (also see Chap. 17). The distal apex of the femoral triangle becomes the superior aspect of the adductor canal. The canal ends distally in the leg at the adductor hiatus. The contents of the canal are the superficial femoral vein, the superficial femoral artery, and the saphenous nerve (Video 32.2). The femoral vein courses posterior to the superficial femoral artery within the canal [6]. Within the canal, the superficial femoral artery gives off the descending genicular and saphenous branches [22]. The distance between the entrance and exit of the adductor canal differs by sex. On average the distance between the anterior superior iliac spine and the entrance to the canal is 25 cm in men and 24 cm in women; the average distance from the adductor hiatus to the patella is 9 cm in males and 9.5 cm in females [22]. After the adductor hiatus, the superficial femoral artery becomes the popliteal artery [6, 16, 21]. As the femoral vein ascends through the canal, it receives contributions from minor veins before it joins with the deep femoral vein and the great saphenous vein to become the common femoral vein [21].

It is important to consider the caliber of the recipient vessels and how it compares to the donor vessels in microsurgical reconstruction. As previously mentioned, because of the important role of the superficial vessels in lower extremity circulation, anastomoses must be performed end-to-side. Vessel caliber differs between sexes and also with age. Czyzewska et al. found that there was a statistically significant difference in the caliber of the superficial femoral artery between men and women, with men having larger vessels [23]. This same group found that with age the caliber of the superficial femoral artery increased in both sexes [23]. Femoral vein diameter was found in a study by Fronek et al. to increase in size with the Valsalva maneuver and decrease in size with age, and the vein was significantly smaller in size in Hispanics, African Americans, and Asians compared to non-Hispanic whites [24]. Body mass index (BMI) was also shown to have an effect on vessel location – vessels are located significantly deeper in overweight patients compared to normal weight patients [25]. A similar relationship was shown by Keiler et al. who found that there was a significant positive correlation between femoral vein diameter and BMI, and they also found positional changes in vein diameter with larger diameter in the upright position compared to supine [26]. The vessel diameter of the superficial femoral artery ranges from 2.5 to 9.6 mm [23, 27, 28]. The vessel diameter of the femoral vein ranges from 11.2 to 16.4 mm [24, 26].

Surgical Site Exposure

Literature has shown that an oblique rather than a longitudinal incision is superior for femoral artery exposure at the groin. A transverse incision is associated with decreased incidence of wound infection, wound dehiscence as the incision follows Langer lines, and preservation of lymphatics [29–32]. If the patient has preexisting incisions or lacerations or wounds, then these should be incorporated into the recipient vessel exposure (Video 32.1). If no such areas exist, then thought should be given to using an oblique incision for superficial femoral artery exposure at the groin. Distal defects of the thigh and knee should take into consideration the existing defect.

The patient is placed supine on the operating table. External rotation of the thigh may help ease vessel exposure [29, 33]. An oblique incision that parallels the inguinal ligament (from the anterior superior iliac spine to the symphysis pubis) is planned; this incision can be either inferior or superior to the ligament but should not lie in the groin crease [29, 30]. The incision needs to be large enough to provide adequate vessel exposure and to facilitate microsurgical anastomosis. If a longitudinal incision is required, the incision should be made at the midpoint of a line along the inguinal ligament and a line extending from the anterior superior iliac spine to the medial femoral condyle [31].

Dissection proceeds through skin and subcutaneous tissue, and as the superficial lymphatics are approached they should be carefully divided or preserved to prevent lymphatic disruption [31]. The femoral vessels are located deep in the groin within the fascial covering of the femoral sheath, beneath the sartorius [33]. The femoral vein and deep lymph nodes will be located medial to the artery within the femoral triangle. Also, branches of the common femoral artery; superficial circumflex iliac, superficial epigastric (also see Chap. 19), and superficial and deep pudendal arteries (also see Chap. 44) may be used for an end-to-end anastomoses. In terms of recipient veins, in addition to the saphenous vein, additional venous options include the superficial circumflex iliac vein (SCIV) and the superficial inferior epigastric vein (SIEV). Alternatively, femoral vein can be used in an end-to-side fashion. If superficial femoral artery exposure is needed more distally, the roof of the adductor canal must be incised, and the sartorius and vastus medialis are retracted laterally, and the adductor longus is moved medially [33] (Figs. 32.1 and 32.2). Anastomosis to the superficial femoral artery is performed end-to-side. Venae comitantes travel with the superficial femoral artery, and an appropriate venous anastomosis can be performed based on the caliber of the donor vein, most frequently in an end-to-side manner. Also, the great saphenous vein can be dissected in the medial thigh and transposed to the vicinity for venous anastomosis. In the adductor canal, additionally the descending genicular vessels can offer alternative recipient (also see Chap. 39). Which vessel to be used as recipient depends on multiple factors that include length and caliber of the donor vessels and location of the defect to be reconstructed.

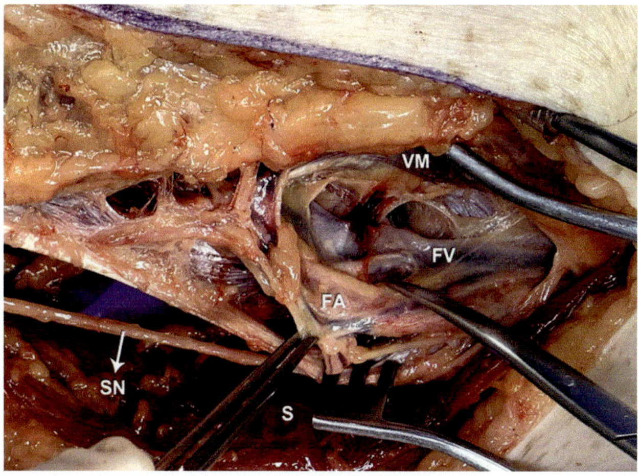

Fig. 32.2 Exposure of the superficial femoral artery (FA) and superficial femoral vein (FV) in the adductor canal. *VM* vastus medialis, *S* sartorius, *SN* saphenous nerve

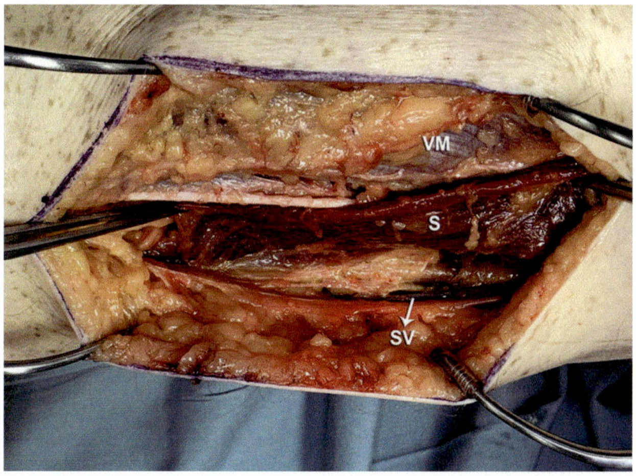

Fig. 32.1 A cadaver dissection for exposure of adductor canal. *S* sartorius, *VM* vastus medialis, *SV* great saphenous vein

Case 1

The patient is a 75-year-old male patient with high-grade undifferentiated pleomorphic sarcoma in the right proximal/medial thigh (Fig. 32.3). He has completed preoperative radiotherapy with 62.5 Gy. Surgery has been timed to allow for a 4-week rest of the soft tissue. Wide local excision of the sarcoma was performed resulting in a large defect with exposed femoral vessels in the femoral triangle (Fig. 32.4). The profunda femoris artery and vein entered the mass and required ligation. The defect was reconstructed using contralateral anterolateral thigh free flap (Fig. 32.5). Arterial anastomosis was performed between the superficial circumflex iliac artery (recipient) and descending branch (flap vessel) in an end-to-end fashion. One venous anastomosis was conducted between the common femoral vein and donor

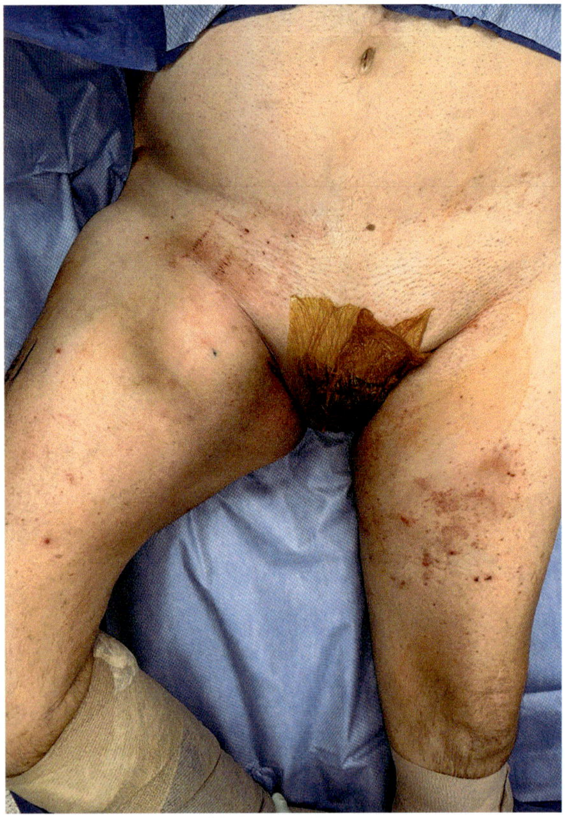

Fig. 32.3 High-grade undifferentiated pleomorphic sarcoma, right proximal/medial thigh

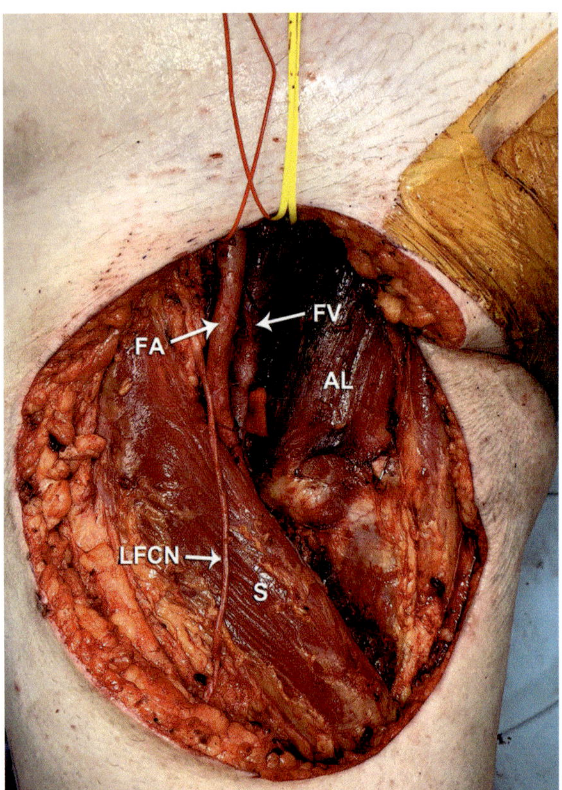

Fig. 32.4 The defect after resection with exposed femoral artery (FA) and femoral vein (FV). *AL* adductor longus, *S* sartorius, *LFCN* lateral femoral cutaneous nerve

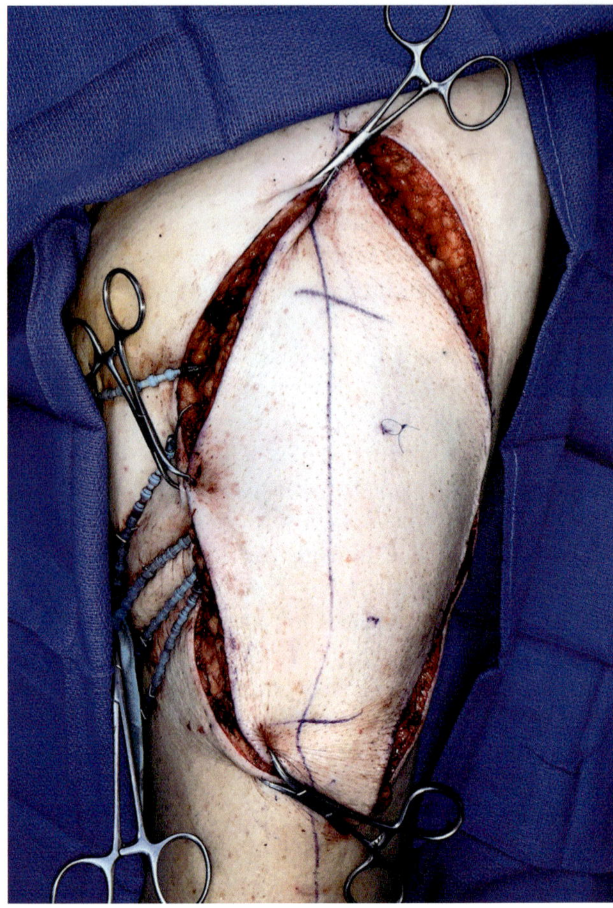

Fig. 32.5 Free anterolateral thigh flap prior to harvest

vein in an end-to-side fashion. The second venous anastomosis was between the superficial circumflex iliac vein and second donor vein using 2.5 mm coupler (Figs. 32.6 and 32.7, Video 32.1).

Case 2

The patient is a 54-year-old male smoker with a history of a motor vehicle accident more than 30 years prior to presentation and a surgical history of open reduction and internal fixation of the right femur and tibia that was complicated by partial right lower extremity paralysis (foot drop, quadriceps wasting, and deficient extensor mechanism) and compartment syndrome requiring decompression and skin grafting. He subsequently sustained a fall 7 years prior to presentation related to his partial paralysis that resulted in patella tendon rupture and chronic patella alta and eventually resulted in a chronic knee wound. He had multiple debridements and courses of intravenous antibiotics performed at another institution. At presentation he was being managed with oral antibiotics and negative pressure wound therapy. On exam there was visible communication of the 4 × 7 cm wound with the knee joint (Fig. 32.8). Knee joint

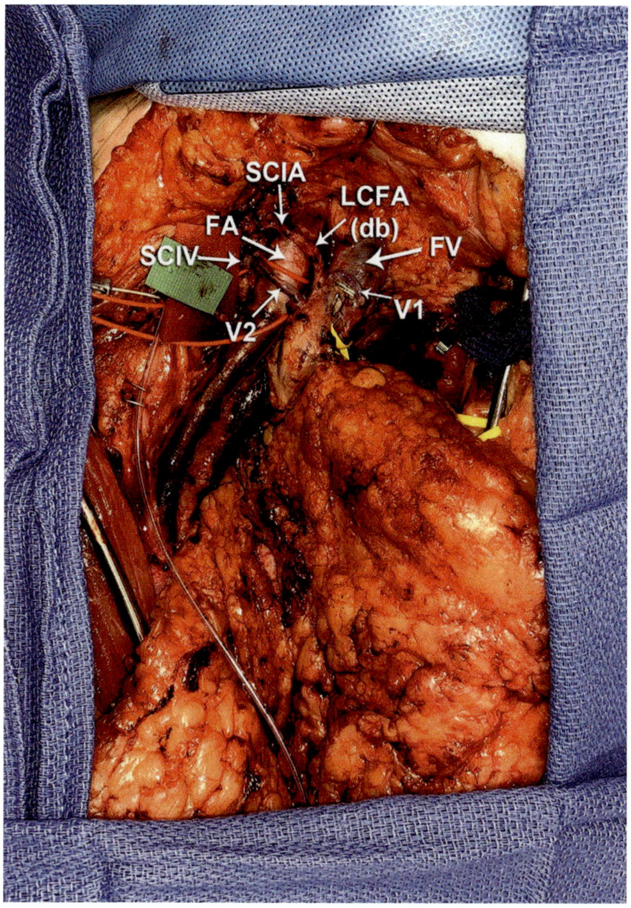

Fig. 32.6 Arterial anastomosis was performed between the superficial circumflex iliac artery (SCIA) (recipient) and descending branch (db) (flap vessel) in an end-to-end fashion. One venous anastomosis was conducted between the common femoral vein (FV) and donor vein (V1) in an end-to-side fashion. The second venous anastomosis was between the superficial circumflex iliac vein (SCIV) and second donor vein (V2) using 2.5 mm coupler

aspiration performed by the orthopedic surgery team revealed *Haemophilus parainfluenzae* and *Staphylococcus epidermidis*. He was subsequently taken by the orthopedic team for serial operative debridements until wound cultures were negative. Pathology did not show osteomyelitis. He remained on intravenous antibiotics per the infectious disease service.

One week later the patient was taken to the operating room for reconstruction. A contralateral free anterolateral thigh flap was raised. Initial exploration of the descending branch of the lateral circumflex femoral vessels and the posterior tibial vessels revealed vessels that were unusable, likely because of trauma and multiple previous surgeries. Attention was then turned to the superficial femoral vessels.

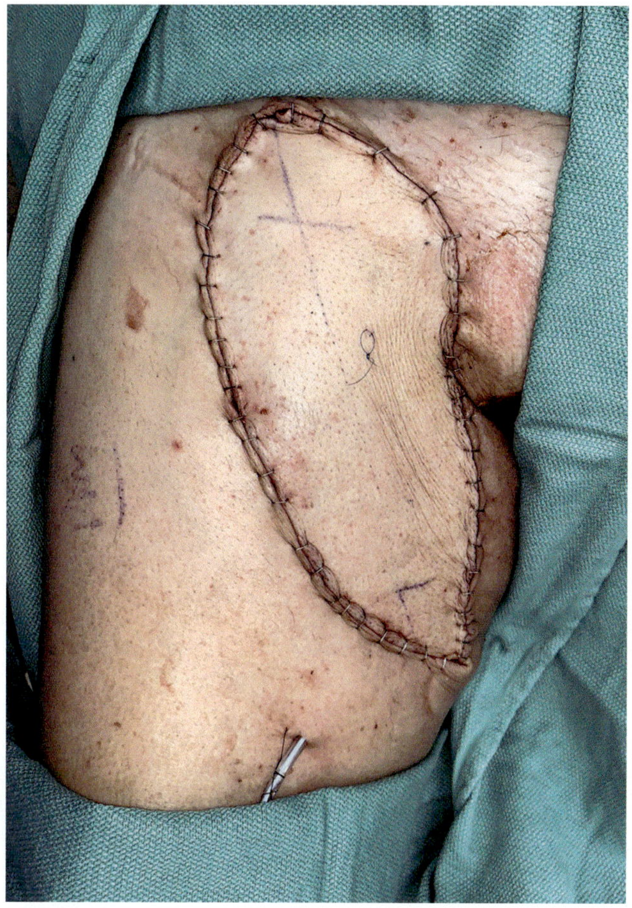

Fig. 32.7 Inset of free anterolateral thigh flap after microvascular anastomoses

A sub-sartorius approach in the distal thigh was used to expose the femoral vessels. End-to-side anastomosis was performed between the superficial femoral vessels and the flap vessels. The flap was inset, and all wounds were closed. In follow-up the patient maintained adequate coverage of the previous knee wound (Fig. 32.9) and was able to ambulate successfully.

Discussion

The superficial femoral artery has been well described in the literature as a donor vessel for flap reconstruction [34–38], but it has also been described for use as a recipient vessel in microsurgical reconstruction. About the knee there are many different flaps described that have used the superficial femoral artery as a recipient [39]. Hierner et al.

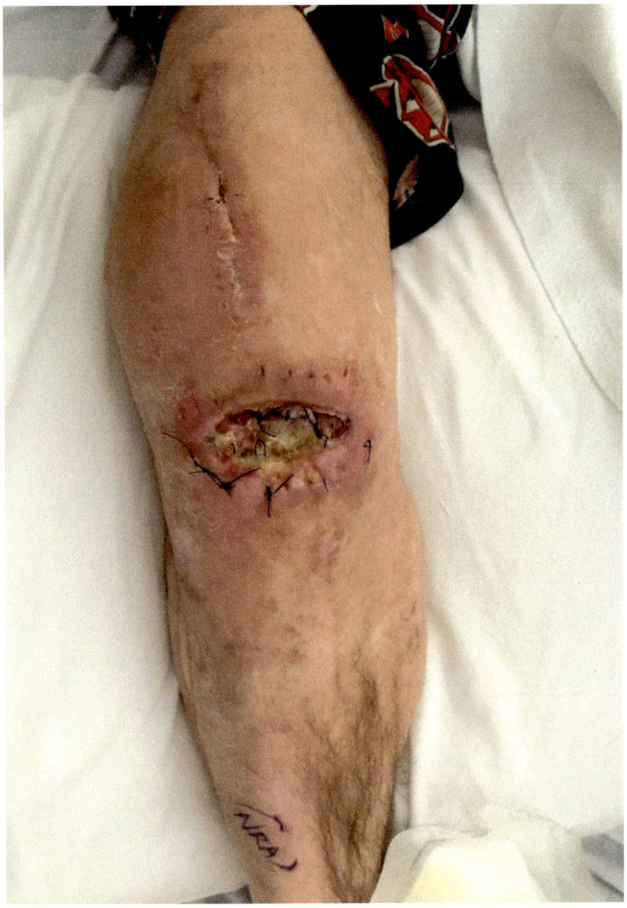

Fig. 32.8 The knee defect

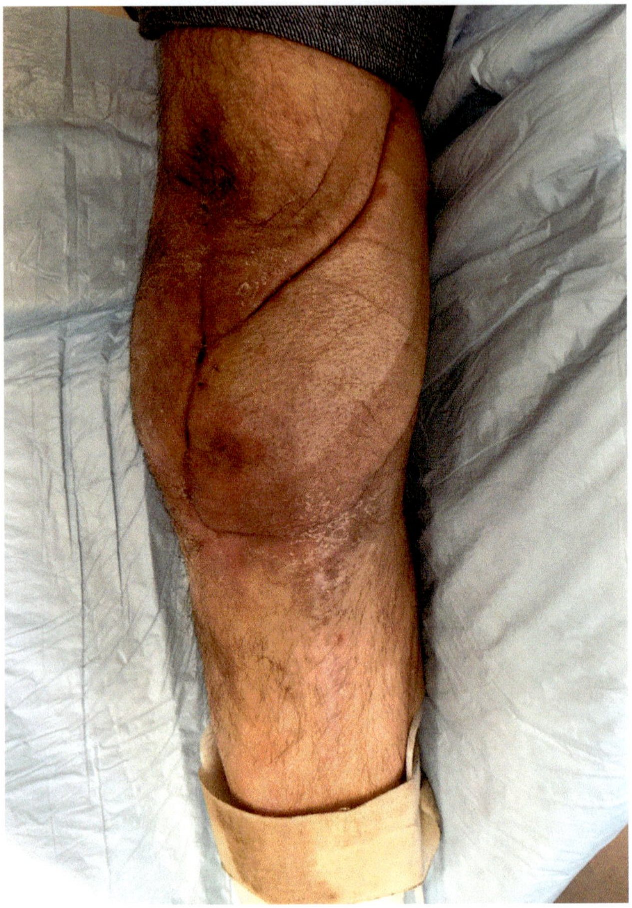

Fig. 32.9 Microsurgical reconstruction was performed using free anterolateral thigh flap after a serial of debridements. Microvascular anastomoses were performed in an end-to-side fashion between the femoral vessels and flap pedicle

describe their series of 14 patients in whom they performed free myocutaneous latissimus dorsi flap reconstruction after total knee arthroplasty with good results [40]. Peters et al. report a similar case of using a latissimus dorsi free flap for lower limb trauma in which the superficial femoral artery was used as a recipient, but postoperatively the artery thrombosed and resulted in complete flap loss [41]. It is important to keep this in mind when selecting the superficial femoral as a recipient. Herrera et al. have described using a consistent muscular branch of the superficial femoral artery to the sartorius muscle as a recipient vessel for reconstruction around the knee and proximal tibia [42]. In this cadaveric study, the authors found that this arterial branch had a mean diameter of 1.5 mm and can be found on average 13 cm proximal to the medial epicondyle of the femur, entering the sartorius on its deep surface. The venae comitantes that travel with this branch were on average 1.2 mm; alternatively the saphenous vein can be used for venous outflow [42].

Another indication for use of the superficial femoral vessels as recipient vessels is phalloplasty defects, both congenital and traumatic. Perovic et al. describe using a free musculocutaneous latissimus dorsi flap for congenital, iatrogenic, and traumatic penile defects in adults and children [43]. The authors used the femoral artery and saphenous vein as recipient vessels, and they reported no flap loss [43]. Similarly, these vessels can be used as recipients in masculinizing gender confirmation surgery during phalloplasty. Several authors, including Safa and colleagues, advocate for radial forearm phalloplasty using an end-to-side anastomosis to the superficial femoral artery and saphenous vein [44, 45] (also see Chap. 44).

Conclusion

The superficial femoral artery has an important role in providing blood flow to the lower extremity, and its total sacrifice would result in critical limb ischemia. This vessel and its branches may be used for microsurgical reconstruction of defects of the perineum, thigh, and knee and for phalloplasty defects or reconstruction. The superficial femoral artery can be identified proximally in the groin in the femoral triangle or distally in the thigh in the adductor canal. Caution must be used in patients at high risk for peripheral arterial disease to ensure patency of the vessels. Because of its critical role, use of this vessel requires end-to-side arterial anastomosis. The venae comitantes that travel with the artery or branches of the saphenous vein may be used for venous outflow.

References

1. Wei FC, Mardini S. Free style flaps. In: Wei FC, Mardini S, editors. Flaps and reconstructive surgery. China: Elsevier Inc; 2009. p. 617–24.
2. Perlstein TS, Krichavsky. Peripheral artery disease. In: Antman EM, Sabatine MS, editors. Cardiovascular therapeutics: a companion to Braunwald's heart disease. Philadelphia: Elsevier Inc; 2013. p. 539–550.
3. Moosavi J. Peripheral artery disease. In: Maleki M, Alizadehasl A, Haghjoo M, editors. Practical cardiology. St. Louis: Elsevier Inc; 2018. p. 367–75.
4. Ouriel K. Peripheral arterial disease. Lancet. 2001;358(9289):1257–64. https://doi.org/10.1016/S0140-6736(01)06351-6.
5. Lee GK, Fox PM, Riboh J, Hsu C, Saber S, Rubin GD, et al. Computed tomography angiography in microsurgery: indications, clinical utility, and pitfalls. Eplasty. 2013;13:e42.
6. Swift H, Bordoni B. Anatomy, bony pelvis and lower limb, femoral artery [Updated 2020 Aug 10]. In: StatPearls [Internet]. Treasure Island (FL): StatPearls Publishing; 2020 Jan-. Available from: https://www.ncbi.nlm.nih.gov/books/NBK538262/.
7. Yu SH, Hwang JH, Kim JH, Park S, Lee KH, Choi ST. Duplication of superficial femoral artery: imaging findings and literature review. BMC Med Imaging. 2020;20(99).https://doi.org/10.1186/s12880-020-00500-4.
8. Hapugoda S, Hsu CC, Kwan GNC, Watkins TW, Rophael JA. Duplication of the superficial femoral artery: comprehensive review of imaging literature and insight into embryology. Acta Rad Open. 2016; https://doi.org/10.1177/2058460116659098.
9. Kwon JH, Shin JH. Hypoplastic superficial femoral artery combined with connection of the deep femoral artery to the popliteal artery. Radiol Case Rep. 2018;13(1):39–42. https://doi.org/10.1016/j.radcr.2017.10.028.
10. Buckley JG, Levitt RG, Zuckerman DA. Hypoplastic superficial femoral artery associated with bilateral persistent sciatic arteries: a diagnostic pitfall. Cardiovasc Intervent Radiol. 1992;15:240–3. https://doi.org/10.1007/BF02733930.
11. Shehzad KN, Monib S, Mensa M, Halawa MO. Bilateral persistent sciatic arteries complicated by unilateral acute lower limb ischaemia. J Surg Case Rep. 2019. 2019;4:rjz119. https://doi.org/10.1093/jscr/rjz119.
12. Van Hooft IM, Zeebregts CJ, van Sterkenburg SMM, de Vries WR, Reijnen MMPJ. The persistent sciatic artery. Eur J Vasc Endovasc Surg. 2009;37(5):585–91. https://doi.org/10.1016/j.ejvs.2009.01.014.
13. Brancaccio G, Falco E, Pera M, Celoria G, Stefanini T, Puccianti F. Symptomatic persistent sciatic artery. J Am Coll Surg. 2004;198(1):158. https://doi.org/10.1016/j.jamcollsurg.2003.06.008.
14. Lekehal B, Taberkant M, Sefiani Y, Mekouar T. El Mesnaoui, Benjelloun a et al. aneurysm of a persistent sciatic artery: five case reports. J Mal Vasc. 2001;26(1):60–4.
15. Kritsch D, Hutter HP, Hirschl M, Katzenschlager R. Persistent sciatic artery: an uncommon cause of intermittent claudication. Int Angiol. 2006;25(3):327–9.
16. Wheeless C. Femoral artery. In Wheless' textbook of orthopedics. 2015. http://www.wheelessonline.com/ortho/femoral_artery. Accessed 12 Sep 2020.
17. Gocmen-Mas N, Aksu F, Edizer M, Magden O, Tayfur V, Seyhan T. The arterial anatomy of the saphenous flap: a cadaveric study. Folia Morphol (Warsz). 2012;71(1):10–4.
18. Garcia-Pumarino R, Franco JM. Anatomical variability of descending genicular artery. Ann Plast Surg. 2014;73(5):607–11. https://doi.org/10.1097/SAP.0b013e318276d964.
19. Basinger H, Hogg JP. Anatomy, abdomen and pelvis, femoral triangle [Updated 2020 Jul 27]. In: StatPearls [Internet]. Treasure Island (FL): StatPearls Publishing; 2020 Jan-. Available from: https://www.ncbi.nlm.nih.gov/books/NBK541140/.
20. Ebraheim N, Whaley J, Stirton J, Hamilton R, Andrews K. Femoral triangle anatomy: review, surgical application, and novel mnemonic. J Orthop Res Ther. 2017;129. https://doi.org/10.29011/2575-8241.000139.
21. Migirov A, Vilella RC. Anatomy, abdomen and pelvis, adductor canal (subsartorial, Hunter's canal) [Updated 2020 Sep 13]. In: StatPearls [Internet]. Treasure Island (FL): StatPearls Publishing; 2020 Jan. Available from: https://www.ncbi.nlm.nih.gov/books/NBK556046/.
22. Thiayagarajan MK, Kumar SV, Venkatesh S. An exact localization of adductor canal and its clinical significance: a cadaveric study. Anesth Essays Res. 2019;13(2):284–6. https://doi.org/10.4103/aer.AER_35_19.
23. Czyzewska D, Ustymowicz A, Krysiuk K, Witkowski P, Zonenberg M, Dobrzycki K et al. Ultrasound assessment of the caliber of the arteries in the lower extremities in healthy persons – the dependency on age, sex and morphological parameters of the subjects. J Ultrason. 2012;12(51):420–7. https://doi.org/10.15557/JoU.2012.0030.
24. Fronek A, Criqui MH, Denenberg J, Langer RD. Common femoral vein dimensions and hemodynamics including Valsalva response as a function of sex, age, and ethnicity in a population study. J Vasc Surg. 2001;33(5):1050–6. https://doi.org/10.1067/mva.2001.113496.
25. Seyahi N, Kahveci A, Altiparmak MR, Serdengecti K, Erek E. Ultrasound imaging findings of femoral veins in patients with renal failure and its impact on vascular access. Nephrol Dial Transplant. 2005;20(9):1864–7. https://doi.org/10.1093/ndt/gfh942.
26. Keiler J, Seidel R, Wree A. The femoral vein diameter and its correlation with sex, age and body mass index - an anatomical parameter with clinical relevance. Phlebology. 2019;34(1):58–69. https://doi.org/10.1177/0268355518772746.
27. Spector KS, Lawson WE. Optimizing safe femoral access during cardiac catheterization. Catheter Cardiovasc Interv. 2001;53(2):209–12. https://doi.org/10.1002/ccd.1150.
28. Lorbeer R, Grotz A, Dorr M, Volzke H, Lieb W, Kuhn J, et al. Reference values of vessel diameters, stenosis prevalence, and arterial variations of the lower limb arteries in a male population sample using contrast-enhanced MR angiography. PLoS One. 2018;13(6):e0197559. https://doi.org/10.1371/journal.pone.0197559.
29. Chester JF, Butler CM, Taylor RS. Vascular reconstruction at the groin: oblique or vertical incisions? Ann R Coll Surg Engl. 1992;74(2):112–4.

30. Caiati JM, Kaplan D, Gitlitz D, Hollier LH, Marin ML. The value of the oblique groin incision for femoral artery access during endovascular procedures. Ann Vasc Surg. 2000;14(3):248–53. https://doi.org/10.1007/s100169910042.
31. Cantreras M, Baptista-Silvs JC, do Carmo Novaes F, Cacione DG. Transverse versus vertical groin incision for femoral artery approach. Cochrane Database Syst Rev. 2020;4(4):CD013153. https://doi.org/10.1002/14651858.CD013153.pub2.
32. Tremblay C, Grabs D, Bourgouin D, Bronchti G. Cutaneous vascularization of the femoral triangle in respect to groin incisions. J Vasc Surg. 2016;64(3):757–64. https://doi.org/10.1016/j.jvs.2015.04.385.
33. Velmahos G, Gelbard R. Femoral artery injuries. In: Demetriades D, Inaba K, Velmahos, editors. Atlas of surgical techniques in trauma. Cambridge: Cambridge University Press; 2015. p. 303–336.
34. El-Hadi H, Morris S, Alkhawaji A. The superficial femoral artery flap: a 3-dimensional anatomical study. Plast Surg (Oakv). 2017;25(3):188–93. https://doi.org/10.1177/2292550317716125.
35. Koshima I, Hosoda M, Inagawa K, Moriguchi T, Orita Y. Free medial thigh perforator-based flaps: new definition of the pedicle vessels and versatile application. Ann Plast Surg. 1996;37(5):507–15. https://doi.org/10.1097/00000637-199611000-00009.
36. Mojallal A, Boucher F, Shipkov H, Saint-Cyr M, Braye F. Superficial femoral artery perforator flap: anatomical study of a new flap and clinical cases. Plast Reconstr Surg. 2014;133(4):934–44. https://doi.org/10.1097/PRS.0000000000000005.
37. Ratanshi I, McInnes CW, Islur A. The proximal superficial femoral artery perforator flap: anatomic study and clinical cases. Microsurgery. 2017;37(6):581–8. https://doi.org/10.1002/micr.30155.
38. Mohan AT, Zhu L, Morsy M, Sur YJ, Michalak GJ, Lachman N et al. Reappraisal of perforasomes of the superficial femoral, descending genicular, and saphenous arteries and clinical applications to locoregional reconstruction. Plast Reconstr Surg. 2019;143(3):613e–27e. https://doi.org/10.1097/PRS.0000000000005395.
39. Fang T, Zhang W, Lineaweaver WC, Zhang F. Recipient vessels in the free flap reconstruction around the knee. Ann Plast Surg. 2013;71(4):429–33. https://doi.org/10.1097/SAP.0b013e31824e5e6e.
40. Hierner R, Reynders-Frederix P, Bellemans J, Stuyck J, Peeters W. Free myocutaneous latissimus dorsi flap transfer in total knee arthroplasty. J Plast Reconstr Aesthet Surg. 2009;62(12):1692–700. https://doi.org/10.1016/j.bjps.2008.07.038.
41. Peters T, Fischer P, Lahoda L, Niederbichler AD, Alkandari Q, Vogt P. The free latissimus dorsi flap as primary free flap and crane flap with secondary pedicled transfer. J Reconstr Microsurg. 2008;24(2):73–7. https://doi.org/10.1055/s-2008-1064922.
42. Herrera FA, Lee CK, Kiehn MW, Hansen SL. The distal superficial femoral arterial branch to the sartorius muscle as a recipient vessel for soft tissue defects around the knee: anatomic study and clinical applications. Microsurgery. 2009;29(6):425–9. https://doi.org/10.1002/micr.20620.
43. Perovic SV, Djinovic R, Bumbasirevic M, Djordjevic M, Vukovic P. Total phalloplasty using a musculocutaneous latissimus dorsi flap. BJU Int. 2007;100(4):899–905.; discussion 905. https://doi.org/10.1111/j.1464-410X.2007.07084.x.
44. Safa B, Lin WC, Salim AM, Deschamps-Braly JC, Poh MM. Current concepts in masculinizing gender surgery. Plast Reconstr Surg. 2019;143(4):857e–71e. https://doi.org/10.1097/PRS.0000000000005453.
45. Gottlieb LJ. Radial forearm. Clin Plastic Surg. 2018;45(3):391–8. https://doi.org/10.1016/j.cps.2018.03.009.

Popliteal Vessels and Branches

33

Sarah N. Bishop, DeAsia D. Jacob, Richard L. Drake, and Raffi Gurunian

Introduction

The popliteal vessels provide a broad area of recipient targets for limb salvage for flap coverage of the thigh, knee, or leg. There are several named vessel branches that can be anastomosed to. Unnamed branches can be used as recipient vessels as well as the popliteal vessels themselves. Named and unnamed branches may be anastomosed in an end-to-end fashion. If the popliteal vessels are used directly, then the popliteal vessels should be anastomosed in an end-to-side technique to continue perfusion distally to the leg.

Preoperative Assessment

Patients requiring flaps for limb salvage may have a multitude of etiologies. Lower extremity limb salvage is most often required in the setting of peripheral vascular disease or trauma; however, tumors, infection, or neuropathic ulcers are also inciting factors [1, 2].

Supplementary Information The online version of this chapter (https://doi.org/10.1007/978-3-030-75389-4_33) contains supplementary material, which is available to authorized users.

S. N. Bishop (✉) · R. Gurunian
Department of Plastic Surgery, Cleveland Clinic, Cleveland, OH, USA

Cleveland Clinic Lerner College of Medicine, Case Western Reserve University, Cleveland, OH, USA
e-mail: bishops@ccf.org; gurunir@ccf.org

D. D. Jacob
Department of Plastic Surgery, Cleveland Clinic, Cleveland, OH, USA

R. L. Drake
Department of Anatomy, Cleveland Clinic Lerner College of Medicine, Case Western Reserve University, Cleveland, OH, USA
e-mail: DRAKER@ccf.org

For patients with peripheral vascular disease or trauma, an appropriate vascular workup should be obtained to not only ensure that the popliteal vessels and its branches are patent and not injured but to assess the overall perfusion to the leg and ability to heal. It may be necessary for vascular procedures to be performed to improve the overall perfusion to the leg prior to a flap being performed. One should also note that vascular surgery may also ligate or block branches, and care should be taken in assessing the altered surgical anatomy when choosing recipient targets.

The initial vascular workup for patients with peripheral vascular disease is the ankle brachial index (ABI), pulse volume recording (PVR), and arterial duplex. If there are significant concerns, then additional imaging should be taken with computed tomography angiogram (CTA), or a formal angiogram can be performed. The use of CTA can be helpful in assessing the surrounding anatomy to the defect and is noninvasive except for the use of IV contrast. A formal angiogram can be helpful to more accurately diagnose the patency of the vasculature and can also treat vascular lesions with angioplasty or stenting.

Patients with concern for venous insufficiency should have venous duplexes that specifically assess for venous insufficiency. If venous reflux is seen, then a vascular surgeon can be consulted to treat with radiofrequency ablation or localized vein stripping.

Patients with trauma or infection need to have the appropriate amount of debridement performed to obtain a healthy wound bed. Trauma should also take into account the zone of injury. The zone of injury has been described as the inflammatory territory that extends beyond the wound bed and is thought to have increased rate of free flap failure due to microvascular thromboses [3, 4]. To avoid the zone of injury, substantial proximal dissections and/or vein grafting was used [5]. However, the concept of using recipient vessels far away from the zone of injury has been challenged. Healthy

R. Gurunian, R. Djohan (eds.), *Recipient Vessels in Reconstructive Microsurgery*, https://doi.org/10.1007/978-3-030-75389-4_33

recipient vessels *subjacent* to the wound bed have since been found to be safe and reliable [6].

Patients that require flaps after an oncologic resection have special concerns. Patients may be malnourished or hypercoagulable. Furthermore, these patients often have had preoperative radiation. Vessels that have been in a radiated bed can still be used for microvascular anastomosis, but special care must be taken as these vessels will be friable and easily damaged. In the case that the intended vessels are found not to be reliable, the operative team should be prepared for a different recipient site which may also require additional vein grafting for microvascular anastomoses.

Lower limb salvage is often coupled with orthopedic surgery, and the position of the external fixator device may inhibit the ability to expose specific vessels. Often the reconstructive surgeon will be asked to cover knee arthroplasties. It should be discussed with the orthopedic surgeon preoperatively if an articulating or non-articulating device will be placed. If a non-articulating device is implanted, then the patient will not be able to frog-leg in the supine position which can change the reconstructive surgeon's choices. If a non-articulating spacer will be placed, then the reconstructive surgeon can request to dissect out the recipient vessels before, choose a different recipient location, or accept that a position change may be necessary.

There are a multitude of causes for a patient needing flaps for limb salvage. Each etiology carries its own set of understanding and planning for safe recipient vessel targets.

Applied Anatomy

The popliteal artery supplies the lower thigh, knee, and upper leg area and is a continuation of the superficial femoral artery (see Chap. 32). The popliteal artery transitions from being the superficial femoral artery at the adductor hiatus of the adductor magnus muscle and travels posteriorly to the knee and ends at the lower border of the popliteus muscle where it bifurcates into the anterior tibial artery and the tibioperoneal trunk (which then bifurcates into the posterior tibial artery and peroneal artery) (See Chap. 35). There are some variations of the terminal aspect of the popliteal artery including where the popliteal vessel terminates into the anterior tibial and peroneal with a diminutive or absent posterior tibial artery.

There are three sections of the popliteal artery with corresponding surgical approaches. The popliteal artery is divided into the suprageniculate, midpopliteal, and infrageniculate sections. The "genicular" refers to the knee as in the Greek *genu* translating as knee. The suprageniculate popliteal artery gives rise to the superior medial genicular artery and the superior lateral genicular artery as well as unnamed superior muscular branches within the lower portion of the adductor magnus and hamstring muscles. The superior muscular branches will anastomose with the profunda femoris. The superior medial genicular artery is a small branch that runs around and above the medial epicondyle of the femur and supplies portions of the quadriceps femoris muscles and the knee joint. The superior lateral genicular artery runs below the biceps femoris tendon and around the lateral condyle of the femur and supplies portions of the quadriceps muscles and the knee joint.

The midpopliteal portion of the popliteal artery will give rise to the single and small middle genicular artery and the sural vessels. The middle genicular artery arises posterior to the knee joint and punctures the oblique popliteal ligament and supplies the synovial membrane and ligaments of the knee joint. The sural vessels (or inferior muscular arteries) have two branches: the medial sural and lateral sural which branch off of the midpopliteal area. The medial sural artery is a well-described recipient vessel for microvascular surgery and is discussed in more detail in a subsequent Chapters [7–9] (see Chap. 40).

The infrageniculate popliteal artery gives rise to the inferior medial genicular artery and the inferior lateral genicular artery as well as cutaneous branches that course between the two heads of the gastrocnemius muscles. The inferior medial genicular artery courses around the medial condyle of the tibia and supplies the proximal portion of the tibia and the knee joint. The inferior lateral genicular artery runs laterally around the fibular head and supplies the knee. All four of the superior and inferior medial and lateral genicular arteries form a complex anastomosis to each other anterior to the knee and supply the four quadrants of the popliteal fossa (Figs. 33.1 and 33.2). The supe-

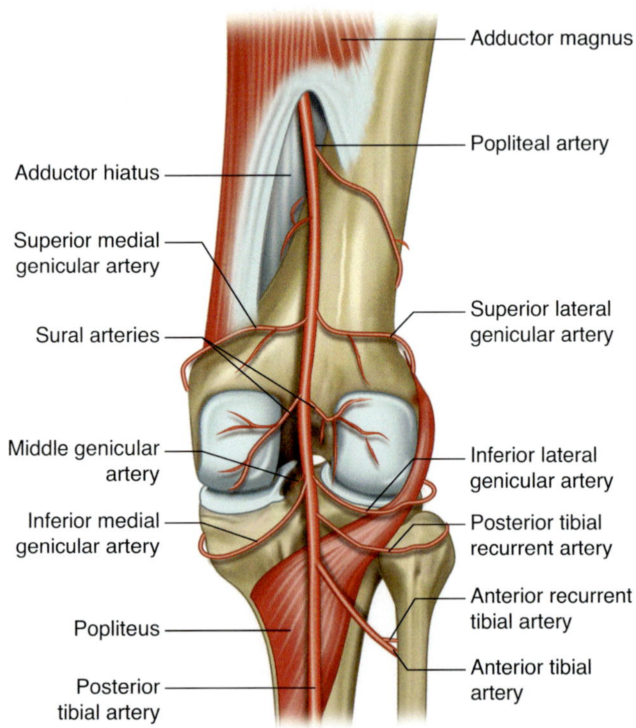

Fig. 33.1 Illustration of popliteal artery branches: posterior view

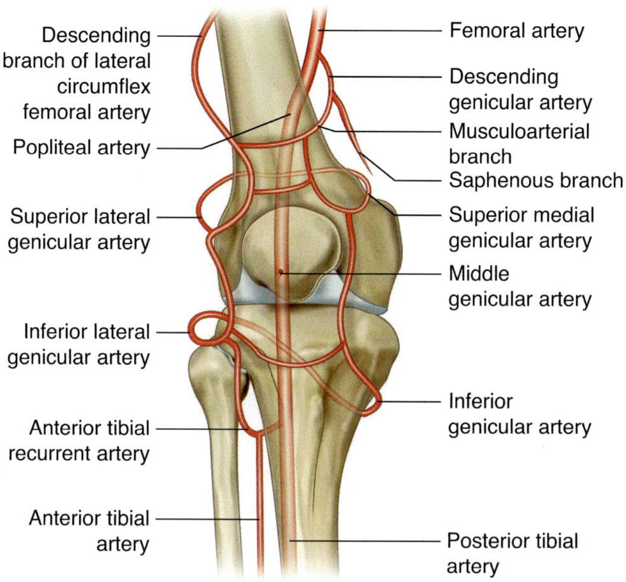

Fig. 33.2 Illustration of popliteal artery branches: anterior view

rior lateral genicular artery also anastomoses with the lateral circumflex femoral artery.

The descending genicular artery or highest genicular artery should also be discussed although technically it is a branch off of the superficial femoral artery (SFA or femoral artery) (see Chaps. 32 and 39). The descending genicular branches off of the femoral artery right before the SFA turns into the popliteal artery just prior to the entrance into the adductor hiatus. The descending genicular artery branches into a saphenous branch (which anastomoses with the medial inferior genicular artery) and the musculo-articular branch (which anastomoses with the medial superior genicular artery and the anterior recurrent tibial artery).

Surgical Site Exposure

The supragenicular and infragenicular popliteal sections are exposed most easily through medial approaches, whereas the midpopliteal portion is exposed through a posterior approach.

Suprageniculate Popliteal Artery Exposure

The suprageniculate portion is typically approached through a medial incision with the patient in the supine position with the leg externally rotated and the knee slightly flexed (Fig. 33.3). The medial incision is made along the anterior border of the sartorius muscle in the distal third of the thigh. The sartorius muscle fascia is incised, the muscle is retracted posteriorly, and the vastus medialis muscle is retracted anteriorly. There is a thick fascial band between the adductor tendon and semimembranosus muscle that potentially have to be divided for adequate exposure (Fig. 33.4). There are fascial adhesions between the medial intermuscular septum and the adductor magnus tendon that require division to expose the adductor hiatus. The medial superior genicular artery will be encountered here as well as the saphenous branch of the femoral nerve. A fibrous sheath will envelope the popliteal vessels. After excising the fibrous sheath, the artery will be medial to the paired veins (Video 33.1).

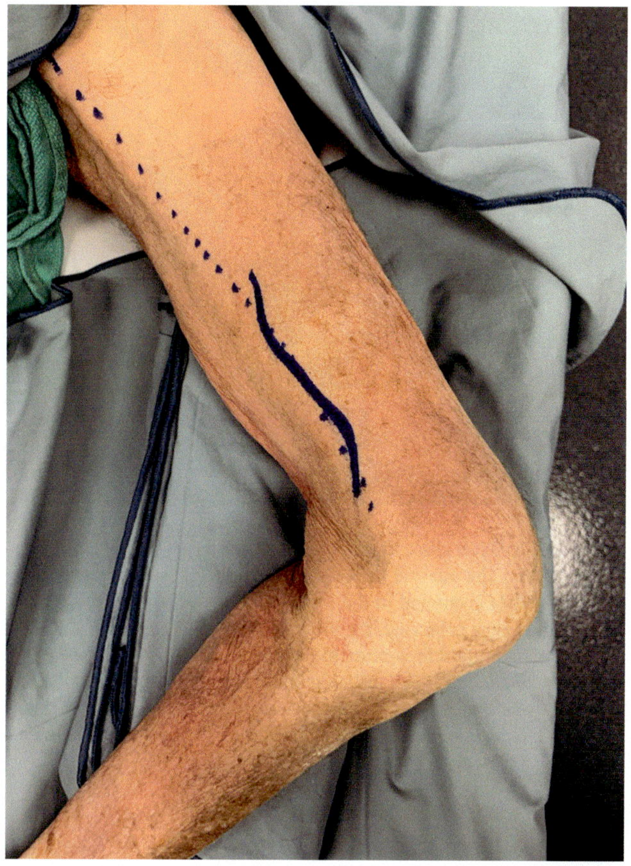

Fig. 33.3 The suprageniculate (proximal portion of the popliteal artery) portion is typically approached through a medial incision with the cadaver or patient in the supine position with the leg externally rotated and the knee slightly flexed. The incision (the solid blue line) runs from the adductor tubercle of the femur distally toward the midpoint of the inguinal ligament (dashed blue line), ending at the junction of the middle and distal thirds of the thigh

The medial exposure is the most facile and common approach for exposing the suprageniculate artery. However, if there has been prior surgery such as a vascular bypass, then taking advantage of the lateral approach can be used [10]. The patient stays in a supine position but with the leg internally rotated. An incision is made in the distal third of the thigh between the biceps femoris muscle and the iliotibial tract. The incision is continued through the fascia latae where the iliotibial tract and lateral intermuscular septum meet. Once the lateral intermuscular septum is incised, the popli-

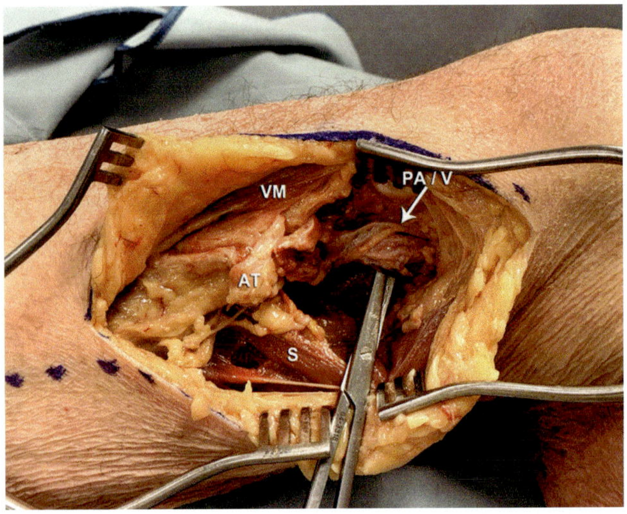

Fig. 33.4 Cadaver dissection for exposure of the suprageniculate popliteal vessels. The interval between the sartorius muscle and the vastus medialis (VM) is entered in the distal third of the thigh. The sartorius muscle (S) fascia is incised, the muscle is retracted posteriorly, and the vastus medialis muscle is retracted anteriorly and laterally. There is a thick fascial band between the adductor tendon (AT) and semimembranosus muscle that are divided for adequate exposure of the popliteal vessels. Division of the AT facilitates the exposure. *PA/V* popliteal artery and vein

teal artery can be palpated within the popliteal fat. There is a "loophole" where the short head of the biceps femoris ends above its insertion on the lateral femoral condyle leaving several centimeters of avascular space where the popliteal vessels can be reached [11]. The popliteal vessels are immediately posterior to the femur, and the tibial and peroneal nerves will lie further posterior and adherent to the hamstring muscles.

Midpopliteal Popliteal Artery Exposure

The midpopliteal exposure is preferably performed in a prone position with gentle flexion of the knee. Traditionally, an S-shaped incision which begins with a longitudinal incision medially hugging the lateral border of the hamstring muscles in the thigh, continuing horizontally across the popliteal fossa, and then ending with a vertical incision in the upper leg laterally along the lateral border of the gastrocnemius muscles (Fig. 33.5). The S-shaped incision is used to avoid a flexion contracture; however, if a flap will be placed within this space, then the S-shaped incision can be modified. Once the skin is incised, the small saphenous vein will be encountered in the subcutaneous space. The deep fascia is then incised, and the medial sural nerve should be identified and preserved (see Chap. 40). Within the midline, the tibial nerve is identified and retracted medially followed by medial retraction of the peroneal nerve which can be found along the biceps femoris

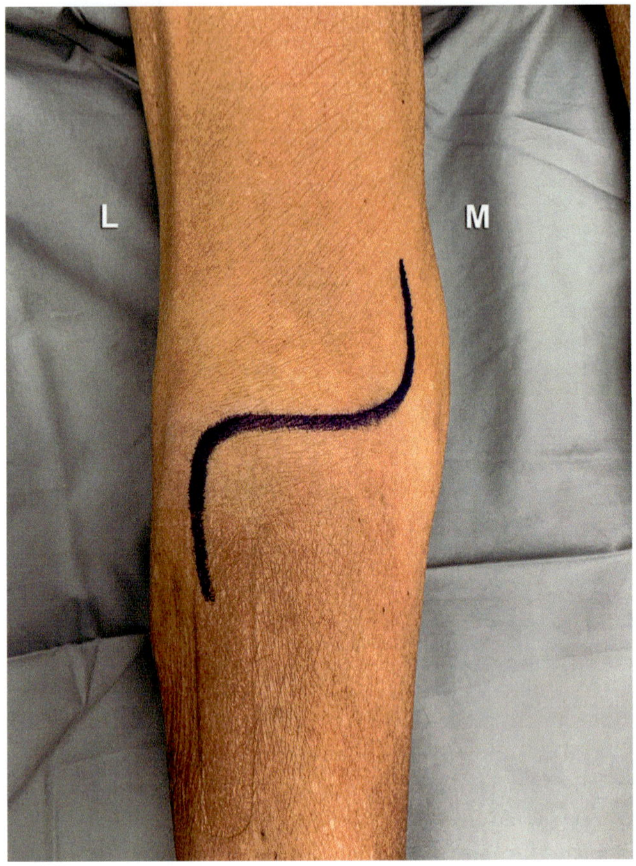

Fig. 33.5 Lazy S skin incision for exposure of the popliteal vessels through posterior approach in a cadaver (*M* medial, *L* lateral)

tendon and the fibular neck. The popliteal vessels should be found within a sheath with the artery medial and anterior to the vein (Fig. 33.6, Video 33.1). If more distal length is needed, the two heads of the medial and lateral gastrocnemius muscles can be divided.

Surgical exposure of the middle portion of the popliteal vessels through medial approach is also possible, albeit difficult. The skin incision used for exposure of the suprageniculate portion of the popliteal vessels can be extended distally over the medial knee, or a separate skin incision is performed (Fig. 33.7). The greater saphenous vein and the sartorius are identified. The deep fascia is divided between the sartorius and medial hamstring tendons. While dissecting between them, the saphenous vessels and nerve are seen emerging between the sartorius and gracilis at the knee joint at a subcutaneous tissue and running distally with the greater saphenous vein. Common tendon of gracilis, semimembranosus, and semitendinosus is divided for exposure (Fig. 33.8, Video 33.1). The medial head of the gastrocnemius muscle can be detached from the medial condyle of the femur. Adequate attachment should be left to facilitate later suturing and to avoid injuring the synovial membrane of the knee joint in actual patient.

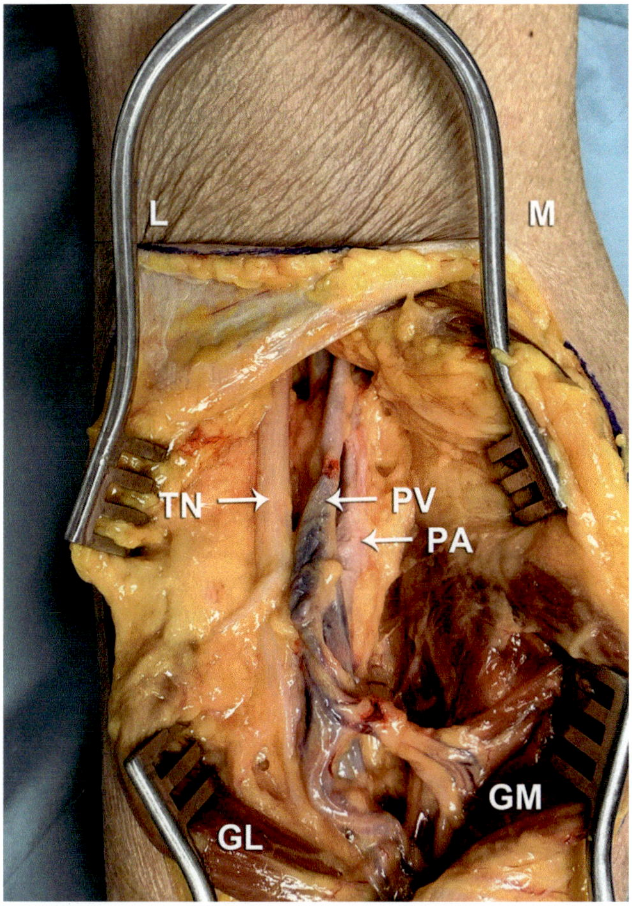

Fig. 33.6 Exposure of popliteal vessels through posterior approach (*M* medial, *L* lateral, *GM* medial head of the gastrocnemius muscle, *GL* lateral head of the gastrocnemius muscle, *PA* popliteal artery, *PV* popliteal vein, *TN* tibial nerve)

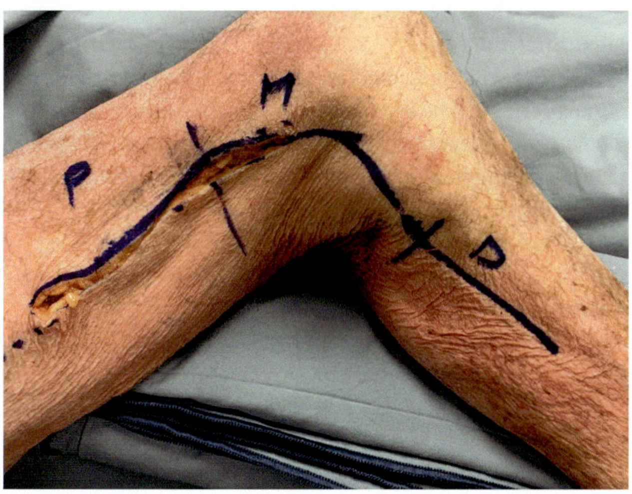

Fig. 33.7 The skin incision in the distal thigh (*P* proximal), in the medial knee (*M* middle), and in the proximal medial leg (*D* distal) for surgical exposure of the popliteal vessels in the supragenicul ate, mid-popliteal, and infrageniculate regions through medial approach

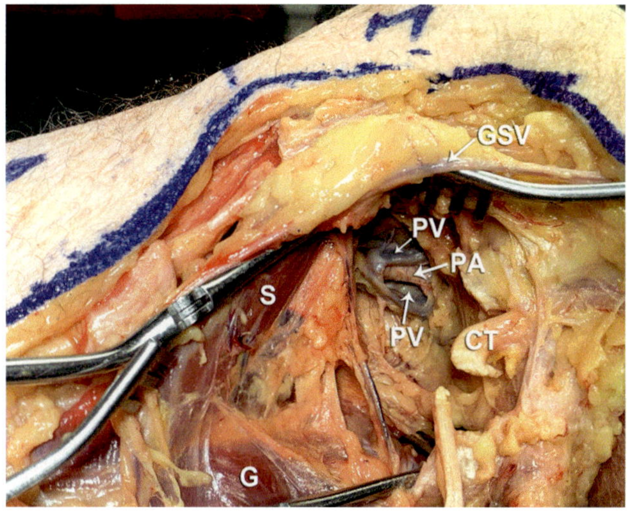

Fig. 33.8 Surgical exposure of middle portion of the popliteal vessels through medial approach in a cadaver: Dissection between the sartorius and the gracilis. Common tendon (CT) of gracilis, semimembranosus, and semitendinosus is divided for exposure. The medial head of the gastrocnemius muscle can be detached from the medial condyle of the femur. Adequate attachment should be left to facilitate later suturing and to avoid injuring the synovial membrane of the knee joint in actual patient. (*S* sartorius, *G* gracilis, *PA* popliteal artery, *PV* popliteal vein, *GSV* great saphenous vein)

Infrageniculate Artery Exposure

The infrageniculate popliteal artery as the suprageniculate popliteal artery can be exposed via medial and lateral incisions. The medial incision provides access through a supine position with the knee flexed to 30°, hip externally rotated, and a bump placed underneath the knee (Fig. 33.7). A vertical incision is made about 1 cm posterior to the medial border of the tibia extending from the lower border of the knee to the midpoint of the leg. The great saphenous vein is found within this location and should be preserved. The deep fascia is incised along the posterior edge of the tibia gaining access into the deep posterior compartment. The medial head of the gastrocnemius muscle is retracted posteriorly to expose the popliteal vessels (Video 33.1). Once the neurovascular sheath is incised, the popliteal vein should be encountered first. The popliteal vein is usually paired with crossing veins. The tendons of the semitendinosus, semimembranosus, and gracilis muscles can be divided to increase the proximal exposure. Dissection of the medial attachments of the soleus muscle to the tibia will facilitate more distal exposure of the tibioperoneal trunk and the anterior tibial vessels (Fig. 33.9).

The infrageniculate popliteal vessels can also be exposed through a lateral approach [10]. The patient may still be in the supine position with the leg internally rotated and the knee flexed. The incision is placed vertically over the head of the fibula or just posterior to it. The biceps femoris tendon is

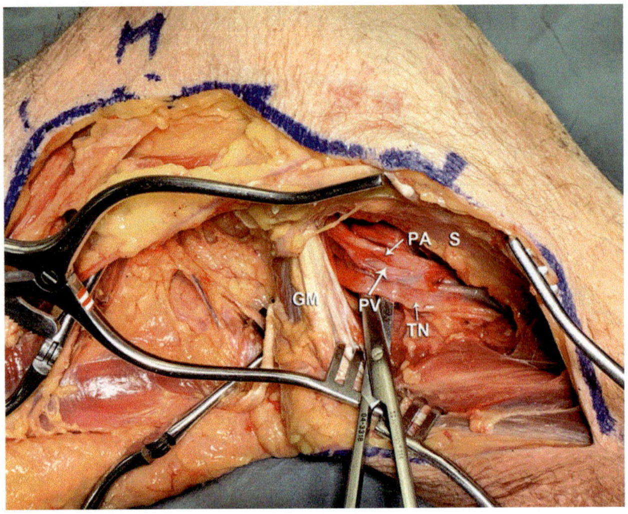

Fig. 33.9 Surgical exposure of the infrageniculate portion of the popliteal vessels through medial approach in a cadaveric dissection. An incision is made from the adductor tubercle of the femur via the medial condyle of the tibia extending along the posteromedial border of the tibia distally. The deep fascia is incised along the posterior edge of the tibia gaining access into the deep posterior compartment. The medial head of the gastrocnemius muscle is retracted posteriorly to expose the popliteal vessels. Once the neurovascular sheath is incised, the popliteal vein should be encountered first. The popliteal vein is usually paired with crossing veins. The tendons of the semitendinosus, semimembranosus, and gracilis muscles can be divided to increase the proximal exposure. Dissection of the medial attachments of the soleus muscle to the tibia will facilitate more distal exposure of the tibioperoneal trunk and the anterior tibial vessels. *GM* medial head of the gastrocnemius muscle, *S* soleus, *PA* popliteal artery, *PV* popliteal vein, *TN* tibial nerve

seen as it inserts on the fibular head. The common peroneal nerve is seen posterior to the biceps femoris tendon and then coursing anteriorly around the fibular neck. The upper one third of the fibula needs to be removed to gain access to the popliteal vessels from the lateral approach. The biceps femoris tendon is first divided, and common peroneal nerve and its branches are retracted carefully. All of the muscular and ligamentous attachments to the upper fibula are removed to enable removal of the bone. Alternatively the fibular periosteum can be incised and dissected from the fibular bone and the bone removed with a saw. The popliteal vessels are found deep to the fibular periosteum. The popliteal artery will be encountered first prior to the vein. The anterior tibial artery and tibioperoneal trunk can also be exposed by furthering the dissection distally.

Discussion

The popliteal vessels and their branches offer multiple recipient options. As discussed above, there are multiple named branches of the popliteal artery. However, there are several unnamed muscular branches that may be of sufficient size and be used in microvascular surgery. Many of the vessels can be expendable depending on the particular procedure, and anastomoses can be performed in an end-to-end fashion. However, if the popliteal vessels and their termination into the anterior tibial artery, posterior tibial and peroneal artery are used directly, and then an end-to-side anastomosis should be considered to continue end flow to the distal leg and foot.

Many of the popliteal branches have been described for use as recipient vessels in microvascular surgery. The superior genicular arteries both medial and lateral can be used [12]. The superior medial genicular artery is often small which can signal that the highest or descending genicular artery (see Chap. 39) is larger [13]. However, the superior medial genicular has been described as a recipient for knee coverage [14, 15] (see Chap. 39). The superior lateral genicular artery can also be used prior or after dividing into a superficial and deep branch.

The middle genicular artery is generally small but can be of sufficient size of 2–4 mm for microsurgery. However, it has a short intra-articular course and can become kinked if the knee is flexed [16]. There may be certain situations if the patient's knee has a non-articulating spacer that does not allow for bending of the knee that would lead to a successful anastomosis. However, in most situations, another recipient vessel may prove to be more optimal.

The inferior genicular arteries can potentially be used; however, their use has not been described as much as the other popliteal branches have.

Hong and Koshima described supermicrosurgical techniques using random suprafascial perforators [17]. As these perforators are not anatomically reliable, imaging with Doppler, CTA or magnetic resonance angiography is necessary. Using these perforators takes expert technique and should be undertaken by the experienced supermicrosurgeon.

The descending genicular, lateral circumflex femoral, and sural arteries can be used and have been frequently described. Their use is described in more detail in Chap. 39 for the descending genicular, in Chaps. 30 and 31 for the lateral circumflex femoral, and in Chap. 40 for sural vessels.

Conclusion

There are multiple options for recipient vessels from the popliteal artery and the popliteal branches with multiple exposures, be it lateral, medial, supine, or prone. One should always take into account the prior surgeries, specific needs of the patient, characteristics of the defect, intraoperative positioning, flap donor site, microsurgical flap and its pedicle characteristics, and planned postoperative course when selecting the appropriate recipient vessel for microvascular anastomosis.

References

1. Bradley L, Kirker SG. Secondary prevention of arteriosclerosis in lower limb vascular amputees: a missed opportunity. Eur J Vasc Endovasc Surg. 2006;32(5):491–3.
2. Nance ML. National Trauma Data Bank 2015 Annual Report. American College of Surgeons 2015;66.
3. Francel TJ, Vander Kolk CA, Hoopes JE, Manson PN, Yaremchuk MJ. Microvascular soft-tissue transplantation for reconstruction of acute open tibial fractures: timing of coverage and long-term functional results. Plast Reconstr Surg. 1992;89(3):478–87. discussion 88–9
4. Francel TJ. Salvage of the massively traumatized lower extremity. Clin Plast Surg. 1992;19(4):871–80.
5. Arnez ZM. Immediate reconstruction of the lower extremity–an update. Clin Plast Surg. 1991;18(3):449–57.
6. Isenberg JS, Sherman R. Zone of injury: a valid concept in microvascular reconstruction of the traumatized lower limb? Ann Plast Surg. 1996;36(3):270–2.
7. Hallock GG. The medial approach to the sural vessels to facilitate microanastomosis about the knee. Ann Plast Surg. 1994;32(4):388–93.
8. Beumer JD, Karoo R, Caplash Y, Semmler JG, Taylor J. The medial sural artery as recipient vessel and the impact on the medial gastrocnemius. Ann Plast Surg. 2011;67(4):382–6.
9. Johnson PE, Harris GD, Nagle DJ, Lewis VL. The sural artery and vein as recipient vessels in free flap reconstruction about the knee. J Reconstr Microsurg. 1987;3(3):233–41.
10. Veith FJ, Ascer E, Gupta SK, Wengerter KR. Lateral approach to the popliteal artery. J Vasc Surg. 1987;6(2):119–23.
11. Wind GGaRJV. Anatomic exposures in vascular surgery. 3rd ed. Lippincott Williams & Wilkins. 2013;Ch 17 Popliteal Artery, p. 464.
12. Fang T, Zhang EW, Lineaweaver WC, Zhang F. Recipient vessels in the free flap reconstruction around the knee. Ann Plast Surg. 2013;71(4):429–33.
13. Cormack GC, Lamberty BG. Cadaver studies of correlation between vessel size and anatomical territory of cutaneous supply. Br J Plast Surg. 1986;39(3):300–6.
14. Park S, Eom JS. Selection of the recipient vessel in the free flap around the knee: the superior medial genicular vessels and the descending genicular vessels. Plast Reconstr Surg. 2001;107(5):1177–82.
15. Rees-Lee JE, Khan U. Superior medial genicular artery (SMGA): a recipient vessel for free-flap reconstruction of anterior and medial knee defects. J Plast Reconstr Aesthet Surg. 2011;64(12):1727–9.
16. Salaria H, Atkinson R. Anatomic study of the middle genicular artery. J Orthop Surg (Hong Kong). 2008;16(1):47–9.
17. Hong JP, Koshima I. Using perforators as recipient vessels (supermicrosurgery) for free flap reconstruction of the knee region. Ann Plast Surg. 2010;64(3):291–3.

Anterior Tibial Vessels and Dorsalis Pedis

34

Philip S. Brazio and Gordon K. Lee

Introduction

The anterior tibial (AT) artery and vein are a useful target for traumatic, oncologic, and diabetic lower extremity salvage. They are located deep within the anterior compartment and give off multiple perforators to anterior compartment muscles. These characteristics can make surgical access more challenging than the posterior tibial vessels; therefore, detailed knowledge of the surgical anatomy is necessary to maximize the AT's utility in microvascular reconstruction of the lower extremity.

Preoperative Assessment

Choice of recipient vessel in the lower extremity is frequently dictated by vascular trauma or insufficiency concomitant to the defect, superimposed on the usual considerations of vessel caliber, location, and length. Preoperative imaging is often helpful, if not necessary, for reliable use of the AT. A pencil Doppler signal in the DP with compression of the posterior tibial at the ankle can be sufficient to confirm patency. A computed tomographic angiogram may already be available from initial assessments in trauma. This will delineate not only the relative patency of each vessel to the foot but the extent of surrounding bone and soft tissue trauma. Careful appraisal of the soft tissues surrounding vessels in trauma can help define the quality of inflow, outflow, and vessel walls.

In patients with concomitant baseline vascular insufficiency, a dynamic study is most useful. Contrast angiography is commonly used to determine relative flow rates of target vessels and residual vascular supply to the foot. Traditional angiography has several problems, including invasiveness, contrast nephropathy, and at some institutions the difficulty of obtaining the study in a timely fashion. A noninvasive, targeted duplex ultrasound can overcome these limitations and also characterize venous flow. Difficulties with duplex ultrasonography may be encountered if there is significant edema, gas, or bone fragmentation in the defect, if the defect itself is large, or if there is a bulky splint or external fixator limiting access.

Applied Anatomy

The AT artery and its venae comitantes originate from the popliteal artery in the deep posterior compartment of the leg and immediately veer anteriorly to pass over the soleal arch, between the two heads of the tibialis posterior muscle and over the upper border of the interosseous membrane. The artery supplies all the muscles of the anterior compartment and has close relations to them. In the upper two thirds of its course, the AT lies between the interosseous membrane and tibialis anterior muscle. In the upper third, it apposes these and the extensor digitorum longus (EDL) and in the middle third the extensor hallucis longus (EHL) (Figs. 34.1 and 34.2). In the distal third (and sometimes more proximally), it leaves the surface of the interosseous membrane and becomes more superficial, coursing closer to the surface of the tibia [1].

As it traverses deep to the superior extensor retinaculum (transverse talar ligament) in the upper ankle, the AT is also crossed by the EHL tendon from lateral to medial. It nests between the EHL and EDL tendons as it crosses the ankle, overlying the tibiotalar joint capsule. The AT emerges from under the extensor tendons as the dorsalis pedis

Supplementary Information The online version of this chapter (https://doi.org/10.1007/978-3-030-75389-4_34) contains supplementary material, which is available to authorized users.

P. S. Brazio · G. K. Lee (✉)
Plastic and Reconstructive Surgery, Stanford University, Palo Alto, CA, USA

R. Gurunian, R. Djohan (eds.), *Recipient Vessels in Reconstructive Microsurgery*, https://doi.org/10.1007/978-3-030-75389-4_34

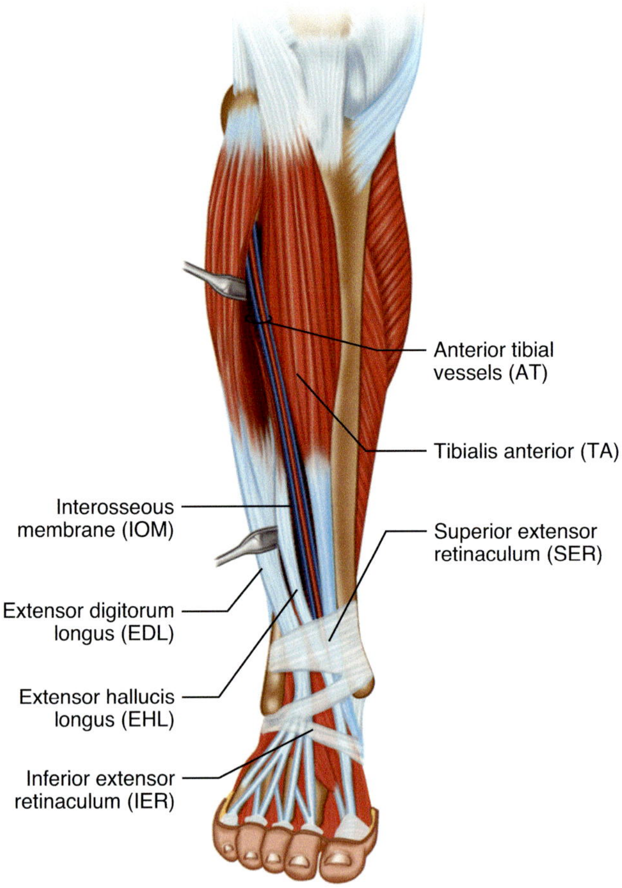

Fig. 34.1 Illustration: Anterior tibial vessels (AT): surface anatomy and markings. The AT follows a line from the head of the fibula head to a point midway between the malleoli. In the upper two thirds of its course, the AT lies between the interosseous membrane (IOM) and tibialis anterior muscle (TA). In the upper third, it apposes these and the extensor digitorum longus (EDL) and in the middle third the extensor hallucis longus (EHL). *SER* superior extensor retinaculum, *IER* inferior extensor retinaculum

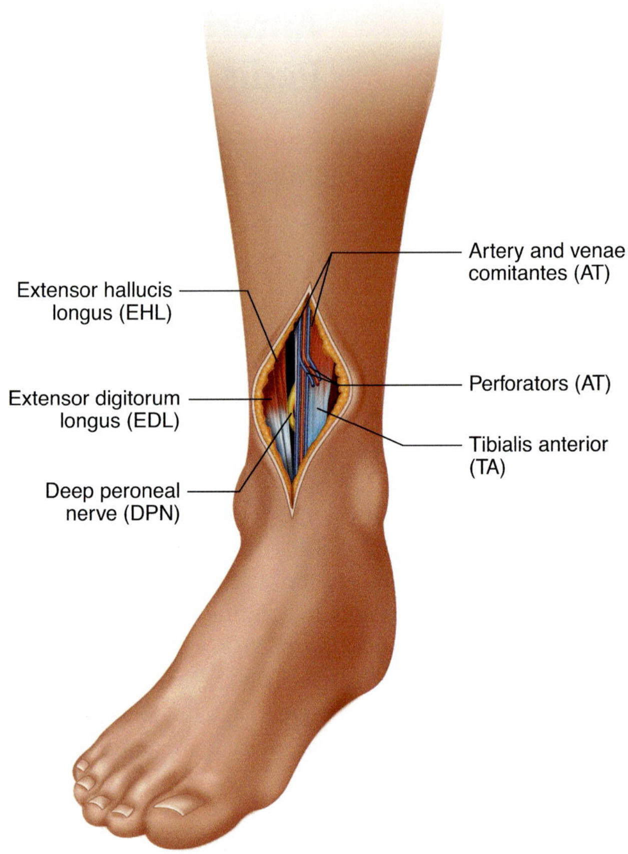

Fig. 34.2 Illustration of exposure of anterior tibial artery and venae comitantes between TA, tibialis anterior muscle and EDL, extensor digitorum longus and EHL, extensor hallucis longus. *DPN* deep peroneal nerve

(DP). The DP continues to follow the lateral border of the EHL tendon as it crosses deep to the inferior extensor retinaculum (cruciate crural ligament) and is then joined laterally by the extensor hallucis brevis muscle. Its terminal branches are the first dorsal metatarsal artery and the deep plantar artery [1].

The AT artery has two venae comitantes. Its diameter is 4–6 mm proximally and 2–3 mm just above the ankle. Throughout its course multiple muscular branches arise anteriorly, laterally, and medially into the anterior compartment muscles and overlying skin. Although there are few deep branches piercing the interosseous membrane, awareness of these can be crucial. The deep peroneal nerve joins course with the AT vessels near the middle of the leg and lies posterior and lateral to the artery [1].

Surgical Site Exposure

Anterior Tibial Artery

The patient may be positioned supine or in partial lateral decubitus, with a pillow or bump under the knee. The course of the AT follows a line from the head of the fibula head to a point midway between the malleoli (Fig. 34.1). The incision is made over the lateral edge of the tibialis anterior muscle or, if this is not palpable one, fingerbreadth lateral to the tibia. The incision is carried through the deep fascia to expose the plane between the EHL and the tibialis anterior muscle. As dissection proceeds, self-retaining retractors are placed proximally and distally to expose the interval between the muscles or tendons. Multiple branches radiate from the AT into the anterior compartment muscles and should be ligated with clips or bipolar electrocautery. In a hostile field, these can be traced retrograde toward the neurovascular bundle. The vessels can be identified in the interval between muscle bellies as a bundle encased in a layer of fat (Fig. 34.2). Care must be taken to avoid injury to the accompanying deep peroneal nerve, which can cause foot drop [2]. Dissection of a longer segment of pedicle facilitates anastomosis by delivering the cut end of the recipient vessels more superficially (Video 34.1).

The distal-most portion of the AT, despite its proximity to the skin, can be less convenient for recipient vessel anastomosis because of the crossing of the EHL tendon and superior extensor retinaculum. The EHL tendon can be retracted to the side for anastomosis, but the superior extensor retinaculum can cause compression or kinking of the pedicle unless partially divided. If distal access to the recipient vessels is required, the proximal DP may represent a better target (Fig. 34.3).

Dorsalis Pedis Artery

The DP pulse is palpable in the first metatarsal interspace between the EHL and EDL tendons. An incision is made directly overlying the artery, through the skin and thin subcutaneous fat. Depending on the level, the extensor retinaculum may overlie the artery. In this situation the artery will lie deeper than would be immediately apparent, and the extensor retinaculum may require partial division (Fig. 34.4). The retinaculum should not be fully divided, to prevent bowstringing of the extensor tendons. The tarsal branch of the deep peroneal nerve runs medial to the artery and branches extensively in the proximal foot and should be preserved. The artery itself is between 1 and 2 mm in diameter but easily enters into vasospasm. Therefore, care must be taken to minimize manipulation, and the vessel caliber and inflow should only be assessed after pharmacological or mechanical maneuvers to resolve the spasm. The venae comitantes are less distinct at this level and may have the appearance of a venous plexus neighboring the artery.

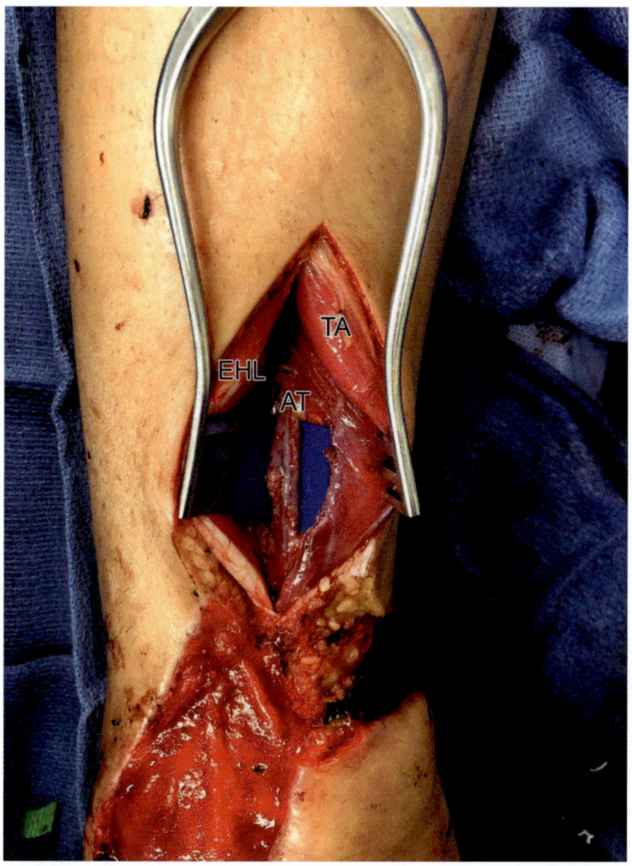

Fig. 34.3 Actual patient photo: Surgical exposure of the AT, anterior tibial vessels between TA, tibialis anterior and EHL, and extensor halluces longus in distal lower leg, demonstrating the principle of beginning the dissection proximally, well away from the wound

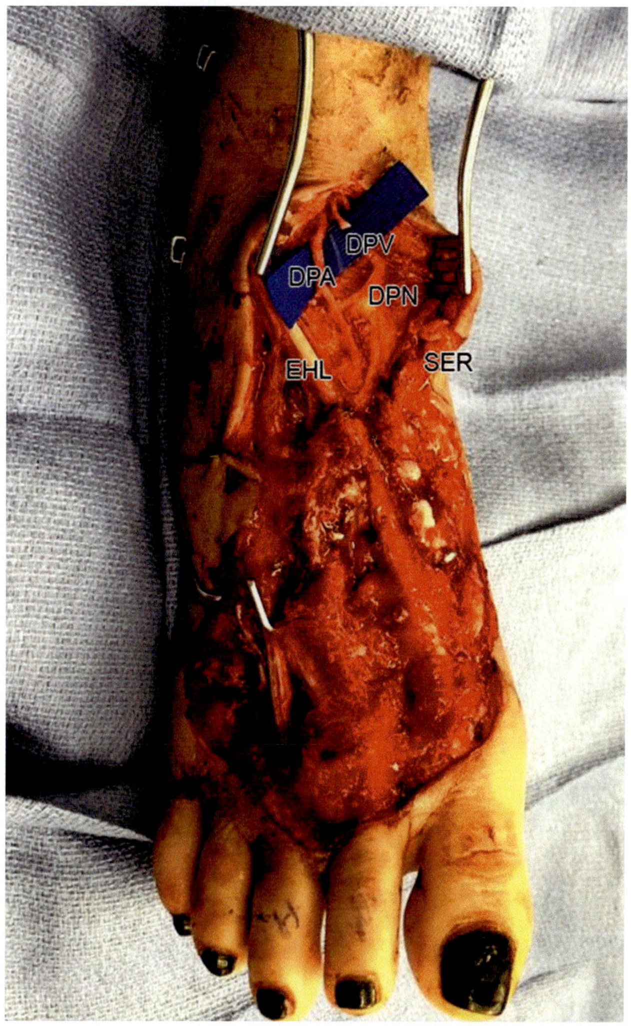

Fig. 34.4 Actual patient photo: Surgical exposure of dorsalis pedis artery (DPA) following partial division of superior extensor retinaculum (SER), including an adjacent stump of dorsalis pedis vein (DPV), underlying deep peroneal nerve branches (DPN), and extensor hallucis longus tendon (EHL) retracted laterally

Discussion

Target Vessel Selection

Because of their ease of dissection, as well as availability from much of the circumference of the lower leg, the posterior tibial vessels may be given preference over the AT in the absence of other factors. The AT or its terminal branch, the dorsalis pedis (DP), may be preferred if the PT is unavailable (due to interruption or surrounding zone of injury causing difficult dissection and unreliable outflow) or if pedicle reach is a priority due to a short flap pedicle or very anterior defect.

Anterior tibial vessels that are interrupted by a defect and do not continue to the foot may represent ideal candidates for end-to-end anastomosis, as no further distal vascular supply needs to be sacrificed. Caution must be taken in high-velocity ballistic or automotive trauma, however, when there may be a zone of blunt injury that extends proximal to the defect and renders the vessels unusable, even close to their origin deep in the anterior compartment.

Considerations for Zone of Injury and Defect Location

When the AT vessels traverse a distal defect, edema, friability, fibrosis, and scar (in the case of subacute or chronic wound reconstruction) can make the dissection difficult. In this case the incision should be generously extended and the dissection started at least 5–10 cm proximal to the defect to approach and identify the vessels within enter virgin planes (Fig. 34.3).

Conversely, in the traumatized leg with a proximal defect but with an intact AT artery distally, the distal artery can be a more suitable target for free tissue transfer than the proximal artery. While the arterial inflow is simple to evaluate clinically, maneuvers such as flushing the vein may not be sensitive enough to guarantee adequate outflow. In these cases the dissection of the pedicle should be confined distal to the zone of injury, rather than tracing the vein proximally to examine it. Proximal dissection would inevitably require the ligation of numerous venous branches that communicate with the posterior tibial or superficial systems, compromising the outflow. Limiting the dissection to the distal vessel preserves these collaterals, helping to ensure outflow even in the absence of an intact proximal AT vein.

References

1. Standring S, editor. Gray's anatomy: the anatomical basis of clinical practice. 41st ed. New York: Elsevier; 2015.
2. Sadri A, Bodansky DMS, Shokrollahi K. Recipient vessels for microsurgery. In: Shokrollahi K, Whitaker I, Nahai F, editors. Flaps: practical reconstructive surgery. 1st ed. New York: Thieme; 2017.

Tibioperoneal Trunk and Posterior Tibial Artery

35

Sarah N. Bishop, Richard L. Drake, DeAsia D. Jacob, and Raffi Gurunian

Introduction

The lower extremity offers multiple recipient sites for microvascular anastomosis. The tibioperoneal trunk offers a large reliable vessel that can be anastomosed in an end-to-side fashion. As the tibioperoneal trunk divides into the posterior tibial and peroneal arteries, the tibioperoneal trunk should not be anastomosed in an end-to-end technique so as to keep the lower extremity distally perfused. The posterior tibial artery offers multiple locations throughout its course for anastomosis. Both end-to-side and end-to-end anastomoses can be used if there are still other major vessels providing sufficient blood flow to the entire lower extremity. This chapter will discuss the exposures and uses of the tibioperoneal trunk and the upper, middle, and lower exposures of the posterior tibial artery.

Supplementary Information The online version of this chapter (https://doi.org/10.1007/978-3-030-75389-4_35) contains supplementary material, which is available to authorized users.

S. N. Bishop (✉) · R. Gurunian
Department of Plastic Surgery, Cleveland Clinic, Cleveland, OH, USA

Cleveland Clinic Lerner College of Medicine, Case Western Reserve University, Cleveland, OH, USA
e-mail: bishops@ccf.org; gurunian@ccf.org

R. L. Drake
Department of Anatomy, Cleveland Clinic Lerner College of Medicine, Case Western Reserve University, Cleveland, OH, USA
e-mail: DRAKER@ccf.org

D. D. Jacob
Department of Plastic Surgery, Cleveland Clinic, Cleveland, OH, USA

Preoperative Assessment

The preoperative assessment for exposure of vessels in the lower extremity is discussed in more detail in Chap. 33. Reconstruction of the lower extremity can have a multitude of etiologies including peripheral vascular disease, trauma, tumors, infection, or neuropathic ulcers [1, 2]. A thorough understanding of the inciting events that lead to the defect is crucial as well as a thorough debridement and preparation of the wound bed. Preoperative imaging may be necessary in the setting of trauma to assess for any vascular injury. If there is any concern for peripheral vascular disease, then noninvasive studies at the very least should be performed with ankle brachial index (ABI), pulse volume recording (PVR), and arterial duplex. If the vascular studies are not normal, then a computed tomography angiogram (CTA) or a formal angiogram can further delineate the anatomy. Lower extremity reconstruction is often performed in the setting of limb salvage, and so a thorough discussion of the risks and benefits of limb salvage compared to amputation should be discussed as well as the expected postoperative course and rehabilitation.

Applied Anatomy

The tibioperoneal trunk and posterior tibial vessels diverge from the popliteal vessels (also see Chaps. 33 and 34). Traditionally the popliteal branches (anterior tibial artery, posterior tibial artery, and peroneal artery) have been termed a trifurcation. Although there are three major branches of the popliteal artery, it is not truly a trifurcation, except in 3% of the population [3]. Rather, the popliteal artery branches in two different bifurcations. The anterior tibial artery and the tibioperoneal trunk bifurcate off of the popliteal vessel. The tibioperoneal trunk then bifurcates again 2–3 cm distally into the posterior tibial and peroneal arteries.

R. Gurunian, R. Djohan (eds.), *Recipient Vessels in Reconstructive Microsurgery*, https://doi.org/10.1007/978-3-030-75389-4_35

There are significant fascial layers within the leg that divide the compartments into anterior, lateral, superficial posterior, and deep posterior compartments. The interosseous membrane divides the anterior from the posterior. A secondary septum connects the tibia and fibula which divides the deep and superficial posterior compartments. Only the anterior and deep posterior compartments contain the prominent popliteal branches. The anterior tibial artery resides in the anterior compartment, and the posterior tibial artery and peroneal artery are located within the deep posterior compartment. The posterior tibial and peroneal artery feed the superficial posterior compartment and the lateral compartment via perforating branches.

Although only two of the four compartments house major blood vessels, there are major nerves within three of the compartments. The tibial nerve is sometimes incorrectly called the posterior tibial nerve as it resides within the deep posterior compartment and lies in the bundle containing the posterior tibial vessels and supplies the posterior compartment flexor muscles. The tibial nerve is not called the posterior tibial nerve as there is no anterior tibial nerve. The nerve that lies within the anterior tibial vessels bundle in the anterior compartment is the deep peroneal nerve which supplies the anterior compartment extensor muscles. The deep peroneal nerve and the superficial peroneal nerve are terminal branches of the common peroneal nerve. The superficial peroneal nerve supplies the peroneal longus and brevis muscles within the lateral compartment enabling eversion of the foot.

The significant fascial interactions within the leg divide the leg into compartments which can lead to retention of pressure that can build up after trauma or ischemia or any event that can lead to increases in intercompartmental pressures. It is important to have a thorough understanding of the specific compartments to enable fasciotomies to release disabling pressure if necessary to avoid muscle necrosis and nerve damage.

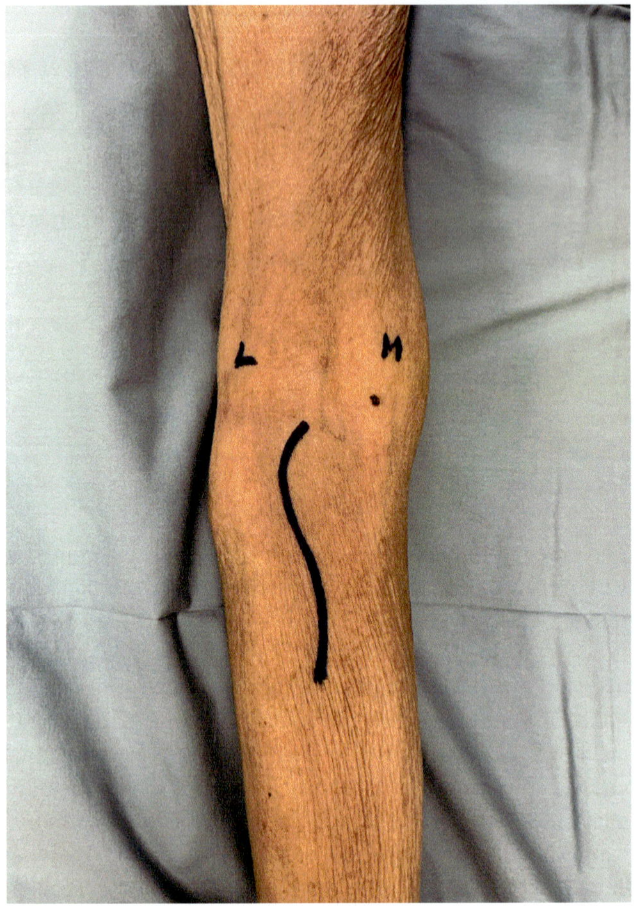

Fig. 35.1 Outline of the skin incision for exposure of the tibioperoneal trunk and its tributaries through the posterior approach. *M* medial, *L* lateral. The cadaver was positioned prone with the left knee in full extension

Surgical Site Exposure

Tibioperoneal Trunk and Posterior Exposure of the Posterior Tibial Artery

The tibioperoneal trunk can be exposed as described below in the upper posterior tibial artery exposure, or the tibioperoneal trunk can be exposed via a posterior incision. This posterior incision can also be extended to expose the entire length of the posterior tibial artery. The patient is placed prone with the knee in full extension. A longitudinal or curvilinear incision is made that extends from the level of the knee joint along the posterior midline of the calf (Fig. 35.1). The small saphenous vein should be preserved and can be used in microvascular anastomoses if necessary. The small saphenous vein lies initially posteriorly behind the lateral malleolus, then lateral to the Achilles tendon, and finally midline as it ascends to the popliteal fossa. The small saphenous vein lies within the subcutaneous space along the surface of the fascia before penetrating the fascia to converge with the popliteal vein. The incision should start superiorly within the popliteal fossa, and exposure of the infragenicular popliteal artery is performed as described in Chap. 33. The deep fascia will be excised, and the two heads of the gastrocnemius muscle will be identified with the popliteal artery residing within these two heads. The tibial nerve is the most superficial structure and should be retracted laterally and preserved. The popliteal vein will be seen next followed by the popliteal artery as the most deep structure. By following the popliteal vessels distally the anterior tibial artery, tibioperoneal trunk, and its bifurcating vessels, the posterior tibial artery and peroneal artery will be exposed (Figs. 35.2 and 35.3). The exposure can be further aided by dividing the raphe of the gastrocnemius muscles and the origin of the soleus muscle on the tibia. A separate longitudinal incision

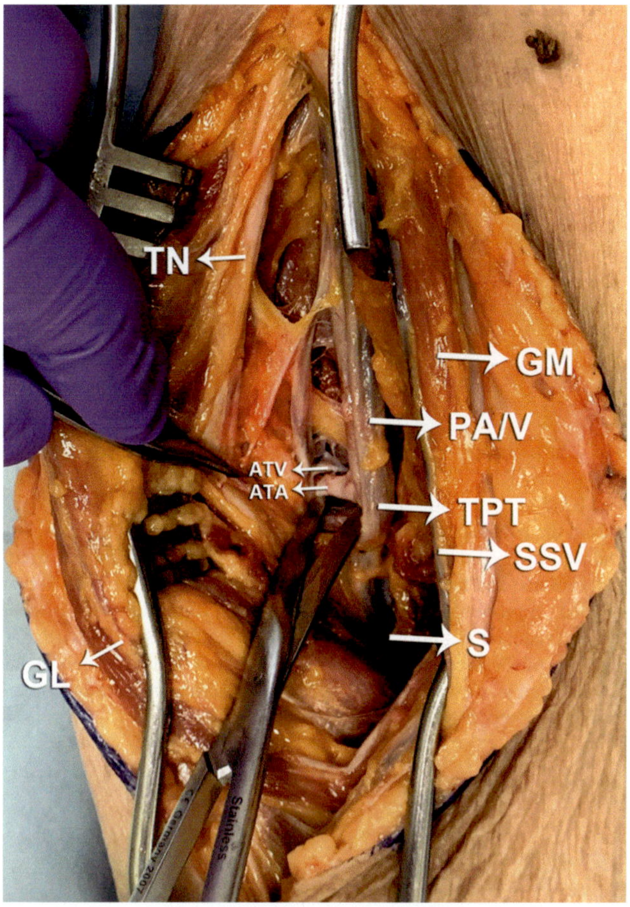

Fig. 35.2 Exposure of the tibioperoneal trunk (TPT) and the anterior tibial vessels. *SSV* small saphenous vein, *GM* gastrocnemius medial head, *GL* gastrocnemius lateral head, *S* soleus, *TN* tibial nerve, *PA/V* popliteal artery and vein, *ATA* anterior tibial artery, *ATV* anterior tibial vein. Note that the soleus is split to expose the TPT

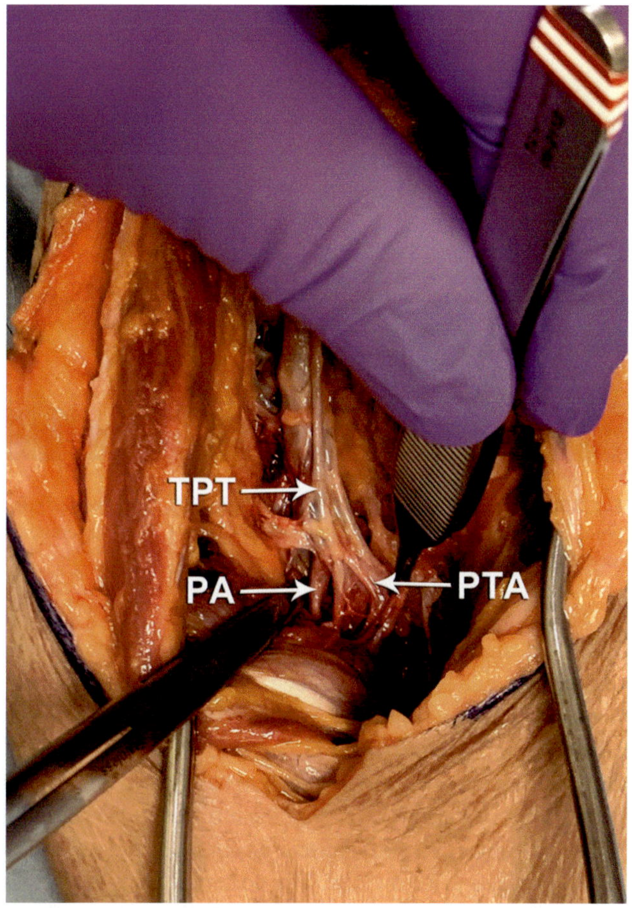

Fig. 35.3 Further dissection of the tibioperoneal trunk (TPT) distally to expose the peroneal artery (PA) and posterior tibial artery (PTA)

can be made to expose the posterior tibial artery in the distal third of the leg. The deep fascia will be encountered which separates the superficial and deep posterior compartments. The posterior tibial artery will then be located on the medial surface of the flexor digitorum longus muscle. The tibial nerve will be anterior to the posterior tibial artery at this level (Video 35.1).

Upper Posterior Tibial Artery and Tibioperoneal Trunk Exposure

Both the tibioperoneal trunk and the upper posterior tibial artery just distal to its takeoff from the tibioperoneal trunk can be exposed through a proximal medial incision. The exposure of the proximal posterior tibial artery is similar to that of exposure of the infrageniculate popliteal artery. The patient is supine with the leg externally rotated and the knee flexed. A roll to support the lateral knee is placed. The incision is made approximately 2 cm behind the medial border of the tibia and extended from middle of the knee to 10–15 cm distally (Fig. 35.4). The saphenous vein and nerve should be

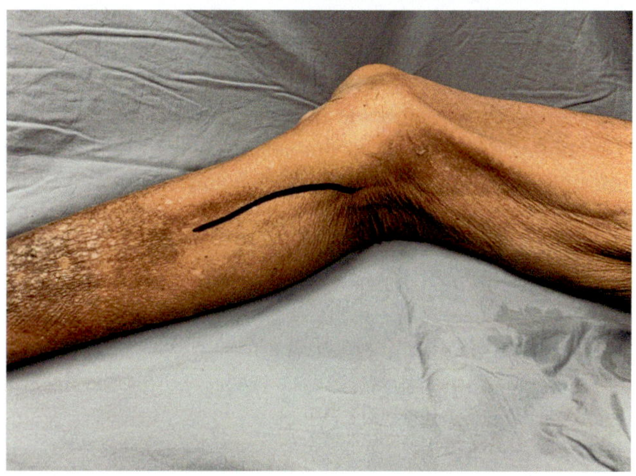

Fig. 35.4 The skin incision for exposure of tibioperoneal trunk using the medial approach. The cadaver was positioned supine with the right thigh abducted and externally rotated and the knee flexed

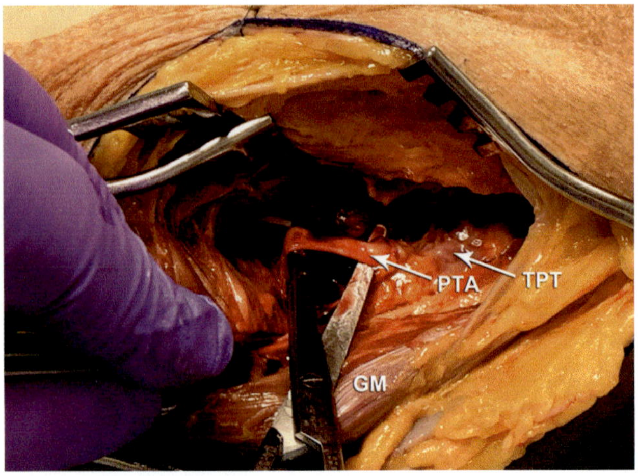

Fig. 35.5 Exposure of the tibioperoneal trunk (TPT) and the posterior tibial artery (PTA) through the medial approach. *GM* gastrocnemius medial head

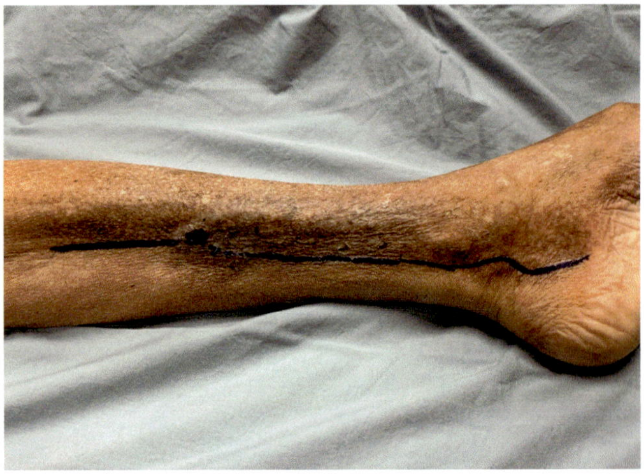

Fig. 35.6 The skin incision for the exposure of the posterior tibial vessels in the mid-leg and distal leg posterior to the medial malleolus. The cadaver was positioned supine with the left thigh abducted and externally rotated and the knee slightly flexed. The incision typically is performed approximately 2 cm posterior to the tibia and extends approximately 1 cm posterior to the medial malleolus. The length and location of the incision is determined based on which portion of the posterior tibial vessels need to be exposed taking the location of the defect to be reconstructed into consideration

identified and preserved. If vein grafting is needed or an additional vein for microvascular anastomosis, the saphenous vein can be considered. After the skin and subcutaneous tissue are incised, the deep fascia will follow. The medial head of the gastrocnemius muscle will be exposed and should be retracted posteriorly to expose the infragenicular popliteal artery. The medial soleal muscle origin attachments on the tibia will need to be divided. The posterior tibial artery lies deep to the soleal muscles and proximally lies between flexor digitorum longus and tibialis posterior muscles (Fig. 35.5). However, more distally in the leg the posterior tibial artery will lie directly posterior to the flexor digitorum muscle. Below the soleus both the tibioperoneal trunk and the anterior tibial artery will be seen. The anterior tibial artery is the first branch of the popliteal artery which will dive through the interosseous membrane into the anterior compartment. The tibioperoneal trunk continues after the anterior tibial artery takeoff and will typically divide into the medial posterior tibial artery and the lateral peroneal artery after 2.5 cm [3] (Figs. 35.2 and 35.3). The anterior tibial vein may need to be divided to gain adequate exposure. The tibial nerve will run with the posterior tibial artery and should be preserved. Both the tibioperoneal trunk and the posterior tibial artery should be anastomosed in an end-to-side fashion to preserve flow to the foot (Video 35.1).

Middle Posterior Tibial Artery Exposure

Exposure for the middle posterior tibial artery has the same positioning as for the upper posterior exposure. The patient is supine, the leg externally rotated, and knee flexed with a bump placed for knee support (Fig. 35.6). Again a longitudinal incision is made 2 cm posterior to the medial border of

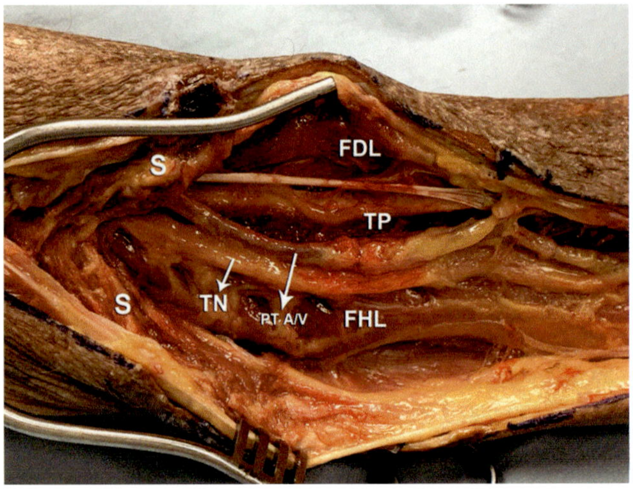

Fig. 35.7 Exposure of the posterior tibial vessels at the level of middle third. After the deep fascia is divided and soleus muscle is detached from the tibia or split, the neurovascular structures are dissected. *S* soleus, *FDL* flexor digitorum longus, *FHL* flexor hallucis longus, *TP* tibialis posterior, *TN* tibial nerve, *PT A/V* posterior tibial artery and vein

the tibia from the upper leg distally for 10 cm. The incision is made through the skin, subcutaneous tissue (avoiding the greater saphenous vein), deep fascia, and finally dividing the soleus attachments to the tibia. After the soleus is retracted posteriorly, a space can be made between the soleus and the flexor digitorum longus muscles. The posterior tibial vessels will lie on the posterior surface of the tibialis posterior muscle (Fig. 35.7). Care should always be taken to spare the tibial nerve within the neurovascular bundle. There will be a surrounding venous plexus that can be used for microvascular anastomoses (Video 35.1).

Lower Posterior Tibial Artery Exposure

The lower posterior tibial artery is most easily exposed with the patient in supine position and the leg placed in a frog-leg position with the leg externally rotated and the knee flexed. The posterior tibial artery is at its most superficial course distally and is therefore often chosen as a microvascular recipient in this location. A longitudinal incision is made 1–2 cm posterior to the medial edge of the tibia and curved obliquely around the medial malleolus. The saphenous vein and nerve should be preserved. After the skin and subcutaneous tissue are divided, the flexor retinaculum will need to be divided to expose the neurovascular bundle. If the fascia is excised more proximally on the lower leg opening, the deep fascia will expose the deep posterior compartment as the superficial and deep posterior compartments fuse in the distal third of the leg. The neurovascular bundle will lie between the flexor digitorum longus tendons anteriorly and the flexor hallucis longus tendon posteriorly (Fig. 35.8, Video 35.1). The flexor digitorum longus will be a tendon starting within the distal third of the leg, whereas the flexor hallucis longus will be muscular within the leg transitioning to a tendon at the level of the malleolus. The flexor digitorum longus tendon can be mobilized and retracted anteriorly to aid in exposure. To aid in identification, the flexor hallucis longus tendon can be visualized by moving the great toe up and down as the flexor hallucis longus inserts onto the base of the distal phalanx of the great toe. The medical school acronym "Tom, Dick and Harry" (tibialis posterior, flexor digitorum longus, flexor hallucis longus) or the more extensive "Tom, Dick and very nervous Harry (tibialis posterior, flexor digitorum longus, posterior tibial artery, posterior tibial vein, tibial nerve, flexor hallucis longus) refers to the anatomy of the tendons at the medial malleolus under the flexor retinaculum from anterior to posterior within the tarsal tunnel.

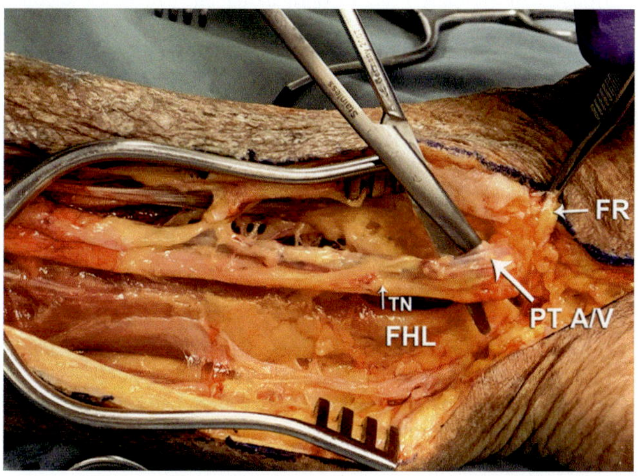

Fig. 35.8 The exposure of the posterior tibial artery and vein (PT A/V) in the distal leg and posterior to the medial malleolus. The neurovascular structures run between flexor hallucis longus (FHL) posteriorly and flexor digitorum longus anteriorly. The flexor retinaculum (FR) is opened up partially in this case for exposure. *TN* tibial nerve

The posterior tibial artery distally will terminate into the medial and lateral plantar arteries after it dives under the abductor hallucis muscle which will need to be divided to expose the bifurcation. The medial plantar artery is noted to be much smaller than the lateral plantar artery. The medial plantar artery is typically between 1 and 2, cm and perforators to the medial plantar flap will be found arising between the flexor hallucis brevis and abductor hallucis muscles.

The lateral plantar artery, after coming off the posterior tibial artery, runs between the flexor digitorum brevis muscle and the quadratus plantae muscle.

Discussion

The tibioperoneal trunk is a major vessel ultimately dividing into the posterior tibial and peroneal vessels and as such should not be sacrificed with an end-to-end anastomosis to preserve blood flow to the leg distally. End-to-side anastomosis can be considered if no other options are available.

The posterior tibial artery presents a plethora of options for microvascular anastomosis throughout its extensive course and has been widely described as a recipient vessel for microvascular anastomosis. Additionally, any small muscular branches that arise from the posterior tibial artery can also be considered for microvascular anastomoses if of sufficient caliber. Perforators can have many advantages such as limiting extensive dissections and maintaining axial flow to the distal extremity, and in the vasculopathic patient perforators may have adequate flow, whereas the major blood vessels may not due to extensive atherosclerosis [4–7]. However, perforator anastomoses do require a supermicrosurgical skillset.

Many have assessed lower extremity reconstruction and the safety of certain recipient vessels. Park et al. proposed an algorithm for recipient vessel selection in microvascular surgery [8]. Their experience comes from 50 consecutive lower extremity free flaps and discusses key points such as the recipient vessel selection being more important than the type of flap selected and that the most important factors in recipient vessel selection are the vascular status of the lower extremity and the injury site. Park et al. felt that the anterior tibial artery was an easier vessel compared to the posterior tibial artery for microvascular anastomoses. However, Nemoto et al. preferred the posterior tibial vessels in open fractures as it is less frequently injured than the anterior tibial vessels [9]. Godina et al., Bowen and Manktelow, as well as Chen et al. were also concerned that an unrecognized injury to the anterior tibial artery could occur and therefore advocated the use of the posterior tibial vessels [10–12]. Chen et al. looked at a series of 126 Gustilo type III open fractures of the tibia that required free flaps for coverage in Chang Gung [12]. They found that the anterior tibial was much more frequently injured and that if the posterior tibial artery was injured, it was often injured in conjunction with the anterior tibial artery requiring revascularization of the leg. There were six free flap failures, all of which were end-to-end anastomoses to the anterior tibial artery. For patients requiring free flaps in the lower extremity after trauma, Chen et al. advocated using the posterior tibial vessels in an end-to-side fashion.

End-to-end microvascular anastomoses are often preferred by microsurgeons for technical reasons. End-to-end and end-to-side techniques have shown equivalent flap success rates [13–15]. Godina and Hong et al. have preferred end-to-side techniques for flow preservation, less arterial spasm, and less flow aberrations from anastomotic mismatches [4, 16]. Also if end-to-end techniques are used, it is preferred to be used in a muscle flap as a muscle flap has less resistance than a skin flap and can adequately receive the higher blood flow [4, 17–19]. Acland advocates the use of the "cobra-head anastomosis" for his end-to-side technique where a long arteriotomy is made on both the recipient artery and the flap artery with minimal trimming of the flap artery edges [20]. The resultant anastomoses will resemble a cobra's head which he states leads to better eversion and less disturbance in the luminal blow flow, increase in anastomotic diameter, and resultantly less thrombus formation. Furthermore, if there is any concern about the vascular status of the lower extremity, then an end-to-side technique or flow-through technique should be performed. Intraoperatively the posterior tibial artery can be clamped and the perfusion to the lower extremity assessed with clinical exam and the use of a Doppler to confirm a signal on the plantar arch to aid in determining if an end-to-end anastomosis can be safely performed.

There are many branches throughout the course of the posterior tibial artery that can be safely performed for microvascular anastomoses. The soleal muscular branches off of the posterior tibial and peroneal arteries have been safely described [21]. Muramatsu et al. described using the posterior tibial artery or branches of the posterior tibial artery through the tibial tunnel as a safe and short route for microvascular anastomosis [22].

The posterior tibial artery terminal branches of the medial and lateral plantar artery can be used for free flap recipient vessels too. The lateral plantar artery is noted to be larger than the medial plantar artery, and 15–20% of the time the dominant blood supply to the plantar arterial arch comes from the lateral plantar artery [23, 24]. Chen and Scaglioni describe the lateral plantar artery as a recipient vessel for lateral plantar forefoot reconstruction and found it to be a sizeable vessel with an easy dissection [25]. Even the lateral calcaneal artery has been described as a recipient for free flaps [26].

Both the tibioperoneal trunk and the posterior tibial artery provide an extensive array of opportunities for free flap reconstructive recipient vessels. Many surgeons use the posterior tibial artery as their preferred recipient vessel in lower extremity reconstructions. There are many branches of the posterior tibial artery that can be used for microvascular surgery, and the decision to perform an end-to-side versus an end-to-end anastomosis for recipient vessels in the lower extremity should be made on a case-by-case basis making sure that end-line flow is preserved throughout the lower extremity.

References

1. Bradley L, Kirker SG. Secondary prevention of arteriosclerosis in lower limb vascular amputees: a missed opportunity. Eur J Vasc Endovasc Surg. 2006;32(5):491–3.
2. Nance M. National Trauma Data Bank 2015 annual report. Am College Surg 2015;66.
3. Colborn GL, Lumsden AB, Taylor BS, Skandalakis JE. The surgical anatomy of the popliteal artery. Am Surg. 1994;60(4):238–46.
4. Hong JP, Park CJ, Suh HP. Importance of vascularity and selecting the recipient vessels of lower extremity reconstruction. J Reconstr Microsurg. 2021;37(1):83–8.
5. Suh HS, Oh TS, Lee HS, Lee SH, Cho YP, Park JR, et al. A new approach for reconstruction of diabetic foot wounds using the angiosome and supermicrosurgery concept. Plast Reconstr Surg. 2016;138(4):702e–9e.
6. Suh HP, Kim Y, Suh Y, Hong J. Multidetector computed tomography (CT) analysis of 168 cases in diabetic patients with Total superficial femoral artery occlusion: is it safe to use an anterolateral thigh flap without CT angiography in diabetic patients? J Reconstr Microsurg. 2018;34(1):65–70.
7. Suh HS, Oh TS, Hong JP. Innovations in diabetic foot reconstruction using supermicrosurgery. Diabetes Metab Res Rev. 2016;32(Suppl 1):275–80.
8. Park S, Han SH, Lee TJ. Algorithm for recipient vessel selection in free tissue transfer to the lower extremity. Plast Reconstr Surg. 1999;103(7):1937–48.
9. Nemoto M, Ishikawa S, Kounoike N, Sugimoto T, Takeda A. Free flap transfer to preserve main arterial flow in early reconstruction of open fracture in the lower extremity. Plast Surg Int. 2015;2015:213892.
10. Godina M, Arnez ZM, Lister GD. Preferential use of the posterior approach to blood vessels of the lower leg in microvascular surgery. Plast Reconstr Surg. 1991;88(2):287–91.
11. Bowen V, Manktelow RT. Complications and unsatisfactory results in the microsurgical reconstruction of lower extremities. Microsurgery. 1993;14(3):196–202.
12. Chen HC, Chuang CC, Chen S, Hsu WM, Wei FC. Selection of recipient vessels for free flaps to the distal leg and foot following trauma. Microsurgery. 1994;15(5):358–63.
13. Samaha FJ, Oliva A, Buncke GM, Buncke HJ, Siko PP. A clinical study of end-to-end versus end-to-side techniques for microvascular anastomosis. Plast Reconstr Surg. 1997;99(4):1109–11.

14. Albertengo JB, Rodriguez A, Buncke HJ, Hall EJ. A comparative study of flap survival rates in end-to-end and end-to-side microvascular anastomosis. Plast Reconstr Surg. 1981;67(2):194–9.
15. Cho EH, Garcia RM, Blau J, Levinson H, Erdmann D, Levin LS, et al. Microvascular anastomoses using end-to-end versus end-to-side technique in lower extremity free tissue transfer. J Reconstr Microsurg. 2016;32(2):114–20.
16. Godina M. Preferential use of end-to-side arterial anastomoses in free flap transfers. Plast Reconstr Surg. 1979;64(5):673–82.
17. Takanari K, Kamei Y, Toriyama K, Yagi S, Torii S. Differences in blood flow volume and vascular resistance between free flaps: assessment in 58 cases. J Reconstr Microsurg. 2009;25(1):39–45.
18. Sasmor MT, Reus WF, Straker DJ, Colen LB. Vascular resistance considerations in free-tissue transfer. J Reconstr Microsurg. 1992;8(3):195–200.
19. Ono M, Takanari K, Toriyama K, Yagi S, Ebisawa K, Sawamura H, et al. Effects of tissue component volumes on vascular resistance in free flaps. J Reconstr Microsurg. 2017;33(1):32–9.
20. Acland RD. Refinements in lower extremity free flap surgery. Clin Plast Surg. 1990;17(4):733–44.
21. Haddock N, Garfein ES, Reformat D, Hecht E, Levine J, Saadeh P. Perforator vessel recipient options in the lower extremity: an anatomically based approach to safer limb salvage. J Reconstr Microsurg. 2010;26(7):461–9.
22. Muramatsu K, Shigetomi M, Ihara K, Kawai S. Microvascular anastomosis through the tibial tunnel: a new technique in free-tissue transfer to the leg. Microsurgery. 2004;24(4):293–7.
23. Vann H. A note on the formation of the plantar arterial arch of the human foot. Anatomical Record. 1943;85(83).
24. Kalicharan A, Pillay P, Rennie C, Haffajee MR. The anatomy of the plantar arterial arch. Int J Morphol. 2015;33(1):36–42.
25. Chen YC, Scaglioni MF. The lateral plantar artery as recipient vessel for microsurgical lateral plantar forefoot reconstruction: case report. Int Microsurg J. 2017;1(2):2.
26. Chang H, Kwon SS, Minn KW. Lateral calcaneal artery as a recipient pedicle for microsurgical foot reconstruction. J Plast Reconstr Aesthet Surg. 2010;63(11):1860–4.

Peroneal Vessels

36

Nicholas T. Haddock and Austin Hembd

Introduction

Recipient vessel selection is one of the most critical decisions toward maximizing the success of lower extremity microsurgical free-flap reconstruction [1–3]. This decision is based on location of defect, zone of injury, status of the three main vessels in the lower leg, preexisting peripheral vascular disease, length of available donor, and ease of dissection or microsurgical tissue transfer. The anterior and posterior tibial vessels are more commonly utilized and described due to their ease of dissection and access for lower extremity wounds [3, 4]. However, trauma, oncologic resection, peripheral vascular disease, and anatomical variation can all limit ideal donor vessel selection. The peroneal vessels, like the posterior tibial system, are deeper and more protected from the anterior blunt trauma that commonly occurs in open Gustilo fracture patterns. This is why several large series have found far fewer peroneal artery disruptions than anterior tibial artery disruptions in this patient population [1, 3].

Moreover, in the setting of the growing understanding and utilization of perforator flaps in the lower extremity, it is advantageous for the reconstructive microsurgeon to be able to identify and utilize the consistent peroneal perforators for recipient microsurgical anastomoses if needed [5–11]. This is particularly true in the difficult setting of lower extremities with single vessel inflow to the foot, where other options are limited to end-to-side anastomoses, A-V loops, and vein grafts. This chapter will review pertinent surgical anatomy and exposure of the peroneal vessels along with its cutaneous and soleus perforators, pertinent physical examination, and a discussion of innovative, alternative uses of this uncommonly utilized vessel in the setting of extremity salvage.

Supplementary Information The online version of this chapter (https://doi.org/10.1007/978-3-030-75389-4_36) contains supplementary material, which is available to authorized users.

N. T. Haddock (✉) · A. Hembd
Department of Plastic Surgery, UT Southwestern Medical Center, Dallas, TX, USA
e-mail: Nicholas.Haddock@UTSouthwestern.edu; Austin.Hembd@PHHS.org

Anatomy of the Peroneal Vessels and Perforators

The tibioperoneal trunk, the continuation of the popliteal vessels after the branch point of the anterior tibial artery and vein, typically gives rise to the peroneal artery roughly 6–8 cm distal to the fibular head as it courses into the deep posterior leg compartment [8, 12]. The peroneal artery then travels 4–5 cm further before inserting into the FHL muscle [12]. At this level, it has a diameter of about 3–4 mm. Distal to the proximal third of the leg, it then courses parallel and in close proximity to the fibula, providing blood supply to it and the overlying skin before terminating as an anterior perforating branch and a lateral calcaneal artery approximately 6 cm proximal to the tip of the lateral malleolus. Along its course it sends muscle branches and musculocutaneous perforators to the soleus, tibialis posterior, peroneus brevis, peroneus longus, and flexor hallucis muscles. Of note, the proximal fibular epiphysis, fibular head, and overlying skin are not in the angiosome of the peroneal artery and instead in the vascular territory of the inferior lateral geniculate artery, the anterior tibial artery, or the common tibioperoneal trunk.

There are typically about 4–5 perforating branches of the peroneal artery to the skin from its origin to its terminal branches [8, 11]. While there are varying reports of the percentage of muscular versus septocutaneous perforators, generally the musculocutaneous perforators dominate in the superior two-thirds of the leg. They arise from within 3 cm of the posterior border of the fibula, with an average of 1.8 cm [8]. The external diameter of all of the perforators averaged together is 0.6 mm, but this includes the smaller diameter septocutaneous perforators along the posterior intermuscular

R. Gurunian, R. Djohan (eds.), *Recipient Vessels in Reconstructive Microsurgery*, https://doi.org/10.1007/978-3-030-75389-4_36

septum that are well known from a long-standing experience with the fibula osteocutaneous flap.

The sizes of the proximal perforators to the soleus muscle are larger and can potentially be more suitable matches for microsurgical free tissue transfer. On average there are 3–4 soleus muscle branches from the peroneal vessels. The most proximal perforator is around 1.7 mm in diameter, branched prior to the insertion of the FHL, and was about 24 cm proximal from the lateral malleolus [11]. In another MRA study, the mean length between the peroneal artery origin (which itself is typically 6–8 cm distal to the fibular head) and the first peroneal muscle perforator was 7–8 cm [12]. The second and third perforators to the soleus are found to branch within the proximal FHL muscle. These are around 1.4 mm in diameter and about 7 cm distal to the origin of the peroneal artery and 13 cm cephalad to the lateral malleolus [11]. Other studies have found similar results, with Wong et al. dissecting 20 cadaver limbs and found 90% having one or more musculocutaneous perforators between 0.8 and 1.5 mm in diameter within 6 cm of the middle third and lower third junction of the fibula [13]. In addition, Schaverien et al. found peroneal artery perforators emerging through the posterior intermuscular septum to the skin from the soleus and peroneus longus muscles proximally and between the FHL and peroneus brevis distally. They found a cluster of perforators most commonly between 13–18 cm proximal to the lateral malleolus and thus corresponding to the middle third of the fibula, along with 93% of other lower extremity studies [5] (Fig. 36.1).

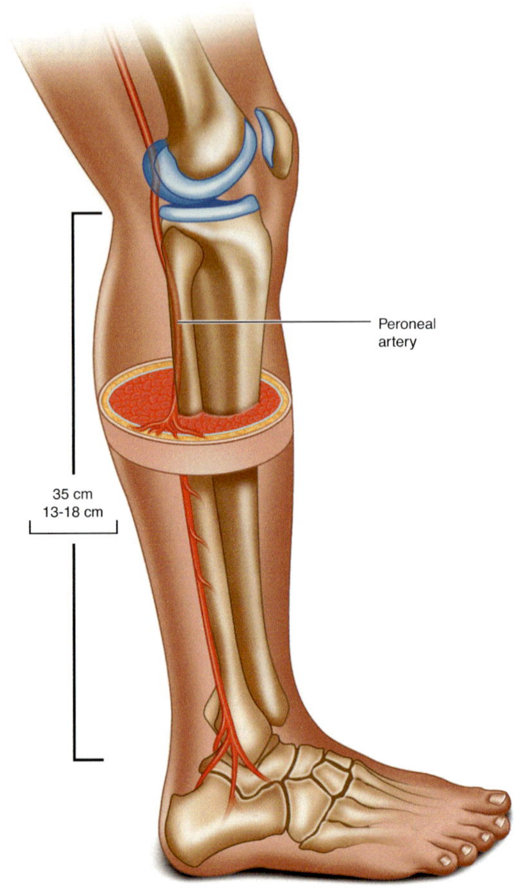

Fig. 36.1 Depicted is the course of the popliteal artery branching from the tibioperoneal trunk, running in the deep posterior compartment and supplying the fibula and surrounding musculature, and terminating at the distal ankle as the lateral calcaneal artery. The average distance between the fibular head and the lateral malleolus is around 35 cm, and the area of maximal peroneal skin perforator density lies between 13 cm and 18 cm proximal to the lateral malleolus

Preoperative Assessment

The need for preoperative vascular imaging is a long-debated topic in lower extremity reconstructive microsurgery. Some publications have reported a high success rate in patients with physical exam only and found angiography is beneficial in patients without palpable pedal pulses [14, 15]. Alternatively, Duymaz et al. showed a 29% incidence of single-vessel arterial occlusion on preoperative CTA of traumatized lower extremities undergoing reconstructive planning [16]. Additionally, 64% of limbs with normal pulses or Doppler exams had arterial injuries found on CTA imaging. Perhaps it is more important for planning chronic lower extremity wound coverage in vasculopathy or diabetic patients, as endovascular interventions can be performed simultaneously where necessary [17].

A possible reason for the discrepancy in these types of studies is that simply performing distal pedal pulse exams or checking for audible Doppler signals can be confounded by the rich collateral and anastomotic system in the lower leg and foot. Therefore, we believe that the most accurate information from a physical exam can come from performing a lower extremity Allen test (LEAT) to isolate individual vessel contribution to the foot [18]. To perform, a handheld Doppler is used to identify the first dorsal metatarsal artery in the first web space, while compression is placed on the dorsalis pedis and posterior tibial arteries. If there is a persistent signal, then there is collateral flow through the peroneal system, although because the peroneal artery collaterals are proximal to the point of compression, this is rare. If the signal dissipates, then pressure on the dorsalis pedis or posterior tibial artery is released in alternating fashion to see which, if not both, allow resumption of a distal signal and therefore indicate if the foot is reliant on either vessel.

In our experience, we typically only get preoperative angiographic imaging studies if there are absent pulses and if there is a history of severe vascular disease, causing ischemic tissue loss or requiring revascularization, or orthopedic trauma including Gustilo IIIB or IIIC fracture types. Even in these high-risk patients, if possible, we always perform a preoperative and intraoperative LEAT before deciding to perform any end-to-end anastomosis. We often find that this physical exam accurately guides decision-making for recipient vessels in the majority of our lower extremity reconstructions.

Surgical Exposures

Lateral Approach to Peroneal Artery Perforators Cutaneous perforators of the peroneal vessels in the middle and distal thirds of the leg course through the posterior intermuscular septum that separates the lateral and posterior compartments. This anatomy is well known to reconstructive microsurgeons harvesting the fibula as a free osteocutaneous flap. These cutaneous perforators can be utilized as recipient vessels and propeller flaps for lower extremity coverage. As microvascular recipient vessels, the peroneal perforators to the soleus muscle are of more reliable quality and diameter for adequate size and match to the pedicle diameters of most free flaps. As detailed above, the most proximal, and largest, soleus perforator is about 24 cm proximal to the lateral malleolus, roughly 10–13 cm distal to the fibular head, and proximal to the peroneal artery and vein insertion to the FHL muscle. Therefore, an exploratory longitudinal incision can be made corresponding to this area (largely the middle third of the leg) just posterior the palpable fibula. Dissection proceeds posterior to the intermuscular septum, and the middle portion of the soleus is then carefully separated off the fibula. In this plane peroneal artery perforators are identified coursing into the soleus muscle from an anterior to posterior direction (see Video 36.1). These perforators can be dissected toward their origin for additional length. In this region, the small saphenous vein can be utilized as additional venous outflow if required (Figs. 36.2 and 36.3).

Medial Approach to the Peroneal Artery While the medial approach to the peroneal vessels is uncommon in reconstructive microsurgery, it has been used in vascular surgery as an approach to the peroneal, posterior tibial, and popliteal systems. Because the posterior tibial vessels are readily accessible from the medial aspect of the lower leg, the medial approach to the peroneal vessels would likely only be utilized in the event of an unknown vascular anomaly with an atretic posterior tibial artery or if the posterior tibial vessels were in the zone of injury in an anteromedial soft tissue defect. If the lower leg defect is more anterior or anterolateral, then approaching the peroneal perforators from a lateral approach as described above is more straightforward [11]. However, if a medial approach is made to the posterior tibial vessels and they are unusable, then the same incision can be utilized to expose the peroneal vessels. To this one must dissect past the tibial nerve and posterior tibial vessels, anterior to the soleus and flexor hallucis longus muscles, while remaining in the deep posterior compartment. The peroneal vessels are then found with blunt dissection past the flexor

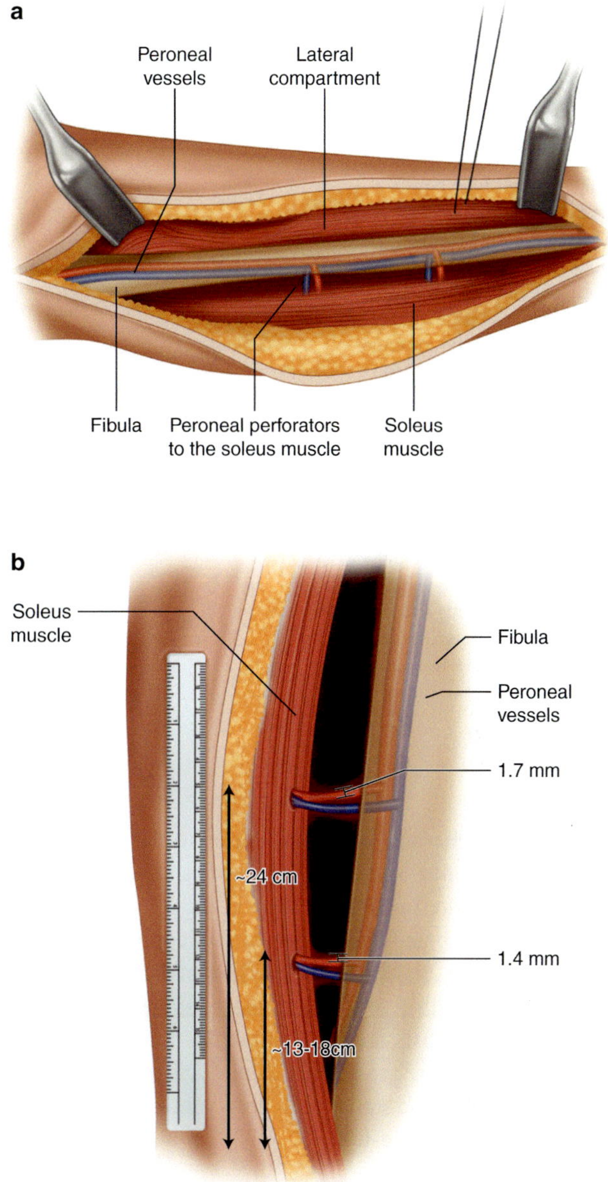

Fig. 36.2 (**a**) Lateral view of leg with lateral muscular compartment and superficial posterior compartments dissected off the lateral spine of the fibula. The muscular perforators from the peroneal vessels can be seen entering the soleus muscle from the source peroneal vessels that lay directly medial to the fibula. (**b**) The interval between the superficial posterior compartment and the posterior aspect of the fibula is entered after freeing these muscles from the fascial attachments to the lateral aspect of the fibula. The peroneal vessels have a proximal most muscular perforator, an average of 1.7 mm in diameter, which can be seen coursing into the soleus on an average of 24 cm proximal to the lateral malleolus. A second direct soleus muscular perforator, an average of 1.4 mm in diameter, can generally be found 13–18 cm proximal to the lateral malleolus. This latter distance is also the highest density of peroneal cutaneous perforators as well. These can alternatively be utilized as recipient vessels or to perfuse a free flap from the lateral leg

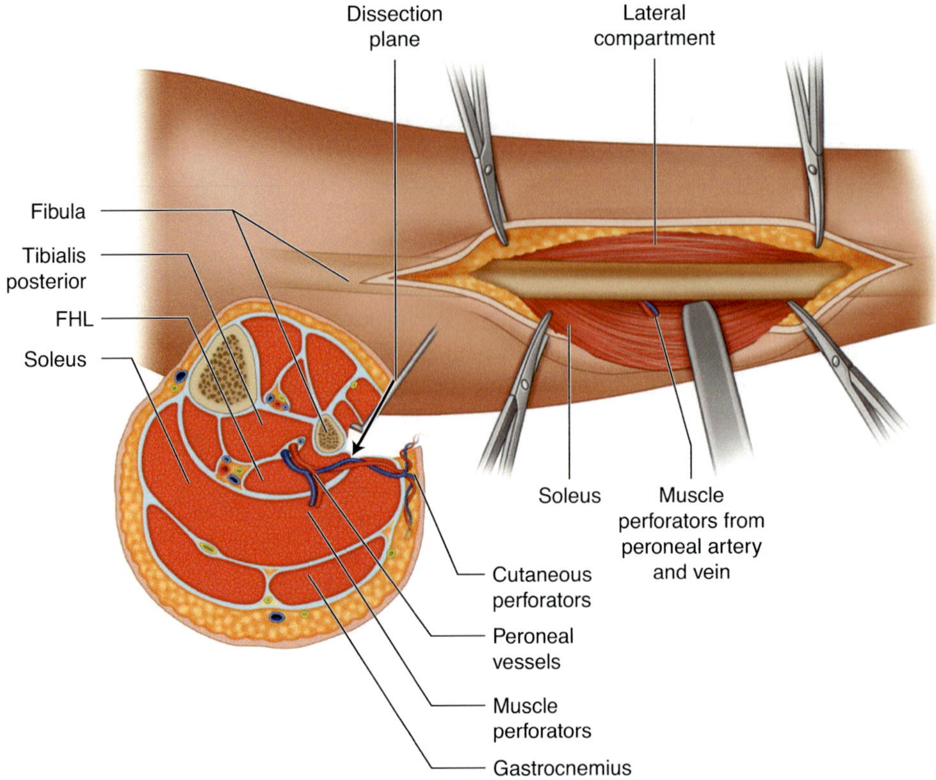

Fig. 36.3 *Above.* Lateral aspect of the leg with peroneal perforator supplying the soleus and superficial posterior compartment. *Below.* Cross-sectional anatomy of the leg. Depicted is the course of the peroneal artery and its perforators, which can send branches along the posterior intermuscular septum between the superficial posterior and lateral muscular compartments to supply the skin. This will be encountered first and examined for adequacy as recipient vessels. If one continues the plane of dissection between the soleus and the flexor hallucis longus (FHL), then large muscular perforators from the peroneal vessels to the soleus and gastrocnemius muscles can be visualized coming from an anterior to posterior direction

digitorum longus and tibialis posterior to the interval that houses the peroneal vessels. These vessels are in close proximity to the posterior tibial vessels in the middle and distal thirds of the leg, and knowledge of this approach can save another incision, dissection, or need for pedicle lengthening or vein grafts with free tissue transfer [19]. One benefit of free flap anastomosis medially on the lower leg, however, is the proximity to the greater saphenous vein as an additional outflow option in the setting of a deep venous thrombosis or free flap venous congestion.

Discussion

Pedicled FHL Flap with the Peroneal Vessels for Middle/Proximal Third Leg and Knee Coverage While upper third and knee defects can often be treated with pedicled muscle flaps such as the gastrocnemius or local perforator flaps like the medial sural artery perforator flap, large oncological or traumatic defects can often be either too large for these options or include these commonly used pedicles in the zone of injury. In these cases, free tissue transfer can be indicated, particularly for the lateral aspect of the knee where the gastrocnemius is smaller and loses length and mobility around the fibula.

Previously established as a local muscle option in the lower extremity [19], Sailon et al. further described using the pedicled anterograde FHL flap as a local coverage option for small lateral knee or upper third lower extremity defects [12]. Perhaps the most interesting and innovative use for this muscle flap is that the muscle can provide coverage of a rotated peroneal artery and vein pedicle. This provides an anterograde recipient site for subsequent free tissue transfer around the knee. A case report from this study described a traumatic posterior knee dislocation that interrupted the popliteal vessels and requiring an interposition saphenous vein graft. With concern for integrity of the sural arteries and a large anterior soft tissue defect, the FHL was taken along with the peroneal vessels, and a free rectus abdominis flap was used to close the defect [12].

If gastrocnemius or medial sural artery flaps cannot be reliably used or will not cover the defect area around the knee, this flap provides a small amount of soft tissue coverage laterally as well as a readily available recipient vessel. We would prefer this approach to other commonly cited alternatives to the gastrocnemius flaps such as the distally based ALT flap, which we find unreliable and do not regularly consider it as a viable coverage option.

Fibula Flow-Through Flaps In a concept similar to the pedicled FHL flap above, the peroneal vessels can be great recipient artery and vein option for microsurgical anastomosis after a fibula flap is performed. When a large three-dimensional head and neck or extremity defect requires a vascularized bone flap and a second free flap for additional skin or soft tissue bulk, the distal end of the fibula flap can provide a recipient vessel. On rare occurrences the skin paddle that is normally supplied by septocutaneous perforators from the peroneal artery instead arises from the posterior tibial vessels [20]. Parr et al. described the anastomoses of the fibula skin paddle to the distal peroneal vessels, and the resulting improved degree of freedom and length that is achieved [21]. In lower extremity combined tibial bone and soft tissue defects, Jeng et al. performed elegant single-stage reconstruction with ipsilateral pedicled fibula bone segment and soft tissue coverage with free tissue transfer to the distal peroneal vessels [22]. This enables a large degree of freedom of where the fibular graft can be designed as it does not necessitate being placed under the septocutaneous skin perforators.

Utilizing the distal continuation of the peroneal vessels for microsurgical transfer in conjunction with a free or pedicled fibula flap can thus be a powerful and useful tool in the vessel-depleted head and neck or complex extremity defects for creative single-stage reconstruction.

Fitting Peroneal Vessels and Perforators into the Recipient Vessel Algorithm

The peroneal vessels are rarely discussed in lower extremity recipient vessel algorithms due to their deep location and the difficulty of access for microsurgical tissue transfer [1–2, 23]. However, their location can provide protection, particularly from blunt anterior-directed forces common in open tibial injuries. In a retrospective review of 191 lower extremity trauma patients with abnormal angiograms, it was found that the total number of peroneal artery disruptions was 15.7%, nearly half the incidence of anterior tibial artery injuries [3]. After performing a lower extremity Allen test and understanding which vessels are imperative for foot perfusion, we generally agree with the algorithm set forth by Yazar and Chi-Hung Lin [1]. In this algorithm, the anterior or posterior tibial vessels are utilized that are adjacent to the defect in the leg with three-vessel runoff. If there is an injured vessel, the proximal or distal end of that vessel is an attractive next option if convenient for the defect location, and it does not require too a large distance (and therefore pedicle length) to escape the zone of injury. In the single-vessel leg, we prefer end-to-end anastomoses to an injured vessel or end-to-side to the single patent vessel. In some situations a large zone of injury or vasculopathy makes utilizing the injured/occluded vessel difficult, but performing end-to-side anastomoses to the single patent vessel risks perfusion of the foot if technical issues or thrombosis occurs. These factors must be carefully considered and individualized.

In our experience, end-to-side anastomoses in the setting of atherosclerosis and calcifications prove even more challenging. In these chronic patients, or those with acute traumatic injuries along the anterolateral aspect of the lower leg and a large zone of injury to the anterior tibial vessels, the lateral approach to the soleal perforators as described above can potentially be a safer and more facile option for microsurgical free tissue transfer. Therefore, while undoubtedly a less common option, understanding the locations and approaches to the peroneal vessels and its muscle or cutaneous perforators can aid the reconstructive microsurgeon in extremity salvage.

References

1. Yazar S, Lin C. Selection of recipient vessel in traumatic lower extremity. J Reconstr Microsurg. 2012;28(03):199–204.
2. Park S, Han S, Lee T. Algorithm for recipient vessel selection in free tissue transfer to the lower extremity. Plast Reconstr Surg. 1999;103(7):1937–48.
3. Haddock N, Weichman K, Reformat D, Kligman B, Levine J, Saadeh P. Lower extremity arterial injury patterns and reconstructive outcomes in patients with severe lower extremity trauma: a 26-year review. J Am Coll Surg. 2010;210(1):66–72.
4. Pu L, Levine J, Wei F. Reconstructive surgery of the lower extremity. St. Louis: Quality Medical Publ; 2013.
5. Schaverien M, Saint-Cyr M. Perforators of the lower leg: analysis of perforator locations and clinical application for Pedicled perforator flaps. Plast Reconstr Surg. 2008;122(1):161–70.
6. Hong J. The use of supermicrosurgery in lower extremity reconstruction: the next step in evolution. Plast Reconstr Surg. 2009;123(1):230–5.
7. Kim C, Naidu S, Kim Y. Supermicrosurgery in peroneal and soleus perforator-based free flap coverage of foot defects caused by occlusive vascular diseases. Plast Reconstr Surg. 2010;126(2):499–507.
8. Heitmann C, Khan F, Levin S. Vasculature of the peroneal artery: an anatomic study focused on the perforator vessels. J Reconstr Microsurg. 2003;19(3):157–62.
9. Iorio M, Cheerharan M, Olding M. A systematic review and pooled analysis of peroneal artery perforators for fibula Osteocutaneous and perforator flaps. Plast Reconstr Surg. 2012;130(3):600–7.
10. Seo S, Kim K, Yoon C. Extended scope of the use of the peroneal perforator flap in lower limb reconstruction. J Reconstr Microsurg. 2015;31(09):654–9.
11. Haddock N, Garfein E, Reformat D, Hecht E, Levine J, Saadeh P. Perforator vessel recipient options in the lower extremity: an anatomically based approach to safer limb salvage. J Reconstr Microsurg. 2010;26(07):461–9.
12. Sailon A, Reformat D, Hecht E, Garfein E, Spector J, Levine J, et al. The proximally based peroneal vascular bundle. Ann Plast Surg. 2009;62(5):556–9.
13. Wong C, Tan B, Wei F, Song C. Use of the soleus musculocutaneous perforator for skin paddle salvage of the fibula Osteoseptocutaneous flap: anatomical study and clinical confirmation. Plast Reconstr Surg. 2007;120(6):1576–84.
14. Isenberg J, Sherman R. The limited value of preoperative angiography in microsurgical reconstruction of the lower limb. J Reconstr Microsurg. 1996;12(05):303–6.

15. Lutz B, Wei F, Machens H, Rhode U, Berger A. Indications and limitations of angiography before free-flap transplantation to the distal lower leg after trauma: prospective study in 36 patients. J Reconstr Microsurg. 2000;16(3):0187–92.
16. Duymaz A, Karabekmez F, Vrtiska T, Mardini S, Moran S. Free tissue transfer for lower extremity reconstruction: A study of the role of computed angiography in the planning of free tissue transfer in the posttraumatic setting. Plast Reconstr Surg. 2009;124(2):523–9.
17. Janhofer D, Lakhiani C, Kim P, Akbari C, Naz I, Tefera E, et al. The utility of preoperative arteriography for free flap planning in patients with chronic lower extremity wounds. Plast Reconstr Surg. 2019;143(2):604–13.
18. Haddock N, Garfein E, Saadeh P, Levine J. The lower-extremity Allen test. J Reconstr Microsurg. 2009;25(07):399–403.
19. Hughes L, Mahoney J. Anatomic basis of local muscle flaps in the distal third of the leg. Plast Reconstr Surg. 1993;92(6):1144–54.
20. Tan B, Wong C. An anomalous septocutaneous perforator to the skin paddle of the fibula osteocutaneous flap originating from the posterior tibial artery. J Plast Reconstr Aesthet Surg. 2009;62(5):690–2.
21. Parr J, Adams B, Wagels M. Flow-through flap for salvage of fibula osseocutaneous vascular variations: a surgical approach and proposed modification of its classification. J Oral Maxillofac Surg. 2014;72(6):1197–202.
22. Jeng S, Kuo Y, Wei F, Wang J, Chen S. Concomitant ipsilateral Pedicled fibular transfer and free muscle flap for compound Tibial defect reconstruction. Ann Plast Surg. 2001;47(1):47–52.
23. Chen H, Chuang C, Chen S, Hsu W, Wei F. Selection of recipient vessels for free flaps to the distal leg and foot following trauma. Microsurgery. 1994;15(5):358–63.

Recipient Vessels: Femur Reconstruction

37

Margaret S. Roubaud, Matthew M. Hanasono, and Edward I. Chang

Introduction

Taylor and colleagues [1] described the first vascularized fibula transplant in 1974. Since that time, numerous studies have documented the safety and reliability of the free fibula flap as a vascularized bone graft for different osseous defects. In particular, the free fibula has become the gold standard of long bone reconstruction of extremities, with single and double strut techniques described.

Free fibula reconstruction of the femur is possible after oncologic, traumatic, and infectious etiologies of bony loss. One of the key determinants of successful reconstruction is appropriate graft positioning and pedicle orientation toward recipient vessels. In the thigh, branches of the common femoral, deep femoral, and superficial femoral vasculature are excellent recipients due to their caliber and high flow.

Preoperative Assessment

When planning free fibula reconstruction of the femur, the reconstructive surgeon must consider the anatomy of the defect and the vascular status of the lower extremity. In particular, the selection of optimal recipient vessels will depend highly on the location of the femur deficit. Furthermore, the necessary bone length and orientation of the pedicle are dependent on the vascular status of both the donor and recipient site.

Prior to any operative intervention, the resecting and reconstructive surgeon should evaluate the femoral deficit. Defects at the femoral head and neck will require anastomoses far more proximal than others and will rely on the common femoral and superficial femoral branches. Midshaft defects frequently require anastomosis to the first through third perforating branches from the deep femoral system, if available. More distal defects may require anastomoses to the superficial femoral system at the transition to the popliteal. Of importance, distal defects are more likely to require arteriovenous (AV) loop or end-to-side anastomoses to keep the popliteal artery open to the remaining lower extremity.

Assessment of the vascular system of lower extremity is pertinent prior to any intervention. The authors recommend a thorough clinical exam prior to any radiographic or interventional studies. The common femoral artery should be easily palpable at the groin within the femoral triangle. Weak pulses in this area, assuming normotension of the patient, should prompt workup for femoral artery stenosis or significant calcification. Distal pulses, including the dorsalis pedis and posterior tibial, should be assessed for distal runoff. Bounding pulses at the dorsalis pedis suggest patency of the vascular system from the groin to toes, although weak or non-palpable pulses should warrant further investigation. The patient's extremity should be checked for visible trauma and previous surgical scars. In cases of extensive traumatic injury, vascular deficits should be assumed until proven otherwise.

Several clinical studies are available to help assess the vascular status of the extremity. Duplex doppler sonography gives real-time information regarding the patency and flow of arteries and veins within the extremity and poses minimal risk to the patient. However, the preferred methods of assessment, when possible, are computed tomography angiography (CTA) or magnetic resonance angiography (MRA) with contrast. These methods give critical three-dimensional information regarding the patency and spatial position of pertinent vessels. Finally, the gold standard of vascular imaging remains interventional angiography, which can provide real-time flow and three-dimensional information regarding vasculature status. The authors recommend interventional

M. S. Roubaud (✉) · M. M. Hanasono · E. I. Chang
Department of Plastic Surgery, The University of Texas MD Anderson Cancer Center, Houston, TX, USA
e-mail: MSRoubaud@mdanderson.org; MHanasono@mdanderson.org; eichang@mdanderson.org

R. Gurunian, R. Djohan (eds.), *Recipient Vessels in Reconstructive Microsurgery*, https://doi.org/10.1007/978-3-030-75389-4_37

lateral leg and used to reach recipient vessels if none are readily available near the defect.

When a defect is associated with radiation or severe traumatic injury, finding vessels outside of the area of concern is warranted. In this case, dissection of a proximal vessel is advised. In the femoral triangle, there are a multitude of branches supplying the abdomen and upper thigh that can be utilized, including the deep and superficial inferior epigastrics, superficial circumflex iliacs, and the pudendal system. Saphenous vein interposition or AV loop grafting can transverse large distances and provide blood supply to flaps in vessel-depleted regions. Distal vessels can be used alternatively, although they must be thoroughly investigated for adequate flow past the traumatized region. Depending on the distance to the available recipients, the recipient vessels can be accessed by direct defect extension or tunneling.

One important consideration when performing vascularized fibula reconstruction of the femur is the use of additional soft tissue flaps, when necessary. In the authors' experience, many intercalary defects of the femur are associated with soft tissue loss as well, either due to radiation or traumatic injury. In these instances, the combination of soft tissue flap, such as a free latissimus dorsi or anterolateral thigh, can achieve bony and soft tissue reconstruction simultaneously. Furthermore, with advanced microsurgical techniques, the fibula may be "piggybacked" onto side branches of the soft tissue flap and thereby avoid the need for vein grafting or multiple anastomoses to support each flap. Others have described this technique as well with success [27, 28].

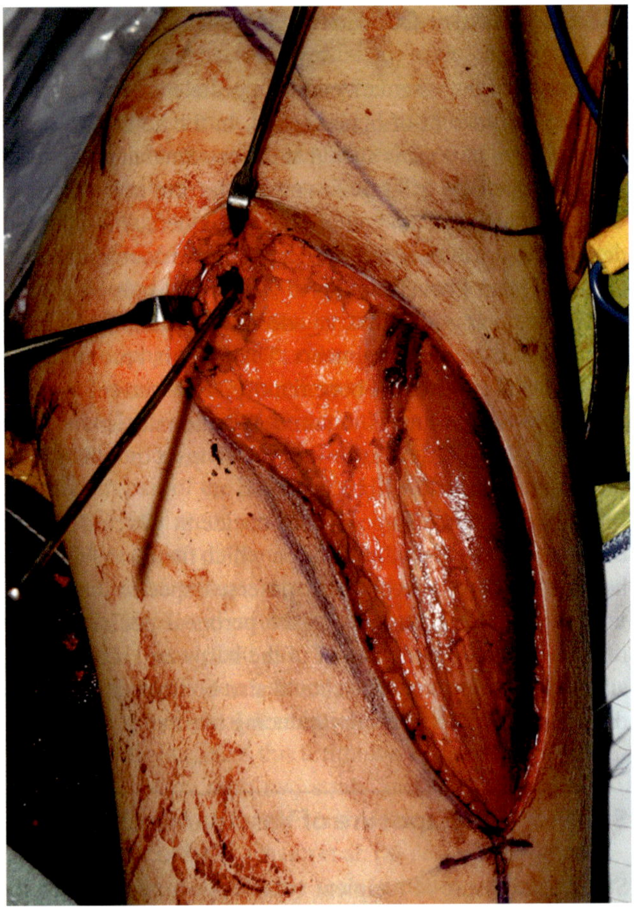

Fig. 37.2 Exposure of the left femoral neck. A lateral incision was made, and the reamer is seen in the medullary cavity of the femoral neck

Case Example

WM is a 12-year-old male with history of polyostotic fibrous dysplasia. He developed medial groin pain while participating in sports and was diagnosed with a non-displaced pathologic fracture of the right femoral neck. Orthopedic surgery requested femoral neck reconstruction with vascularized fibula and the time of open reduction and internal fixation.

The femoral neck was accessed by a lateral approach (Fig. 37.2). The femoral neck underwent core decompression with up to an 18 mm reamer. The ascending, descending, and transverse branches of the LCFA were identified. The descending branch had the greatest length. Therefore, it was ligated distally and rotated clockwise. An 8-cm-long fibula free flap was harvested from the ipsilateral leg (Fig. 37.3). The distal fibula was placed into the femoral neck core with the pedicle facing anterosuperior (Fig. 37.4). The proximal fibula was burred for precise fit in the core. The peroneal vessels anastomosed end-to-end to the descending branch of the LCFA. X-rays demonstrate placement of the fibula intraoperatively (Fig. 37.5) with healing at 1 year postoperatively (Fig. 37.6a, b).

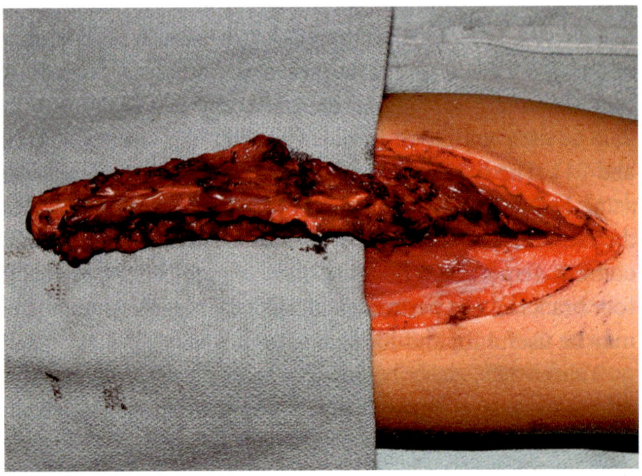

Fig. 37.3 A fibula osseous free flap was harvested from the left lower extremity based on the peroneal artery and vein

Summary

The free fibula flap, either single or double-barreled, is the

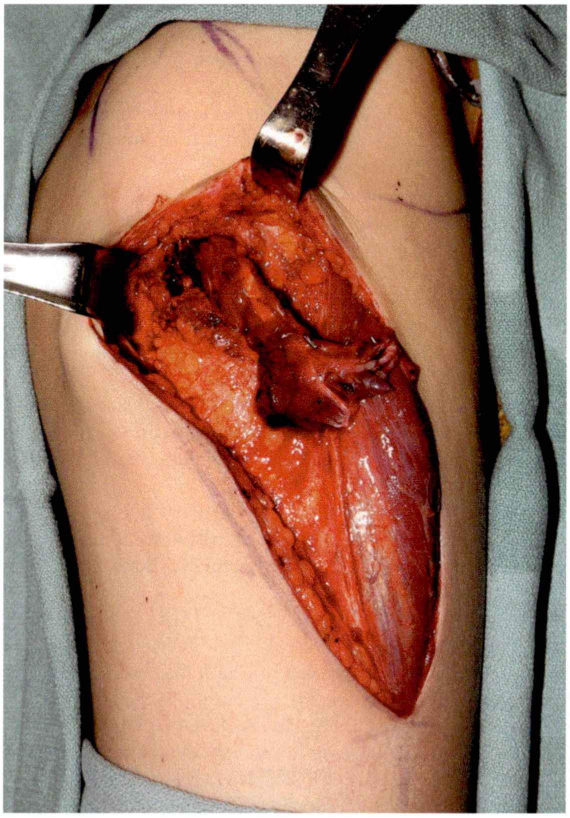

Fig. 37.4 The fibula being placed in an intercalary manner down the femoral neck. The vascular pedicle can be seen anastomosed to the descending branch of the LCFA

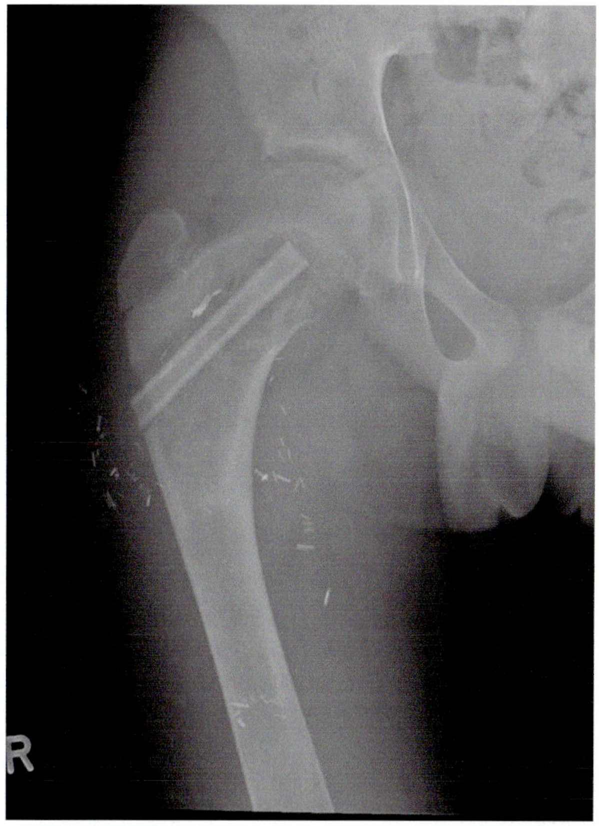

Fig. 37.5 Intraoperative radiograph confirming position of the fibula

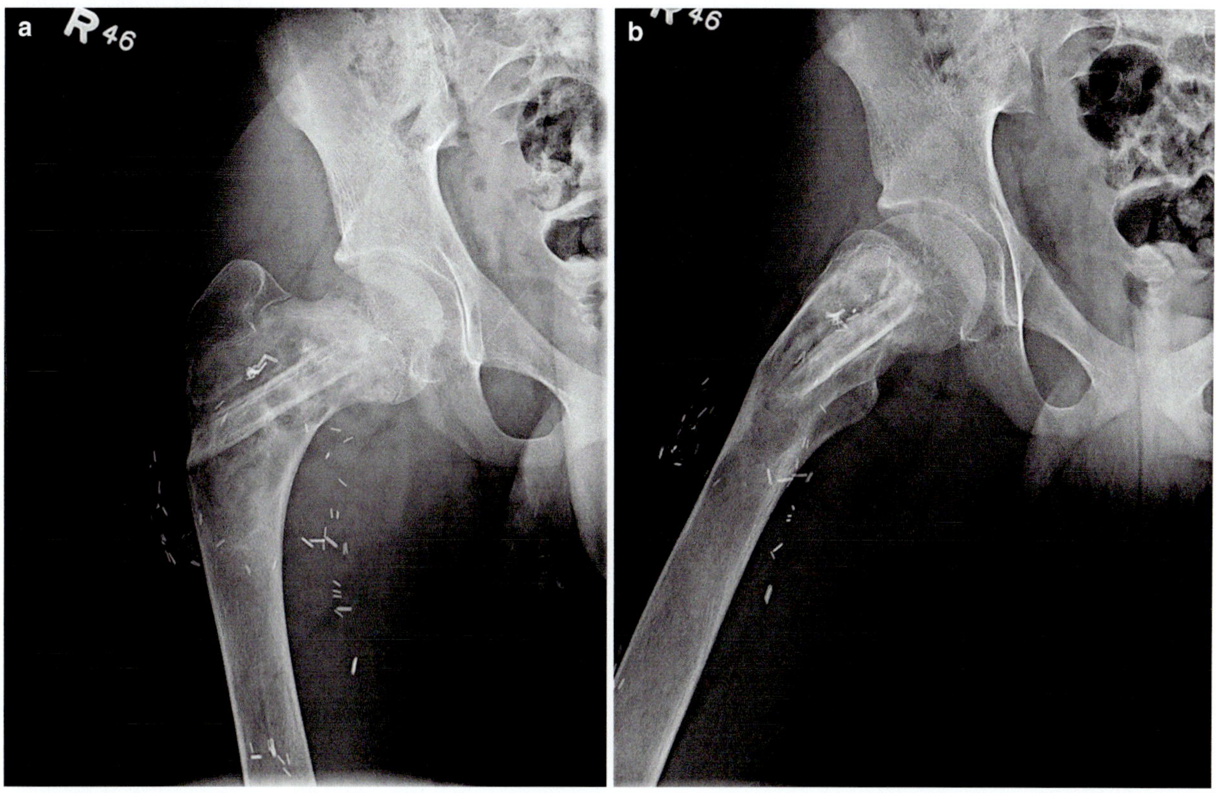

Fig. 37.6 Anterior-posterior (**a**) and oblique (**b**) postoperative radiographs showing bony healing of the femoral neck and an intact fibula free flap. Surgical clips trace the path of the vascular pedicle

gold standard of reconstruction for large defects of the femur. The femoral vasculature, including the superficial and deep systems, is rich in high-flow branches including segmental perforators to the muscle. At the proximal femur, the ascending and descending branches of the lateral circumflex femoral artery are most commonly utilized. In the mid-shaft, the LCFA and segmental branches to the deep thigh musculature are readily available. In the distal femur, the genicular and sural arteries are valuable recipients. In all three areas, end-to-side anastomoses are possible but technically more difficult. AV grafting to more proximal vessels in the femoral triangle is recommended when locoregional blood supply is diminished.

References

1. Taylor GI, Miller GDH, Ham TJ. The free vascularized bone graft: clinical extension of microvascular techniques. Plast Reconstr Surg. 1974;55:533.
2. Feldesman MR, Kleckner JG, Lundy JK. The femur/stature ratio and estimates of stature in mid and late-pleistocene fossil hominids. Am J Phys Anthr. 1990;83:359–72.
3. Ide Y, Matsunaga S, Harris J, O'Connell D, Seikaly H, Wolfaardt J. Anatomical examination of the fibula: digital imaging study for osseointegrated implant installation. J Otolaryngol Head Neck Surg. 2015;44:1.
4. Hou SM, Liu TK. Reconstruction of skeletal defects in the femur with "two-strut" free vascularized fibular grafts. J Trauma. 1992;33:840–5.
5. Wei FC, Chen HC, Chuang CC, Noordhoff MS. Fibular osteoseptocutaneous flap: anatomic study and clinical application. Plast Reconstr Surg. 1986;78:191–200.
6. Guo F. Observation of the blood supply to the fibula. Arch Orthop Trauma Surg. 1981;98:147–51.
7. Jupiter JB, Bour CJ, May JW. The reconstruction of defects in the femoral shaft with vascularized fibular bone transfers. J Bone Joint Surg. 1987;69:365–74.
8. Chang MC, Lo WH, Chen CM, Chen TM. Treatment of large skeletal defects in the lower extremities using double-strut, free vascularized fibular bone grafting. Orthopedics. 1999;22:739–44.
9. de Boer HH, Wood MB. Bone changes in the vascularized fibular graft. J Bone Joint Surg Br. 1989;71:374–8.
10. Jones NF, Swartz WM, Mears DC, Jupiter JB, Grossman A. The "double-barrel" free vascularized fibular bone graft. Plast Reconstr Surg. 1988;81:378–85.
11. Enneking WF, Eady JL, Burchardt H. Autogenous cortical bone graft in the reconstruction of segmental skeletal defects. J Bone Joint Surg Am. 1980;62:1039–58.
12. Weiland AJ, Phillips TW, Randolph MA. Bone grafts: a radiologic, histologic, and biomechanical model comparing autografts, allografts, and free vascularized bone grafts. Plast Reconstr Surg. 1984;74:368–79.
13. Nishida Y, Tsukushi S, Wasa J, Urakawa H, Toriyama K, Kamei Y, et al. Vascularized fibular flaps enhance histological repair in pasteurized autogenous bone graft. Ann Plast Surg. 2011;67:416–20.
14. Dautel G, Duteille F, Merle M. Use of the osteocutaneous "double-barrel fibular flaps" in limb reconstruction: four clinical cases. Microsurgery. 2001;21:340–4.
15. Chen CM, Disa JJ, Lee HY, Mehrara BJ, Hu QY, Nathan S, et al. Reconstruction of extremity long bone defects after sarcoma resection with vascularized fibula flaps: a 10-year review. Plast Reconstr Surg. 2007;119:915–24.
16. Capanna R, Bufalini C, Campanacci M. A new technique for reconstruction of large metadiaphyseal bone defects: a combined graft (allograft shell plus vascularized fibula). Orthop Traumatol. 1993;2:159.
17. Zaretski A, Amir A, Meller I, Leshem D, Kollender Y, Barnea Y, et al. Free fibula long bone reconstruction in orthopedic oncology: a surgical algorithm for reconstructive options. Plast Reconstr Surg. 2004;113:1989–2000.
18. Chang DW, Weber KL. Use of vascularized fibula bone flap and intercalary allograft for diaphyseal reconstruction after resection of primary extremity bone sarcomas. Plast Reconstr Surg. 2005;116:1918–25.
19. Li J, Wang Z, Guo Z, Chen GJ, Fu J, Pei GX. The use of allograft shell with intramedullary vascularized fibula graft for intercalary reconstruction after diaphyseal resection for lower extremity bony malignancy. J Surg Oncol. 2010;102:368–74.
20. Shankhdhar VK, Yadav PS, Puri A, Kasat A, Dushyant J, Raghu RB, et al. Free fibula flap for lower limb salvage after tumour resection. Indian J Plast Surg. 2019;51:274–82.
21. Weichman KE, Dec W, Morris CD, Mehrara B, Disa JJ. Lower extremity osseous oncologic reconstruction with composite microsurgical free fibula inside massive bony allograft. Plast Reconstr Surg. 2015;136:396–403.
22. Venkatramani H, Sabapathy SR, Dheenadayalan J, Devendra A, Rajasekaran S. Reconstruction of post-traumatic long segment bone defects of the lower end of the femur by vascularized fibula combined with allograft (modified Capanna's technique). Eur J Trauma Emerg Surg. 2015;41:17–24.
23. Donati D, Di Liddo M, Zavatta M, Manfrini M, Bacci G, Picci P, et al. Massive bone allograft reconstruction in high-grade osteosarcoma. Clin Orthop. 2000;377:186.
24. Hornicek FJ, Gebhardt MC, Tomford WW, Sorger JI, Zavatta M, Menzner JP, et al. Factors affecting nonunion of the allograft-host junction. Clin Orthop. 2001;382:87.
25. Yajima H, Tamai S, Mizumoto S, Inada Y. Vascularized fibular grafts in the treatment of osteomyelitis and infected non-union. Clin Orthop. 1993;293:256–64.
26. Tu Y, Chen Z, Lineaweaver WC, Zhang F. Different recipient vessels for free microsurgical fibula flaps in the treatment of avascular necrosis of the femoral head. Ann Plast Surg. 2017;79:583–9.
27. Yazar S, Lin CH, Wei FC. One-stage reconstruction of composite bone and soft tissue defects in traumatic lower extremity injuries. Plast Reconstr Surg. 2004;114:1457–66.
28. McKnight AJ, Lewis VO, Rhines LD, Hanasono MM. Femur-fibula-fillet of leg chimeric free flap for sacral-pelvic reconstruction. J Plast Reconstr Aesth Surg. 2013;66:1784–7.

Recipient Vessels: Tibia Reconstruction

38

Meenakshi Rajan, Matthew Joy, L. Scott Levin, and Stephen J. Kovacs III

Introduction

Critical-size tibial bone defects with overlying soft tissue deficits are a major challenge for reconstructive surgeons [1–4]. Complex tibial bone defects larger than 6 cm, complicated by extensive soft tissue and segmented bone, may challenge the limits of distraction osteogenesis and bone grafting techniques [5–7]. In these situations, it becomes necessary to consider the use of vascularized bone grafts, either free or pedicled, to achieve a functional limb [8–15].

Anatomy of the Fibula Flap

The fibula resides posterior and lateral to the tibia and associates with all of the four leg compartments along its course. Though not a weight bearing bone, it contributes to the structure and stability of the knee and ankle joints at the fibular head proximally and lateral malleolus distally [16]. The fibula also serves as the origin of eight different muscles in the leg residing in all four leg compartments. There are dense attachments along the length of the bone to the anterior and posterior intermuscular septae as well as the interosseous membrane which must be carefully divided during flap harvest [17]. The fibula's length, cortical bone thickness, cross-sectional triangular shape, and diameter make it uniquely well suited for reconstruction of segmental defects of the tibia [16, 17].

The vascular supply of the flap derives from the peroneal artery and vein which run adjacent to the bone in the deep posterior compartment between the tibialis posterior and flexor hallucis longus muscles [18]. Blood supply to the fibula is provided by the nutrient artery located just proximal to the midpoint of the bone and supplying the endosteal system, as well as numerous smaller branches to the periosteum along the length of the bone [19]. The common peroneal nerve wraps around the posterior aspect of the fibular head and courses anteriorly around the fibular neck in the subcutaneous plane [16]. Just distal to the fibular neck, the nerve divides into the superficial peroneal nerve which tracks distally in the lateral compartment and the deep peroneal nerve which enters the anterior compartment and travels with the anterior tibial artery [18]. Care must be taken to avoid injury to the common and superficial peroneal nerves, particularly during proximal flap and pedicle dissection.

Flap Dissection

Most often the contralateral fibula is utilized for tibial reconstruction, particularly in the setting of trauma when the ipsilateral fibula is expected to be within the zone of injury

Supplementary Information The online version of this chapter (https://doi.org/10.1007/978-3-030-75389-4_38) contains supplementary material, which is available to authorized users.

M. Rajan (✉)
Department of Plastic Surgery, Cleveland Clinic, Cleveland, OH, USA
e-mail: RAJANM@ccf.org

M. Joy
Division of Plastic Surgery, Department of Surgery, University of Pennsylvania, Philadelphia, PA, USA
e-mail: Matthew.Joy@pennmedicine.upenn.edu

L. S. Levin · S. J. Kovacs III
Division of Plastic Surgery, Department of Surgery, University of Pennsylvania, Philadelphia, PA, USA

Department of Orthopaedic Surgery, University of Pennsylvania, Philadelphia, PA, USA
e-mail: scott.levin@uphs.upenn.edu; stephen.kovach@uphs.upenn.edu

R. Gurunian, R. Djohan (eds.), *Recipient Vessels in Reconstructive Microsurgery*, https://doi.org/10.1007/978-3-030-75389-4_38

(Fig. 38.1). Additionally, this facilitates a two-team approach for concurrent flap harvest and recipient site preparation. The patient is positioned supine with additional padding under the hip on the side of flap harvest to better expose the lateral leg. Care should be taken to ensure proper padding and pressure offloading and a urinary catheter placed due to the expected duration of this procedure. The bilateral lower extremities are prepared with chlorhexidine and draped such that both legs can be easily manipulated during the procedure for both flap harvest and subsequent inset (Fig. 38.2). On the donor leg, the entire fibula is palpated and outlined, marking along the anterior and posterior borders as well as around the head proximally and lateral malleolus distally. It is essential to measure, mark, and preserve 6 cm of bone proximally to protect the common peroneal nerve as well as distally to protect the tibiofibular syndesmosis and superficial peroneal nerve. If an osteocutaneous flap is planned, a skin paddle is marked as a longitudinally oriented ellipse centered over the posterior border of the fibula and peroneus muscle tendons distally which correspond to the position of the posterior intermuscular septum. Typically, the skin paddle is designed over the distal most aspect of the planned fibula harvest. This allows for proximal bone shortening which lengthens the free vascular pedicle relative to the bony portion of the flap. A handheld Doppler probe can also be used to identify and mark cutaneous perforators in this area prior to designing the cutaneous portion of the flap. Prior anatomic studies by Wei et al. [17] in 1986 and Yoshimura et al. [20] in 1983 and describe the anatomy of the perforating vessels to the lateral skin island with musculocutaneous vessels more commonly encountered in the proximal aspect of the leg and septocutaneous vessels found more distally [17, 20].

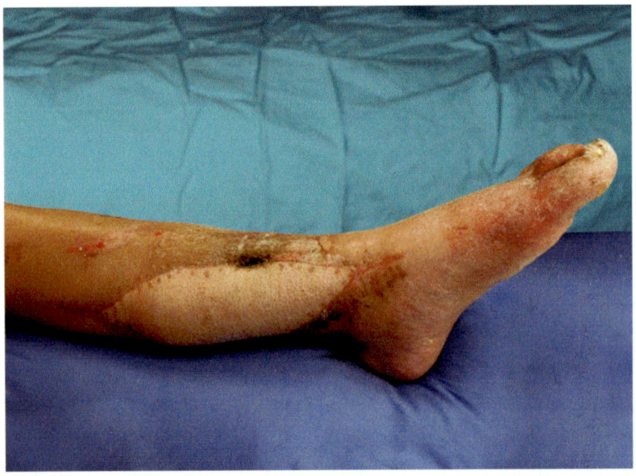

Fig. 38.1 Preoperative image shows healed lower extremity with previous free flap using posterior tibial vessels. The patient needs tibial bone reconstruction for a segmental defect

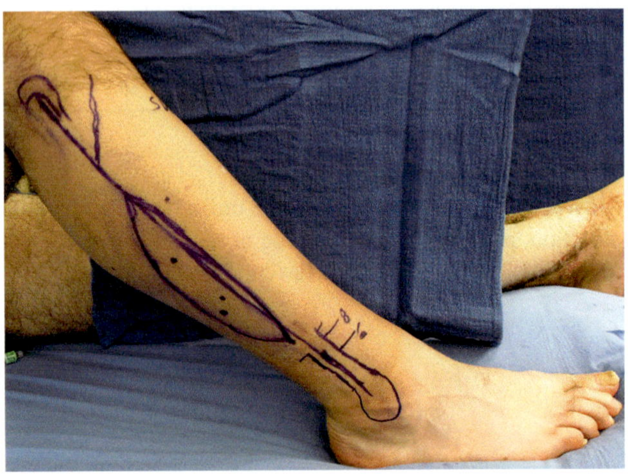

Fig. 38.2 Preoperative markings of the fibula flap using the contralateral leg: the fibula is palpated and outlined, marking along the anterior and posterior borders as well as around the head proximally and lateral malleolus distally. It is essential to measure, mark, and preserve 6 cm of bone proximally to protect the common peroneal nerve as well as distally to protect the tibiofibular syndesmosis and superficial peroneal nerve

The dissection can be carried out with or without a tourniquet. There are advantages and disadvantages to either option, which is at the discretion of the surgeon. A longitudinal incision is made along the posterior border of fibula and anterior aspect of the designed skin paddle. The anterior aspect of the skin paddle dissection is carried down to the fascia overlying the lateral compartment. The fascia is incised and skin paddle elevated in the subfascial plane from anterior to posterior to the posterior intermuscular septum. At this point the septocutaneous perforating vessels should be identified and protected. Once the vessels are identified, the posterior incision of the skin paddle is made and elevated again in the subfascial plane now from posterior to anterior until the other side of the posterior intermuscular septum is reached. Now with the skin paddle elevated on its septocutaneous blood supply, attention is turned to elevation of the fibula itself. The lateral compartment muscles are reflected anteriorly, leaving a very thin layer of muscle attached to the fibula to protect the periosteum and its blood supply to the fibula. Care is taken during this portion of the dissection to protect the superficial peroneal nerve along its course in the lateral compartment. This maneuver exposes the anterior intermuscular septum which can be divided sharply using scissors or with low-energy electrocautery taking care not to injury the underlying anterior tibial vessels and deep peroneal nerve. Once in the anterior compartment, the foot extensor musculature can be bluntly separated from the fibula to expose the interosseous membrane. Blunt dissection in this area also protects the anterior tibial neurovasculature. With the interosseous membrane exposed and the anterior tibial vessels and deep peroneal nerve protected, the interosseous membrane is divided sharply along the entire length of the planned fibula harvest. The peroneal artery and associated venae comitantes are carefully dissected off the distal fibula and protected. A right-angle clamp can then be used to encircle the distal fibula in the subperiosteal plane. It is essential to stay in this plane to avoid any chance of injury to the peroneal vessels. A thin malleable retractor can then be passed back through this space, following the right-angle clamp in the same subperiosteal plane in preparation for the distal osteotomy. The authors prefer to use an oscillating saw and copious saline irrigation for osteotomy of the fibula. After completing the distal osteotomy, the proximal cut is made following the same steps of passing a clamp and then malleable retractor around the fibula in the subperiosteal plane to protect the proximal pedicle as well as the branches of the peroneal nerve. At this point the flap should be able to be mobilized and elevated laterally. If the osteotomized fibula is not able to be retracted laterally out of the wound, that suggests either an incomplete osteotomy or incomplete division of the interosseous membrane. Next attention is turned to dissection of the peroneal vessels at the distal end of the flap. With gentle spreading and careful dissection through the deep posterior compartment musculature, the pedicle is identified between the tibialis posterior and flexor hallucis longus muscles. With the bone retracted, the distal pedicle can be ligated and divided (Fig. 38.3). The final flap elevation is then carried out from distal to proximal, following directly over the peroneal vessels and carefully dissecting and dividing the flexor hallucis longus muscle attachments of the posterior compartment muscles. Care is taken to identify muscular perforating branches off the pedicle into these muscles. In many cases, perforating vessels to the soleus muscle in particular can be quite large and should be carefully dissected and ligated prior to division. Proceeding

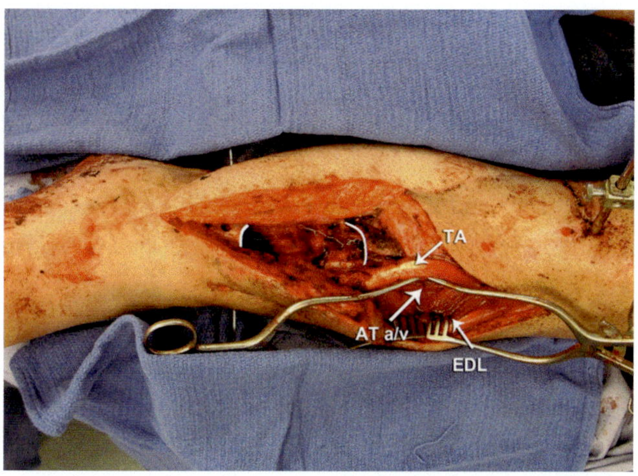

Fig. 38.3 The anterior tibial artery and associated venae comitantes are preferred as recipient vessels given their proximity to the tibia. *TA* tibialis anterior muscle, *EDL* extensor digitorum longus, *AT a/v* anterior tibial artery and vein. Curved white lines indicate the proximal and distal edges of the tibia and the bone defect in between

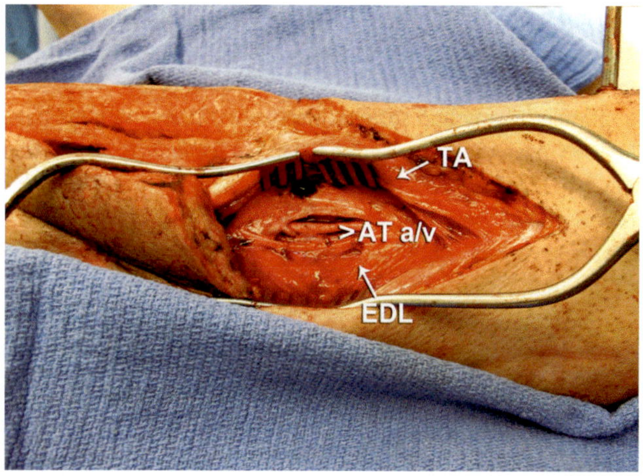

Fig. 38.4 The selected anterior tibial recipient vessels are carefully dissected and exposed in the extensor compartment, ideally outside the zone of injury. Dissection is carried down between tibialis anterior (TA) and extensor digitorum longus (EDL) for exposure of anterior tibial vessels. *AT a/v* anterior tibial artery and vein

proximally with the pedicle dissection, the tibioperoneal trunk is identified and carefully dissected around the takeoff of the peroneal vessels as this is the proximal limit of the vascular pedicle.

Once the flap elevation is complete, the flap can be either be left in situ or harvested and taken to the back table for separation of the proximal pedicle from the fibula and shortening of the fibula bone to the desired length for tibia reconstruction (Fig. 38.4). An intravenous bolus dose of heparin is administered prior to flap harvest. The authors generally prefer to harvest the flap prior to these steps as manipulation of the flap, subperiosteal stripping, and additional osteotomies are often easier to perform on the back table with the flap completely free. When preparing the flap for reconstruction of intercalary defects of the tibia, the authors will add 2 cm of length in addition to the defect to allow for 1 cm overlap of the fibula within the medullary canal of the proximal and distal tibia segments.

Preparation of the Recipient Site and Flap Inset

In the case of immediate reconstruction, as in the case of sarcoma defects, the tibial defect is often already exposed following either resection in the case on oncologic defects or serial debridement in the case of trauma. The wound should be irrigated with copious sterile saline solution and any additional debridement of soft tissue or bone carried out as needed. In the case of traumatic defects of the tibia, prior to flap inset, the proximal and distal aspects of the fracture site are debrided using a powered burr to smooth any sharp or irregular contours and debride back to healthy bleeding bone. The anterior tibial artery or the posterior tibial and associated venae comitantes are the preferred recipient vessels given their proximity to the tibia (Fig. 38.5). The applied anatomy and surgical exposure of these vessels have been extensively discussed in Chap. 34 for anterior tibial and in Chap. 35 for posterior tibial vessels. Therefore, the reader is referred to these chapters for details.

These vessels may be directly involved especially in case of traumatic injuries and thus it is essential to perform preoperative angiography, either by CT scan or formal angiography, to determine vessel patency and assist in selection of the recipient vessels. The selected recipient vessels (in this case the anterior tibial artery) are carefully dissected and exposed, ideally outside the zone of injury (Fig. 38.6). The accompanying video shows the dissection of the anterior tibial artery in a cadaver (Video 38.1). There should be a low threshold for the utilization of autologous vein graft as either an arteriovenous loop or interposition graft to allow for tension free anastomosis outside the zone of injury as much as possible.

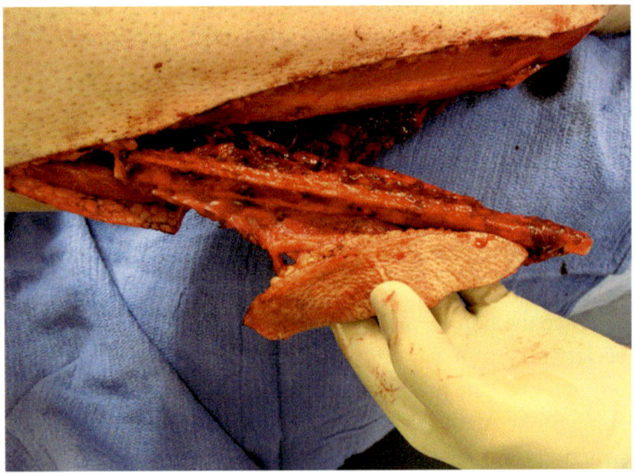

Fig. 38.5 Dissection of the fibula osteocutaneous flap is complete with distal and proximal osteotomies. It will be inset into the intramedullary canal of the tibia essentially as a living intramedullary nail for at least 2–5 cm to ensure appropriate overlap of tibia and fibula

Next the fibula flap is inset bridging the tibial defect and secured in place by adjusting external fixation devices as needed (Fig. 38.7). It is essential to ensure appropriate bone flap position and stability prior to microvascular anastomosis as the flap should not be manipulated after this step of the procedure. The fibula is inset into the intramedullary canal of the tibia essentially as a living intramedullary nail for at least 2–5 cm to ensure appropriate overlap of tibia and fibula. The authors' preference is to perform an end-to-end venous anastomosis between the donor peroneal vein and one of the recipient vena comitantes and an end-to-side arterial anastomosis between the donor peroneal artery and the selected recipient artery. The donor artery is spatulated widely and positioned over the recipient artery in situ to mark the arteriotomy site. All anastomoses should be performed under absolutely no tension, and there should be a very low threshold to utilize interposition vein grafts as needed to achieve this goal. With the recipient artery clamped proximally and distally, a longitudinal arteriotomy is made using a number 11 blade, and a small strip of the artery wall is resected prior to performing the anastomosis. Microvascular anastomoses are then completed in the standard fashion using a coupler device for the end-to-end venous anastomosis and hand-sewn technique for the end-to-side arterial anastomosis. At this point, patency of arterial inflow and venous outflow is confirmed, and then attention is turned to wound closure.

If an osteocutaneous flap was performed, the skin paddle is inset under minimal tension during closure of the leg wounds ensuring that the septum is also not under tension.

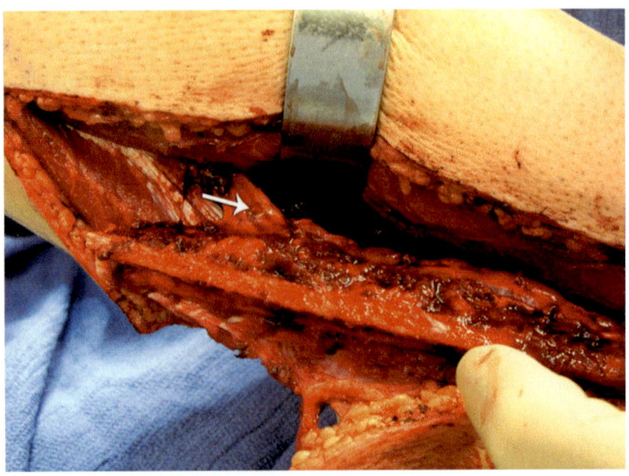

Fig. 38.6 Once the flap elevation is complete, the flap can be either be left in situ or harvested and taken to the back table for separation of the proximal pedicle from the fibula and shortening of the fibula bone to the desired length for tibia reconstruction. Arrow indicates the peroneal vessels

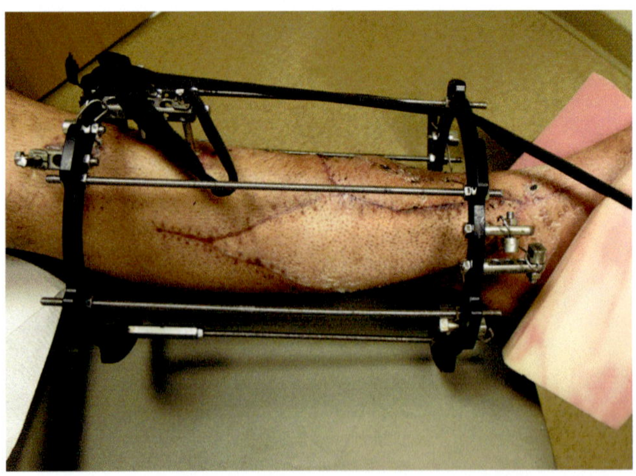

Fig. 38.7 Postoperative photo: The fibula flap was inset bridging the tibial defect and secured in place by adjusting external fixation devices as needed

Perfusion to the skin paddle should be assessed after wound closure. Closed suction drains are utilized, taking care not to position the internal portion of the drain on or adjacent to the microvascular anastomoses. Minimal dressings are applied to allow for easy postoperative flap monitoring, and no circumferential dressings should be applied as limb and flap edema can increase significantly in the days following surgery resulting in compression of the reconstructive limb even from loosely placed wraps at the time of surgery.

Postoperative Care

Following free flap reconstruction, the patient is admitted or transferred to the intensive care unit or other advanced care unit with nursing staff that are trained for or experienced in postoperative flap monitoring. The authors' typical protocol for flap monitoring is hourly flap checks for the first 48 h after surgery, either via clinical and handheld Doppler exam of an osteocutaneous flap or monitoring via an implantable Doppler device for bone-only buried flaps. Flap checks are then decreased in frequency to every 2, 4, and 8 h at 48, 72, and 96 h from surgery, respectively. The reconstructed limb should remain elevated at or above heart level with careful padding and positioning to avoid any pressure points or extrinsic compression of the limb particularly at the level of the anastomoses and flap skin paddle. The authors' typical protocol involves strict limb elevation for 2–3 weeks with only brief dependent positioning for transfers as necessary. This is followed by a progressive limb dangling protocol starting with 15 min of dangling four times daily and gradually increasing duration and frequency of dangling over the course of several weeks. For initiation of any progressive dangling protocol, it is advised that an experienced clinician examine the flap or limb at the time of the first trial of dangling to confirm that the flap or reconstructed limb does not become significantly congested or edematous when placed in a dependent position.

Conclusion

The free fibula is particularly suited to address large intercalary defects when soft tissue coverage is also required, because the flap can be harvested with muscle and skin. The free fibula has an advantage of potentially achieving a one-stage bone and soft tissue reconstruction [21, 22]. Tibial vessels are reliable recipient options for revascularization of the fibula flap. Patient comorbidities, prior surgeries, zone of injury, characteristics (location and length) of the tibia defect, and the proximity of reliable tibial vessels in relation with the bone defect should be taken into account when selecting the appropriate recipient vessel.

References

1. Banic A, Hertel R. Double vascularized fibulas for reconstruction of large tibial defects. J Reconstr Microsurg. 1993;9(6):421–8. https://doi.org/10.1055/s-2007-1006751.
2. Bibbo C, Bauder AR, Nelson J, et al. Reconstruction of traumatic defects of the tibia with free fibula flap and external fixation. Ann Plast Surg. 2020;85(5):516–21. https://doi.org/10.1097/SAP.0000000000002240.
3. Li J, Wang Z, Guo Z, Chen G, Li S, Pei G-X. The use of massive allograft with intramedullary fibular graft for intercalary reconstruction after resection of tibial malignancy. J Reconstr Microsurg. 2011;27(1):37–46. https://doi.org/10.1055/s-0030-1267381.
4. Schwarz GS, Disa JJ, Mehrara BJ, Healey JH, Cordeiro PG. Reconstruction of oncologic tibial defects in children using vascularized fibula flaps. Plast Reconstr Surg Published online. 2012; https://doi.org/10.1097/PRS.0b013e318230e463.
5. Cavadas PC, Landín L, Ibáñez J, Nthumba P. Reconstruction of major traumatic segmental bone defects of the tibia with vascularized bone transfers. Plast Reconstr Surg. 2010;125(1):215–23. https://doi.org/10.1097/PRS.0b013e3181c495b3.
6. Chang DW, Weber KL. Use of a vascularized fibula bone flap and intercalary allograft for diaphyseal reconstruction after resection of primary extremity bone sarcomas. Plast Reconstr Surg. 2005;116(7):1918–25. https://doi.org/10.1097/01.prs.0000189203.38204.d5.
7. Zhen P, Liu X-Y, Lu H, Li X-S. Fixation and reconstruction of severe tibial shaft fractures with vascularized fibular grafting. Arch Orthop Trauma Surg. 2011;131(1):93–9. https://doi.org/10.1007/s00402-010-1121-4.
8. Zhen P, Hu YY, Luo ZJ, Liu XY, Lu H, Li XS. One-stage treatment and reconstruction of gustilo type III open tibial shaft fractures with a vascularized fibular osteoseptocutaneous flap graft. J Orthop Trauma. Published online. 2010; https://doi.org/10.1097/BOT.0b013e3181d88a07.
9. Zaretski A, Amir A, Meller I, et al. Free fibula long bone reconstruction in orthopedic oncology: a surgical algorithm for reconstructive options. Plast Reconstr Surg. 2004;113(7):1989–2000. https://doi.org/10.1097/01.prs.0000122213.82011.c5.
10. Wang X, Li Y, Guo J. Repairing chronic osteomyelitis complicated by long bone defect in tibia with free segmented-fibula transplantation. Zhongguo xiu fu chong jian wai ke za zhi = Zhongguo xiufu chongjian waike zazhi = Chinese J reparative Reconstr Surg. 2007;21(3):278–81.
11. Shankhdhar VK, Yadav PS, Puri A, et al. Free fibula flap for lower limb salvage after tumour resection. Indian J Plast Surg. 2018;51(3):274–82. https://doi.org/10.4103/ijps.IJPS_113_17.
12. Mateev M, Huang C, Imanaliev A, Ono S, Hyakusoku H, Ogawa R. Combining the external fixation and microsurgical osteoseptocutaneous flap transplantation methods for limb salvage. Eplasty. 2012;12:e16.
13. Özaksar K, Sügün TS, Toros T, Gürbüz Y, Kayalar M, Özerkan F. Free vascularized fibular grafts in type 3 open tibia fractures. Acta Orthop Traumatol Turc. 2012;46(6):430–7. https://doi.org/10.3944/aott.2012.2876.
14. Chung DW, Han CS, Lee JH. Reconstruction of composite tibial defect with free flaps and ipsilateral vascularized fibular transposition. Microsurgery. 2011;31(5):340–6. https://doi.org/10.1002/micr.20884.
15. Lee KS, Park JW. Free vascularized osteocutaneous fibular graft to the tibia. Microsurgery. 1999;19(3):141–7. https://doi.org/10.1002/(sici)1098-2752(1999)19:3<141::aid-micr4>3.0.co;2-w.
16. Beppu M, Hanel DP, Johnston GH, Carmo JM, Tsai TM. The osteocutaneous fibula flap: an anatomic study. J Reconstr Microsurg. 1992;8(3):215–23. https://doi.org/10.1055/s-2007-1006703.

17. Wei FC, Chen HC, Chuang CC, Noordhoff MS. Fibular osteoseptocutaneous flap: anatomic study and clinical application. Plast Reconstr Surg. 1986;78(2):191–200. https://doi.org/10.1097/00006534-198608000-00008.
18. Abou-Foul AK, Fasanmade A, Prabhu S, Borumandi F. Anatomy of the vasculature of the lower leg and harvest of a fibular flap: a systematic review. Br J Oral Maxillofac Surg. 2017;55(9):904–10. https://doi.org/10.1016/j.bjoms.2017.08.363.
19. Taylor GI, Miller GD, Ham FJ. The free vascularized bone graft. A clinical extension of microvascular techniques. Plast Reconstr Surg. 1975;55(5):533–44. https://doi.org/10.1097/00006534-197505000-00002.
20. Yoshimura M, Shimamura K, Iwai Y, Yamauchi S, Ueno T. Free vascularized fibular transplant. A new method for monitoring circulation of the grafted fibula. J Bone Joint Surg Am. 1983;65(9):1295–301.
21. Yazar S, Lin C-H, Wei F-C. One-stage reconstruction of composite bone and soft-tissue defects in traumatic lower extremities. Plast Reconstr Surg. 2004;114(6):1457–66. https://doi.org/10.1097/01.prs.0000138811.88807.65.
22. Guo Q-F, Xu Z-H, Wen S-F, et al. Value of a skin island flap as a postoperative predictor of vascularized fibula graft viability in extensive diaphyseal bone defect reconstruction. Orthop Traumatol Surg Res. 2012;98(5):576–82. https://doi.org/10.1016/j.otsr.2012.03.009.

Medial Superior and Descending Genicular Vessels

39

Jonathan M. Bekisz, Carter J. Boyd, and Pierre B. Saadeh

Introduction

The medial superior and descending genicular vessels are key members of an intricate anastomotic plexus surrounding the knee joint. The pair have a well-described history as the source vessels for various composite and chimeric flaps arising from the region of the medial femoral condyle. However, there is also an evolving understanding and appreciation of their utility as recipients targets in microvascular free tissue reconstruction of the middle third of the lower extremity.

Preoperative Assessment

Each microsurgical free tissue transfer merits a thorough review of the patient's health status and anatomical considerations related to the defect and proposed flap. Decisions surrounding the flap type, defect size, defect location, vessel length, and vessel caliber are critical for success in the perioperative period as well as obtaining good long-term results. The genicular artery system has been described as viable recipient vessels for defects at the knee, among other vessels. The superior medial genicular vessel is more commonly used for posterior defects, while anterior defects are more well suited for anastomosis to the descending genicular vessels [1]. Assessment of the vessels can be performed preoperatively with the assistance of Doppler ultrasound, computed tomography angiography, or magnetic resonance angiography. The final decision of which vessels should be used requires an integration of these imaging modalities along with careful intraoperative visualization of the vasculature.

Jonathan M. Bekisz and Carter J. Boyd contributed equally with all other contributors.

J. M. Bekisz · C. J. Boyd
NYU Grossman School of Medicine, New York, NY, USA
e-mail: Jonathan.Bekisz@nyulangone.org; Carter.Boyd@nyulangone.org

P. B. Saadeh (✉)
Hansjörg Wyss Department of Plastic Surgery at NYU Grossman School of Medicine, Plastic Surgery Service – Bellevue Hospital Center, New York, NY, USA
e-mail: pierre.saadeh@nyulangone.org

Applied Anatomy

Medial Superior Genicular Artery

In a cadaveric study of 19 lower limbs, Yamamoto and associates traced the anatomy of the superior medial genicular artery. The vessel was present in all specimens, and its origin was on average 5.2 cm (3.5–6.5 cm) superior to the knee joint branching medially from the popliteal artery [2, 3]. Mean caliber of the vessel was 0.78 mm in diameter (range 0.38–1.4 mm) [3]. The superior medial genicular artery descends inferiorly behind the adductor magnus tendon, semimembranosus muscle, and semitendinosus muscle. The vessel supplies the distal most aspect of the vastus medialis muscle and feeds into the osteoarticular branch of the descending genicular artery contributing to the medial femoral condyle perforators [1, 3].

Descending Genicular Artery

The descending genicular artery has more length and larger caliber than the medial superior genicular artery [2]. The descending genicular artery originates proximal to the medial superior genicular artery branching medially from the superficial femoral artery just prior to the adductor hiatus [1, 2]. This origin is on average 13.7 cm proximal to the knee with a mean vessel diameter of 1.5 mm (range 1–2 mm). The artery was present in 17 of 19 specimens and runs along the posterior aspect of the medial intermuscular septum either deep or lateral to the adductor magnus tendon. The descending genicular artery has three terminal branches including

R. Gurunian, R. Djohan (eds.), *Recipient Vessels in Reconstructive Microsurgery*,
https://doi.org/10.1007/978-3-030-75389-4_39

the saphenous, muscular, and osteoarticular branches that supply the subcutaneous and cutaneous tissue, vastus medialis muscle, and superior femoral condyle, respectively [2, 3]. The descending genicular artery is paired with venae comitantes that follow a similar course and can be considered for free tissue transfer venous drainage along with the greater saphenous vein [4].

Surgical Site Exposure

Medial Superior Genicular Artery

Exposure of the medial superior genicular artery begins by identifying the popliteal artery in the popliteal fossa [1]. When approaching via the posterior surface of the knee, dissection should first be carried through the skin and subcutaneous tissue to the popliteal fascia. Upon incising the fascia and gaining access to the popliteal fossa, the artery is positioned anterior to the popliteal vein and the tibial nerve [5, 6]. The vessel sits deep to the semimembranosus muscle, and thus retracting the muscle allows for visualization of the medial superior genicular artery and its venae comitantes, which branch off the popliteal artery at a point roughly in line with the superior aspect of the femoral condyle. With the vessel identified, it can be prepared for microvascular anastomosis by clearing any attachments in the anterior and medial directions, ligating branching vessels as needed [1]. (Figs. 39.1 and 39.2) (also see Chap. 40 and Video 40.1).

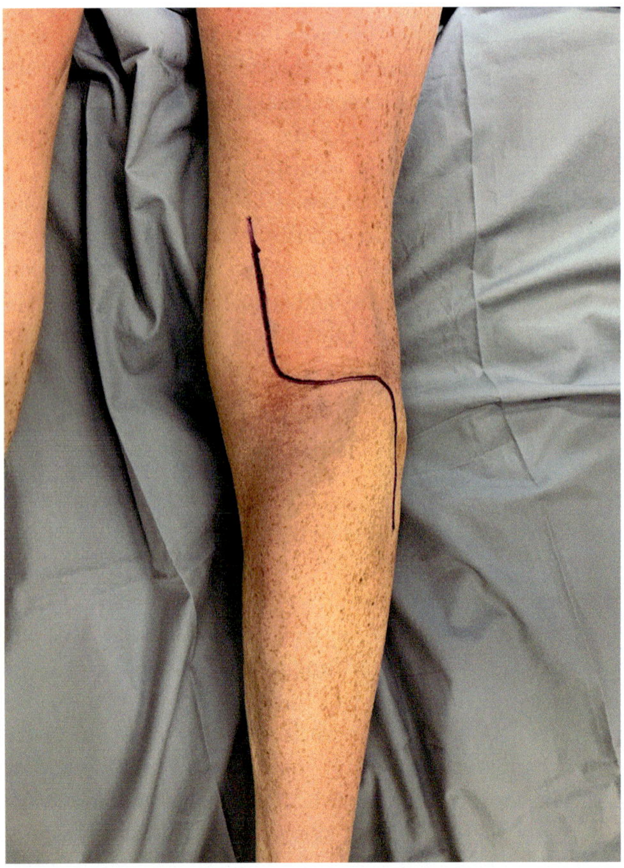

Fig. 39.1 Cadaveric dissection: Posterior popliteal approach for exposure of the medial superior genicular vessels

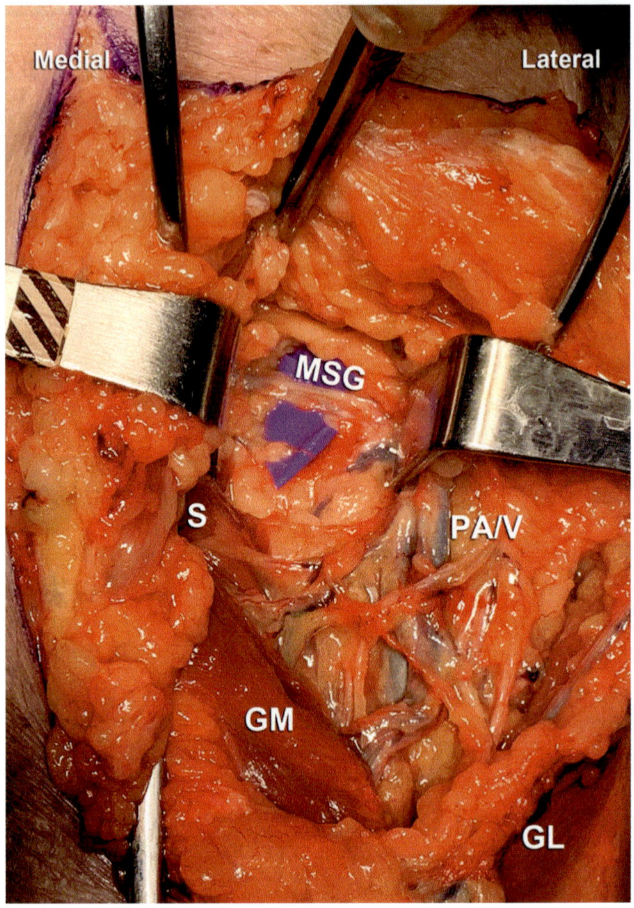

Fig. 39.2 Cadaveric dissection: Exposure of the medial superior genicular vessels with the semimembranosus muscle retracted medially (*S* semimembranosus, *GM* gastrocnemius medial head, *GL* gastrocnemius lateral head, *PA/V* popliteal artery and vein, *MSG* medial superior genicular vessels)

Descending Genicular Artery

The descending genicular artery is accessed via an incision on the medial surface of the distal thigh. Both vertical [1] and curvilinear [4] incisions have been described, with placement recommended slightly anterior to the medial condyle of the femur. Dissection should be carried down to the interval between the vastus medialis and sartorius muscles. At this point, two approaches can be pursued to visualize the descending genicular artery. The fascia of the vastus medialis can be incised and reflected posteriorly,

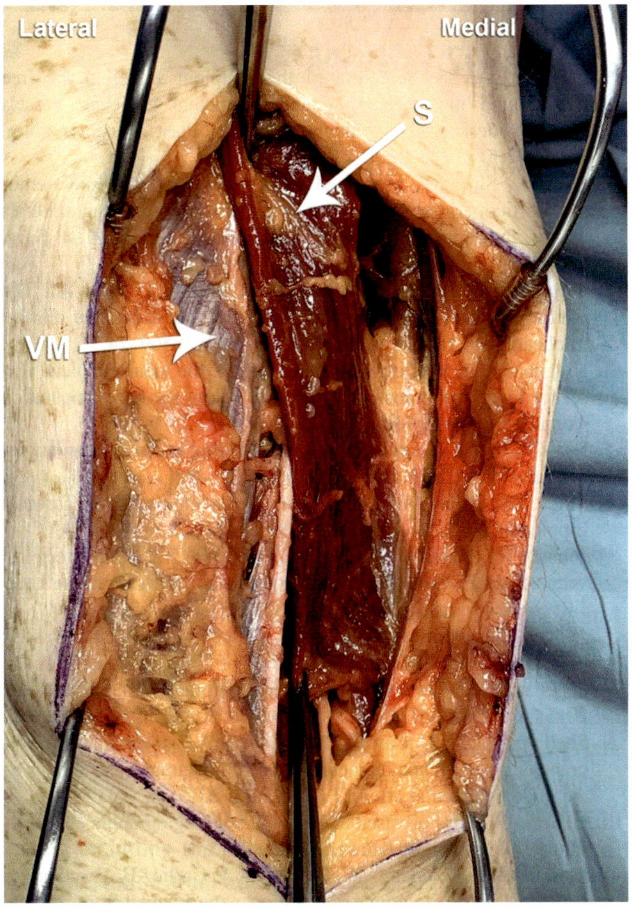

Fig. 39.3 Cadaveric dissection: Skin incision over the medial thigh is carried down to vastus medialis (VM) and sartorius (S) muscles

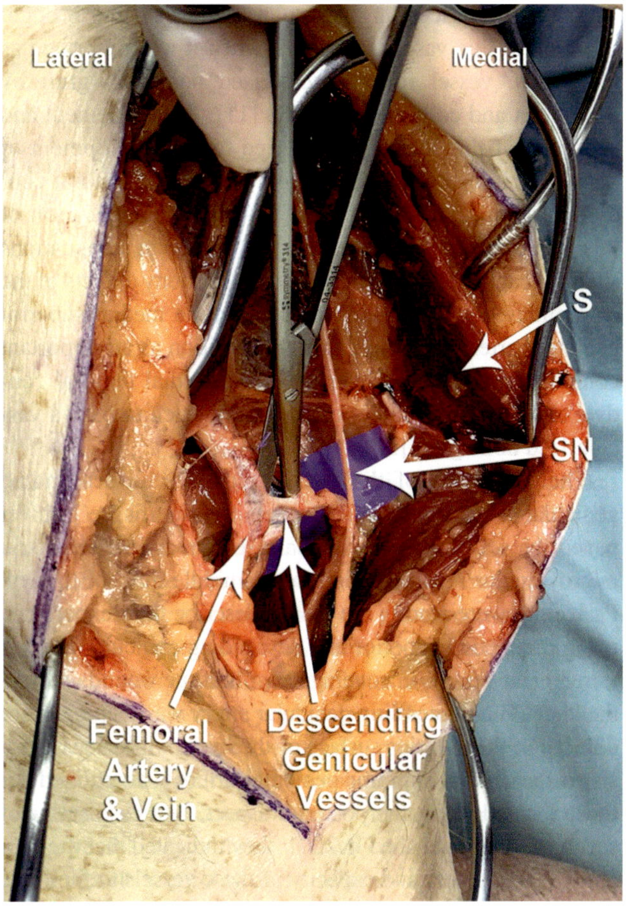

Fig. 39.4 Sartorius muscle (S) retracted medially and vastus muscle laterally to dissect the femoral vessels in the adductor canal. The descending genicular vessels are dissected off the femoral vessels (*SN* saphenous nerve)

while the underlying muscle is pulled forward, bringing the vessels into view below [4]. Alternatively, the sartorius can be retracted in a medial direction, revealing the descending genicular artery and its venae comitantes just behind the vastus medialis [1] (Figs. 39.3 and 39.4). Distal division of the artery is suggested at a point proximal to the periosteum of the medial femoral condyle. The length and mobility necessary for anastomosis, up to about 8–9 cm, can be obtained by tracing the vessel proximally toward its origin from the superficial femoral artery near the adductor hiatus, skeletonizing the vessel, and obtaining control of any side branches along the way [4].

Discussion

Closure and coverage of defects in the middle third of the leg poses a unique reconstructive challenge. The risks of exposure of the knee joint and proximal tibia demand that wounds be addressed in a timely fashion. However, the region is notorious for a lack of excess soft tissue and limited tissue pliability. Therefore, proper management often necessitates pedicled or free tissue transfer. When microvascular reconstruction is employed, the common femoral and popliteal systems have long been established as robust and reliable recipient vessel options in this region [7, 8]. In recent years, the network of genicular vessels, namely, the descending or highest genicular artery and the medial superior genicular artery, has gained favor as an alternative anastomotic target.

The genicular vessels include six arteries that make up a complex anastomotic network in the region of the knee. Five of these arise from the popliteal artery: the medial and lateral superior genicular arteries, middle genicular artery, and medial and lateral inferior genicular arteries [9]. The descending, or highest, genicular artery arises from the superficial femoral artery and subsequently gives off saphenous and articular branches that anastomose with the medial inferior and medial superior genicular arteries, respectively [10]. The latter of these pairings continues to supply a vascular plexus around the medial femoral condyle [3].

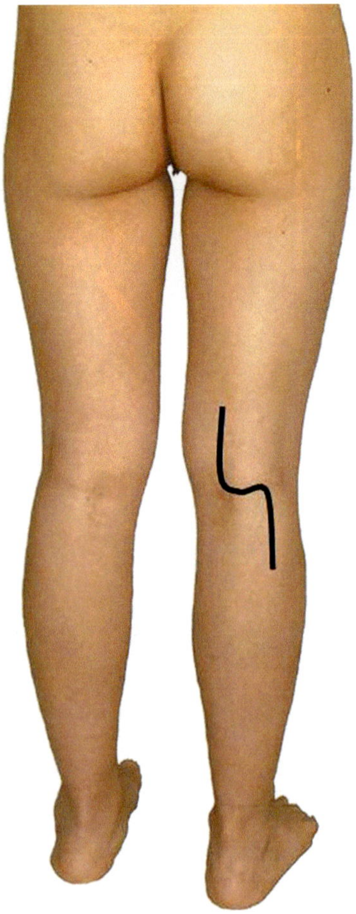

Fig. 40.4 Wide exposure using the posterior approach to the medial sural vessels follows a transverse line in the popliteal fossa corresponding to the knee joint, which curves upward medially along the course of the medial hamstring muscles, then downward laterally toward the lateral head of the gastrocnemius muscle

the knee flexed and hip externally rotated. If a thigh tourniquet is used, exsanguination should not be done to insure that all veins remain filled and obvious. A subfascial longitudinal exploratory incision is first made to confirm the exact location of the perforator (Fig. 40.6). Just as with any perforator flap, the usual tedious intramuscular dissection of the perforator back to its origin from a medial sural branch requires careful control of side branches to maintain hemostasis (Fig. 40.7). This dissection is completed when the medial sural vein and artery are of sufficient caliber to match that of the flap as apropos and can actually be continued back to their origin from the popliteal vessels if necessary [24]. If the vein is inadequate, a nearby subcutaneous branch or the greater saphenous vein itself may be sought.

Discussion

The medial sural vessels represent alternative if a recipient vascular site is needed around the knee [11, 12]. Unlike some other branches of the major vessels of the thigh, these will always be present and always of reasonable caliber. An end-to-end microanastomosis can always be done with good exposure, as these vessels can be brought up somewhat from the depths of the popliteal space. In addition, this will also avoid using an end-to-side anastomosis to the popliteal vessels, which could be technically challenging.

The medial approach to the popliteal fossa probably is the simplest for finding the extramuscular course of the medial sural vessels [12] and best if the patient must be in a supine position to allow access to the more common anterior lower leg injures requiring simultaneous debridement or flap insetting. Postoperative external pressures on microanastomosis here will be better avoided, particularly when compared to the posterior approach. That, of course, would be imperative if a prone position were mandatory [11]. The newest option is the intramuscular perforator approach to the medial sural vessels which would be just like raising the pedicle of any perforator flap. That in itself requires a more difficult microsurgical dissection [25] than the other approaches. Rarely, the purported medial sural musculocutaneous perforator chosen with this approach may turn out to be a median [superficial] sural perforator that might have insufficient dimensions even with more proximal dissection [26]. In addition, access to the cornucopia of vein options as found with either the medial or posterior approach would not be readily available. However, the detachment of muscles or tendons or even injury to the tibial nerve will be avoided with maximum function preservation. As time marches on, the new generation of supermicrosurgeons may even use the perforator alone for a perforator-to-perforator microanastomosis!

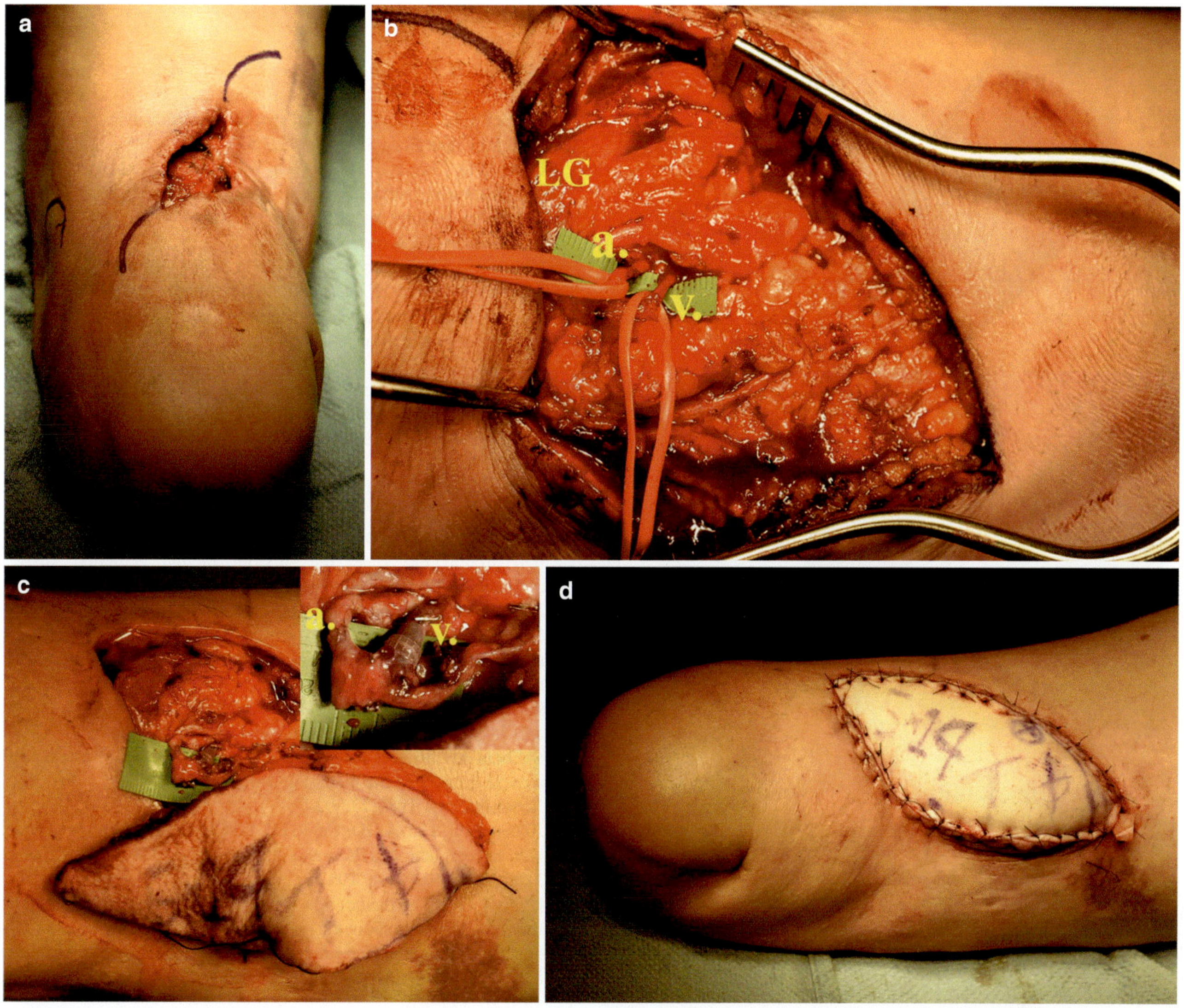

Fig. 40.5 (**a**) Wound dehiscence involving chronic atrophic scar of popliteal space in below-knee amputation stump, (**b**) posterior approach to the medial sural artery [a.] and vein [v.] seen in vessel loops. Incidental exposure of lateral gastrocnemius muscle [LG] verified level of dissection in this scarred region, (**c**) profunda artery perforator free flap chosen to resurface the defect using medial sural vessels recipient site [microgrid] with flap artery anastomosed in end-to-end fashion to medial sural artery [a.] and vein coupled to medial sural vein [v.] as seen in enlarged view, (**d**) early successful flap revascularization

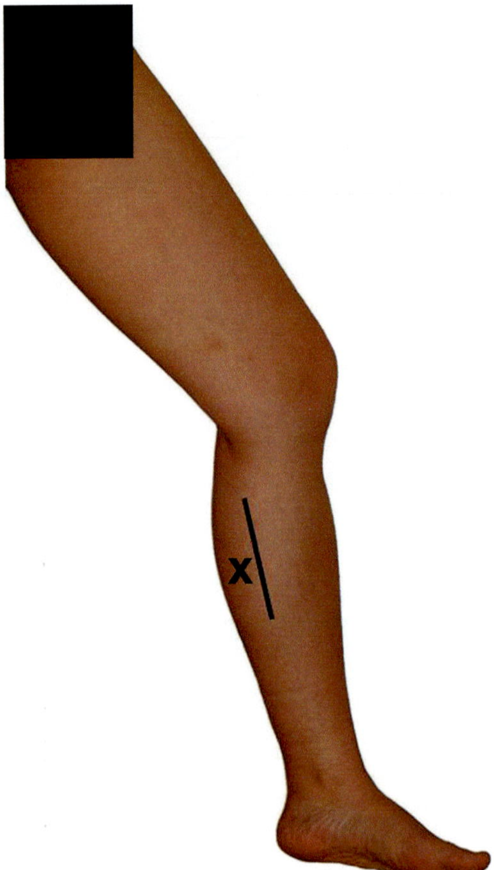

Fig. 40.6 The intramuscular perforator approach to the medial sural vessels first requires a longitudinal exploratory incision over the medial head of the gastrocnemius muscle, centered in the proximity of a suspected musculocutaneous perforator "x"

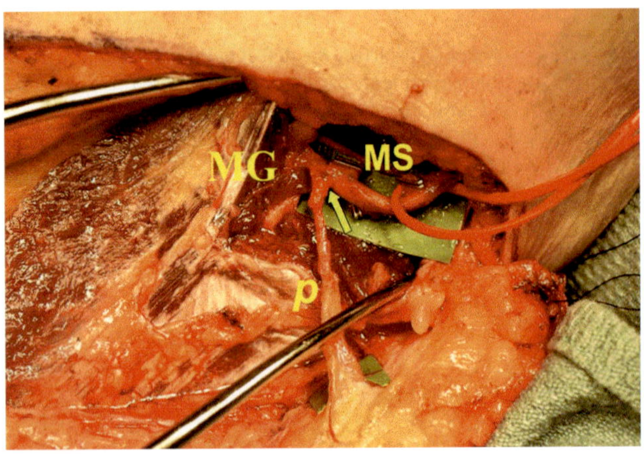

Fig. 40.7 Dissection of medial sural musculocutaneous perforator [*p*] through medial gastrocnemius muscle [MG] will lead to a branch of the medial sural vessels [MS, here encircled in vessel loop] that can be further dissected toward the vascular hilum until the desired caliber is reached to serve as a recipient site

References

1. McCraw JB, Fishman JH, Sharzer LA. The versatile gastrocnemius myocutaneous flap. Plast Reconstr Surg. 1978;62:15–23.
2. Hallock GG. The medial sural (medial gastrocnemius) perforator local flap. Ann Plast Surg. 2004;53:501–5.
3. Chien WH, Chen IC, Tan TS, Tang YW. Salvage of knee joint tumor prosthesis using turnover reverse-flow descending branch of lateral circumflex femoral artery as recipient vessel for the free ALT flap: a case report. J Reconstr Microsurg. 2007;23:505–9.
4. Kim JS, Lee HS, Jang PY, Choi TH, Lee KS, Kim NG. Use of the descending branch of lateral circumflex femoral artery as a recipient pedicle for coverage of a knee defect with free flap: anatomical and clinical study. Microsurgery. 2010;30:32–6.
5. Gao SH, Feng SM, Chen C, Jiao C, Sun LQ, Zhang WL. A new recipient artery for reconstruction of soft-tissue defects in the lower limb with a free anterolateral thigh flap: the reversed descending branch of the lateral femoral circumflex artery. Plast Reconstr Surg. 2012;130:1059–65.
6. Yuen JC, Zhou AT. Free flap coverage for knee salvage. Ann Plast Surg. 1996;37:158–66.
7. Park S, Eom JS. Selection of the recipient vessel in the free flap around the knee: the superior medial genicular vessels and the descending genicular vessels. Plast Reconstr Surg. 2001;105:1177–82.
8. Fang T, Zhang EW, Lineaweaver WC, Zhang F. Recipient vessels in the free flap reconstruction around the knee. Ann Plast Surg. 2013;71:429–33.
9. Keller A, Allen R, Shaw W. The medial gastrocnemius muscle flap: a local free flap. Plast Reconstr Surg. 1984;73:974–6.
10. Salibian AH, Rogers FR, Lamb RC. Microvascular gastrocnemius muscle transfer to the distal leg using saphenous vein grafts. Plast Reconstr Surg. 1984;73:302–7.
11. Johnson PE, Harris GD, Nagle DJ, Lewis VL. The sural artery and vein as recipient vessels in free flap reconstruction about the knee. J Reconstr Microsurg. 1987;3:233–41.
12. Hallock GG. The medial approach to the sural vessels to facilitate microanastomosis about the knee. Ann Plast Surg. 1994;32:388–93.
13. Mathes SJ, Najai F. Classification of the vascular anatomy of muscles: experimental and clinical correlation. Plast Reconstr Surg. 1981;67:177–87.
14. Beumer JD, Karoo R, Caplash Y, Semmler JG, Taylor J. The medial sural artery as recipient vessel and the impact on the medial gastrocnemius. Ann Plast Surg. 2011;67:382–6.
15. Ghosh MM. The gastrocnemius vessels as recipient vessels for lower limb free-tissue transfer. Plast Reconstr Surg. 2003;112:936–7.
16. Tsetsonis CH, Kaxira OS, Laoulakos DH, Spiliopoulou CA, Koutselinis AS. The arterial communications between the gastrocnemius muscle heads: a fresh cadaveric study and clinical implications. Plast Reconstr Surg. 2000;105:94–8.
17. Arnold PG, Mixter RC. Making the Most of the gastrocnemius muscles. Plast Reconstr Surg. 1983;72:38–48.
18. Strauch B, Yu HL. Atlas of microvascular surgery. New York: Thieme Medical Publishers; 1993. p. 244–85.
19. Cavadas PC, Sanz-Giménez-Rico JR, Gutierrez-de la Cámara A, Navarro-Monzonís A, Soler-Nomdedeu S, Martínez-Soriano. The medial sural artery perforator free flap. Plast Reconstr Surg. 2001;108:1609–15.
20. Dusseldorp JR, Pham QJ, Ngo W, Gianoutsos M, Moradi P. Vascular anatomy of the medial sural artery perforator flap: a new classification system of intra-muscular branching patterns. J Plast Reconstr Aesthet Surg. 2014;67:1267–75.

21. Godina M, Arnez ZM, Lister GD. Preferential use of the posterior approach to blood vessels of the lower leg in microvascular surgery. Plast Reconstr Surg. 1991;88:287–91.
22. Kosutic D, Pejkovic B, Anderhuber F, Vadnjal-Donlagic S, Zic R, Gulic R, Krajnc I, Solman L, Kocbek L. Complete mapping of lateral and medial sural artery perforators: anatomical study with Duplex-Doppler ultrasound correlation. J Plast Reconstr Aesth Surg. 2012;65:1530–6.
23. Daar DA, Abdou SA, Cohen JM, Wilson SC, Levine JP. Is the medial sural artery perforator flap a new workhorse flap? A systematic review and meta-analysis. Plast Reconstr Surg. 2019;143:393e–403e.
24. Smith ML, Molina BJ, Dayan E, Kim JN, Kagen A, Dayan JH. Use of distal medial sural vessels as recipient vessels in free tissue transfer. J Recon Microsurg. 2017;33:59–62.
25. Georgescu AV, Matei I, Ardelean F, Capota I. Microsurgical non-microvascular flaps in forearm and hand reconstruction. Microsurgery. 2007;27:384–94.
26. Hallock GG. Anatomic basis of the gastrocnemius perforator-based flap. Ann Plast Surg. 2001;47:517–22.

Part VI

Miscellaneous Special

Recipient Vessels for Vascularized Lymph Node Transplant

41

Fatma Betul Tuncer and Graham Schwarz

Introduction

Vascularized lymph node transplant (VLNT) for treatment of lymphedema was proposed by Hung-Chi Chen in a canine model in 1990 [1]. Hung-Chi Chen and Corinne Becker reported the first clinical use of VLNT in the early 1990s [2–4]. Since then, many more vascularized lymph node flaps such as supraclavicular, submental, axillary, omental, inguinal, and lateral thoracic lymph node flaps have been described [5–11]. Recipient sites (orthotopic vs heterotopic, distal vs proximal, single vs double) have greatly varied between different surgical groups [12]. For example, in upper extremity lymphedema, some surgeons have performed VLNT to the wrist [4], whereas others have preferred the axilla [7]. At the time of this writing, no consensus has been reached regarding the optimal recipient site for VLNT in the upper or lower extremity. Our goal in this chapter is to highlight the most common recipient vessels for VLNT and describe the surgical technique for their exposure.

Preoperative Assessment

Physical examination of the planned recipient site, including palpation of the peripheral pulses, should be performed preoperatively. Advanced imaging (CT or MRI angiography) of recipient vessels is usually not required for healthy patients and atraumatic extremities. The course of selected recipient arteries such as radial recurrent artery, radial artery, and dorsalis pedis artery can be easily mapped out on the skin using handheld Doppler. This also helps planning of the incisions.

F. B. Tuncer
Department of Plastic Surgery, Cleveland Clinic, Cleveland, OH, USA

Division of Plastic Surgery, University of Utah, Salt Lake City, UT, USA
e-mail: fatma.tuncer@hsc.utah.edu

G. Schwarz (✉)
Department of Plastic Surgery, Cleveland Clinic, Cleveland, OH, USA
e-mail: SCHWARG@ccf.org

Anatomy and Surgical Technique

Axilla

The subscapular system may be used as recipient vessels for transplantation of the lymph node flap to the axilla. Orthotopic placement has been used most commonly in cases where lymphatic injury and tissue fibrosis have occurred due to previous axillary surgery or radiation. The subscapular artery, the largest branch of the axillary artery, passes inferiorly and posteriorly along its lower margin to the inferior angle of scapula, gives off circumflex scapular artery, and continues inferiorly as the thoracodorsal artery (also see Chap. 12) [13]. Either of these arteries with their accompanying veins can be used for vascular anastomosis (Fig. 41.1). When possible, anastomosis should be made proximal to the takeoff of the serratus branch should the need for future latissimus dorsi flap reconstruction arise.

An incision can encompass an existing scar, or a new transverse incision just below the axillary hair bearing skin can be made for patients who do not have a history of axillary surgery. Subcutaneous scar should be completely and safely removed within the anatomic borders of the axilla, until normal subcutaneous fat is encountered. This includes lysis of scar associated with the axillary vein and thoracodorsal vessels with attention to careful preservation of nerves.

Proximal Forearm

The proximal forearm may be used as a recipient site when there is predominantly forearm lymphedema or as a second recipient site for double lymph node transplant. The

R. Gurunian, R. Djohan (eds.), *Recipient Vessels in Reconstructive Microsurgery*,
https://doi.org/10.1007/978-3-030-75389-4_41

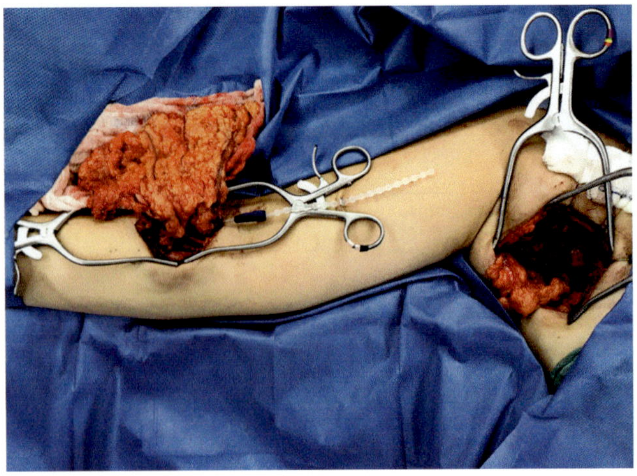

Fig. 41.1 The gastroepiploic lymph node flap was divided into two flaps following its harvest, and they were transferred to the axilla and forearm. The arterial anastomoses were performed to the thoracodorsal artery and radial recurrent artery, respectively. Proximal and distal ends of the gastroepiploic vein were anastomosed to two different veins in each location to prevent venous congestion

recurrent radial artery is a good option as a recipient vessel at this level because its location is consistent and end-to-side anastomosis to a major artery is avoided. Preoperatively, the cephalic vein and radial artery can be mapped out on the skin using handheld Doppler, and the incision can be planned in between these two landmarks (Fig. 41.2). A 6–8 cm long longitudinal incision is made near the antecubital fossa on the radial side of the volar forearm. The cephalic vein and superficial nerves, located in the subcutaneous fat, should be protected. The muscular fascia of the forearm is incised. The recurrent radial artery is the first branch of the radial artery after its bifurcation from the brachial artery. It is located between the brachioradialis and pronator teres muscles, anterior to biceps brachii tendon (also see Chaps. 24 and 25, Fig. 24.4, Fig. 25.3 and Video 25.1). It ascends between branches of the radial nerve, lying on the supinator muscle and then between brachioradialis and brachialis muscles [13]. The branches that go into brachioradialis are divided. The dissection stops after achieving 2–3 cm of arterial length. Therefore, the superficial and deep branches of the radial nerve are not encountered. Venous anastomosis can be performed to venae comitantes of the radial artery or to a superficial vein (e.g., cephalic vein or its tributaries). Subcutaneous fat, often fibrotic from disease, is carefully excised to create a pocket large enough for the inset of the lymph node flap (Fig. 41.1).

Other groups have also described VLNT to the medial site of the elbow with anastomosis to the ulnar artery (end to side), anterior recurrent ulnar artery (end to end), and basilic vein [14]. Johnson et al. reported a case series of flow-through omental flap in the forearm, using the gastroepiploic artery and vein between the radial artery and one of its venae comitantes [15].

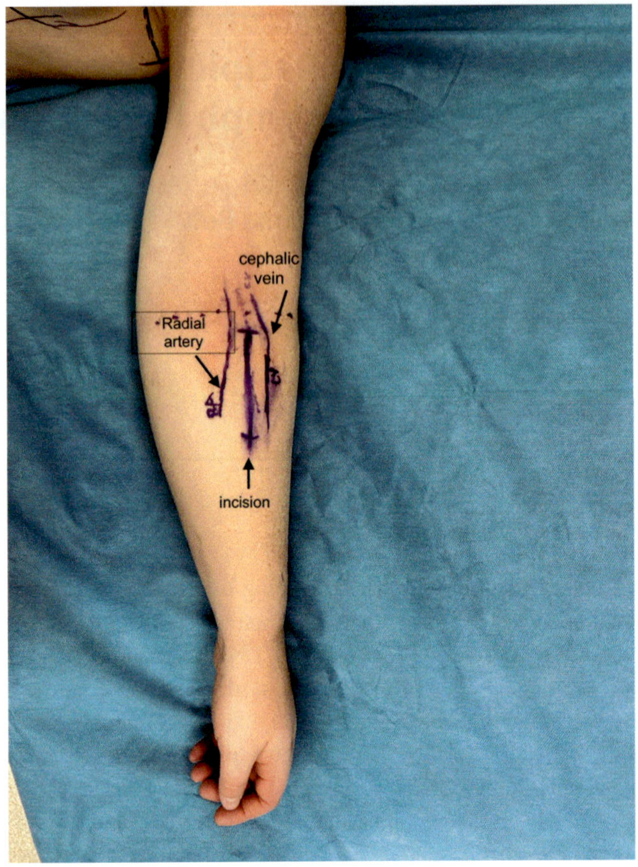

Fig. 41.2 Preoperative marking for the radial artery and cephalic vein

Wrist

Radial artery is the recipient vessel of choice when VLNT is performed to the wrist and can be located distal to the wrist crease in the anatomical snuffbox, between extensor pollicis brevis (EPB), abductor pollicis longus (APL) (medially), and extensor pollicis longus (EPL) (laterally) (Fig. 41.3) (also see Video 25.3). The cephalic vein, also located in the anatomical snuffbox, may be used for venous outflow. Access to this part of the radial artery maintains safety by preserving distal perfusion through the palmar branch. Doppler ultrasound can be performed to perform vascular mapping. A transverse S incision is made on the dorsum of the wrist. Superficial radial nerves are carefully preserved. The branch of the radial artery in anatomical snuffbox is dissected between extensor and abductor tendons of the thumb. The distal end of the artery is divided before it dives into the first dorsal interosseous muscles and rerouted above the EPL and APL tendons to prevent compression of the anastomosis during thumb movements.

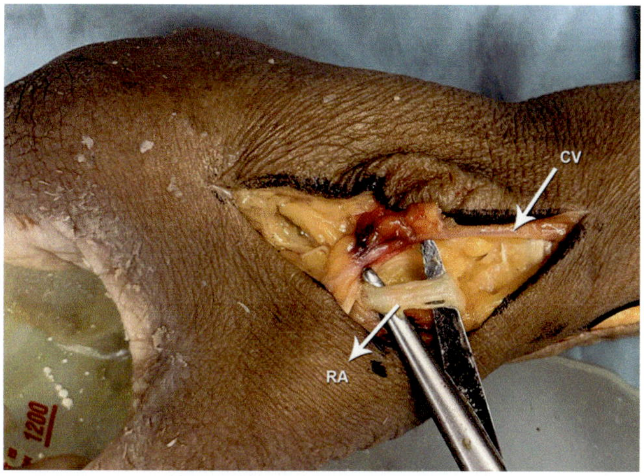

Fig. 41.3 The radial artery (RA) in the anatomical snuffbox. Superficial vein(s) such as cephalic vein (CV) and dorsal digital branches of the radial nerve should be protected during dissection

The radial artery can also be prepared more proximally for end-to-side anastomosis. A pocket is created on the dorsal wrist for partial inset of the flap. The risk of compression to the pedicle is high if the flap were to be inset completely. One side of the flap is inset, and the opposite site can be covered with split thickness skin graft [14].

Thigh

Lymphatic vessels are concentrated on the medial thigh, and lymph node transfer into this region may theoretically increase the chance of lymphangiogenesis [16]. Vascularized lymph node flaps can be placed in the medial thigh using the gracilis flap pedicle (medial circumflex femoral artery and vein) or profunda artery perforator which may be larger [7]. These recipient vessels are exposed when the patient is in the frog-leg position. An incision is made along the posterior border of the adductor longus muscle. Adductor longus fascia is incised, and both profunda artery perforator and the gracilis pedicle can be observed between the adductor longus and gracilis muscles. The profunda artery perforator is located inferior to the gracilis pedicle. It might be found over the adductor magnus muscle but more frequently runs inside the muscle necessitating intramuscular dissection. The greater saphenous vein is located anterior to the incision and should be protected. A posterior branch of the greater saphenous vein can be preserved for additional venous anastomosis.

Most of the lower extremity lymphedema cases are caused by deep pelvic lymph node dissections and radiation due to gynecological cancers. Because anatomical continuity of the lymphatic system could not be restored inside the pelvis, lymph node transplantation is often performed distal to the lymphatic defect. However, the groin can still be a recipient site for VLNT following melanoma or vulvar cancer-related inguinal lymph node dissections. The branches of the femoral artery in the femoral triangle, such as superficial circumflex iliac artery and superficial inferior epigastric artery, are good alternatives for VLNT to the groin.

Lower Leg

The popliteal fossa is a diamond-shaped structure, superiorly bounded by semitendinosus, semimembranosus (medially), and biceps femoris muscles (laterally). Two heads of the gastrocnemius muscle mark the inferior border. In this fossa, the popliteal artery, which is located anterior to the tibial nerve, gives off the medial sural artery, lateral sural artery, and superior and inferior genicular arteries. The medial sural artery is commonly used as a recipient vessel at this location (also see Chap. 40 and Video 40.1). Exposure of the popliteal artery in supine position is technically difficult, and the medial sural artery can be dissected in frog-leg position. A line between midpoint of the popliteal fossa and posterior aspect of the medial malleolus is drawn. An 8 cm incision is made over the medial gastrocnemius muscle extending to the midpoint in the popliteal fossa but below the flexion crease. The medial sural artery perforator is usually located on this line about 8 cm distal to midpoint of the popliteal fossa when the knee is flexed in the frog-leg position [17]. Once identified, it is traced to the main artery [7]. Small saphenous vein or medial sural vein can be used for venous anastomosis. A window of deep investing muscle fascia and a portion of the subcutaneous fat is excised to allow room for the lymph node flap. Care must be taken to preserve the greater saphenous vein and sural nerve [18].

The descending genicular artery can be an alternative recipient vessel at this location (also see Chap. 39) [19].

Ankle

The anterior tibial artery originates from the popliteal artery at the lower border of the popliteus muscle. It passes from the posterior compartment to anterior compartment of the leg through the interosseous membrane. It descends inferiorly between the tibialis anterior (medially) and extensor hallucis longus together with anterior tibial vein and deep peroneal nerve (also see Chap. 34). At the ankle level, the anterior tibial artery passes deep to the extensor retinaculum midway between lateral and medial malleoli and becomes the dorsalis pedis artery.

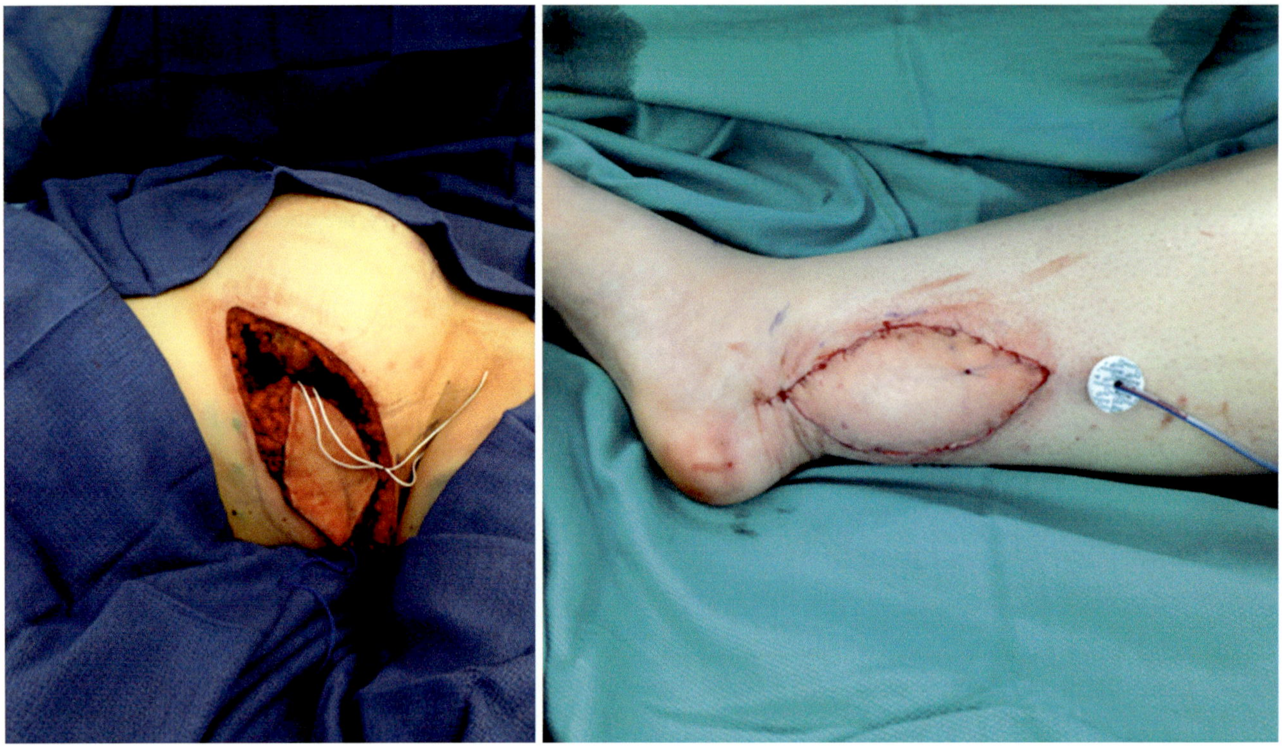

Fig. 41.4 The lateral thoracic artery lymph node flap (left) to the lower leg was anastomosed to the posterior tibial artery (right) for lower extremity lymphedema

The incision is planned over the anterior tibial and dorsalis pedis artery by using a handheld Doppler. An S-shaped incision is made on the dorsum of the ankle. The skin envelope is undermined for flap inset. The anterior tibial artery is found between tendons of the extensor hallucis longus and tibialis anterior. It is wise to target recipient vessels a few centimeters above the ankle joint to avoid compression or kinking of the vessels with movements of the ankle [19].

Another recipient vessel in this location is the posterior tibial artery, which runs in the deep posterior compartment of the leg between flexor digitorum longus (medially) and tibialis posterior (laterally) [20] (Fig. 41.4) (also see Chap. 35). It lies more superficial distally, medial to the Achilles tendon and posterior to the medial malleolus. In order to expose the posterior tibial artery, an incision is made on the medial side of the calf. The plane between the flexor digitorum longus and soleus muscle is found. The plantaris tendon is located between the soleus and gastrocnemius muscles and indicates a wrong plane for exposure of the posterior tibial vessels [21].

Venae comitantes of the anterior or posterior tibial arteries as well as the great saphenous vein can be used for venous anastomosis depending on the caliber, orientation, and length of flap vein(s). The great saphenous vein lies in the subcutaneous plane, anterior to the medial malleolus. It ascends superomedially behind the medial femoral condyle and drains into the common femoral vein. Venae comitantes can be diminutive in lymphedematous extremities due to constant compression. Although superficial veins are usually thick and fibrotic in these patients, they may be preferable to comitant veins [19]. Duplex ultrasound or other venous studies can be performed preoperatively to examine valvular competence of the veins of the lower extremity.

Discussion

Vascularized lymph node transplant has been adopted as a useful method to treat lymphedema. The choice of recipient site varies greatly depending on the operating surgeon's view on the mechanism of VLNT [22]. In Cheng's theory, the transferred nodal tissue has the ability to take up lymphatic fluid and shunt that fluid into the recipient vein [19]. Increased pressure gradient between the interstitial space and venous system facilitates the shunting of lymph fluid [19]. Surgeons who perform VLNT to a distal location (e.g., wrist, ankle) propose that placing the flap in the distal limb may facilitate pumping and absorption function of the transplanted lymph node because lymph is usually pools in the most dependent portion of the extremity due to gravitational forces (hydrostatic theory) [4, 6, 23]. Supporters of a proximal recipient site (e.g., axilla) posit that orthotopic transplantation of lymph nodes reestablishes the normal anatomy and bridges the defect caused by lymphadenectomy [7]. Good results have been achieved with both types.

Table 41.1 Vascularized lymph node transplantation (VLNT) can be performed proximally or distally in the extremity. Advantages and disadvantages of each approach is summarized

	Advantages	Disadvantages
Proximal VLNT	Orthotopic transplantation Good cosmetic outcome Axillary/groin scar release	Difficult dissection due to previous surgeries and radiation Flap monitoring may be limited/not possible (in case of buried flaps) Possible limited treatment effect on the distal extremity
Distal VLNT	Flap monitoring Easier dissection (not affected by surgery or radiation) Possible lymphatic catchment due to gravity	Poor cosmesis (unsightly appearance, debulking may be required at a later stage) Need for skin graft

There is no study until to date which shows superiority of one approach to another. There are advantages and disadvantages to both techniques, and these are summarized in Table 41.1.

The level of extremity affected the most by lymphedema, the lymphographic pattern of disease, patients' cosmetic concerns, and the presence of constricting scar in the lymphadenectomy site should be considered in selection of the recipient site. Dissection can be challenging in previously radiated sites (e.g., axilla, groin), and care must be taken not to injure critical structures inside the axilla or groin. Release of scar secondary to lymph node dissection and radiation alone may decompress obstructed lymphatics and the axillary vein. This in combination with replacement of vascularized tissue might, in itself, improve lymphatic drainage.

Another consideration is multilevel lymph node flap transfer to the same extremity. Anecdotally, some patients who had lymph node transfer to the axilla showed volume reduction in the upper arm and had further benefit from a second lymph node flap at the elbow. Reverse was also shown that the patients who had VLNT to wrist further benefited from a second lymph node flap at the elbow. HC Chen's group demonstrated feasibility of dividing gastroepiploic (omental) lymph node flaps into two and insetting at distal and mid-level levels of the extremity [22]. They reported double omental lymph node transfer at the level of elbow and wrist for the upper limb or the level of knee and ankle for the lower limb [22]. Similarly, Kenworthy et al. reported both transfer of a divided omental lymph node flap to the axilla and proximal forearm for upper limb and to medial thigh and knee for lower limb lymphedema [7]. Double recipient site VLNT were also shown to be feasible with flaps other than the gastroepiploic [24].

For distal and mid-level recipient sites, careful dissection at the subcutaneous plane is necessary to avoid injury to superficial sensory nerves in all of the recipient sites. Fat and fascia are removed to accommodate the flap. A skin paddle may be needed. Flaps transferred to the distal recipient sites usually require skin grafting. Secondary debulking procedure can be done after 3–6 months to improve the cosmetic outcome and function (Table 41.1).

Conclusion

Vascularized lymph node transplantation is an effective procedure for the treatment of fluid predominant lymphedema. Optimal recipient sites for lymph node transplant will remain in question until we have a better understanding of how VLNT works under different clinical scenarios and until controlled studies that compare different recipient sites are performed.

References

1. Chen HC, O'Brien BM, Rogers IW, Pribaz JJ, Eaton CJ. Lymph node transfer for the treatment of obstructive lymphoedema in the canine model. Br J Plast Surg. 1990;43(5):578–86. https://doi.org/10.1016/0007-1226(90)90123-h.
2. Becker C, Hidden G, Godart S, Maurage H, Pecking A. Free lymphatic transplant. Eur J Lymphol Rel Prob. 1991;6:25–77.
3. Becker C, Assouad J, Riquet M, Hidden G. Postmastectomy lymphedema: long-term results following microsurgical lymph node transplantation. Ann Surg. 2006;243(3):313–5. https://doi.org/10.1097/01.sla.0000201258.10304.16.
4. Lin C-H, Ali R, Chen S-C, et al. Vascularized groin lymph node transfer using the wrist as a recipient site for management of postmastectomy upper extremity lymphedema. Plast Reconstr Surg. 2009;123(4):1265–75. https://doi.org/10.1097/PRS.0b013e31819e6529.
5. Maldonado AA, Chen R, Chang DW. The use of supraclavicular free flap with vascularized lymph node transfer for treatment of lymphedema: a prospective study of 100 consecutive cases. J Surg Oncol. 2017;115(1):68–71. https://doi.org/10.1002/jso.24351.
6. Cheng M-H, Huang J-J, Huang J-J, et al. A novel approach to the treatment of lower extremity lymphedema by transferring a vascularized submental lymph node flap to the ankle. Gynecol Oncol. 2012;126(1):93–8. https://doi.org/10.1016/j.ygyno.2012.04.017.
7. Kenworthy EO, Nelson JA, Verma R, Mbabuike J, Mehrara BJ, Dayan JH. Double vascularized omentum lymphatic transplant (VOLT) for the treatment of lymphedema. J Surg Oncol. 2018;117(7):1413–9. https://doi.org/10.1002/jso.25033.
8. Barreiro GC, Baptista RR, Kasai KE, et al. Lymph fasciocutaneous lateral thoracic artery flap: anatomical study and clinical use. J Reconstr Microsurg. 2014;30(6):389–96. https://doi.org/10.1055/s-0034-1372482.
9. Coriddi M, Skoracki R, Eiferman D. Vascularized jejunal mesenteric lymph node transfer for treatment of extremity lymphedema. Microsurgery. 2017;37(2):177–8. https://doi.org/10.1002/micr.30037.
10. Ciudad P, Manrique OJ, Date S, et al. Vascularized appendicular lymph node transfer for treatment of extremity lymphedema: a case

report. Microsurgery. 2018;38(5):553–7. https://doi.org/10.1002/micr.30134.
11. Sapountzis S, Singhal D, Rashid A, Ciudad P, Meo D, Chen H-C. Lymph node flap based on the right transverse cervical artery as a donor site for lymph node transfer. Ann Plast Surg. 2014;73(4):398–401. https://doi.org/10.1097/SAP.0b013e31827fb39e.
12. Scaglioni MF, Arvanitakis M, Chen Y-C, Giovanoli P, Chia-Shen Yang J, Chang EI. Comprehensive review of vascularized lymph node transfers for lymphedema: outcomes and complications: comprehensive review vascularized lymph node transfer. Microsurgery. 2018;38(2):222–9. https://doi.org/10.1002/micr.30079.
13. Gray H. Gray's Anatomy. New York: Barnes&Noble; 2010.
14. Cheng M-H, Chen S-C, Henry SL, Tan BK, Chia-Yu Lin M, Huang J-J. Vascularized groin lymph node flap transfer for postmastectomy upper limb lymphedema: flap anatomy, recipient sites, and outcomes. Plast Reconstr Surg. 2013;131(6):1286–98. https://doi.org/10.1097/PRS.0b013e31828bd3b3.
15. Johnson AR, Bravo MG, Granoff MD, et al. Flow-through omental flap for vascularized lymph node transfer: a novel surgical approach for delayed lymphatic reconstruction. Plast Reconstr Surg Glob Open. 2019;7(9):e2436. https://doi.org/10.1097/GOX.0000000000002436.
16. Nelson JA, Mehrara BH, Dayan JH. Vascularized lymph node transfer to the Profunda artery perforator pedicle: a reliable proximal recipient vessel option in the medial thigh. Plast Reconstr Surg. 2017;140(2):366e–367e. https://doi.org/10.1097/PRS.0000000000003559.
17. Al-Himdani S, Din A, Wright TC, Wheble G, Chapman TWL, Khan U. The medial sural artery perforator (MSAP) flap: a versatile flap for lower extremity reconstruction. Injury. 2020; https://doi.org/10.1016/j.injury.2020.02.060.
18. Dayan JH, Ayala JM, Koshima I. Lymphedema: microsurgical reconstruction. In: Flaps and reconstructive surgery. 2nd ed. Philadelphia; 2017. pp. 40–60. http://www.clinicalkey.com/#!/content/book/3-s2.0-B9780323243223000080. Accessed 21 April 2020.
19. Henry SL, Cheng M-H. Recipient site selection in vascularized lymph node flap transfer. In: Principles and practice of lymphedema surgery. Philadelphia; 2016. pp. 113–121. https://www-clinicalkey-com.ccmain.ohionet.org/#!/content/book/3-s2.0-B9780323298971000139. Accessed 31 March 2020.
20. Koide S, Lin C-Y, Chen C, Cheng M-H. Long-term outcome of lower extremity lymphedema treated with vascularized lymph node flap transfer with or without venous complications. J Surg Oncol. 2020;121(1):129–37. https://doi.org/10.1002/jso.25602.
21. Pannucci CJ, Johnson TS, Levin LS. Clinical anatomy and recipient vessel selection and exposure in the lower extremity. In: Flaps and reconstructive surgery. 2nd ed. Philadelphia; 2017. pp. 115-137. http://www.clinicalkey.com/#!/content/book/3-s2.0-B9780323243223000134. Accessed 20 April 2020.
22. Ciudad P, Manrique OJ, Date S, et al. Double gastroepiploic vascularized lymph node tranfers to middle and distal limb for the treatment of lymphedema. Microsurgery. 2017;37(7):771–9. https://doi.org/10.1002/micr.30168.
23. Ciudad P, Sabbagh MD, Agko M, et al. Surgical management of lower extremity lymphedema: a comprehensive review. Indian J Plast Surg. 2019;52(1):81–92. https://doi.org/10.1055/s-0039-1688537.
24. Ito R, Lin MC-Y, Cheng M-H. Simultaneous bilateral submental lymph node flaps for lower limb lymphedema post leg Charles procedure. Plast Reconstr Surg Glob Open. 2015;3(9):e513. https://doi.org/10.1097/GOX.0000000000000489.

Arteriovenous Loop Graft for Lower Extremity Reconstruction

42

Chih-Hung Lin and Victor Chien

Introduction

Free flap reconstruction of the lower extremity has been a central area to the advent of microsurgical reconstruction since the days of Godina, with a specific focus on the importance of microvascular anastomoses between healthy recipient and donor vessels. The concept of zone of injury was popularized in the 1980s. Attempts were subsequently made to quantify the zone of injury [1].

The theoretical importance of positioning any microvascular anastomoses outside of the inflammatory milieu found within such zones has long been a central tenet of reconstructive microsurgery insofar as it is described in a CME article by Heller et al. in 2001 [2].

Although a subsequent critical review of the literature by Loos et al. [3] in 2010 showed the difficulty in objectively and reproducibly defining the boundaries of any particular zone of injury, the principle of anastomosing healthy recipient and donor vessels remains the same. This chapter provides an overview of methods available to the reconstructive surgeon when local recipient vessels are unavailable in the lower extremity.

A particular challenge in lower extremity reconstruction is the identification and availability of healthy recipient vessels within the effected limb that are accessible to the donor or flap vessels. As lower extremity reconstruction is often done with the goal of limb salvage, reconstructive surgeons assume the added pressure of avoiding the functional, psychosocial, and life expectancy costs associated with extremity amputation.

In the setting of a paucity of healthy recipient vessels from trauma, radiation, or peripheral vascular disease, additional maneuvers must be considered. The concept of the microsurgical vascular loop, introduced by Threlfall et al. [4] in 1982 and popularized by Grenga [5] in 1987, is a useful and versatile tool for facilitating free tissue transfer to defects lacking adequate vessels for microsurgical anastomosis.

Data from our center suggest AV loops are feasible ways to expand the indications for limb salvage in the absence of adequate local recipient vessels [6]. Additional studies have further illustrated characteristics that must be considered to maximize success in these difficult salvage procedures.

Two primary operative and planning considerations appear to play crucial roles in the success of an attempted reconstruction, namely, the achievable length of any grafting or loop procedure without compromising flap perfusion, and whether to stage the reconstruction in the setting of a loop procedure.

Graft Length and Perfusion Pressure

Any discussion of graft length has at its center the goal of locating any microvascular anastomoses outside of the inflammatory microenvironment of any zone of injury associated with the surgical or traumatic defect. A coequal consideration involves whether the resultant perfusion of the transferred tissue is sufficient and is effected by both flow dynamics and available perfusion pressures.

Various studies have shown success in lower extremity microvascular reconstruction with loop or graft lengths of up to 20–30 cm. The vascular conduits have length (L) and internal diameter (r), through which the blood flows. When the pressure in the inlet and outlet is unequal, respectively, this pressure difference (ΔP) drives the force for blood flow. Flow friction develops with certain degree of resistance between streaming blood viscosity and the stationary vascular walls. The perfusion pressures at the site of the pedicle anastomosis are paramount in planning for the inclusion of an interval segmental graft. In other words, there is a relative relationship between vascular flow, pressure difference, and resistance which can be explained using the basic flow equation:

C.-H. Lin (✉) · V. Chien
Chang Gung Memorial Hospital, Taoyuan, Taiwan
e-mail: chihhung@cgmh.org.tw

R. Gurunian, R. Djohan (eds.), *Recipient Vessels in Reconstructive Microsurgery*,
https://doi.org/10.1007/978-3-030-75389-4_42

$$\text{Flow} = \frac{\text{Pressure difference}}{\text{Resistances}}, \text{or } Q = \frac{\Delta P}{R}$$

where Q = flow rate (volume/time), ΔP = pressure difference (mm Hg), and R = resistance to flow (mm Hg × time/volume).

Blood is a non-Newton solution because it has intrinsic viscosity from the inclusion of blood cell components and serum. Besides the vessel is not a straight water pipe that aggravates the resistance in the vascular conduit. Therefore, the importance of this perfusion pressure is suggested in considerations of free tissue transfers based off of vascular bypass grafts in extremities with an otherwise overwhelming burden of atherosclerotic disease.

Staging

An additional consideration with regard to operative planning is the timing of reconstruction and the utilization of these perfusion-extending interventions. Sequence and timing of perfusion-extending procedures remain unsettled.

Several approaches for extending an adequate perfusion between the recipient vessels and donor flap vessels have been suggested. These include either direct interposition vein grafting, single stage, or delayed arteriovenous vascular loop utilization. Various risks and benefits have been ascribed to each of these approaches. Direct interposition graft and single stage AV loop are similar in the physiology dynamics for perfusion as long as a high inflow arterial pressure is supplied to overcome the resistance of vascular length.

On the other hand, the staged AV loops may encounter several obstacles when used for the vascular conduits. Different from the trunk, the lower extremity has a limited circumferential girdle. In addition, fibrosis from ischemic limb or swelling/fibrosis from trauma may have compression tension on the vascular wall resulting in kinking, twisting, or distortion of vascular loop. Furthermore, when an external fixator is required for the fracture fixation, such as Hoffman or Ilizarov pins, it will have spatial hindrance for the route of the vascular loop (Fig. 42.1).

In case of staged AV loop procedure, a continuous arterial shearing stress will impose mechanical impingement of the turning loop area. The greater curvature may develop vein

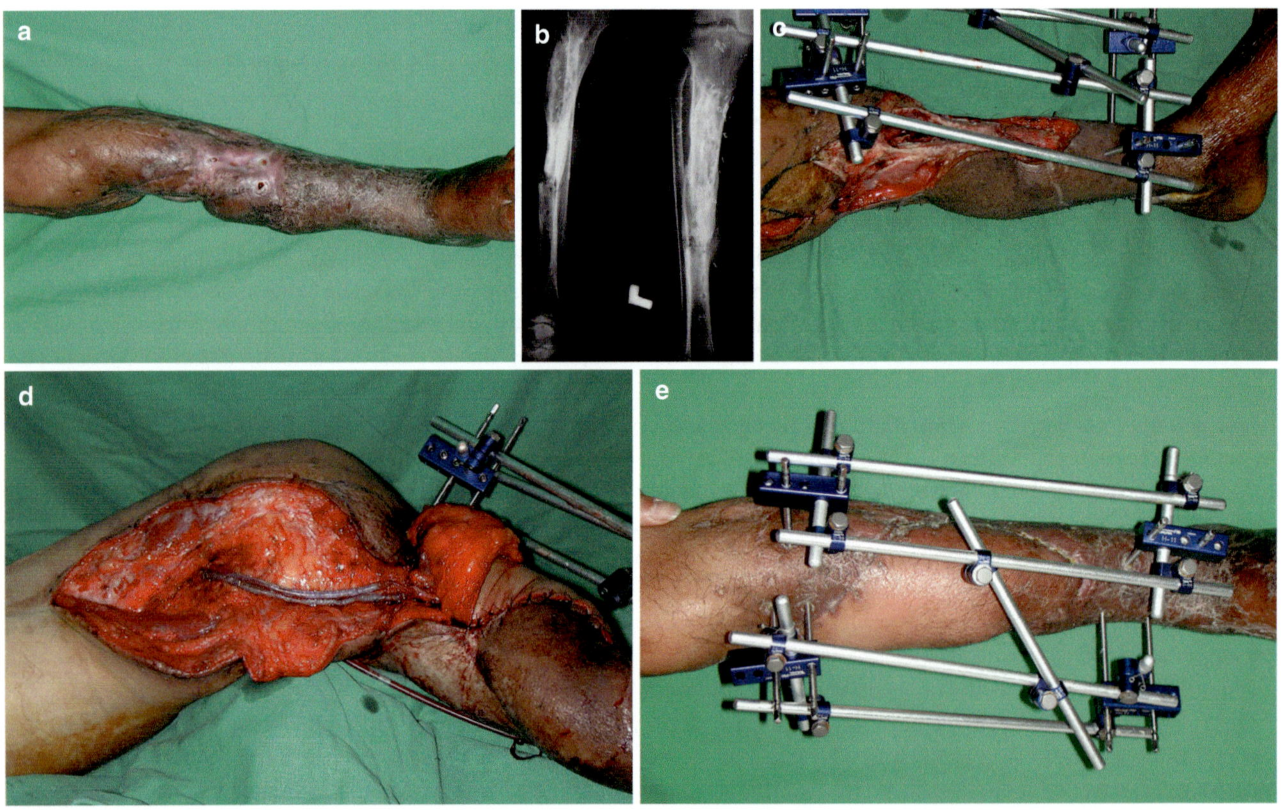

Fig. 42.1 (**a**) Patient underwent free left latissimus dorsi and skin graft for left tibial open fracture. He subsequently sustained left tibial chronic osteomyelitis with extensive lower leg fibrosis and chronically draining sinus. (**b**) Left tibial chronic osteomyelitis. (**c**) Extensive fibrosis and external fixator made the limb short of soft tissue to accommodate staged AV loop. (**d**) Single-stage AV loop was used for free flap transfer. (**e**). 2 months after right latissimus dorsi myocutaneous flap

graft hypertrophy by arterialization, while the lesser curvature may suffer from lipid accumulation and atherosclerotic change. These adverse effects imposed on the greater and lesser curvatures may result in narrowing of the vascular loop on the turning zones. These changes and the patency of the blood flow cannot be assessed reliably by handheld Doppler [7, 8].

Technical Considerations

The following technical considerations are based on our experience of 65 microvascular free tissue transfers that required long vein grafts (>20 cm for the arterial defects) to bridge either arterial defects only or both arterial and venous vascular gaps at Chang Gung Memorial Hospital from 1992 to 2001 [6].

The great saphenous veins were used as vein grafts. The contralateral great saphenous vein or a pedicled ipsilateral great saphenous vein was harvested and flushed from its distal end with a heparin solution (5000 units/500 mL saline, using a 10 mL syringe) while occluding the proximal end with a vascular clamp. The dilated vein was then checked for any leaking side branches, which were then hemoclipped or suture ligated. The newly created vascular conduits were then used as recipient vessels for the microsurgical flap. Anticoagulation therapy was routinely initiated following the creation of the AVF [6]. The regimen consisted of dextran 40 and heparin (5000unit/500 mL) running at 20 mL/h (heparin; 200 U/h) for 7 days. For complicated single-stage cases with a high concern for flap survival and for cases requiring exploration for thrombosis, the dextran/heparin drip rate was increased to 30 mL/h [6]. For the two-stage cases, the intravenous anticoagulation was replaced with aspirin (300 mg/day) till the scheduled free tissue transfer.

Surgical Technique

Arterial and venous gap connected with a looped vein graft (AVF) followed by free tissue transfer in the same stage or another stage: this approach is required when exploration for vessels reveals no adequate artery or vein near the defect. Thus, a long vein graft is used to bridge the gap between the flap and recipient arteries and veins. Whenever possible, the ipsilateral great saphenous vein is used as a pedicled graft (leaving the proximal end intact). When the ipsilateral great saphenous vein is not available, the contralateral great saphenous vein is used as a free graft. Either way, the vein is used to create an arteriovenous fistula.

After the vein graft is harvested, its distal end is placed near the arterial stump. The outflow end of either the contralateral vein graft or the pedicled ipsilateral vein graft is clamped, and the vein graft is flushed and then dilated with a heparin solution. Using a hydraulic pressure is a gentle non-traumatic method to dilate the vascular conduit, which may allow the surgeon to check leakage from branches and prevent vessel twisting. During vascular anastomosis, the vein graft conduit is filled and dilated with heparin solution, and no blood stasis inside the lumen exists. Both ends of the heparin solution filled AV loop are clamped and anastomosed to the clamped inflow recipient artery and clamped outflow recipient vein. After both ends of the AV loop are repaired, all four clamps are released simultaneously (Fig. 42.2).

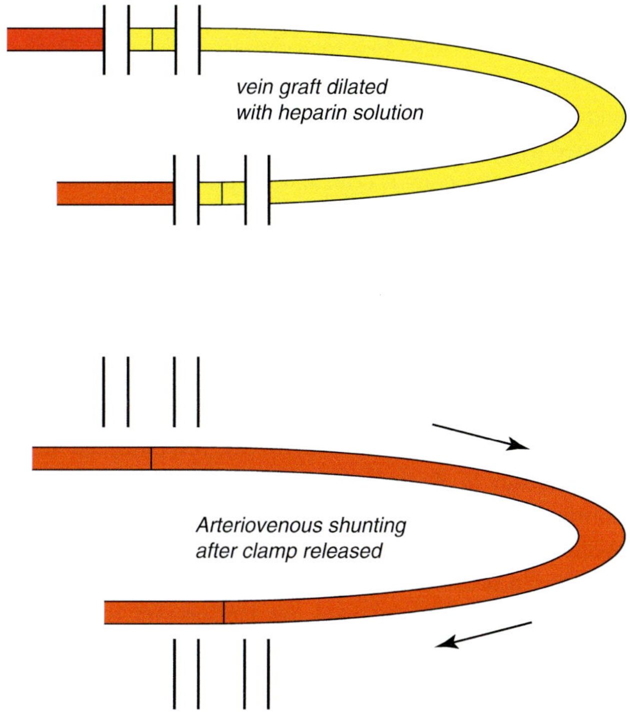

Fig. 42.2 Schematic illustration of the saphenous vein graft for creating the AV loop. The outflow end of either the contralateral vein graft or the pedicled ipsilateral vein graft is clamped, and the vein graft is flushed and then dilated with a heparin solution. During the procedure of vascular anastomosis, the vein graft conduit is filled and dilated with heparin solution. No blood stasis inside the lumen exists. Both ends of the vein graft are anastomosed to the artery and vein, and all clamps (double vertical lines) were released simultaneously

Single-Stage Procedure A significant arterial and venous deficiency for free tissue flap revascularization, this vascular gap requires the connection with vein graft. The AV loop can be used to bridge the arterial inflow and venous outflow in order to shorten the ischemic time during free tissue transfer in a single stage. Some patients may need simultaneous bypass grafting to revascularize the distal extremity (end-to-end fashion). Then, the flap pedicle can be anastomosed to the graft in an end-to-side manner.

In the single stage technique, an arteriovenous loop is created and allowed to perfuse for a period of at least 1 h. During that time, flap harvest ensues. The flap is temporarily inset, and the AV loop is divided at a point that accommodates the desired length of the artery and vein of the flap. The sequence of events at this point is critical to optimizing final outcome. After dividing the AV loop, arterial perfusion is checked for optimal flow, and then a microvascular clamp is applied about 5 cm proximal to the anastomosis between the native artery and the vein graft. The intraluminal blood distal to the clamp is flushed out with heparin solution either through a side branch or by transluminal injection using an angiocatheter. The arterial side vein graft is clamped distally and dilated. This helps prevent a "myogenic response," an inherent tendency of the vascular smooth muscle to maintain a constant developed tension despite changes in pressure [9]. According to Laplace's law (T (tension) = $P \times r$), a sudden increase in pressure (P) would tend to stretch the vascular smooth muscle and increase the tension, yet the muscle responds by contracting to a smaller diameter (r), and the tension decreases back toward control. Then, preparation of the venous side is performed. The graft is flushed with heparin solution and dilated, and a clamp is placed proximal to the distal venous side vein graft (Fig. 42.3). Both the artery and vein of the microsurgical flap are anastomosed to the divided ends of the AV loop graft. During this entire period, the vein grafts are filled and dilated with heparin solution. All clamps are released after all the vascular anastomoses are complete (Fig. 42.3).

Two-Stage Procedure Arterial and venous gap bridged with an AV loop with a period of maturation time (vein grafting and microsurgical flap performed in two separate stages). After creating the looped arteriovenous fistula, the turning point of the loop is placed near the defect for subsequent use as recipient vessels (Fig. 42.3). After a maturation period, which is randomly selected based on patient's condition and operating schedule availability, the patient is brought back to the operating room for the second stage reconstruction. Although examination of the AV loop with a Doppler probe preoperatively may confirm patency, upon exploration this may not be the case. The AV loop is found and tested for patency during surgery. The loop is cut at the turning point, and routine arterial and venous anastomoses are performed between the flap vessels and the divided ends of the AV loop graft. If the vessel is thrombosed, then the fistula is abandoned. However, if the thrombus is on the arterial side of the vein graft proximal to the turning point, there may be cases where thrombectomy may be performed or the arterial side vein graft can be replaced with another vein graft for arterial inflow, and the venous side AV loop can then be used as outflow recipient vessel for the flap.

Flow Characteristics

The choice between direct interposition vein grafting and construction of a temporary arteriovenous loop as the most efficacious and durable techniques to extending the perfusion options to the reconstructive surgeon remains unsettled with studies alternatively showing superiority of one method over the other or no difference. While a randomized controlled trial remains the gold standard for clarifying this question, we propose a hypothesis based on the laws of fluid dynamics that we believe explain the superiority of direct interposition grafting based on our institutional experience.

Construction of an arteriovenous loop requires the use of a loop or curving line of the arteriovenous construct. This by definition must have a circular configuration at its distal most aspect, the diameter of which must lay within the anatomic confines of the area to be reconstructed.

The presence of an artificial loop within the construct alters the flow dynamics at this point and, we believe, creates differential flow rates between the greater and lesser curvatures which, when coupled with the mechanical properties of the less-elastic vein graft and the increased distance the otherwise pulsatile flow must travel through a capacitance vessel, creates a microenvironment in the lesser curve which is relatively more pro-thrombotic. Blood flow through a vessel at any given time is effected with multiple factors that include pressure difference, diameter, viscosity, and length of vessel. It would be noteworthy to remember the Hagen-Poiseuille equation [10]. Poiseuille's law is written as ($Q = \Delta P \pi r^4/8\ \eta l$) ($Q$, blood flow; P, pressure difference; r, diameter of vessel; η, viscosity; l, length of vessel).

According to this equation, the longer the vein graft, the more resistance will be created with resultant reduced blood flow. The pressure and radius are on the numerator side, i.e., high pressure and high vascular diameter will provide more blood flow at a given vascular graft length. In particular, the diameter plays an important role. For instance, a 4 mm vein graft provides more blood flow than a 2 mm vessel, i.e., by 4^4 versus 2^4 times. In case of AV loop construct, lower flow rate at the lesser curvature of the AV loop may create suboptimal conditions. Therefore, it would necessary to use a large-caliber vein graft as well as a donor artery with high pressure inflow for free flap perfusion. Our preference is to use the great saphenous vein graft and superficial femoral artery (end to side) (Figs. 42.1 and 42.4).

In Situ Venous Drainage

Demiri et al. [11] advocated for the use of in situ lesser saphenous venous drainage in appropriate microvascular reconstruction in the lower extremity given the dual deep and

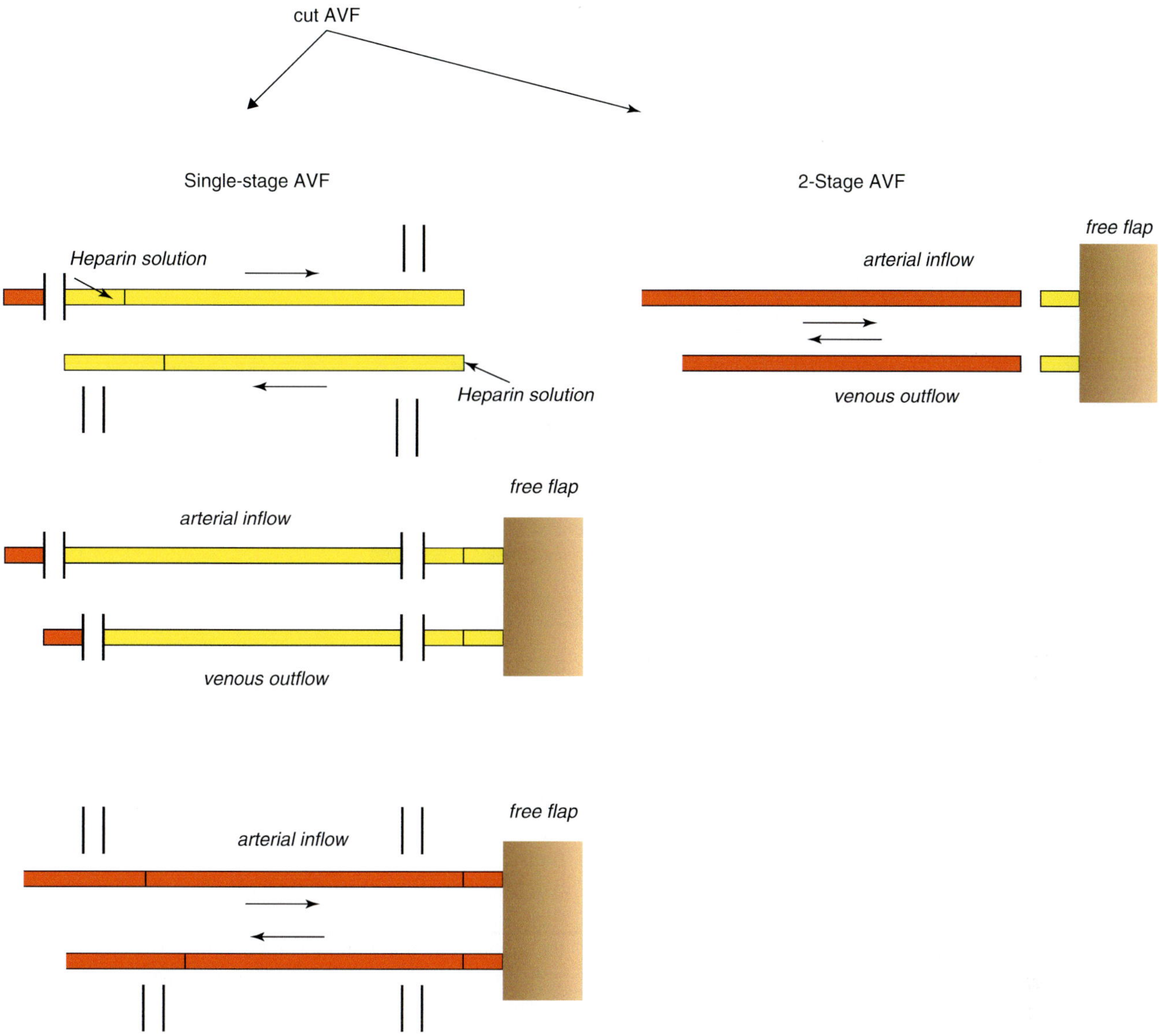

Fig. 42.3 Schematic illustration of divided AV loop graft in single (left) and two stage (right) reconstruction. Both the artery and vein of the flap are anastomosed to the divided ends of the AV loop. During this entire period, the vein grafts are filled and dilated with a heparin solution. After all vascular anastomoses are complete, all clamps (double vertical lines) are released. In the two-stage procedure, the looped arteriovenous fistula with a long maturation time and arterial and venous pedicle of the flap are anastomosed to the divided ends of the AV loop (right)

superficial drainage of the lesser saphenous system. This approach was initially popularized by Vlastou and Earle in 1988 [12].

Further technical considerations include choosing the greater saphenous versus the lesser saphenous vein as a conduit and whether to utilize an in situ conduit reconstruction versus an ex vivo reconstruction.

Discussion

Various approaches for extending an adequate perfusion zone to within reach of a donor or flap vessel have been suggested. These include direct interposition vein grafting, single-stage arteriovenous loop utilization, and delayed arteriovenous loop utilization. Various risks and benefits have been ascribed to each of these approaches.

Variable outcomes have been reported for the use of interposition vein grafts (IVG) for free flap anastomosis, which historically have been associated with an increased risk for postoperative complications [13]. However, more recent studies on large patient cohorts indicate that IVGs yield success rates greater than 95% in primary reconstructions [14]. Whether the use of IVGs has an impact on outcomes of microsurgical lower extremity reconstructions in patients with PVD has been poorly investigated. Henn et al. [15] reviewed venous bypass versus arteriovenous loops for recipient vessels in lower extremity microvascular recon-

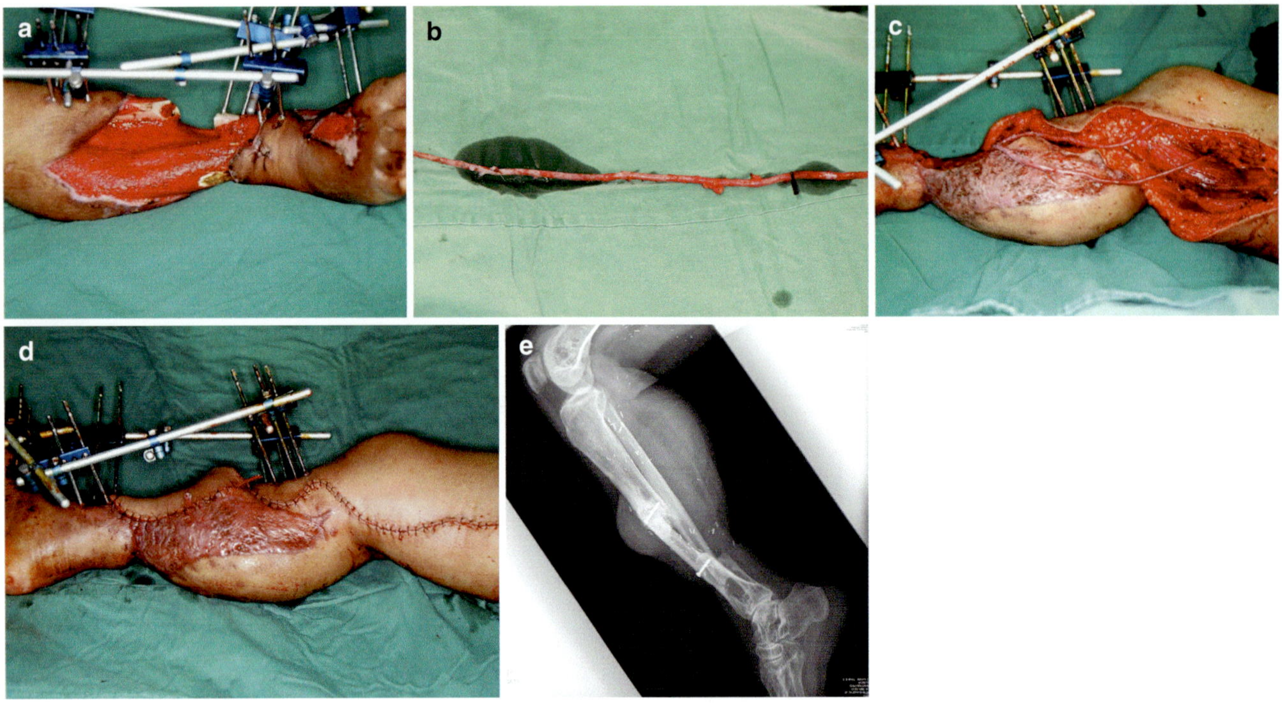

Fig. 42.4 (**a**) Right tibial composite defect with traumatized anterior and posterior tibial arteries. (**b**) Contralateral great saphenous vein graft inflated with heparin solution. (**c**) Single-stage AV loop between superficial femoral artery and ipsilateral great saphenous vein. (**d**) Revascularized fibular flap. (**e**) Fibula bone hypertrophy after bone union

struction in patients with peripheral vascular disease and found matched-pair analysis of 22 patients with PVD undergoing free flap reconstructions of the lower extremity with end-to-side anastomosis to an autologous venous bypass or an AV loop. Postoperative complications including thromboses did not show significant differences between the groups. Flap failures were absent in both groups. Momeni et al. [16] demonstrated that the placement of AV loops for primary reconstruction in traumatic defects does not increase postoperative complications. Angel et al. [17] reported successful use of the interposition arteriovenous loop graft in free tissue transfers.

The study by Inbal et al. [18] favored planned use of vein grafts as transposition and arteriovenous loops over interposition vein grafts. Different findings in different studies underscore the fact that there are multiple variables involved in complex microsurgical reconstructions, and hence it is hard to draw definitive conclusions in term of superiority of vein grafts versus AV loop. Therefore, the decision to use vein grafts in the form of transposition, arteriovenous loop, or interposition should be individualized according to the specifics of microsurgical flap reconstruction. The principles of microsurgery along with optimal technique and expertise are required for the best possible outcome.

Timing of AV loop placement in relation to the microsurgical flap transfer remains a controversial issue in the literature. A meta-analysis of 35 small case series found a significantly higher rate of major complications and flap failures in reconstructions in which loop placement and free flap transfer had been carried out in two separate surgeries compared to one-stage procedures [19]. The shearing stress on the turning point of the AV loop can create arterialization on the greater curvature and thrombosis on the lesser curvature which may result in vascular pathogenic deterioration.

On the other hand, Marchesini et al. [20] investigating the role of the arteriovenous loop for free flap reconstruction demonstrated the efficacy and feasibility of a two-step intervention in acute posttraumatic events. They suggested a single-step procedure should be preferred in chronic situation and oncologic reconstruction.

Our institutional data also suggest one-stage arteriovenous fistulae (AVF) is associated with lower reexploration rates and better free flap success; two-stage AVF patients are associated with higher graft occlusion and limb amputation rates. The findings in the study by Silva et al. [21] investigating the role of arteriovenous vascular loops in microsurgical reconstruction of the extremities also favor the single-stage reconstruction. However, a recent analysis of 103 AV loop reconstructions by Henn's group, however, did not find any differences in postoperative outcomes with respect to the timing of AV loop placements [22].

Direct vein grafting versus temporary arteriovenous loop reconstruction are viable methods to extend adequate recipient vessel perfusion pressures to within reach of standard pedicle lengths for various fasciocutaneous, muscle, or myocutaneous free tissue flaps to render an otherwise hostile lower extremity and otherwise limited to amputation adequate for limb salvage. Though these methods are typically avoided in standard microsurgical reconstruction, review of the literature suggests that these maneuvers are not only feasible but also safe, with comparable limb salvage rates when compared to primary microsurgical reconstruction.

Certainly, these maneuvers should be limited to patients with severe injury and utilized in situations where standard methods of limb salvage are rendered insufficient due to available recipient options for flap perfusion and where the alternative is amputation. In effect, these maneuvers extend the indications for limb salvage.

In our experience, the principle of maximizing pre-conduit starting pressures by either using the superficial femoral artery or popliteal artery and utilizing sizable great saphenous vein grafting as conduit to have high blood flow by high pressure and large diameter vascular conduit in single-stage arteriovenous loop utilization is an important consideration in maximizing the success of this technique. The theoretical advantage of an arteriovenous loop, whether with a transposition component or not compared to an interposition vein graft, is that it allows physical distention of the vein before anastomosis which ensures patency, prevents twists or kinks, and allows for the checks before flap harvest, minimizing ischemia time. Transposition arteriovenous loops are considered to have an additional advantage due to fewer anastomosis sites.

Further studies should be conducted to further elucidate the indications for direct interposition vein grafting versus immediate or delayed arteriovenous loop utilization. Outcomes will likely depend on clarification of achievable perfusion pressures given differences in pre-conduit starting pressures and conduit characteristics including configuration, diameter, expansibility, length, and their effect on flap perfusion pressures.

Conclusions

Extended long vein grafts are frequently used when free tissue transfer is required and only poor-quality vessels are available in the vicinity of the wound. Arteriovenous fistulas are used when both an arterial and venous gap are present. Allowing for a long maturation time seems to increase the risk of thrombosis of this loop due to kinking, compression, or thrombosis at the curvature resulting from blood flow alterations. Laws of physics dictate that large-caliber conduits and high inflow pressures provide high flow. Increasing the length of these grafts necessarily causes a decrease in flow pressure. For this reason, large-caliber grafts such as the greater saphenous vein are used. Measures need to be taken to avoid a large mismatch between any of the vessels to avoid turbulence at the sites of anastomoses. To compensate for a potential decrease in flow, large-diameter vessels with high flow rates are used as proximal donor vessels whenever possible.

In our experience, one-stage reconstructions with large-caliber grafts, anastomosed to proximal, large-caliber recipient vessels and anastomosed to a sizable donor flap pedicle with little size mismatch were paramount to a high success rate to this difficult reconstructive problem.

More research must be done to fully quantify the relative risk of locating a microsurgical anastomosis within a zone of injury. But beyond these concerns, the use of these adjunct maneuvers can expand the indications for limb salvage in vessel-depleted sites where the alternative is amputation.

References

1. Isenberg JS, Sherman R. Zone of injury: a valid concept in microvascular reconstruction of the traumatized lower limb? Ann Plast Surg. 1996;36(3):270–2.
2. Heller L, Levin LS. Lower extremity microsurgical reconstruction. Plast Reconstr Surg. 2001;108(4):1029–41; quiz 1042.
3. Loos MS, Freeman BG, Lorenzetti A. Zone of injury: a critical review of the literature. Ann Plast Surg. 2010;65(6):573–7.
4. Threlfall GN, Little JM, Cummine J. Free flap transfer—preliminary establishment of an arteriovenous fistula: a case report. Aust N Z J Surg. 1982;52(2):182–4.
5. Grenga TE, Yetman RJ. Temporary arteriovenous shunt prior to free myoosseous flap transfer. Microsurgery. 1987;8(1):2–4.
6. Lin CH, Mardini S, Lin YT, Yeh JT, Wei FC, Chen HC. Sixty-five clinical cases of free tissue transfer using long arteriovenous fistulas or vein grafts. J Trauma. 2004;56(5):1107–17.
7. Cunningham KS, Gotlieb AI. The role of shear stress in the pathogenesis of atherosclerosis. Lab Investig. 2005;85(1):9–23.
8. Slager CJ, Wentzel JJ, Gijsen FJ, Schuurbiers JC, van der Wal AC, van der Steen AF, Serruys PW. The role of shear stress in the generation of rupture-prone vulnerable plaques. Nat Clin Pract Cardiovasc Med. 2005;2(8):401–7.
9. Klitzman B. Microvascular determinants of blood flow. J Reconstr Microsurg. 1987;4(1):77–80.
10. https://en.wikipedia.org/wiki/Hagen%E2%80%93Poiseuille_equation
11. Demiri EC, Hatzokos H, Dionyssiou D, Megalopoulos A, Pitoulias G, Papadimitriou D. Single stage arteriovenous short saphenous loops in microsurgical reconstruction of the lower extremity. Arch Orthop Trauma Surg. 2009;129(4):521–4.
12. Vlastou C, Earle AS. Short saphenous vein grafts as an aid to microsurgical reconstruction of the lower extremity. J Reconstr Microsurg. 1988;4(2):145–54.
13. Khouri RK, Shaw WW. Reconstruction of the lower extremity with microvascular free flaps: a 10-year experience with 304 consecutive cases. J Trauma. 1989;29(8):1086–94.
14. Nelson JA, Fischer JP, Grover R, Kovach SJ, Low DW, Kanchwala SK, Levin LS, Serletti JM, Wu LC. Vein grafting your way out of trouble: examining the utility and efficacy of vein grafts in microsurgery. J Plast Reconstr Aesthet Surg. 2015;68(6):830–6.
15. Henn D, Bigdeli AK, Horsch M, Weiß C, Kühner C, Hirche C, Schmidt VJ, Kneser U. Venous bypass grafts versus arteriovenous loops as recipient vessels for microvascular anastomosis in lower

extremity reconstructions: a matched-pair analysis. Microsurgery. 2020;40(1):12–8.

16. Momeni A, Lanni MA, Levin LS, Kovach SJ. Does the use of arteriovenous loops increase complications rates in posttraumatic microsurgical lower extremity reconstruction?-a matched-pair analysis. Microsurgery. 2018;38(6):605–10.
17. Angel MF, Chang B, Clark N, Wong L, Ringelman P, Manson PN. Further clinical use of the interposition arteriovenous loop graft in free tissue transfers. Microsurgery. 1993;14(8):479–81.
18. Inbal A, Silva AK, Humphries LS, Teven CM, Gottlieb LJ. Bridging the gap: a 20-year experience with vein grafts for free flap reconstruction. The odds for success. Plast Reconstr Surg. 2018;142(3):786–94.
19. Knackstedt R, Aliotta R, Gatherwright J, Djohan R, Gastman B, Schwarz G, Hendrickson M, Gurunluoglu R. Single-stage versus two-stage arteriovenous loop microsurgical reconstruction: a meta-analysis of the literature. Microsurgery. 2018;38(6):706–17.
20. Marchesini A, Senesi L, De Francesco F, Pangrazi PP, Campodonico A, Politano R, Riccio M. Efficacy of the arteriovenous loop for free flap reconstruction in patients with complex limb trauma: case series and literature review. Medicina (Kaunas). 2020;56(11):632.
21. Silva GB, Veronesi BA, Torres LR, Imaguchi RB, Cho AB, Nakamoto HA. Role of arteriovenous venous loops in microsurgical reconstruction of the extremities. Acta Ortop Bras. 2018;26(2):127–30.
22. Henn D, Wähmann MST, Horsch M, Hetjens S, Kremer T, Gazyakan E, Hirche C, Schmidt VJ, Germann G, Kneser U. One-stage versus two-stage arteriovenous loop reconstructions: an experience on 103 cases from a single center. Plast Reconstr Surg. 2019;143(3):912–24.

43 Recipient Vessels for Spine and Posterior Trunk Reconstruction

Alexander F. Mericli

Introduction

The posterior trunk is regarded by many microsurgeons as one of the few "watershed" areas for microsurgical reconstruction, with no readily available recipient vessels. In general, if the flap does not possess a sufficiently long pedicle, either a vein graft or arteriovenous (AV) loop will be required. Whereas posterior trunk reconstruction is associated with superficial wounds with exposed bone or hardware, spinal reconstruction is conducted deep within the posterior trunk and is therefore associated with an entirely different set of recipient vessel options. Patients who require a vascularized bone flap to supplement their spinal reconstruction are rare, with such cases representing only a small percentage of all spine operations. Although an oncologic resection is the most common indication, other spinal defects necessitating a bone flap may result from vertebral osteomyelitis, trauma, or progressive symptomatic spinal deformity [1–9].

Vertebral defects greater than 4 cm reconstructed with nonvascularized bone graft are associated with a 50% nonunion rate [10–13]. This is a serious complication, often resulting in spinal instability and potential subsequent neurologic sequelae [14, 15]. Vascularized bone flaps in the spine are an independent predictor of union and have also been shown to increase the union rate and improve its durability in these challenging wounds [1–8].

Ultimately, the advantages conferred by the use of vascularized bone for spinal reconstruction are entirely dependent upon the ability to revascularize the transferred osseous unit. As such, recipient vessel identification is a very important component of these cases and one upon which the overall success of the reconstruction is highly contingent. Microvascular reconstruction along the spine and posterior trunk is notorious for its difficulty due to limited exposure, the proximity to vital neurovascular structures, and the paucity of adequate recipient vessels.

Preoperative Planning

Thoughtful preoperative planning is imperative for the successful spine or posterior trunk free tissue transfer. Several unique factors must be considered:

- Since these surgeries are typically multidisciplinary affairs, in what order will the different surgical services be present during the surgery and how will this impact the plastic surgeon?
- Should the surgery be staged over a number of days? If so, at what stage should the flap be harvested? Should it be harvested and banked for later transfer, or should it be harvested and transferred during the same stage?
- Can the flap be raised while the wound is being debrided or the tumor being resected?
- From where will the flap be harvested?
- Will a position change be needed between flap harvest and revascularization? If so, the recipient vessels should be identified and fully prepared prior to ligating the pedicle, in order to minimize ischemia time.
- If a prolonged ischemia time is a possibility – such as when repositioning is required between flap harvest and revascularization – then an ice water bath should be available to reduce the flap's metabolic rate while it is ischemic.

Although a dedicated CTA or MRA is not recommended for the singular purpose of vessel detection, if preoperative imaging has been performed for another indication, the reconstructive surgeon should take advantage of it in order to identify potential recipient vessel options.

If possible, the plastic surgeon should choose a flap that can be harvested without requiring an intraoperative position change. Soft tissue flaps that can be reliably harvested in the

A. F. Mericli (✉)
Department of Plastic Surgery, The University of Texas M.D. Anderson Cancer Center, Houston, TX, USA
e-mail: AFMericli@mdanderson.org

R. Gurunian, R. Djohan (eds.), *Recipient Vessels in Reconstructive Microsurgery*,
https://doi.org/10.1007/978-3-030-75389-4_43

prone position include the latissimus dorsi (LD), thoracodorsal artery perforator (TDAP), scapular/parascapular, profunda artery perforator (PAP), superior gluteal artery perforator (SGAP), and inferior gluteal artery perforator (IGAP). Osseous flaps that can be harvested prone include the scapular and fibular free flaps.

The recipient vessels should be identified and prepared prior to flap ischemia. If a vein graft is needed, then the vein graft should be harvested and anastomosed to the recipient artery and vein as a flow-through AV loop and allowed to perfuse and dilate while the flap is being harvested and transferred to the recipient site. This strategy works to further limit ischemia time because only one set of microvascular anastomoses needs to be performed to restore flap perfusion.

Applied Anatomy: Posterior Trunk

Recipient vessel options are related to the defect location, with the most accessible vessels available along the posterior neck and superior thoracic spine/posterior chest wall (Fig. 43.1). For the posterior neck, branches of the external carotid are options as are the transverse cervical vessels [16] (also see Chap. 6). For the posterior chest wall, branches from the subscapular system are most amenable; these include the circumflex scapular, serratus branch, and the thoracodorsal vessels. Intercostal perforating vessels are also potentially available and are located variably along the entire posterior thorax, between the latissimus dorsi muscle and chest wall [17, 18]. Options for inferior thoracic, lumbar, and

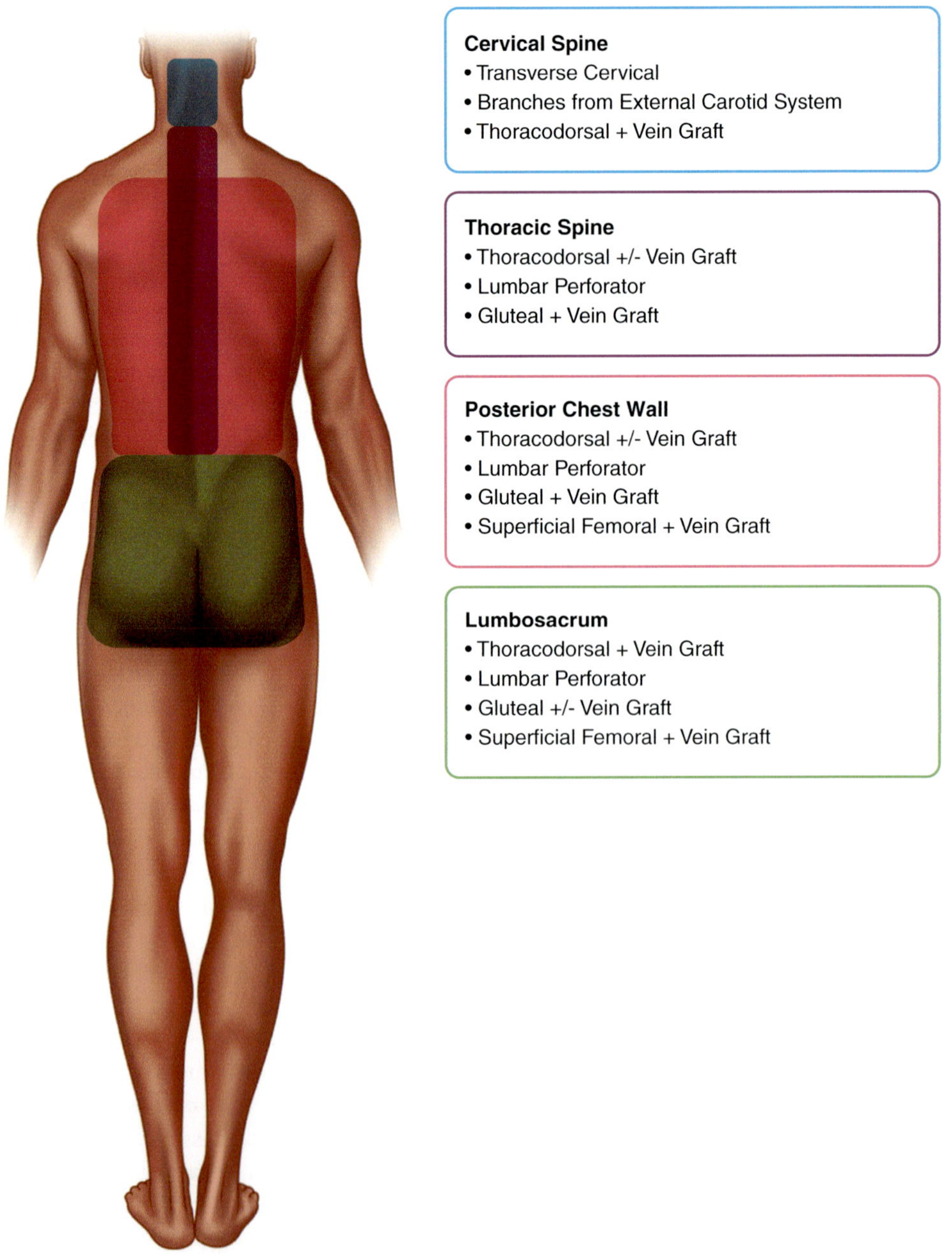

Fig. 43.1 Diagram depicting recipient vessel options for posterior trunk free tissue transfer, according to defect location

sacral defects include the superior and inferior gluteal vessels (Chaps. 22 and 23).

The subscapular artery, which emerges from the axillary artery, is 2–3 mm in diameter and short in length (1–3 cm). It is typically accompanied by one vein (3–4 mm diameter). As the subscapular artery travels inferiorly through the axilla, it branches into the circumflex scapular artery and the thoracodorsal artery. The circumflex scapular artery travels through the triangular space to emerge superficial to the scapula where it becomes a cutaneous vessel perfusing the area of the scapular and parascapular fasciocutaneous flaps. After the circumflex scapular artery branch point, the thoracodorsal artery continues inferiorly for 2–3 cm before it gives off one or two branches to the serratus anterior muscle. The thoracodorsal artery then travels another 3–5 cm inferiorly before terminating in the latissimus dorsi muscle. In general, the thoracodorsal, serratus branch, and circumflex scapular arteries are each accompanied by one or two suitable recipient veins measuring 2.5–3.5 mm in diameter.

Both the superior and inferior gluteal arteries are terminal branches of the internal iliac artery. They exit the pelvis superior and inferior to the pyriformis muscle, respectively, supplying the upper and lower half of the gluteus maximus muscle and overlying skin and subcutaneous tissue. After it exits the greater sciatic foramen, above the pyriformis muscle, the superior gluteal artery is 2–3 mm in diameter and 2–3 cm in length. This is the most optimal location for a microvascular anastomosis, as the vessels become significantly smaller as they travel distally. At this point the vessels are located deep to the gluteus maximus muscle and gluteus medius muscle, but superficial to the gluteus minimus (Fig. 43.2). The point at which the inferior gluteal vessels emerge from the pelvis, inferior to the pyriformis muscle, is in close proximity to posterior femoral cutaneous nerve of the thigh. The sciatic nerve is immediately deep to the inferior gluteal vessels at this location, and great care must be taken to not disturb this important structure.

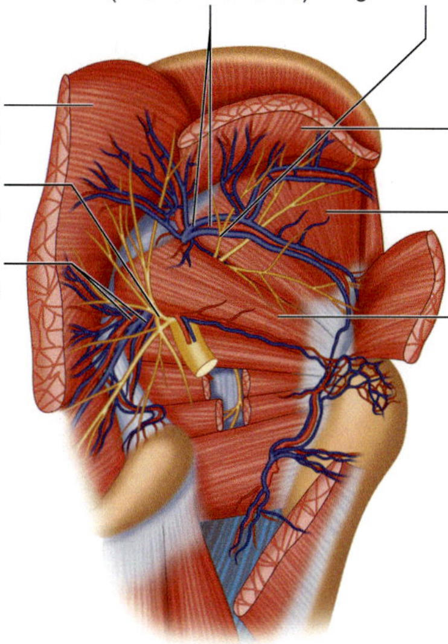

Fig. 43.2 Associated anatomy of the superior and inferior gluteal vessels

Applied Anatomy: Spine

Cervical spine defects necessitating a free tissue transfer rarely present considerable difficulty, considering the numerous high-quality, easily accessible recipient vessels in this area. Any external carotid artery branch, such as the facial vessels (2–3 mm diameter) or lingual vessels (2–2.5 mm diameter), as well as the transverse cervical (2–3 mm diameter), is a potential option.

The choices are significantly more limited along the thoracic spine. Ideally, a thoracic segmental artery can be identified along with an accompanying vein. These vessels branch directly from the aorta and travel posteriorly along the vertebral body (Fig. 43.3). Both the artery and vein are 2–2.5 mm in diameter. Most commonly, microsurgery along the thoracic spine is performed through the thoracotomy that was used to obtain anterior spinal exposure. This approach provides access to the thoracic segmental vessels for end-to-end anastomosis, as well as to the aorta for an end-to-side anastomosis. Venous options include the accompanying thoracic segmental vein, the azygous vein (for right-sided approaches), or the hemiazygos vein (for left-sided approaches). Occasionally, the thoracic spine will be approached by the spine surgeon through a midline sternotomy. This approach provides access to additional recipient vessels, notably the internal mammary artery and vein(s), which most microsurgeons are familiar with, given their utility for breast reconstruction. The internal mammary vessels can be dissected away from the musculoskeletal chest wall in order to provide adequate length to reach any thoracic spine defect [19].

Recipient options in the thoracolumbar and lumbar spine are also problematic. The approach to these vessels is through the same incision used to expose the anterior spine, usually a thoraco-phrenico-laparotomy or lumbotomy. The thoracic and lumbar segmental vessels – as they emerge from the aorta and inferior vena cava – are the first choice but are often deep within the body cavity and therefore exceedingly difficult to reach. Furthermore, they are thin-walled and easily damaged. The gastroepiploic vessels via the omentum are another option; the omentum can be transposed to a posterior extraperitoneal location adjacent to the spine, in close proximity to the vertebral defect. The common, external, and internal iliac vessels are often exposed and available for end-to-side anastomosis for lumbosacral spinal defects.

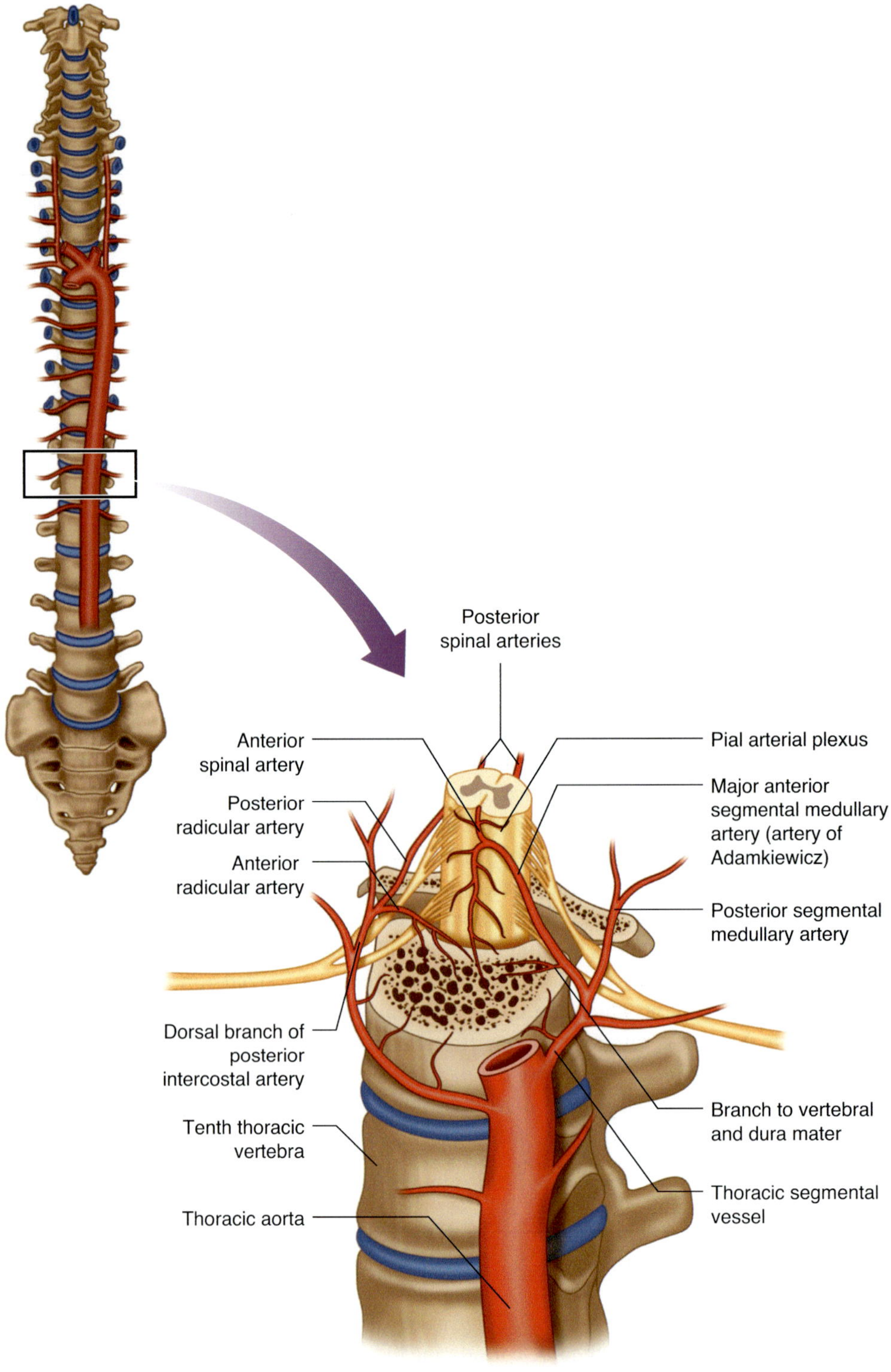

Fig. 43.3 Illustration demonstrating the relationship between the thoracic vertebra, aorta, and segmental vasculature. Each thoracic or lumbar segmental artery is 2–2.5 mm and can serve as a reliable recipient. If a vertebrectomy is being performed, the spine surgeon should carefully elevate the segmental vessels away from the vertebral body so that they are not injured during the extirpative portion of the surgery

Surgical Technique

Posterior Neck

The surgical technique for exposure and dissection of the external carotid artery and its branches can be reviewed in-depth in the head and neck section of this text book (also see Chaps. 2, 3 and 5). Soft tissue defects along the posterior neck, such as exposed hardware or bone, will likely require a longer recipient vessel/pedicle length than bony defects. As such, a vein graft or AV loop is necessary to reach the more anteriorly located external carotid branches. This will necessitate the patient being positioned in the lateral decubitus, in order to access the recipient vessels, perform the microanastomosis, and inset the flap without a position change.

Posterior Chest Wall

The subscapular vascular axis is considered the first-line recipient vessel system for defects along the posterior chest wall. These vessels can be accessed from the prone or decubitus positions. If the axilla has not been dissected as part of the defect, the subscapular axis is approached through a transverse incision between the anterior and posterior axillary folds, immediately inferior to the axillary hair line. The lateral border of the pectoralis major muscle is defined, and the axillary fat is entered directly posterior to this. The lateral thoracic vein is typically first encountered and should be spared for a potential outflow source. Spreading in the axillary fat just posterior to the origin of the lateral thoracic vein usually reveals the proximal portion of the thoracodorsal vessels and nerve. The thoracodorsal vessels can be dissected superiorly to identify the serratus anterior branch, the circumflex scapular branch, and the subscapular source vessel. Self-retaining retractors are useful for this dissection; with proper retraction, it is unnecessary to remove any of the lymphatic tissue. The thoracodorsal vessels should be circumferentially dissected from where they enter the latissimus dorsi muscle to where they emerge from the subclavian; the entire subscapular vascular axis can then be transposed posteriorly and medially in order to place these recipient vessels in closer proximity to the posterior chest wall defect. If the thoracodorsal vessels are found to be unusable due to prior surgery, the circumflex scapular vessels should be examined since they are not usually injured by previous axillary surgery.

Soft Tissue Defects Along the Lumbar Back and Sacral Area

The gluteal vessels are the first-line recipient vessel option for soft tissue defects along the lumbosacral posterior trunk. These vessels can be accessed from the prone or decubitus positions; anatomic landmarks are helpful. With the hip subtly flexed and internally rotated, a line is drawn from the posterior superior iliac spine (PSIS) to the posterior superior angle of the greater trochanter. The point of emergence of the superior gluteal artery from the upper part of the greater sciatic foramen corresponds to the junction of the upper and middle thirds of this line (also see Chap. 22). A second line is drawn from the PSIS to the outer part of the ischial tuberosity; the junction of the lower and middle third marks the location of where the inferior gluteal vessels exit from the pelvis, inferior to the piriformis muscle (also see Chap. 23).

Cervical Spine

The recipient vessel approach for cervical spine bony defects is determined by the exposure used by the spine surgeon. An anterolateral approach is favored to expose the vertebral body and reach recipient vessels for vertebral defects inferior to C3. For high defects involving C1, C2, or the suboccipital condyles and skull base, a combined dorsal, lateral, and trans-oral approach is often necessary. If an anterior trans-oral mandible-splitting pharyngotomy approach was used, then the facial and lingual vessels may be easily within reach. However, if the external carotid branches are not exposed via this approach, then accessing the facial vessels through a submandibular counter incision may be a better option.

Thoracic Spine

The selection of recipient vessels depends on the approach to the vertebral body and should be carefully planned in conjunction with the spine surgeon. Most commonly, a thoracotomy is performed to gain access to the thoracic vertebral bodies. This provides reasonable access to the spine, but the approach is complicated by the fact that the spine and associated recipient vessels are located deep within a cavity with a very narrow opening. This makes microvascular anastomosis with standard instruments and magnification technology impossible (Fig. 43.4). Special elongated microsurgical instruments are imperative for performing such an anastomosis. Additionally, standard microvascular surgical microscopes have a focal length that is incompatible with a deep thoracotomy cavity. We therefore recommend using a neurosurgical or spinal surgical microscope which has a longer working focal length. The first-line option for recipient arter-

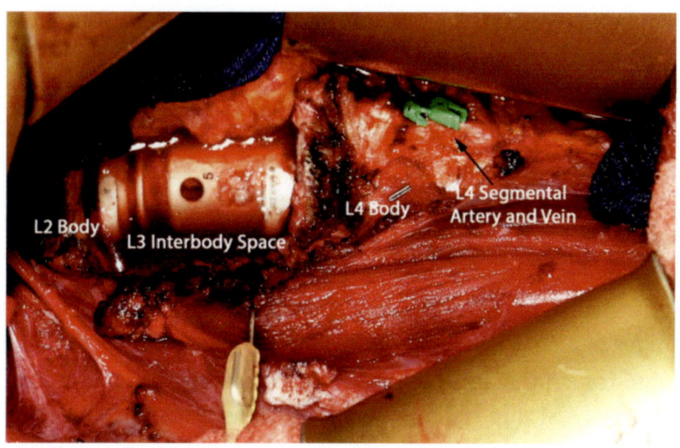

Fig. 43.4 Defect after L3 vertebrectomy for chordoma. An expandable interbody cage is seen in the L3 interbody space. The fibula will be placed alongside the cage to biologically enhance the fusion. The L4 lumbar segmental recipient artery and vein are visualized as they travel from anterior to posterior along the L4 body. The vessels are temporarily occluded with green microvascular clamps

ies and veins along the thoracic spine is the thoracic segmental vessels, emerging from the aorta and traveling to the IVC, respectively. If segmental vessels are not available, an end-to-side anastomosis to the aortal or IVC is another option. In this situation, the aorta can be partially occluded with a Satinsky clamp while still allowing distal perfusion. Care must be taken to ensure that the mesenteric or renal arteries are not occluded when the clamp is applied. Furthermore, once the clamp is applied, dorsalis pedis pulses should be checked to ensure that distal flow is adequate. An arteriotomy is performed with a 2 or 3 mm aortic punch, and the flap's artery is anastomosed to the aorta with interrupted 8-0 Nylon sutures in the standard fashion. The Satinsky clamp is then removed, and distal pulses are checked again. This technique is not recommended in older patients with atherosclerosis and those with aortic disease or prior aortic surgery.

Lumbosacral Spine

Approaches to the anterior lumbosacral spine are either through a lumbotomy or through a midline laparotomy, with the latter being favored for sacrectomy. This is likely to be the most difficult region for microvascular anastomosis due to the depth of the approach. Lumbar segmental vessels are first choice but are difficult to reach, necessitating specialized microsurgical instruments and magnification. In this region, an innovative mind-set is necessary. Through a right-sided approach, the IVC can be reached for an end-to-side anastomosis, but the aorta will be inaccessible. Similarly, for a left-sided approach, the aorta can be reached for an end-to-side anastomosis, but the IVC will be inaccessible. As Winters and colleagues suggest, if no local recipient vessels can be found, a large AV loop saphenous vein transposition can be performed. In this technique, the saphenous vein is identified anterior to the medial malleolus and circumferentially dissected to the saphenofemoral junction. The junction is maintained, and the distal saphenous vein is anastomosed end to side to the femoral artery, creating an AV loop. The loop can then be tunneled into the defect and act as a recipient source [20] (also see Chaps. 18 and 42).

For sacrectomies, both bone and soft tissue flaps are usually necessary [21]. A pedicled vertical rectus abdominis myocutaneous (VRAM) flap can be harvested during the anterior approach, which is performed through a laparotomy. The VRAM flap is banked within the pelvis and re-accessed during the second stage, which is performed in the prone position. The superior epigastric vessels along the superior extent of the VRAM flap can be utilized as recipient vessels for the free bone flap [22]. If the superior epigastric vessels are inadequate, then the internal or external iliac vessels are typically in close proximity and can be accessed in an end-to-side fashion. Vein grafts are commonly needed to reach the iliacs in this situation [21]. Most often, the bone flap is fixated first, prior to performing the anastomosis. Considering this, the reconstructive surgeon must ensure that the recipient vessels will remain easily accessible after fixation of the flap. If the flap itself will obscure the recipient vessels after fixation, then a small AV loop can be made prior to flap fixation to bring the recipient vessels to a more superficial, easily accessible location [23].

Discussion

Considering the limited recipient vessel options along the posterior trunk and spine, it is fortunate that free tissue transfer is not commonly indicated for defects in these anatomic regions. There are a multitude of local and regional paired muscle and myocutaneous flap options along the posterior trunk – such as the paraspinous, latissimus dorsi, and trapezius – as well as a number of fasciocutaneous and perforator flap options. As such, it is only in the direst circumstances (multiple failed flaps, radiation injury, multiple same-site surgeries, etc.) that a free flap is indicated for soft tissue resurfacing, bone coverage, or hardware protection along the back [24]. Regarding the spine, vascularized bone flaps are only truly indicated after a biomechanically destabilizing vertebrectomy in a patient with a normal life expectancy. Examples include extensive vertebral osteomyelitis, failed symptomatic nonunion after an initial attempt with a nonvascularized graft, and oncologic vertebrectomy for primary bone tumors. Symptomatic spinal metastases frequently require a destabilizing vertebrectomy, but due to the limited life expectancy of a patient with metastatic cancer, a hardware-only fusion – without a bone flap – is considered sufficient [1].

In our institutional experience with free tissue transfer for soft tissue defects along the posterior trunk, the most common indication was an oncologic resection (69%) or chronic radiation wound (31%). Nearly 40% of flaps required a vein graft to reach the recipient vessels. Recipient vessel choice was dictated by the location of the defect. The three most common recipient arteries were the subscapular/thoracodorsal (31%), superior or inferior gluteal (19%), and external carotid branch (15%). The three most common recipient veins were the subscapular/thoracodorsal (27%), internal jugular branch or external jugular (23%), and gluteal (19%).

Regarding free fibula flaps for the mobile spine, all cases in our series were primary bone tumors with the most common being a chordoma [1]. Lumbar or thoracic segmental vessels were the most common recipients with vein grafts utilized in up to 25% of anastomoses. Several uncommon recipient vessels were employed in our series, which bear mentioning. In one case which necessitated a splenectomy as a component of the curative oncologic resection, the peroneal artery and vein of the free fibula flap were anastomosed to the splenic artery and vein. In another case, no lumbar or segmental vessels were present along the aorta, and the area of exposed aorta was along the celiac trunk, preventing end-to-side anastomosis. The omentum was transposed through the diaphragm and into the thoracic cavity, placing the gastroepiploic vessels in close proximity to the spine and providing a convenient anastomotic site for the peroneal vessels of the fibula flap. If a recipient vein is not found along the thoracic spine, Winters and colleagues report using the thoracic duct as an outflow source [20, 25]. Although spinal reconstructive microsurgery is uncommon, a multitude of recipient vessels options exist for the creative and innovative plastic surgeon.

In our institutional experience using free fibula flaps to reconstruct the spinopelvic junction after total sacrectomy, the iliacs were the most common recipient vessels [21]. Of ten patients, the internal iliacs were used in three, the superior epigastrics via the VRAM flap in three, the external iliacs in two, and the common iliacs in two. All anastomoses were performed in an end-to-side fashion, and 70% required a vein graft.

Conclusion

Although the indications are few, microvascular reconstruction can be safely and reliably performed for defects associated with the spine and posterior trunk. Due to the limited recipient vessel options, vein grafts and AV loops are common and should be planned for. Specialized elongated microsurgical instruments and a surgical microscope with a longer focal length are imperative for successfully performing free vascularized bone flap reconstruction for spinal defects.

References

1. Mericli AF, Boukovalas S, Rhines LD, et al. Free fibula flap for restoration of spinal stability after oncologic vertebrectomy is predictive of bony union. Plast Reconstr Surg. 2020;145:219.
2. Houdek MT, Rose PS, Bakri K, et al. Outcomes and complications of reconstruction with use of free vascularized fibular graft for spinal and pelvic defects following resection of a malignant tumor. J Bone Joint Surg Am. 2017;99:e69.
3. Moran SL, Bakri K, Mardini S, Shin AY, Bishop AT. The use of vascularized fibular grafts for the reconstruction of spinal and sacral defects. Microsurgery. 2009;29:393–400.
4. Aliano KA, Agulnick M, Cohen B, et al. Spinal reconstruction for osteomyelitis with free vascularized fibular grafts using intra-abdominal recipient vessels: a series of three cases. Microsurgery. 2013;33:560–6.
5. Lee MJ, Ondra SL, Mindea SA, Fine NA, Dumanian GA. Indications and rationale for use of vascularized fibula bone flaps in cervical spine arthrodeses. Plast Reconstr Surg. 2005;116:1–7.
6. Wuisman PI, Jiya TU, Van Dijk M, Sugihara S, Van Royen BJ, Winters HA. Free vascularized bone graft in spinal surgery: indications and outcome in eight cases. Eur Spine J. 1999;8:296–303.
7. Yanamadala V, Rozman PA, Kumar JI, et al. Vascularized fibular strut autografts in spinal reconstruction after resection of vertebral chordoma or chondrosarcoma: a retrospective series. Neurosurgery. 2017;81:156–64.
8. Winters HA, van Engeland AE, Jiya TU, van Royen BJ. The use of free vascularised bone grafts in spinal reconstruction. J Plast Reconstr Aesthet Surg. 2010;63:516–23.
9. Erdmann D, Meade RA, Lins RE, McCann RL, Richardson WJ, Levin LS. Use of the microvascular free fibula transfer as a salvage reconstruction for failed anterior spine surgery due to chronic osteomyelitis. Plast Reconstr Surg. 2006;117:2438–45.
10. Bradford DS, Daher YH. Vascularised rib grafts for stabilization of kyphosis. J Bone Joint Surg Br. 1986;68:357–61.
11. Saraph VJ, Bach CM, Krismer M, Wimmer C. Evaluation of spinal fusion using autologous anterior strut grafts and posterior instrumentation for thoracic/thoracolumbar kyphosis. Spine (Phila Pa 1976). 2005;30:1594–601.
12. Bradford DS, Ganjavian S, Antonious D, Winter RB, Lonstein JE, Moe JH. Anterior strut grafting for the treatment of kyphosis: review of experience with forty-eight patients. J Bone Joint Surg Am. 1982;64:680–90.
13. Lonstein JE, Winter RB. Long multiple struts for severe kyphosis. Clin Orthop Relat Res. 2002;394:130–8.
14. Jenkins DH, Hodgson AR, Yau AC, et al. Stabilization of the spine in the surgical treatment of severe spinal tuberculosis in children. Clin Orthop Relat Res. 1975;110:69–80.
15. Rajasekaran S, Soundarapandian S. Progression of kyphosis in tuberculosis of the spine treated by anterior arthrodesis. J Bone Joint Surg Am. 1989;71:1314–23.
16. Yu P. The transverse cervical vessels as recipient vessels for previously treated head and neck cancer patients. Plast Reconstr Surg. 2005;115(5):1253–8.
17. Lee YJ, Baek SE, Lee J, Oh DY, Rhie JW, Moon SH. Perforating vessel as an alternative option of a recipient selection for posterior trunk-free flap reconstruction. Microsurgery. 2018;38:763–71.
18. Aho JM, Laungani AT, Herbig KS, Wong C, Kirchoff RW, Saint-Cyr M. Lumbar and thoracic perforators: vascular anatomy and clinical implications. Plast Reconstr Surg. 2014;134:635e–45e.
19. Hu H, Winters HAH, Paul RMA, Wuisman PIJM. Internal thoracic vessels used as a pedicle graft for anastomosis with vascularized bone graft to reconstruct C7-T3 spinal defects. Spine. 2007;32:601–5.
20. Winters HAH, Kraak J, Oosterhuis JWA, de Kleuver M. Spinal reconstruction with free vascularised bone grafts; approaches and selection of acceptor vessels. Scand J Surg. 2013;102:42–8.
21. Mericli AF, Boukovalas S, Roubaud MS, Chu CK, Bird J, Lewis VO, Rhines LD, Chang EI, Adelman DM, Hanasono MM. Restoration of spinopelvic continuity with the free fibula flap after limb-sparing oncologic resection is associated with a high union rate and superior functional outcomes. Plast Reconstr Surg. 2020;146(3):650–62.
22. Garvey PB, Clemens MW, Rhines LD, Sacks JM. Vertical rectus abdominis musculocutaneous flow-through flap to a free fibula flap for total sacrectomy reconstruction. Microsurgery. 2013;33:32–8.
23. Agrawal N, MV DF, Bird JE, Mericli AF. Avoiding a hemicorporectomy with bilateral free fibula flaps in a tripod configuration after massive spinopelvic osteosarcoma resection. Microsurgery. 2020;27(2):380–4.
24. Akdeniz Z, Roubaud MS, Kapur SK, et al. Free flap reconstruction of posterior trunk soft tissue defects: single institution experience and systematic literature review. Plast Reconstr Surg. 2020;147(3):728–40.
25. Winters HA. The thoracic duct as a venous receptor vessel for free flap transplantation. Plast Reconstr Surg. 1998;101:872–3.

Recipient Vessels for Genital Reconstruction

44

Alireza Hamidian Jahromi, Deana Shenaq, Jenna Rose Stoehr, and Loren S. Schechter

Introduction

Genital reconstruction, specifically gender affirmation surgery (GAS), has become increasingly linked with microsurgery, such that genital reconstruction without microsurgical expertise is now unimaginable. While advances in microsurgical techniques and instrumentation revolutionized phalloplasty procedures [1, 2], they also translated to advances in transfeminine genital reconstruction, including both peritoneal and intestinal vaginoplasty [3–5]. In addition to gender-affirming surgical procedures, free tissue transfers may also be employed in the reconstruction of inguinal and perineal defects [6].

Multiple recipient vessels are utilized for free tissue transfer in the genital region. The most commonly utilized recipient vessels are the common femoral artery and its branches and the branches of the femoral vein, including the great saphenous vein (GSV) [7–14]. The branches of the common femoral artery include the superficial circumflex iliac artery (SCIA), the superficial inferior epigastric artery (SIEA) (also see Chap. 19), the superficial external pudendal artery (SEPA), and the deep external pudendal artery (DEPA). The common femoral artery divides into the profunda and superficial branches, and the medial and lateral femoral circumflex arteries (MFCA and LFCA) arise as branches from the profunda femoral artery. The LFCA further divides into ascending, transverse, and descending branches (also see Chaps. 30 and 31). The descending branch of the LFCA represents the vascular supply of the anterolateral thigh flap (ALT), but it may also be used as a recipient vessel for free tissue transfer. The superficial femoral artery (SFA) continues distally in the thigh (Table 44.1, Fig. 44.1) (also see Chap. 32). In terms of recipient veins, in addition to the saphenous vein, additional venous options include the superficial circumflex iliac vein (SCIV) and the inferior epigastric veins, both superficial and deep branches (SIEV and DIEV, respectively).

Supplementary Information The online version of this chapter (https://doi.org/10.1007/978-3-030-75389-4_44) contains supplementary material, which is available to authorized users.

A. Hamidian Jahromi · D. Shenaq
Plastic and Reconstructive Surgery Department, Rush University Medical Center, Chicago, IL, USA
e-mail: Deana_Shenaq@rush.edu

J. R. Stoehr
Feinberg School of Medicine, Northwestern University, Chicago, IL, USA
e-mail: jenna.stoehr@northwestern.edu

L. S. Schechter (✉)
Plastic and Reconstructive Surgery Department, Rush University Medical Center, Chicago, IL, USA

The Center for Gender Confirmation Surgery, Weiss Memorial Hospital, The University of Illinois at Chicago, Chicago, IL, USA

Table 44.1 Surgical anatomy of the common femoral artery and its branches

Artery (abbreviation)	Anatomical description	Mean diameter (range)[a]
Common femoral (CFA)	Continuation of external iliac artery	6.6 (3.9–8.9) [29]
Superficial circumflex iliac (SCIA)	First or second branch of CFA (can also arise from common trunk with SIEA)	1.92 (1.2–3) [45]
Superficial inferior epigastric (SIEA)	First or second branch of (can also arise from common trunk with SIEA)	1.6 (0.75–3.5) [32]
Superficial external pudendal (SEPA)	Third branch of CFA	1.2–3.8[b] [46]
Deep external pudendal (DEPA)	Fourth branch of CFA	0.6[c] [47]
Medial femoral circumflex (MFCA)	First branch of DFA (can also arise from CFA)	3.0 (2.0–4.1) [48]
Lateral femoral circumflex (LFCA)	Second branch of DFA (can also arise from CFA)	4.9 (2.4–8.0) [49]
Deep femoral (DFA)	Final branch of CFA	4.9 (2.7–7.6) [29]
Superficial femoral (SFA)	Continuation of CFA	5.2 (2.5–9.6) [29]

[a]Figures are expressed in millimeters
[b]Mean is not available
[c]Range is not available

R. Gurunian, R. Djohan (eds.), *Recipient Vessels in Reconstructive Microsurgery*, https://doi.org/10.1007/978-3-030-75389-4_44

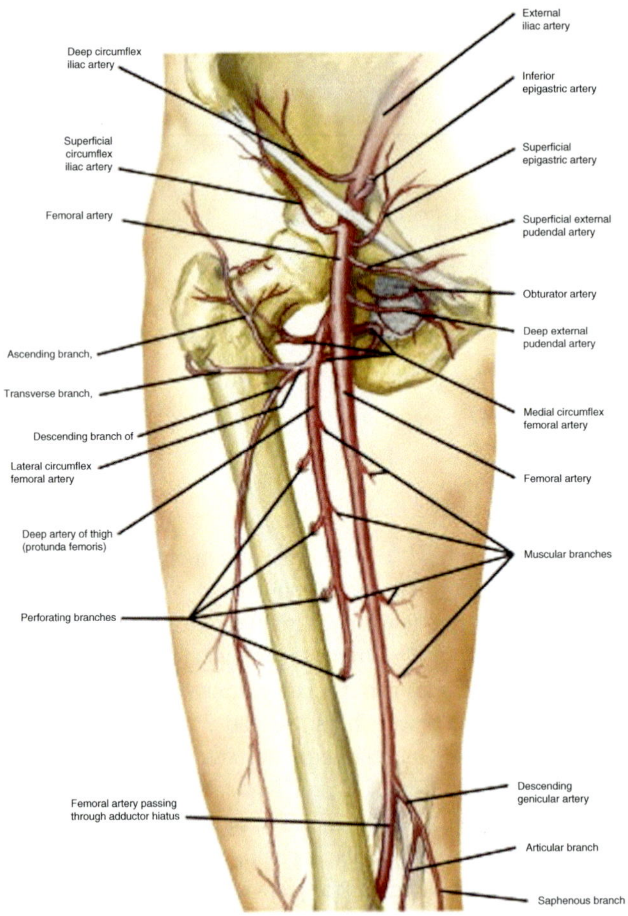

Fig. 44.1 Branches of common femoral artery (reprinted from Netter's Surgical Anatomy and Approaches, Wang JC, Chap. 37: Exposure of the Common Femoral Artery and Vein, Pages 439–448, Copyright 2014, with permission from Elsevier)

Additional options for recipient vessels include the deep inferior epigastric artery (DIEA), a branch of external iliac artery, and its corresponding vein, the DIEV [9, 10, 15–17] (also see Chap. 15). Venous outflow can be accomplished with a single venous anastomosis, but multiple venous anastomoses (minimum two) are often performed in order to augment flap drainage [12]. Arteriovenous (AV) loops (also see Chap. 42), using a saphenous vein graft, can increase recipient vessel length and are particularly advantageous when using a radial forearm free flap (RFFF) (Video 44.1).

Preoperative Assessment

Preoperative assessment and planning are paramount to the success of any free tissue transfer. Understanding the patient's goals and expectations helps to clarify the reconstructive requirements and also facilitates a shared decision-making approach. In addition, the overall health and clinical condition of the patient is assessed by performing a thorough history and physical examination [18].

The history should include information about previous surgeries, including abdominal, pelvic, and genital procedures (i.e., abdominoplasty, inguinal hernia repair, open hysterectomy). Comorbidities, such as increased age, atherosclerotic disease, diabetes, and peripheral vascular disease, may limit microsurgical options. Lifestyle habits that adversely affect the vascular system and/or compromise wound healing, such as tobacco use and nutritional deficiencies, should also be investigated [19]. For individuals taking testosterone, a complete blood count should be obtained prior to surgery. Testosterone may increase the hematocrit, leading to increased coagulability [20]. If patients are polycythemic, testosterone may be discontinued prior to surgery. While it may not be possible to treat all medical conditions within a brief preoperative window, attempts should be made to optimize the patient's condition prior to surgery, especially for elective procedures. A proactive approach may help to avoid selection of recipient arteries with extensive calcifications (which increase the risk of thrombosis) or selection of smaller recipient vessels which can be prone to spasm and may increase the technical difficulty of the anastomosis [21].

Physical examination provides important information that may influence the reconstructive plan. The patient's body habitus and body mass index (BMI) play a role in both flap and recipient vessel choice. Obesity is associated with an increased rate of complications, including dehiscence, delayed wound healing, and flap loss [22, 23], and may also increase the difficulty of accessing recipient vessels in the abdominal and groin regions. A vascular exam, including palpation of femoral, posterior tibial, and dorsalis pedis, should be performed, and when considering a RFF, an Allen's test should be performed (also see Chaps. 25 and 26). However, the reliability of the Allen's test has been called into question. If there is suspicion of an incomplete palmar arch, a color Doppler ultrasound may be useful for further evaluation [24].

Preoperative radiographic and/or sonographic imaging of the recipient vasculature is not routinely obtained when the clinical exam is unremarkable. However, preoperative imaging should be considered if there is a concern, such as vascular insufficiency, significant vascular comorbidities, a history of trauma to the area, and/or an abnormal physical examination. The presence of scars may warrant further evaluation as to the potential for disruption of the vascular anatomy. The choice of imaging studies and/or radiographic evaluation is individualized and depends upon the surgeon's preference and/or institutional testing availability. Imaging studies may include color Doppler ultrasound, computerized tomography angiogram (CTA), magnetic resonance angiography (MRA), or conventional angiography, the latter of which is considered by many as the "gold standard" vascular study.

Applied Anatomy

The anatomy of the lower abdomen, groin, and the upper thigh has been studied extensively. The common femoral artery (CFA) originates as an extension of the external iliac artery (EIA) as it passes beneath the inguinal ligament

(Fig. 44.1). The course of the femoral artery can be approximated at the skin surface by drawing a line connecting the mid-inguinal point (the midpoint between the pubic symphysis and the anterior superior iliac spine (ASIS)) and the adductor tubercle, while the hip is flexed, abducted, and rotated laterally [25, 26]. The mid-inguinal point is considered to be a relatively consistent landmark for the origin of the CFA, as the CFA tends to lie within 1.5 cm of this point [26]. The CFA continues for 4–5 cm distal to the inguinal ligament, giving rise to the superficial circumflex iliac artery (SCIA), the superficial inferior epigastric artery (SIEA), and the superficial and deep external pudendal arteries (SEPA, DEPA). The CFA then bifurcates into the superficial and deep femoral arteries [27]. The average diameter of the CFA is reported as 6.6–9.8 mm, and the diameter increases with age and male sex [28–30].

For many surgeons, the great saphenous vein (GSV) is the preferred venous outflow for genital reconstructive procedures. The GSV originates at the dorsal foot, passes anterior to the medial malleolus, and courses proximally along the medial leg, passing posterior to the medial femoral condyle. It is supplied by the superficial external pudendal vein, the superficial inferior epigastric vein (SIEV), and the superficial circumflex iliac vein (SCIV). The GSV joins the femoral vein at a point approximately 2.5–4.0 cm inferior and lateral of the pubic tubercle [27]. Average GSV diameter is reported as 2.6–3.1 mm [31] but decreases with age. The SIEV and SCIV provide alternative or additional venous outflow tracts.

The deep inferior epigastric vessels are a viable alternative to the femoral system [17]. The DIEA is a branch of the external iliac artery, and it is located just proximal to the inguinal ligament. It courses in a superomedial direction between the peritoneum and the transversalis fascia, giving off multiple peritoneal branches. The DIEA divides into two branches (lateral and medial) prior to entering the rectus abdominus muscle [32]. The lateral and medial branches yield an average of five cutaneous perforators, with diameters ranging from 0.5 to 1.5 mm. The preferred DIEA perforators are usually found within a 6-cm radius lateral and inferior to the umbilicus. When considering the DIEA as a recipient vessel, its diameter (3.5 mm at its origin) is considered a good match for both the radial artery and the descending branch of the LCFA [17]. The DIEV and the GSV are both options for recipient veins.

The descending branch of the LCFA is the arterial pedicle for ALT flap, but it may also be used as a recipient artery for free tissue transfer. The LCFA is one of the main branches of the profunda femoris artery. It passes laterally from its origin, behind the sartorius and rectus femoris muscles, before dividing into ascending, transverse, and descending branches [33]. The descending branch courses between the rectus femoris and vastus lateralis muscles in an oblique fashion to give off multiple musculocutaneous and septocutaneous perforators. In most cases, an appropriate perforator is found within the area of a circle with a 3-cm radius centered at the midpoint of a line drawn between ASIS and the lateral border of the patella [33, 34]. The descending branch of LCFA has an mean pedicle length of 12 cm, proximal diameter of 3.4 mm, and distal diameter of 1.9 mm [35].

Recipient Site Exposure

When performing a single-stage gender-affirming phalloplasty, the patient is initially positioned in dorsal lithotomy (Fig. 44.2) [36]. A dose of antibiotics is given 30–60 min prior to start of the case. For an ALT phalloplasty, a loose,

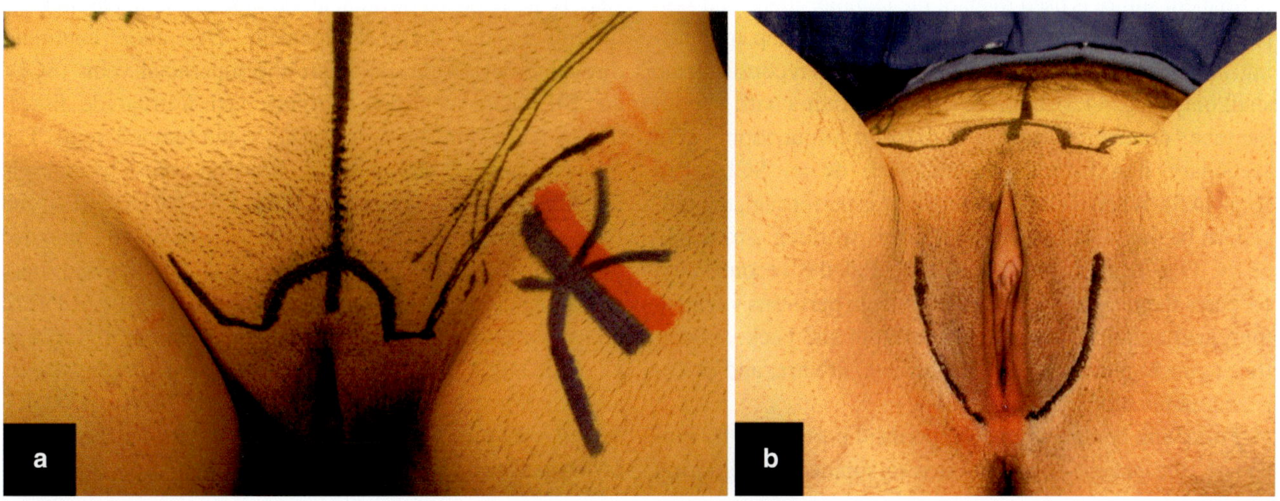

Fig. 44.2 (**a**) (left image). Anterior view of preoperative markings of the recipient site for gender-affirming phalloplasty. The omega-shaped incision over the pubis is the primary donor site incision. The course of the common femoral artery, femoral vein and branches, and ilioinguinal nerve are marked. (**b**) (right image). Perineal view of preoperative markings of the same patient recipient site for gender-affirming phalloplasty. The labial incisions allow for the construction of the scrotum. (©Loren Schechter 2021)

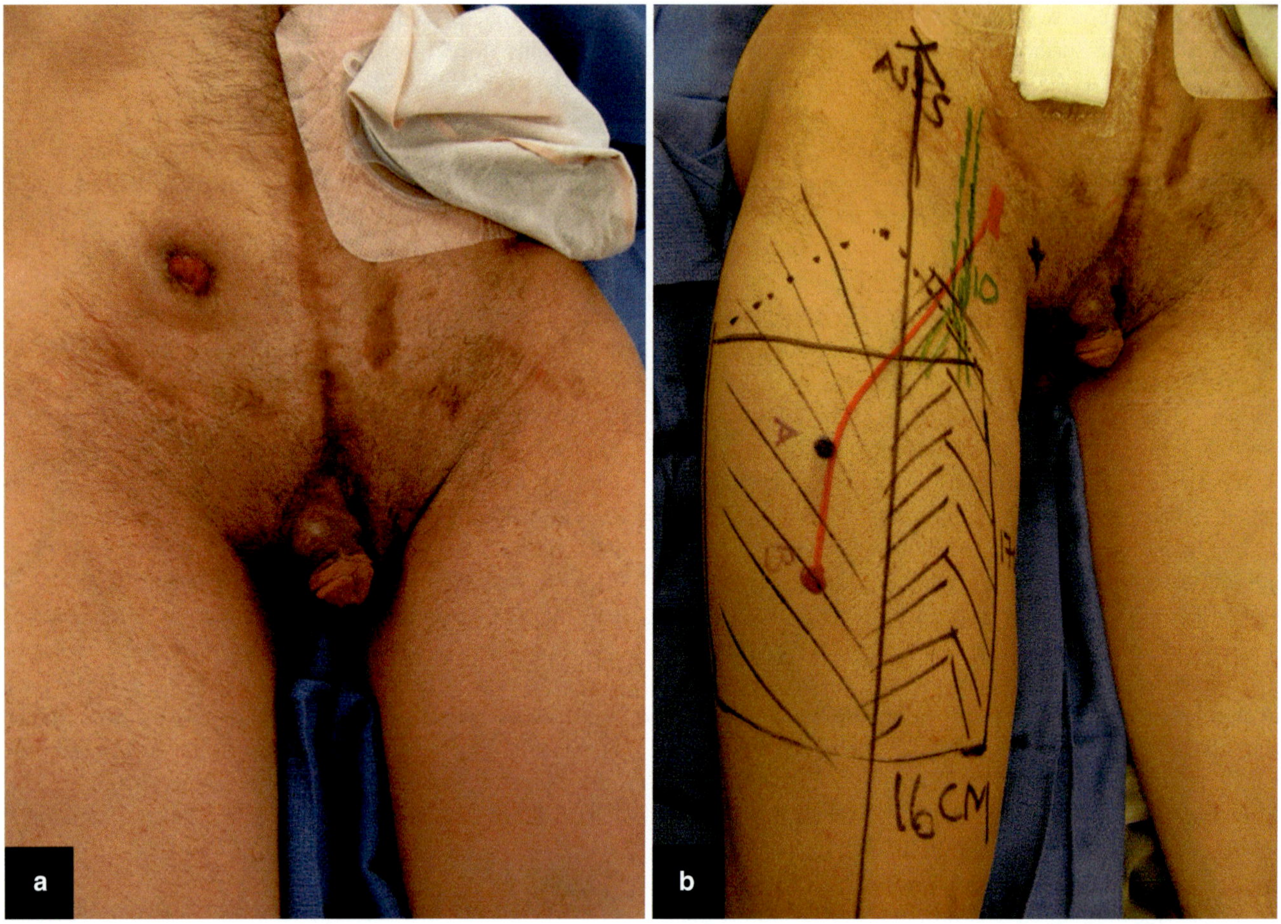

Fig. 44.3 (**a**) (left image). Preoperative photograph of patient with microphallus and exstrophy. (**b**) (right image). Preoperative markings of a pedicled anterolateral thigh (ALT) flap for a shaft-only phalloplasty with a 16 × 17 cm skin paddle (average width: 15–20 cm, depending on subcutaneous thickness). The line from the anterior superior iliac spine (ASIS) to the superolateral border of the patella approximates the intermuscular septum between the rectus femoris and vastus lateralis muscles. The descending branch of the lateral femoral circumflex artery (LCFA) and two cutaneous perforating branches are marked, as well as the lateral femoral cutaneous nerve (marking). (©Loren Schechter 2021)

permanent suture is used to mark the Doppler-identified skin perforator in order to facilitate postoperative flap monitoring. An ALT phalloplasty may be designed to reconstruct the shaft only (Fig. 44.3), both the shaft and urethra with a "double tube" configuration (Fig. 44.4), or in conjunction with a secondary flap for the urethra, such as an SCIA flap (Fig. 44.5). When an RFF phalloplasty is performed, the procedure begins with two surgical teams working simultaneously. One team harvests the RFF, and the second team prepares the recipient site. The latter team performs vaginectomy and colpocleisis (suturing the front and back walls of the vagina together), creates the perineal urethra, and places a suprapubic tube.

Following completion of the perineal portion of the procedure, the patient is repositioned to supine. The recipient vessels are exposed through an oblique incision, parallel and inferior to the inguinal ligament. Dissection continues through Scarpa's fascia, where the superficial veins (SCIV and SIEV) are identified and preserved. Retrograde dissection of these veins leads to the GSV and femoral veins. The femoral sheath is opened [37], allowing access to multiple recipient vessels, including the CFA, SFA, SCIA, SEPA, and DEPA [36]. If the inferior epigastric vessels are the intended recipient vessels, the incision is oriented obliquely and superior to the inguinal ligament. To access the DIEA and DIEV, an incision is made in the anterior rectus fascia. In order to align the DIEA and DIEV with the recipient site, the vessels are either brought through the ilioinguinal ring or through a separate myofasciotomy in the anterior rectus fascia [17] (also see Chap. 15).

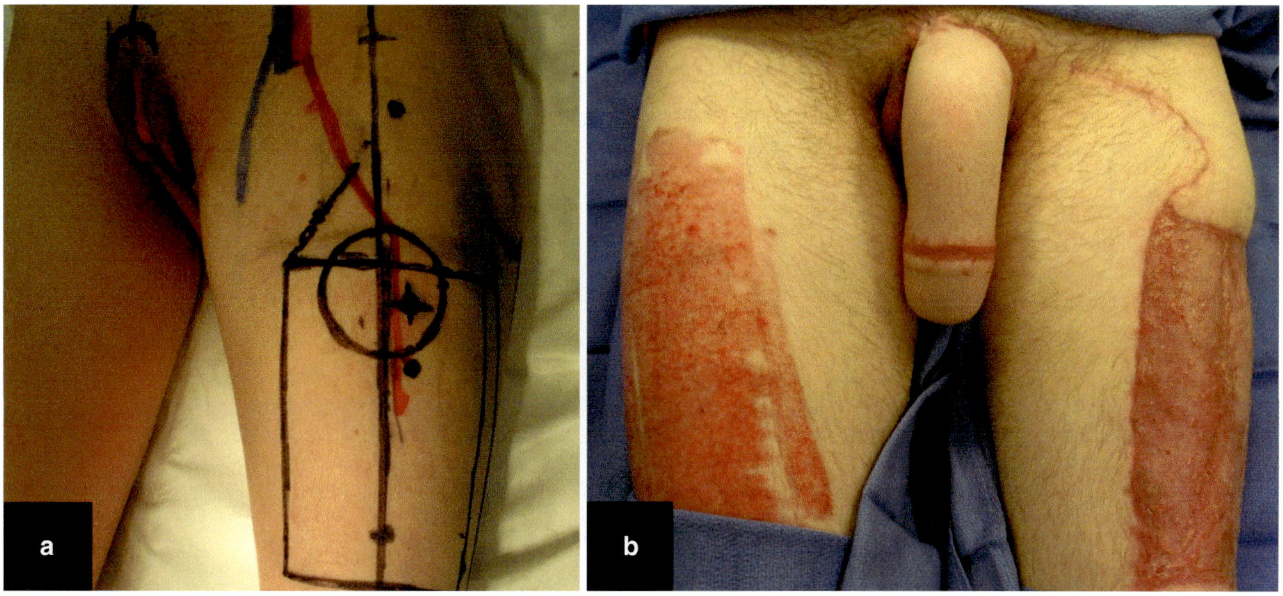

Fig. 44.4 (**a**) (left image). Preoperative photograph of patient for gender-affirming phalloplasty procedure with skin markings for a double tube ALT. The shaft component is 15-cm long. The urethral component is 4-cm wide with a 3-cm-long extension for reaching the perineal urethra. There is an intervening 1–1.5-cm de-epithelialized area between the urethra and shaft. The width of the double tube flap (including the urethra) is typically about 18–22 cm. (**b**) (right image). Postoperative image of the same patient following a double tube ALT gender-affirming phalloplasty. (©Loren Schechter 2021)

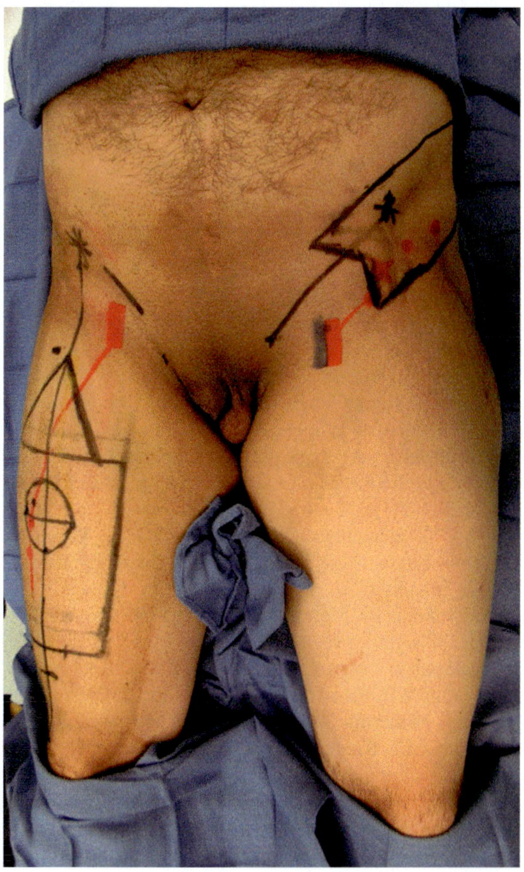

Fig. 44.5 Anterior view of preoperative markings of a patient for a combined anterolateral thigh (ALT) and superficial circumflex iliac artery (SCIA) flap for phalloplasty. Both flap designs and their respective arterial pedicles (descending branch of the lateral femoral circumflex artery for the ALT, SCIA) are marked. The ALT is used to create the shaft, and the SCIA flap is used to create the urethra. (©Loren Schechter 2021)

Discussion

When selecting recipient vessels, the decision depends upon the preoperative assessment, intraoperative considerations, reconstructive requirements, and the surgeon's judgment. While the CFA and SFA are commonly chosen recipient vessels for phalloplasty, consideration should be given as to the risk or presence of atherosclerotic disease. The CFA and SFA have the benefit of allowing for a relatively straightforward dissection that does not violate the abdominal fascia. However, these vessels may elevate the risk of ischemic or embolic vascular complications to the lower extremity.

When selecting the deep inferior epigastric vessels, the dissection requires an incision in the abdominal wall fascia. This may increase the risk of a postoperative hernia or bulge. Proponents of the DIE vessels assert that the size match and the vessel length offer an advantage and may avoid the use of vein grafts [17]. The SIEA and SIEV are alternative options to the DIEA and DIEV. However, the SIEA has a smaller-caliber and less reliable perfusion compared to the DIEA, and some surgeons consider it more prone to spasm [38, 39]. The anatomical variability in the SIEA is another disadvantage. The SIEA may originate from the CFA (in 17% of patients), from a common trunk with the SCIA (in 48% of patients), or it can be absent or hypoplastic (in 35% of patients) [32]. Conversely, the DIEA anatomy, especially near its origin, is relatively consistent. The SIEV offers an option for secondary venous drainage. To date, there has been no direct comparison, either prospectively or retrospectively, of outcomes and complications between the different recipient vessels for phalloplasty procedures.

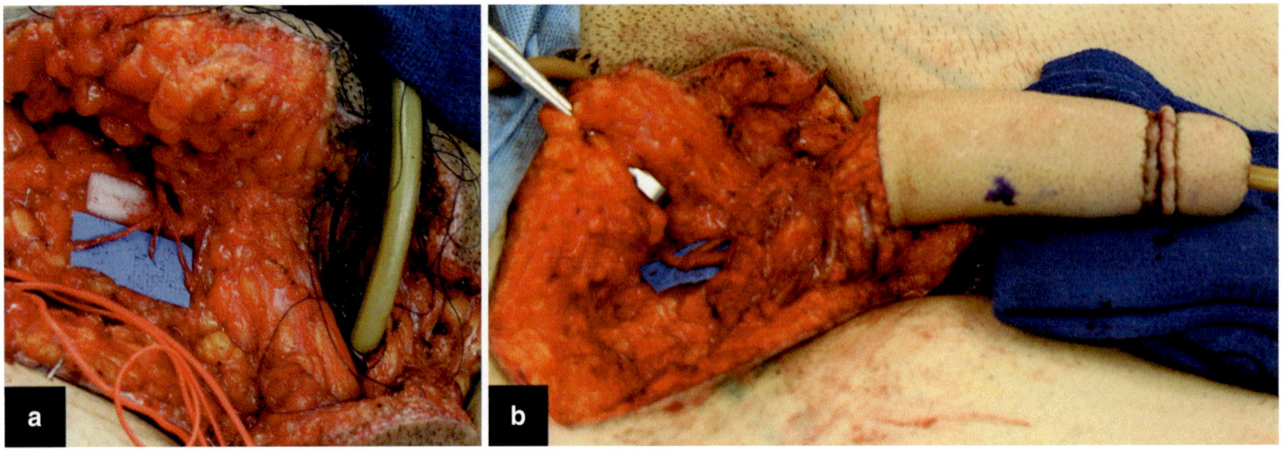

Fig. 44.6 (**a**) (left image). Intraoperative view of phalloplasty procedure showing the recipient site vessels prepared prior to microsurgical anastomosis. (**b**) (right image). Intraoperative view of the phalloplasty using radial forearm free flap after vascular anastomosis and neurorrhaphy, prior to completion of flap inset. (©Loren Schechter 2021)

In regard to venous outflow, some surgeons recommend performing at least two venous anastomoses [12, 40–42]. Other surgeons argue that one venous anastomosis is equally efficacious, requires less operative time, and causes no additional morbidity [43]. It is the authors' preference to utilize two or more veins, as we believe the benefits of additional outflow outweigh increases in operative time.

When selecting recipient vessels, consideration is also given to those donor vessels that will optimize pedicle orientation and flap inset (Fig. 44.6). Although a long pedicle is ideal, caution should be taken to avoid kinking or stretching of the pedicle. This is particularly important when utilizing AV loops; the loop should have a gentle curve with no points of kinking or tension. In an end-to-side anastomosis, the angle which the donor vessel aligns with the larger recipient vessel is also important. An angle that is too acute or too wide can potentiate clot formation.

In certain situations, increased pedicle length may be necessary, which may be accomplished with vein grafts or AV loops. While vein grafts on the arterial limb are of less concern, the authors try to avoid the use of vein grafts on the venous limb as the slower blood flow and extra anastomoses may result in a higher risk of thrombosis. More frequently, the authors prefer to use AV loops. The AV loop is usually created between the GSV and the SFA (Video 44.1) (also see Chap. 18). After determining the necessary pedicle length, the GSV is divided distally and anastomosed in an end-to-side fashion to the SFA. The loop is then divided at a location that provides suitable extension of the arterial and/or venous limbs [44]. Both techniques, vein grafts and AV loops, lengthen the vascular pedicle and allow for improved maneuverability of the transferred tissue.

Genital reconstruction is both challenging and rewarding. The reconstruction of this deeply personal area is immensely significant to patients. Multiple variables, including the reconstructive requirements, the patient's goals and expectations, the available donor tissue, and the accessible recipient vessels, are considered. These procedures require the highest level of technical and surgical expertise, a comprehensive understanding of the anatomy, and the flexibility to alter the operative plans based upon intraoperative findings. As the field of GAS and genital reconstruction continues to flourish, further study and refinement of these techniques will enhance the surgeon's ability to achieve optimal results for their patients.

References

1. Zurada A, Salandy S, Roberts W, Gielecki J, Schober J, Loukas M. The evolution of transgender surgery. Clin Anat. 2018;31(6):878–86.
2. Al-Tamimi M, Pigot GL, Elfering L, Ozer M, de Haseth K, van de Grift TC, Mullender MG, Bouman MB, Van der Sluis WB. Genital gender-affirming surgery in transgender men in the Netherlands from 1989 to 2018: the evolution of surgical care. Plast Reconstr Surg. 2020;145(1):153e–61e.
3. Perovic SV, Stanojevic DS, Djordjevic ML. Vaginoplasty in male transsexuals using penile skin and a urethral flap. BJU Int. 2000;86(7):843–50.
4. Bhaskar V, Sinha RJ, Mehrotra S, Mehrotra CN, Singh V. Long-term outcomes of sigmoid vaginoplasty in patients with disorder of sexual development – our experience. Urol Ann. 2018;10(2):185–90.
5. van der Sluis WB, Pavan N, Liguori G, Bucci S, Bizic MR, Kojovic V, Hess J, Meijerink WJHJ, Mullender MG, Özer M, Smit JM, Buncamper ME, Krege S, Djordjevic ML, Trombetta C, Bouman MB. Ileal vaginoplasty as vaginal reconstruction in transgender women and patients with disorders of sex development: an international, multicentre, retrospective study on surgical characteristics and outcomes. BJU Int. 2018;121(6):952–8.
6. Ahn DK, Kim SW, Park SY, Kim YH. Reconstructive strategy and classification of penoscrotal defects. Urology. 2014;84(5):1217–22.

7. Papadopulos NA, Schaff J, Biemer E. The use of free prelaminated and sensate osteofasciocutaneous fibular flap in phalloplasty. Injury. 2008;39(Suppl 3):S62–7.
8. Zaheer U, Granger A, Ortiz A, Terrell M, Loukas M, Schober J. The anatomy of free fibula osteoseptocutaneous flap in neophalloplasty in transgender surgery. Clin Anat. 2018;31(2):169–74.
9. Felici N, Felici A. A new phalloplasty technique: the free anterolateral thigh flap phalloplasty. J Plast Reconstr Aesthet Surg. 2006;59(2):153–7.
10. Dennis M, Granger A, Ortiz A, Terrell M, Loukos M, Schober J. The anatomy of the musculocutaneous latissimus dorsi flap for neophalloplasty. Clin Anat. 2018;31(2):152–9.
11. Jun MS, Pusica S, Kojovic V, Bizic M, Stojanovic B, Krstic Z, Korac G, Djordjevic ML. Total phalloplasty with latissimus dorsi musculocutaneous flap in female-to-male transgender surgery. Urology. 2018;120:269–70.
12. Spennato S, Burger AE, Schlosshauer T, Kuenzlen L, Rothenberger J, Kuhn S, Kiehlmann M, Radacki I, Sohn M, Rieger UM. Microsurgical phalloplasty in nontranssexual patients – considerations after a retrospective single-center analysis of 23 cases. Urology. 2020;141:154–61. https://doi.org/10.1016/j.urology.2020.03.038.
13. Bluebond-Langner R, Redett RJ. Phalloplasty in complete aphallia and ambiguous genitalia. Semin Plast Surg. 2011;25(3):196–205.
14. Annen AW, Heston AL, Dugi DD III, Dy GW, Bluebond-Langner R, Jensen KK, Berli JU. Masculinizing genital surgery: an imaging primer for the radiologist. AJR Am J Roentgenol. 2020;214(1):W27–36.
15. Fan J, Liu Y, Liu L, Gan C. Aesthetic pubic reconstruction after electrical burn using a portion of hair-bearing expanded free-forehead flap. Aesthet Plast Surg. 2009;33(4):643–6.
16. Dong L, Dong Y, He L, Liu C, Zhang Z, Xiao B, Xia W, Xia W. Penile reconstruction by preexpanded free scapular flap in severely burned patient. Ann Plast Surg. 2014;73(Suppl 1):S27–30.
17. Danker S, Annen AW, Cylinder I, Esmonde NO, Berli JU. Technical description and microsurgical outcomes in phalloplasty using the DIEA and locoregional veins. Plast Reconstr Surg. 2020;146(2):196e–204e. https://doi.org/10.1097/PRS.0000000000007036.
18. Gottlieb LJ, Shenaq DS. Penile (re)construction with the radial forearm free flap. In: Evans GR, editor. Operative plastic surgery. 2nd ed. Oxford University Press; 2019. p. 823–31.
19. Kropp B, Cohn JE, Wang W, Sokoya M, Ducic Y. Free tissue transfer penile reconstruction. Semin Plast Surg. 2019;33(1):24–9.
20. Walker RF, Zakai NA, MacLehose RF, Cowan LT, Adam TJ, Alonso A, Lutsey PL. Association of testosterone therapy with risk of venous thromboembolism among men with and without hypogonadism. JAMA Intern Med. 2019;180(2):190–7.
21. Chen HC, Coskunfirat OK, Ozkan O, Mardini S, Cigna E, Salgado CJ, Spanio S. Guidelines for the optimization of microsurgery in atherosclerotic patients. Microsurgery. 2006;26(5):356–62.
22. Spitz JA, Bradford PS, Aguilar F, Turin SY, Ellis MF. How big is too big: pushing the obesity limits in microsurgical breast reconstruction. Ann Plast Surg. 2018;80(2):137–40.
23. Shin JY, Roh SG, Lee NH, Yang KM. Is obesity a predisposing factor for free flap failure and complications? Comparison between breast and nonbreast reconstruction: systematic review and meta-analysis. Medicine (Baltimore). 2016;95(26):e4072.
24. Agrifoglio M, Dainese L, Pasotti S, Galanti A, Cannata A, Roberto M, Parolari A, Biglioli P. Preoperative assessment of the radial artery for coronary artery bypass grafting: is the clinical Allen test adequate? Ann Thorac Surg. 2005;79(2):570–2.
25. Irani F, Kumar S, Colyer WR Jr. Common femoral artery access techniques: a review. J Cardiovasc Med (Hagerstown). 2009;10(7):517–22.
26. Hunt JA, Harris JP. Is the mid-inguinal point an accurate landmark for the common femoral artery in vascular patients? Aust N Z J Surg. 1996;66(1):43–5.
27. Forsythe RO, Hinchliffe RJ. Vascular anatomy of the lower limb. In: Brennan PA, Standring SM, Wiseman SM, editors. Gray's surgical anatomy. 1st ed. Amsterdam: Elsevier; 2020. p. 577–83.
28. Sandgren T, Sonesson B, Ahlgren R, Lanne T. The diameter of the common femoral artery in healthy human: influence of sex, age, and body size. J Vasc Surg. 1999;29(3):503–10.
29. Spector KS, Lawson WE. Optimizing safe femoral access during cardiac catheterization. Catheter Cardiovasc Interv. 2001;53(2):209–12.
30. Lorbeer R, Grotz A, Dorr M, Volzke H, Lieb W, Kuhn JP, et al. Reference values of vessel diameters, stenosis prevalence, and arterial variations of the lower limb arteries in a male population sample using contrast-enhanced MR angiography. PLoS One. 2018;13(6):e0197559.
31. Zachrisson H, Lindenberger M, Hallman D, Ekman M, Neider D, Lanne T. Diameter and compliance of the greater saphenous vein – effect of age and nitroglycerine. Clin Physiol Funct Imaging. 2011;31(4):300–6.
32. Gangnon A, et al. Deep and superficial inferior epigastric artery perforator flaps. In: Wei F-C, Mardini S, editors. Flaps and reconstructive surgery. Philadelphia: Elsevier; 2017. p. 668–87.
33. Mardini S, et al. Anterolateral and anteromedial thigh flaps. In: Wei F-C, Mardini S, editors. Flaps and reconstructive surgery. Philadelphia: Elsevier; 2017. p. 700–16.
34. Yu P, Selber J. Perforator patterns of the anteromedial thigh flap. Plast Reconstr Surg. 2011;128(3):151e–7e.
35. Zenn MR, Pribaz J, Walsh M. Use of the descending lateral femoral circumflex artery and vein for vascular grafting: a better alternative to an arteriovenous loop. Plast Reconstr Surg. 2010;126(1):140–2.
36. Schechter LS. Surgical therapy for transmen. In: Surgical management of the transgender patient. Philadelphia: Elsevier; 2016. p. 61–105.
37. Pomposelli FB, Prushik S, Shean K. Lower extremity arterial exposure. In: Sidawy AN, Perler BA, editors. Rutherford's vascular surgery and endovascular therapy. 9th ed. Philadelphia: Elsevier; 2019. p. 688–705.
38. Coroneos CJ, Heller AM, Voineskos SH, Avram R. SIEA versus DIEP arterial complications: a cohort study. Plast Reconstr Surg. 2015;135(5):802e–7e.
39. Sarik JR, Bank J, Wu LC, Serletti JM. Superficial inferior epigastric artery: learning curve versus reality. Plast Reconstr Surg. 2016;137(1):1e–6e.
40. Christianto S, Lau A, Li KY, Yang WF, Su YX. One versus two venous anastomoses in microsurgical head and neck reconstruction: a cumulative meta-analysis. Int J Oral Maxillofac Surg. 2018;47(5):585–94.
41. Heidekrueger PI, Ehrl D, Heine-Geldern A, Ninkovic M, Broer PN. One versus two venous anastomoses in microvascular lower extremity reconstruction using gracilis muscle or anterolateral thigh flaps. Injury. 2016;47(12):2828–32.
42. Lee YC, Chen WC, Chen SH, Hung KS, Hsiao JR, Lee JW, et al. One versus two venous anastomoses in anterolateral thigh flap reconstruction after oral cancer ablation. Plast Reconstr Surg. 2016;138(2):481–9.
43. Futran ND, Stack BC Jr. Single versus dual venous drainage of the radial forearm free flap. Am J Otolaryngol. 1996;17(2):112–7.
44. Virasoro R, Jordan GH, McCammon KA. Surgery for benign disorders of the penis and urethra. In: Partin AW, editor. Campbell-Walsh-Wein urology. 12th ed. Elsevier; 2021. p. 1804–42.
45. Sinna R, Hajji H, Qassemyar Q, Perignon D, et al. Anatomical background of the perforator flap based on the deep branch of the superficial circumflex iliac artery (SCIP Flap): a cadaveric study. Eplasty. 2010;10:e11.

46. La Falce OL, Ambrosio JD, Souza RR. The anatomy of the superficial external pudendal artery: a quantitative study. Clinics (Sao Paulo). 2006;61(5):441–4.
47. Giraldo F, Mora MJ, Solano A, Gonzalez C, Smith-Fernandez V. Male perineogenital anatomy and clinical applications in genital reconstructions and male-to-female sex reassignment surgery. Plast Reconstr Surg. 2002;109(4):1301–10.
48. Zlotorowicz M, Szczodry M, Czubak J, Ciszek B. Anatomy of the medial femoral circumflex artery with respect to the vascularity of the femoral head. J Bone Joint Surg Br. 2011;93(11):1471–4.
49. Tansatit T, Wanidchaphloi S, Sanguansit P. The anatomy of the lateral circumflex femoral artery in anterolateral thigh flap. J Med Assoc Thail. 2008;91(9):1404–9.

Index

R. Gurunian, R. Djohan (eds.), *Recipient Vessels in Reconstructive Microsurgery*,
https://doi.org/10.1007/978-3-030-75389-4

MIX
Papier aus verantwortungsvollen Quellen
Paper from responsible sources
FSC® C105338
FSC
www.fsc.org

If you have any concerns about our products,
you can contact us on
ProductSafety@springernature.com

In case Publisher is established outside the EU,
the EU authorized representative is:
Springer Nature Customer Service Center GmbH
Europaplatz 3, 69115 Heidelberg, Germany

Printed by Libri Plureos GmbH
in Hamburg, Germany